ADVANCING
YOUR CAREER

ADVANCING YOUR CAREER

Concepts of Professional Nursing

THIRD EDITION

Rose Kearney-Nunnery, RN, PhD

Vice President for Academic Affairs
Technical College of the Lowcountry
Beaufort, South Carolina
Member and past president
South Carolina Board of Nursing

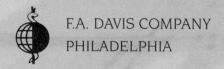

F.A. DAVIS COMPANY
PHILADELPHIA

F. A. Davis Company
1915 Arch Street
Philadelphia, PA 19103

Printed in the United States of America

Last digit indicates print number: 10 9 8 7 6 5 4 3 2
Acquisitions Editor: Joanne P. DaCunha, RN, MSN
Developmental Editor: Caryn Abramowitz
Project Editor: Kristin L. Kern

As new scientific information becomes available through basic and clinical research, recommended treatments and drug therapies undergo changes. The author and publisher have done everything possible to make this book accurate, up to date, and in accord with accepted standards at the time of publication. The author, editors, and publisher are not responsible for errors or omissions or for consequences from application of the book, and make no warranty, expressed or implied, in regard to the contents of the book. Any practice described in this book should be applied by the reader in accordance with professional standards of care used in regard to the unique circumstances that may apply in each situation. The reader is advised always to check product information (package inserts) for changes and new information regarding dose and contraindications before administering any drug. Caution is especially urged when using new or infrequently ordered drugs.

Library of Congress Cataloging-in-Publication Data

Kearney-Nunnery, Rose.
  Advancing your career : concepts of professional nursing / Rose Kearney-Nunnery.–3rd ed.
     p. ; cm.
  Includes bibliographical references and index.
  ISBN 10: 0-8036-1216-8 (alk. paper)
  ISBN 13: 978-0-8036-1216-7
  1. Nursing–Vocational guidance. 2. Career development. 3. Nursing–Vocational guidance–United States. 4. Nursing–Philosophy. I. Title.
  [DNLM: 1. Nursing. 2. Career Mobility. WY 16 K24aa 2005]
  RT82.N85 2005
  610.73′06′9–dc22

2004019401

dedicated to
Helen Kearney

Preface

The nursing profession has undergone major changes in the past decades, and the pace of change seems to accelerate daily. We have entered the millennium while moving from our former role of defending nursing as a profession to our present pivotal role in health care. Focusing on people in their respective environments with their unique health care needs that are addressed through nursing care is vitally important with our rapidly expanding knowledge base and the dynamic changes continually occurring in health care. In essence, our quest in our respective nursing roles is to expand knowledge, become involved within the profession and interdisciplinary, utilize evidence-based practice and expanding technologies, and broaden the vision of professional practice.

This book is directed to the RN student returning to school. The intent is to provide you, the practicing RN, with professional concepts to advance your practice. These concepts build on your prior nursing education, and their application will greatly enhance your professional practice and growth. The aim is to engage you intellectually in an ongoing professional dialogue with your peers, colleagues, and instructors, broaden your professional development, and build on your preexisting knowledge and experiences. You, the RN student, are challenged to delve further into professional education and conceptual practice. The book is written for the adult learner with the characteristics of self-direction, prior experiences, applicability to practice, and motivation to meet the challenge to expand his or her knowledge base.

The third edition has been updated and reorganized and is divided into five sections. As with the first and second editions, each chapter contains chapter objectives, key terms, key points, chapter exercises to assist in meeting each of the chapter objectives, references, online references, and bibliographical sources. Interactive exercises have been extended from the second edition and are provided on an Intranet site to truly engage the reader progressing through the content. The book's Intranet site also houses a clinical scenario bank, thorough glossary of terms, important Internet links, discussion sections, and bonus information on some of the content in the book like research and ethics.

Section I introduces the concepts of professional nursing practice. Chapter 1 focuses on the characteristics of professional nursing as a profession and as a unique professional discipline. Included in this updated chapter is a discussion on the core competencies proposed for all health care professionals. Readers are challenged to develop personal perspectives of professional nursing as a philosophy statement. Coping with returning to school is the theme of Chapter 2. Dr. Bernadette Dorsch Curry's presentation highlights study tips and strategies for success in the arduous process of returning to the student role.

Section II addresses the theoretical bases of nursing practice. First, Chapter 3 presents theory development, description, and use. Terminology is applied to theories from other disciplines and those successfully applied in professional nursing, including Maslow's hierarchy of basic needs, developmental theories, and systems theory. In Chapter 4, Dr. Jacqueline Fawcett and Barbara Swoyer address the evolution of nursing theory. In addition to a discussion of the evolution, vocabulary, and advantages of these nursing models, the chapter presents applications for selecting and using the models as a guide for practice. The bases of nursing theories are followed by discussion of health and illness models that have been successfully used to guide nursing practice (Chapter 5). The theories of health and illness presented include Dunn's high-level wellness, the health belief model, a health promotion model, and a chronic illness model. Focusing on health, the chapter includes issues with levels of prevention and cultural competence. Section II concludes with a focus on evidence-based nursing in Chapter 6, with the view of the research process and the use of evidence of efficacy as a basis for practice. Legal and ethical considerations and utilization and critique of research are highlighted.

Section III features critical components of professional nursing practice. Eight critical components of professional nursing are reviewed: communication, working with groups, critical thinking, teaching and learning, leadership, management in organizations, change, and professional ethics. The first of these critical components is presented by Jacqueline Owers Favret in Chapter 7, with a discussion of communication models, essential ingredients of effective communication, nonverbal communication forms, and specific communication techniques, including communication skills for interdisciplinary practice. Effective communication is broadened in Chapter 8 for use in groups including the characteristics and roles of groups and group leaders and the skills needed for collaboration, coordination, negotiation, and dealing with conflict and difficult people.

Critical thinking is essential to professional nursing practice. In Chapter 9, Drs. Genevieve M. Bartol and Rebecca Parrish trace the historical aspects of critical thinking in nursing, along with the characteristics, measurement, and further development of critical thinking and analysis skills.

Chapter 10 focuses on the teaching and learning process, learning theories and styles, adult learning theory, and learning readiness. Included in this chapter is a discussion on writing behavioral objectives, developing lesson plans, teaching skills and methods, and outcome evaluations.

Drs. Theresa M. Valiga and Sheila C. Grossman address leadership as a critical component of professional nursing practice in Chapter 11. Along with definitions, theories, and styles of leadership, the chapter contains a description of the components of effective leadership.

Understanding organizations and effective management in organizational settings are essential parts of professional practice, as described in Chapter 12. Organizational theory focusing on systems theory, structure and function, culture, and communication skills is applied to a variety of organizational designs with a discussion of selected management theories, delegation principles, and strategies for management situations. Organizations have redefined themselves radically during the past decade. Dealing with change is an involved process. Chapter 13 presents theories of change, the characteristics of change agents, and change in individuals, families, groups, and organizations.

Section III concludes with Chapter 14, "Professional Ethics" by Dr. Joseph T. Catalano. This chapter focuses on basic human rights, the right to privacy and dignity, access to care, informed consent, advance directives, organ procurement, client endangerment, and workplace hazards.

Section IV delves into the concepts needed to provide care as a major activity in professional nursing practice, especially with the emphasis on safety and effective client outcomes. In Chapter 15, Dr. Vicki Budka discusses managing and providing professional nursing care and reviews methods for organizing care activities, including the focus on values and outcomes for client-centered care and interdisciplinary care delivery, use of case management, care maps, documentation, and the use of standardized nomenclatures. Providing care is further challenging as we address at-risk populations and the reduction of health disparities in Chapter 16. National strategies for improving health and reducing health disparities for at-risk population groups are highlighted, including a focus on select populations, like the aging population with quality of healthy life considerations, minority health with identified health disparities, and rural health considerations.

Providing care includes a necessary focus on quality. Quality care is discussed in Chapter 17 by Francoise Dunefsky, who highlights the issues of theoretical models for quality, quality improvement, continuous quality improvement, and quality management. These are presented as important considerations with the accreditation of health care organizations. The use of informatics as one of the core competencies for health care professionals is addressed in Chapter 18 by Dr. Julia Aucoin. Health care information management systems and careers in informatics are discussed along with additional computer applications in professional practice. In Chapter 19, Drs. Cyril F. Chang, Sylvia A. Price, and Susan K. Pfoutz address one of the major issues driving today's health care system: economics. They discuss issues related to types of payers, effectiveness, system reforms, and marketplace considerations.

In response to recent issues relating to protecting the populace, a new chapter has been added on chemical and biologic terrorism. Dr. Robin Vogt presents information on the various methods and agents along with issues and protections in different bioterrorism threat situations.

This section concludes with a presentation of the imperative for nursing to develop both internal and external political efficacy. Chapter 21 has been revised to include both an historical perspective and resources to assist nurses in developing internal political efficacy, which will help the profession in the demonstration of its external efficacy as the political imperative.

Section V confronts the reality of health care and the nursing profession in the 21st century. In Chapter 22, Sister Rosemary Donley addresses the health care agenda and issues debated in both legislative and professional areas that have major implications for the health care of the nation and initiatives for the profession. The final chapter discusses challenges for the future. Topics include driving forces that demand change throughout the health professions and the call for action in the environment with a focus on safety and effective client outcomes.

This book is intended to enhance your professional practice and continued professional development through further education. Your personal characteristics of self-motivation, a thirst for information, and commitment to your clients and the profession will be enhanced as you develop a more conceptual and visionary approach to professional nursing practice. Advance your practice through ongoing education and the concepts basic to professional nursing practice.

Rose Kearney-Nunnery

Acknowledgments

Numerous people have been a large part of this process. Family members, friends, and colleagues have more than tolerated my preoccupation with the profession. My respect is extended to all my professional colleagues for the opportunities they provided for discussion and debate. My particular thanks are extended to all the contributors who have shared their expertise and insights in these pages. Joanne DaCunha, Caryn Abramowitz, and Kristen L. Kern merit particular credit for the completion of this project through their endless encouragement, assistance, enthusiasm, and belief in the potential for our profession. My thanks to my husband Jimmie E. Nunnery, with his political experience, who finally agreed to co-author the chapter on politics in this edition. And a special note of thanks to Helen Kearney, a supportive mother and true friend. I have received endless encouragement from my professional colleagues, friends, and students, all of whom added to this kaleidoscope that has brought the nursing profession to the present with ongoing change in the future. And to all who give to clients of nursing, my endless respect.

Rose Kearney-Nunnery

Contributors

Julia W. Aucoin, DNS, RN, BC
Assistant Professor
University of North Carolina at Greensboro
Greensboro, NC

Genevieve M. Bartol, RN, EdD
Professor Emeritus
The University of North Carolina at Greensboro
School of Nursing
Greensboro, North Carolina

Vicki L. Buchda, RN, MS
Director, Patient Care Resources
Mayo Arizona
Scottsdale, Arizona

Joseph T. Catalano, RN, PhD
Professor
East Central University
Ada, Oklahoma

Cyril F. Chang, PhD
Professor of Economics
Department of Economics
The University of Memphis
Memphis, Tennessee

Bernadette Dorsch Curry, RN, PhD
Chairperson
Mollory College
Rockville Center, New York

Sister Rosemary Donley, RN, PhD, C-ANP,
  FAAN
Executive Vice President
The Catholic University of America
Washington, DC

Francoise Dunefsky, RN, MS, CNAA
Chief Executive Officer
Gateway Community Industries, Inc.
Kingston, New York

Jacqueline Owers Favret, RN, MPH
Assistant Professor of Clinical Nursing
Louisiana State University Health Science
  Center
School of Nursing
New Orleans, Louisiana

Jacqueline Fawcett, PhD, FAAN
Professor
University of Massachusetts
College of Nursing
Boston, Massachusetts

Sheila C. Grossman, RN, PhD
Associate Professor
School of Nursing
Fairfield University
Fairfield, Connecticut

Jimmie E. Nunnery, MA
Distinguished Professor Emeritus
University of South Carolina
Former Member of the South Carolina House
  of Representatives
Member and Secretary of the Medical Military,
  Public and Municipal Affairs Committee
Former Judge, Magistrate Court
  Chester County, South Carolina

Rebecca S. Parrish, RN, PhD
Assistant Professor
The University of North Carolina at Greensboro
Greensboro, North Carolina

Susan K. Pfoutz, RN, PhD
Professor
Department of Nursing
Eastern Michigan University
Ypsilanti, Michigan

Sylvia A. Price, RN, PhD
Professor (Retired)
College of Nursing
University of Tennessee at Memphis
Memphis, Tennessee

Barbara Swoyer, MSN, CRNP
Family Nurse Practitioner
Emkey Arthritis and Osteoporosis Clinic, Inc.
Wyomissing, Pennsylvania

Theresa M. Valiga, RN, EdD
Director of Research
National League for Nursing
New York, New York

Robin S. Vogt, RN, FNP-C, PhD
Medical Staff
Royal Oaks Hospital
Windsor, Missouri
President, Missouri State Board of Nursing
Jefferson City, Missouri

Consultants

Theresa Gallagher Balog, RN, PhD
Assistant Professor of Nursing
Coordinator RN-BSN Nursing Program
Penn State New Kensington
Program Head Nursing
Penn State Commonwealth College
New Kensington, Pennsylvania

Annette Genderman, DEd, MSN, RN
Associate Professor of Nursing
Bloomsburg University
Bloomsburg, Pennsylvania

Holly Evans Madison, RN, MS
Doctoral Student
Southern Vermont College
Bennington, Vermont

CONTENTS

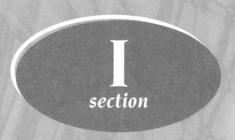

section

Introduction

Rose Kearney-Nunnery

1
chapter

Your Professional Identity

> *The past cannot be changed. The future is yet in your power.*
>
> Mary Pickford, 1893–1979

Chapter Objectives

On completion of this chapter, the reader will be able to:

1. Relate the attributes of a profession to professional nursing practice.
2. Relate the core competencies for health professionals to professional nursing practice.
3. Describe clients of professional nursing practice.
4. Discuss responsibility and accountability in professional nursing practice.
5. Describe ethical responsibilities in professional nursing practice.
6. Discuss the formal and informal educational expectations for professional nursing practice.
7. Develop a personal philosophy of professional nursing.

Key Terms

Theory
Paradigm
Metaparadigm
Person
Environment
Health
Nursing
Authority
Community Sanction
Code of Ethics

Professional Culture
Professional Development
Professional
   Organizations
Educational Background
Core Competencies
Continuing Education
Continued Competency
Communication and
   Publication

Autonomy and Self-
   Regulation
Responsibility
Accountability
Community Service
Theory Use, Development,
   and Evaluation
Evidence-based Practice
Philosophy

As a registered nurse (RN) student pursuing an advanced degree in nursing, you must reevaluate personal and collegial perspectives on what truly constitutes professional practice. You are at a gateway for advancing your nursing practice and the profession. To advance in your professional career, you must broaden and build on your knowledge base. This involves Mezirow's (1991) **theory** of adult development and adult education as transformative learning. This theory proposes that the adult moves from technical and practical learning modes into the reflective learning necessary to understand perceptions of the self and the world. Callin (1996) describes this "perspective transformation" in nursing as requiring the opportunity for reflection, review, and critical thinking. This concept of perspective transformation provides an ongoing process in both personal and professional development.

From the professional standpoint, armed with technical skills and expertise in the practice setting, we chart a course into the conceptual components that embody and expand professional practice. These conceptual tools allow for creativity and refinement within the **paradigm** of professional nursing practice. As a start, consider the concepts that characterize both a profession in general and professional nursing practice specifically.

CHARACTERISTICS OF A PROFESSION

Greenwood (1957) developed a classic work on professionalism in which he proposed five characteristics of a profession. These attributes (Box 1–1) were then applied to the social work discipline to defend its professional status, but they are applicable to any profession, including professional nursing practice.

> **BOX 1–1**
> **CHARACTERISTICS OF A PROFESSION**
>
> - Systematic Theory
> - Authority
> - Community Sanction
> - Ethical Codes
> - Professional Culture
>
> Source: Greenwood, 1957.

Systematic Theory and Knowledge Base

Each profession is guided by systematic theory, on which its knowledge base is built. As Greenwood (1957) noted, "The skills that characterize a profession flow from and are supported by a fund of knowledge that has been organized into an internally consistent system called a body of theory" (p. 46). This system includes theoretical foundations unique to the profession as well as those adapted from other scientific disciplines.

Kerlinger (1986) defines a **theory** as "a set of interrelated constructs (concepts), definitions, and propositions that present a systematic view of phenomena by specifying relations among variables, with the purpose of explaining and predicting the phenomena" (p. 9). This theory base is also referred to as the paradigm used by professionals or the practitioners in a particular scientific community.

Kuhn (1970) has provided us with the well-established definition of a **paradigm** as "universally recognized scientific achievements that, for a time, provide model problems and solutions to a community of practitioners" (p. vii). The paradigm consists of the beliefs and the belief system shared by members of a particular scientific community. When the paradigm is no longer useful in explaining, practicing, and conducting research in that community, the paradigm shifts and a new belief structure is promoted, adopted, and used by its members.

The paradigm is merely the phenomenon of concern that guides nursing practice. In Chapter 4, Fawcett proposes that *conceptual model* and *paradigm* are interchangeable terms relative to the phenomena of nursing. Various nursing paradigms or conceptual models are currently used in practice. The selection is based on the belief structure of the particular nursing community, for example, care of people who are chronically ill and need major assistance with health needs versus the wellness initiatives applicable in occupational settings. The paradigm is determined by the type of nursing, because it meets the health needs of a particular client group in a certain environment or setting.

The **metaparadigm** is the overall concern of nursing common to each nursing model, whether a conceptual model/paradigm or formal theory. Fawcett (1995, 2000) has described the following four requirements for a discipline's metaparadigm: identity, inclusiveness, neutrality, and internationality. First, the metaparadigm must provide an identity for the profession that is distinctly different from that of others. Second, the metaparadigm must address all phenomena of interest to the profession in a manageable and understandable manner. Third, the metaparadigm must be neutral, so that all smaller practice paradigms can fit under the umbrella metaparadigm. And finally, the metaparadigm must be "international in scope and substance" (Fawcett, 1995, p. 6) to represent the profession across national, social, cultural, and ethnic boundaries. The metaparadigm of professional nursing incorporates four concepts: person, environment, health, and nursing, as follows:

- The **person** represents the individual, family, group, or community receiving care, each with unique characteristics.
- The **environment** comprises the physical, social, cultural, spiritual, and emotional climate or setting(s) in which the person lives, works, plays, and interacts.
- **Health** is the focus for the particular type of nursing and specific care provisions needed.
- **Nursing** is defined by its activities, goals, and services.

In any area of professional nursing practice, we can evaluate who the person is as the client or recipient of nursing care, where the person and the caregiver are seen and are influenced by others, why the person needs professional nursing care, and how the professional nurse functions as a provider of care. These concepts are present whether the client is the frail elder in an acute care setting, the expanding family in a birthing center, or an employee group in an occupational setting. Investigate these concepts specific to your own practice setting for an initial view of the systematic theory and knowledge base of your disciplinary paradigm.

Authority

The next characteristic of a professional is **authority**, as viewed by the client. This authority occurs through education and experience, which give the professional the knowledge and skills to make professional judgments. The client perceives the professional as having the knowledge and expertise to assist the client in meeting some need. The professional is therefore viewed as an authority in the area, and his or her judgments are trusted. Authority is the basis for the competence the client perceives and the client-professional relationship.

In the client-nurse relationship, the nurse is perceived as the authority figure whether providing a selected care technique or filling an informational need. The competence and skill demonstrated justify the client's trust in the professional nurse. Benner (1984) has described the following five levels of competency in clinical nursing practice: novice, advanced beginner, competent, proficient, and expert (p. xvii). The higher the levels of competence or expertise clients perceive in any profession, the greater trust or authority they place in the practitioners of that profession. Clients who see nurses as experts in providing needed health care view the profession as having more authority in health-care judgments. On the basis of this perception of authority, society grants the profession and its practitioners certain rights, privileges, and responsibilities.

Community Sanction

Society grants the profession certain powers and obligations to practice the specific profession. Nursing's Social Policy Statement (American Nurses Association [ANA], Nursing's, 2003) attributes professional nursing's authority to a social contract with the community. The professional community is responsible for ensuring safe and effective practice within the discipline. Professional and legal regulation of nursing practice as a **community sanction** occurs through statutes, rules and regulations, definition of practice, and expectations for practitioners. Powers for entry and continuity in the profession are granted through licensure and professional practice parameters dictated in the state practice acts. These laws define a specific practice and provide regulatory powers at the state level for the board, licensing of professionals and protection of title (e.g., RN), general practice standards, approvals for educational programs, and disciplinary procedures.

Definition of practice and specific practice standards are further specified within the professional community through major nursing associations. The American Nurses Association (ANA) has specified a variety of practice standards for the profession, both general and specific to certain practice areas. The ANA has prepared several specialty standards documents jointly with the particular specialty organization to reflect the expectations for specialized professional practice. These standards, which signify the sanction by the community of the nursing profession, are described as "authoritative statements by which the nursing profession describes the responsibilities for which its practitioners are accountable. ...[S]tandards also define the nursing profession's accountability to the public and the outcomes for which registered nurses are responsible" (ANA, 2004, p. 1).

The publication *Nursing: Scope and Standards of Practice* (ANA, 2004), for example, prescribes standards of practice and standards of professional performance. Standards of practice address safe practice and use of the nursing process with the actions of assessment, diagnosis, outcome identification, planning, implementation, and evaluation (ANA, 2004). Standards of professional performance are expected professional roles and behaviors, including quality of practice, education, professional practice evaluation, collegiality, collaboration, ethics, research, resource utilization, and leadership (ANA, 2004, p. 3).

Further standards of specialty practice are provided through the certification process with specialized education, testing, and ongoing learning requirements. Practice standards and expectations have also been developed by the applicable specialty organization. Check the web sites listed on the Intranet for standards of practice expected in selected specialty practice areas.

Another area in which the community grants a profession certain privileges on the basis of professional knowledge and expertise is the education process. Educational programs are both approved at the individual state level, as with the Board of Nursing, and accredited at the national level by the National League for Nursing Accrediting Commission (NLNAC) and the Commission on Collegiate Nursing Education (CCNE). Development, implementation, and evaluation of the organization, curriculum, faculty, students, graduates, facilities, and program resources are important considerations within the accreditation and reaccreditation process. The job of establishing and evaluating these standards is granted to the professional accrediting groups. Here again, the profession is granted the power by the community and has the responsibility to provide the community with practitioners who are appropriately educated for safe and effective practice.

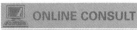

ONLINE CONSULT

ANA Social Policy Statement at
www.nursingworld.org

Greenwood (1957) identified confidentiality as one of the most important professional privileges. Professional nursing enjoys this privilege and conscientiously guards the confidentiality of client information. As discussed in relation to ethical codes, confidentiality is a major consideration in professional nursing practice.

Code of Ethics

A professional abides by a certain code of ethics applicable to the practice area. Developed within the profession, the code addresses general ethical practice issues. As Greenwood (1957) explains, although ethical codes vary among professions, they are uniform in describing client-professional and colleague-colleague relationships (p. 50). The ANA's *Code of Ethics for Nurses* is the ethical standard for professional nursing practice. As the ANA states, the "code makes explicit the primary goals, values, and obligations of the profession" through nine "non-negotiable" provisions (Box 1–2) with interpretative statements (ANA, 2001, p. 5). The interpretative statements promote understanding for appropriate application of the code of ethics in professional practice. The ANA Code embodies both the formal and informal ethical codes referred to by Greenwood. Achieving professional status requires ethical standards for expected behaviors with clients, colleagues, and other professionals.

BOX 1–2
THE CODE OF ETHICS FOR NURSES

1. The nurse, in all professional relationships, practices with compassion and respect for the inherent dignity, worth, and uniqueness of every individual, unrestricted by considerations of social or economic status, personal attributes, or the nature of health problems.
2. The nurse's primary commitment is to the patient, whether an individual, family, group, or community.
3. The nurse promotes, advocates for, and strives to protect the health, safety, and rights of the patient.
4. The nurse is responsible and accountable for individual nursing pratice and determines the appropriate delegation of tasks consistent with the nurse's obligation to provide optimum patient care.
5. The nurse owes the same duties to self as to others, including the responsibility to preserve integrity and safety, to maintain competence, and to continue personal and professional growth.
6. The nurse participates in establishing, maintaining, and improving health-care environments and conditions of employment conducive to the provision of quality health care and consistent with the values of the profession through invididual and collective action.
7. The nurse participates in the advancement of the profession through contributions to practice, education, administration, and knowledge development.
8. The nurse collaborates with other health professionals and the public in promoting community, national, and international efforts to meet health needs.
9. The profession of nursing, as represented by associations and their members, is responsible for articulating nursing values, for maintaining the integrity of the profession and its practice, and for shaping social policy.

Source: Reprinted with permission from the American Nurses Association, *Code of Ethics for Nurses with Interpretive Statements*, ©2001 American Nurses Publishing, American Nurses Association, Washington, DC.

ONLINE CONSULT

Read the *Code of Ethics for Nurses with Interpretative Statements* at
http://www.nursingworld.org/ethics/code/ethicscode150.htm

Professional Culture

The fifth characteristic of a profession is a **professional culture**. Greenwood (1957) described professional culture as the formal and informal groups represented in the profession. *Formal groups* refers to the organizational systems in which the professionals practice, the educational institutions that provide for basic and continued learning, and the professional associations. *Informal groups* are the collegial settings that provide for collaboration, stimulation, and sharing of mutual values. These informal groups exist within each formal group, providing further professional, collegial inclusiveness. These groups and the unique culture of nursing are reinforced in the *Code of Ethics for Nurses*.

Organizational systems in which professional nursing is practiced are diverse and multidimensional. As you will see in later chapters, hospital and home health agency settings are complex parts of a larger system. Professional nursing practice provides a unique culture with the values and norms expected of its practitioners. Organizational philosophies and mission statements provide information on the expressed culture of these settings. Further expression of the professional culture is apparent in the behaviors of professional nurses who practice in these settings.

Formal educational settings for professional nursing practice occur in institutions of higher learning with liberal and specialized learning requirements. In addition, values and norms for continued learning and competency in practice are transmitted as expectations for professional practice. Beyond basic educational practice, **professional development** is provided through continuing education and specialty preparation and continual competency as a professional.

Professional Organizations or associations are a major component of the culture of professional nursing practice, but they vary in purpose or mission and membership. The purpose of some professional organizations, such as the ANA, is to represent the profession globally. Specialty groups, with a more specific focus, promote education, skills, standards, and perhaps certification opportunities for a particular segment of the profession, for example, the American Association of Critical Care Nurses. Each organization has a unique philosophy or mission directed at professional nursing practice.

Professional organizations communicate values and norms in official publications, position statements, and specified practice standards. These organizations promote professional parameters for clinical practice, education, administration, and research. They provide educational opportunities and foster expansion of the knowledge base of individual professionals and the discipline in general. Some organizations focus specifically on the science of the profession. Their purpose is to promote the scholarly aspects of the profession and to build professional skills through education, publications, and conferences. A more global view of practice can be seen in many professional organizations as they reach out to influence public policy.

Consider the organizations that represent professional nursing practice and education listed in Table 1–1. ANA and its state and territorial associations focus mainly on the profession as an entity, with concern for the health of society as well as the welfare of professional nurses through standards, official position statements, political action initiatives, and certification options for specialty practice. Specific to an area of specialty practice, the American Association of Critical Care Nurses, with its worldwide membership, is the largest specialty organization. The National League for Nursing (NLN) has two types of

TABLE 1–1
Characteristics of Selected Professional Organizations

Organization	Focus, Mission, & Membership
American Nurses Association (ANA) and associated constituent state associations and organizational affiliate members Founded 1897 http://www.nursingworld.org	Focus: Professional nursing Mission: "Dedicated to ensuring that an adequate supply of highly-skilled and well-trained nurses is available, the ANA is committed to meeting the needs of nurses as well as health-care consumers. The ANA advances the nursing profession by fostering high standards of nursing practice, promoting the economic and general welfare of nurses in the workplace, projecting a positive and realistic view of nursing, and by lobbying the Congress and regulatory agencies on health-care issues affecting nurses and the public" (ANA, 2003, p. 1). Membership: Individual membership; professional nurses at the state level obtain national and district membership.
American Association of Colleges of Nursing (AACN) Founded 1969 http://www.aacn.nche.edu	Focus: Collegiate nursing education Mission: "The American Association of Colleges of Nursing is the national voice for baccalaureate and graduate-degree nursing education. A unique asset for the nation, AACN serves the public interest by providing standards and resources, and by fostering innovation to advance professional nursing education, research, and practice" (AACN, 2003, p. 1) Membership: Deans and directors of member schools with baccalaureate and higher degree nursing programs
American Association of Critical-Care Nurses (AACN) Founded 1969 http://www.aacn.org	Focus: Specialty care Mission: "Building on decades of clinical excellence, the American Association of Critical-Care Nurses (AACN) provides and inspires leadership to establish work and care environments that are respectful, healing and humane. The key to AACN's success is through its members. Therefore, AACN is committed to providing the highest quality resources to maximize nurses' contribution to caring and improving the healthcare of critically ill patients and their families" (AACN, 2002, p. 1). Membership: Individual membership
National League for Nursing (NLN) and associated constituent leagues Founded 1952 http://nln.org	Focus: Nursing education and community health Mission: To advance quality nursing education that prepares the nursing workforce to meet the needs of diverse populations in an ever-changing health-care environment" (NLN, 2002, p. 1). Membership: Individual and agency (Diploma Programs, Associate Degree Programs, Baccalaureate and Higher Degree Programs) membership

(continued)

TABLE 1–1	
Characteristics of Selected Professional Organizations *(continued)*	
Organization	**Focus, Mission, & Membership**
Sigma Theta Tau International Honor Society of Nursing and member chapters Founded 1922 http://nursingsociety.org	Focus: Nursing scholarship Mission: To serve, support, and improve: Sigma Theta Tau International Honor Society of Nursing provides leadership and scholarship in practice, education, and research to enhance the health of all people. We support the learning and professional development of our members, who strive to improve nursing care worldwide" (Sigma Theta Tau, 2003, p. 1) Membership: Individuals are invited to membership in chartered chapters with selection criteria as baccalaureate or higher degree students, faculty members, or community leaders.

Note: Reference citations in table are from online resources of the respective nursing organizations.

membership, individual and agency, with initiatives related to accreditation of nursing education programs and community health agencies. The American Association of Colleges of Nursing focuses on collegiate education, serving member schools with baccalaureate and higher degree programs through educational standards, programs, policies, research, accreditation, and legislative initiatives directed at high-quality professional education. Sigma Theta Tau, the international honor society for nursing, has a distinctly scientific focus. This organization promotes knowledge development through research, dissemination of scientific information, technology, education, interdisciplinary collaboration, and adaptability for the improvement of the health of people worldwide.

A comprehensive listing of professional organizations and their Website addresses is located on the Intranet site. In addition, useful links to additional resources may be discovered within these sites. Just one word of caution: Website addresses change, as do physical addresses. Try to update your computer browser's address book and "favorites" listing continually with any changes and add new sites that you have found. You will want to add bookmarks in your computer browser as well as keep a hard copy listing of frequently used Websites.

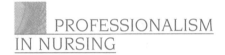

PROFESSIONALISM IN NURSING

The nursing profession is characterized by Greenwood's attributes of a profession. But what of its uniqueness? Miller and associates (1993) have proposed that "nurses must disclaim the traditional analysis of professional and professionalism by other disciplines as the only method to determine definitions and characteristics of professionalism in nursing" (p. 290). They propose the use of a behavioral inventory to assist nurses in attaining higher degrees of professionalism (Miller et al, 1993, p. 294). This behavioral inventory consists of nine categories of professional nursing characteristics (Box 1–3). Consider each of these criteria for professionalism in nursing.

Educational Background

The **educational background** required for professional practice is specified to ensure safe and effective practice. In nursing, the basic education required for entry into the profession varies, with differences among baccalaureate, associate degree, diploma education, and even some entry-level graduate programs. But within each type of educational program, curricula and requirements are guided by general standards.

Although a school's curriculum is developed by its faculty members, certain standards are required for an educational program. Nursing curricula must contain essential content and hours as required by state boards of nursing, higher education boards, professional associations, and national accrediting bodies. Consumers of nursing care can be confused by the different educational routes leading to the title of registered nurse. The Pew Health Professions Commission critically reviewed the various health professions, their regulatory bodies, educational program requirements, and workforce needs to address the changing health-care system. The Commission (1995) then made the following recommendations relative to basic nursing education:

- Recognize value of multiple entry points to professional practice
- Consolidate professional nomenclature, e.g., a single title for each level of nursing preparation/service
- Differentiate practice responsibilities among levels and strengthen existing career ladder programs:

- Associate Degree in Nursing (A.D.N.): entry hospital and nursing home
- Bachelor of Science in Nursing (B.S.N.): hospital care management and community practice
- Master of Science in Nursing (M.S.N.): specialty practice in hospital and independent practice (p. 34).

Ongoing clarification of these areas among professionals and consumers of nursing will have a beneficial effect on the view of nursing as a profession and of individual nurses as true professionals.

As a follow-up to the work of the Pew Commission, two reports from the Institute of Medicine called for changes in education of health professionals. The 2001 report from the Institute of Medicine, *Crossing the Quality Chasm*, proposed 10 rules (Box 1–4) for the health system in the 21st century (Corrigan et al, 2001). A further report following a Health Professions Education Summit led to the identification of five **core competencies** (Box 1–5) for all health professionals to advance these 10 rules with an "overarching vision" that "all health professionals should be educated to deliver patient-centered care as members of an interdisciplinary team,

---

BOX 1-5
CORE COMPETENCIES FOR HEALTH PROFESSIONALS

- Provide patient-centered care.
- Work in interdisciplinary teams.
- Employ evidence-based practice.
- Apply quality improvement.
- Utilize informatics.

Source: Greiner, A.C., & Knebel, E. (eds.). (2003). *Health professions education: A bridge to quality.* Washington, DC: Institute of Medicine.

---

emphasizing evidence-based practice, quality improvement approaches, and informatics" (Greiner and Knebel, 2003, p. 45). To address these competencies in nursing education programs, curriculum must be constantly evaluated for currency, content, and practice opportunities. For example, most nurses will agree that providing patient-centered care is a component of our nursing programs. However, we need to assess carefully whether all programs foster interdiscipinary and evidence-based practice focused on quality improvement and the use of informatics.

Adherence to a Code of Ethics

Adherence to a **code of ethics** is expected in any profession. As illustrated previously, the *Code of Ethics for Nurses with Interpretative Statements* (ANA, 2001) provides the broad guidelines. It is the responsibility of the practicing professional to know these guidelines and practice in accordance with the Code. As Miller and associates (1993) reported, most professional nurse respondents did not have a copy of the ethical code, and many were unfamiliar with the document (p. 293). This problem occurred with the 1985 *Code of Ethics*. The question then becomes, How many nurses are aware of the 2001 revision? To meet this criterion of professionalism, nursing professionals need to demonstrate greater knowledge and understanding of the official ethical code. Periodic review of the nine ethical provisions and their interpretative statements is an important respon-

sibility for all professional nurses. This is especially true when the roles of nurses or clients change, but it is also important for nurses to appreciate fully their professional responsibilities, challenges, and talents when roles are stable.

Participation in Professional Organizations

Participation in the **professional organization** is an important criterion for a profession. Unfortunately, in nursing this is quite a broad area, as is evident from the listing of professional organizations located on the Intranet site. Approximately 10 percent of the more than 2 million nurses in the United States belong to the major professional group ANA. Many nurses prefer to associate with specialty groups that they believe better meet their educational and practice needs.

This brings us to two critical considerations: multiple memberships and activity. Professionals are not limited to membership in one professional association. If all nurses belonged to one official organization representing professional nurses, that organization would have an enormous influence on health care by virtue of these numbers. But because of different disciplinary paradigms, this is not the case. Professionals associate with organizations they view as most appropriate to their belief system views and practice, rather than with organizations they do not perceive as matching their professional practice needs. Yet ANA does represent all nurses in the United States and its territories. The ANA describes its role as follows:

> The American Nurses Association (ANA) is the only full-service professional organization representing the nation's entire registered nurse population. From the halls of Congress and federal agencies to the board rooms, hospitals and other health-care facilities, the ANA is the strongest voice for the nursing profession and for workplace advocacy. (ANA, 2003)

For example, in response to the Institute of Medicine's published report *Crossing the Quality Chasm: A New Health System for the 21st Century* in 2001, the ANA (2002) identified 10 areas of concern demanding action: leadership and planning, delivery systems, legislation/regulatory/policy, professional/nursing culture, recruitment/retention, economic value, work environment, public relations/communication, education, and diversity. This breakdown will have been incorporated into *Nursing's Agenda for the Future* (ANA, 2002) by 2010.

We are beginning to see more collaboration among organizations on key issues. There are now a growing number of organizations that officially affiliate with the ANA, and others are members of a liaison forum (check the ANA Website for a current listing of these affiliates). This movement will further strengthen the profession and create a sense of professional community among nurses. Membership and participation in a major nursing organization are important traits of professionalism for the professional nurse. Active involvement means more than paying dues; it consists of active support of and involvement in the issues addressed by the organization and the profession to promote high-quality health care for the consumer.

Continuing Education

The fourth characteristic of professionalism in nursing involves **continuing education** and **continued competency**. These attributes are crucial to safe, effective, and ethical professional practice. Ongoing improvement and knowledge are the goals of continuing education, which is required for relicensure in some states and recertification in specialty areas. A slowly increasing number of nurses are completing additional education beyond their basic nursing education. But continuing education is more than obtaining required credits, in-service hours, and formal degrees. Remaining current with ideas presented in the nursing and scientific literature is an important component of your continued competency as a professional and for evidence-based practice.

The Internet has made remaining current on issues of concern to the profession more convenient. However, a word of caution is in order: It is important to evaluate the source of information and its validity. Consider whether the information is provided by an organization, an agency, or an individual's own Website and personal perspective.

Identifying your own learning and developmental needs is an expectation and a continual process for competent professional practice. In essence, continuing education for competency involves self-assessment, ongoing learning, and self-evaluation. The focus is on discovery, as in baccalaureate and graduate education. Ongoing learning means that your mind is challenged every day with new ideas, building on a professional knowledge base and skills.

Opportunities for continuing education abound through a variety of formal programs as well as through professional journals and online resources. Many professional organizations have special online services for their members, such as reviews of current literature and care products, bookstores, continuing education programs, e-mail lists, and online discussion forums. Access the resources readily available at *nursingworld.org* and *nurses.com*, to mention only two. Look at resources provided online at Websites of individual specialty groups like AACN and the many others listed on the Intranet site. Publishers also have online resources with special discounts, e-mail updates, associated Websites, discussion groups, and interactive continuing education offerings.

Communication and Publication

Communication and publication were identified as the fifth characteristic of professional nursing. Although Miller and colleagues (1993) reported limited involvement in this area from the subjects in their research study, they did stress that "scholarly writing for publication and communication to others must become a requisite for the professional nurse to maintain and promote professionalism in nursing" (p. 294). This does not necessarily mean that every nurse needs to publish a scholarly article each year. Innovative ideas are communicated in a variety of ways, both within the practice setting and worldwide through publications or on the Internet. Communication among professionals through well-developed and presented memoranda, proposed institutional policies and practices, and reports at the agency level is important and shows professionalism. Sharing with colleagues through specialty, district, or state nurses' association newsletters or publications further promotes professionalism. Consider collaborating with colleagues from other health professions. It is the responsibility of the professional to share innovative ideas that can benefit other professionals. Ideas can be shared though interdisciplinary practice and professional organizations and communicated in professional journals, other publications, and through telecommunications.

Autonomy and Self-Regulation

Autonomy involves independent judgment and self-governing within the scope of one's practice, which changes in response to people's health-care needs. As key professionals in organizational settings, nurses make the time and commitment to ensure that high-quality care and standards are present and upheld. This involves critical thinking, communication, collaboration, and leadership. Important concepts in this area are professional responsibility and accountability. In the *Code of Ethics for Nurses*, **responsibility** is defined as accountability for performance of the duties associated with the professional role, and **accountability** as being answerable to oneself and others for one's judgments and actions in the the course of nursing practice, irrespective of health-care organizations' policies or providers' directives (ANA, 2001, pp. 16–17). In her concept analysis, Wade (1999) defines professional nurse autonomy as "belief in the centrality of the client when making responsible discretionary decisions, both dependently and independently, that reflect advocacy for the client" (p. 311). This is the nurse's accountability to the client. However, as we will see in later chapters, accountability is also extended to the broader population as the profession demonstrates involvement in social policy.

The ANA's *Nursing's Social Policy Statement* (2003) describes **self-regulation** as both personal accountability for the knowledge base for practice and participation in the peer review process (p. 11). Professional responsi-

bility and accountability involve upholding quality standards as well as developing and critically analyzing those standards and the outcomes. Professionals are responsible and answerable to clients for nursing care outcomes. Nurses are actively involved in supervising, delegating, and evaluating others. But their professional status can take the expectations of critical thinking, clinical judgment, expertise, and advocacy beyond a narrowly defined job description or institutional procedure manuals. The regulation of nursing practice includes self-regulation expected of the professional as well as professional regulation through the defined scope of practice, further education, certification, and adherence to the code of ethics. An important component is the peer review process, whether through an annual performance evaluation or of a particular activity or contribution to the literature.

The profession is also regulated through licensure to enter the profession, continuing conpetency requirements, national certification for advanced practice nurses, and the charge of each State Board of Nursing to protect the health and safety of the clients of nursing. An important note here is the focus of the State licensing board versus the state nurses association. The state nurses' association is the advocate for the professionals providing care to clients, as long as the care is provided skillfully, professionally, and ethically. The licensing authority focuses on safe provision of nursing care. This safety is addressed through a defined scope of professional practice, requirements for entry in and continuation in the profession, and disciplinary action in the cases posing danger to clients.

Community Service

Community service was proposed as the seventh characteristic of professionalism in nursing. Nurses are well equipped and talented in this area because of their orientation of service to clients and society at large. Nurses frequently lead health-promoting activities in their employment role, their professional community, and among their families and acquaintances. Consider how residents in a defined community always seem to know who the nurses in the area are and how frequently those nurses are approached with questions or requests to become involved in projects or serve on committees. Also consider how nurses reach out to others with information on health or means to foster wellness in their communities. All these activities consititute community service.

Theory

Although all professions have systematic theory and knowledge on which to base their practice, the eighth characteristic of professionalism in nursing involves greater activity in this process: **theory use, development, and evaluation**. Theory is essential to guiding the practice and research of a profession. Nursing, as a developing and dynamic profession, demands that its professionals develop, refine, and evaluate theory. We not only use theory but are constantly involved in critical analysis of the theory as clients, health-care, and environments change. We are consistently expanding and refining our knowledge base. The challenge is to collect, analyze, and report data on efficacy related to trends in clients' outcomes. These trends, rather than individual cases, provide information that expands and refines the profession's knowledge base. This need for data collection and analysis leads to research, the final characteristic of professional nursing proposed by Miller and associates (1993).

Evidence-Based Practice

Nursing research is much more than leading or participating in a research study. We now look to the core competency of **evidence-based practice** to guide the way we practice. Greiner and Knebel (2003) define evidence-based practice as the integration of the best research with clinical expertise and the client's values for optimum care as well as participation in learning and research activities (pp. 45–46). As found in the interpretative statements of the *Code for Nurses*, "All

nurses working alone or in collaboration with others can participate in the advancement of the profession through the development, evaluation, and application of knowledge in practice" (ANA, 2001, p. 23). Involvement in research, whether by using findings, participating in an investigation, or protecting human subjects, is a characteristic of professionalism in nursing. It adds to our knowledge base, enhances our practice, promotes improved outcomes for our clients, and fosters practice based on evidence of efficacy rather than the tradition of trial and error.

Fulfilling the characteristics described in the nine categories just discussed well is the challenge to professionalism in nursing. Professionalism is an attribute in constant refinement. The degree to which professionals demonstrate professionalism in nursing is apparent in their professional practice and how they define nursing.

> *Research adds to our knowledge base, enhances our practice, promotes improved outcomes for our clients, and fosters practice based on evidence of efficacy rather than the tradition of trial and error.*

YOUR PHILOSOPHY OF NURSING

Virginia Henderson (1897–1996) was an outstanding leader in nursing. Her classic definition of nursing embodied her view of the unique role of the professional nurse as:

> Assisting the individual, sick or well, in the performance of those activities contributing to health or its recovery (or to a peaceful death) that he would perform unaided if he had the necessary strength, will, or knowledge. And to do this in such a way as to help him gain independence as rapidly as possible. (Henderson, 1966, p. 15)

This concrete definition was expanded and applied to nursing practice, education, and research. Henderson's philosophy of nursing was one of caring, assisting, and supporting the person. In her writings, she encouraged every nurse to develop a personal concept of nursing—in essence, his or her philosophy of nursing.

A **philosophy** of nursing presents a particular professional nurse's belief system or worldview of nursing—the nurse's personal definition of nursing. Bevis (1989) defined philosophy as providing a point of view of nature, relationships, and the value of things (p. 34).

As discussed previously, the metaparadigm concept of "the person" relates to nursing clients. Nurses in different practices define "the person" uniquely within the practice, for example, as individuals versus families. The nurse's practice area and client populations also influence the environment, for example, an intensive care unit in an acute care setting or a rural health-care unit located in a community school or modular building. The concept of health also varies, being different for the professional who provides care for trauma victims and the nurse involved with health initiatives in an employee group. Specific nursing roles and the services provided influence the concept of nursing. In addition to the metaparadigm concepts in a personal philosophy of nursing, certain other commonalities are generally apparent. Bevis (1989) identified the following philosophical propositions as generally accepted despite divergent implications and implementation:

1. The individual has intrinsic value and there is worth inherent in human life.
2. Nursing is a rational activity.
3. Nursing's uniqueness is in the way the basic social and biological sciences are synthesized in functions that promote health.
4. The individual nurse-citizen has some control over and responsibility for the political and social milieu in which he/she lives.
5. Nursing is a process with a central subjec-tive purpose, an inherent organization or system, and dynamic creativity. (pp. 43–45)

In addition, consider the following six essential features of professional nursing identified in the ANA's *Nursing's Social Policy Statement* (2003):

1. Provision of a caring relationship tha facilitates health and healing
2. Attention to the range of human experiences and responses to health and illness within the physical and social environments
3. Integration of objective data with knowledge gained from an appreciation of the patient or group's subjective experience
4. Application of scientific knowledge to the processes of diagnosis and treatment through the use of judgment and critical thinking
5. Advancement of professional nursing knowledge through scholarly inquiry
6. Influence on social and public policy to promote social justice (p. 5)

At this point, you should critically analyze your belief system and express your views of nursing. We all have prior experiences that influence our thinking and actions. Try to place those aside and begin to craft your philosophy of nursing. Using these definitions and assumptions, develop your views into a personal philosophy of nursing. Periodically evaluate your philosophy to analyze how your professional practice is enhanced in your ongoing quest for knowledge and expertise in your profession. This is your professional identity.

Key Points

- The following are characteristics of a profession: (1) systematic theory and knowledge base, (2) authority, (3) community sanction, (4) an ethical code, and (5) a professional culture.
- Kerlinger (1986) defines a theory as "a set of interrelated constructs (concepts), definitions, and propositions that present a systematic view of phenomena by specifying relations among variables, with the purpose of explaining and predicting the phenomena" (p. 9). *(continued)*

(continued)

- A paradigm used by professionals in a scientific community consists of the beliefs and the belief system shared by members of that particular community to explain phenomena, practice the profession, and conduct research.

- The metaparadigm of nursing is the overall concern of nursing common to each nursing model, whether a conceptual model/paradigm or formal theory, and it includes the concepts of person, environment, health, and nursing.

- The *Code of Ethics for Nurses* (ANA, 2001) is the ethical standard for professional nursing practice. It identifies expected professional practice behaviors with clients, colleagues, and other professionals within nine provisions with interpretative statements.

- *Autonomy* involves judgment and self-governing within one's scope of practice. This self-governing requires ongoing evaluation of both responsibility and accountability in professional practice. In the ANA's *Code of Ethics for Nurses*, *responsibility* is defined as accountability for performance of the duties associated with the professional role, and *accountability* is being answerable to oneself and others for one's judgments and actions in the course of nursing practice, irrespective of health-care organizations' policies and providers' directives (ANA, 2001, pp. 16–17).

- Miller and associates (1993) have proposed the use of a behavioral inventory to assist nurses in attaining higher levels of professionalism. The following characteristics of professionalism are listed in this inventory: educational background, adherence to the code of ethics, participation in the professional organization, continuing education and competency, communication and publication, autonomy and self-regulation, community service, theory use, development, and evaluation, and involvement in research.

- The five competencies for health professionals are: providing patient-centered care, working in interdisciplinary teams, employing evidence-based practice, applying quality improvement, and using informatics (Greiner and Knebel, 2001).

- A personal philosophy of nursing presents the belief system or world view of nursing for a particular professional nurse. Incorporated into such a philosophy are definitions, values, and assumptions about the metaparadigm concepts of person, environment, health, and nursing.

Thought and Discussion Questions

1. Miller and associates (1993) have proposed that "nurses must disclaim the traditional analysis of professional and professionalism by other disciplines as the only method to determine definitions and characteristics of professionalism in nursing" (p. 290). From what you have read in this chapter and on what you know from the practice setting, can you explain why would they make such a statement? Propose another way to determine the definitions and characteristics of the profession of nursing.

2. Be prepared to participate in a discussion to be scheduled by your instructor on how you demonstrate the five core competencies of health professionals.

3. Explain your views on responsibility and accountability.

4. Describe how you demonstrate continued competency.

5. Review the Chapter Thought located on the first page of the chapter, and discuss it in the context of the contents of the chapter.

Interactive Exercises

1. Locate another definition of *professionalism* or a *profession* online or in the literature. Apply this definition to the nursing profession.

2. Go to the National Council Website at **www.ncsbn.org**, and locate your state's nursing practice act. Analyze the powers, privileges, and responsibilities vested in the profession. Is your state a member of the Nurse Licensure Compact, and what does this compact involve? Be prepared to participate in an online or class discussion to be scheduled by your instructor on how this act directs responsibility and accountability in professional nursing practice.

3. Select at least three professional organizations listed on the Intranet site under "Resources and Links," and access their Websites. Investigate the mission, purposes, major initiatives, membership, and benefits of membership. Discuss the professional culture of the organization and the values related to nursing and health care.

4. Review one of the standards of practice listed in the Bibliography. Identify the legal and ethical responsibilities of practice in this area. Discuss the formal and educational responsibilities for professional practice.

5. For each of the nine ethical provisions of the *Code of Ethics for Nurses* (ANA, 2001), consider the interpretative statements, located on the Website at **www.nursingworld.org/ethics/code/ethicscode150.htm**, and describe how they are applicable to each of the following environments for nursing practice:
   - Acute care in a hospital setting
   - Home care
   - Clinic or occupational health setting

6. Complete the interactive exercise on your nursing philosophy on the Intranet site. Use the exercise to evaluate critically your belief system, express your views on nursing, and begin to craft your personal philosophy. Be prepared to participate in an online or class discussion to be scheduled by your instructor in which you will explain and support your views and identify commonalities between your views and those of your associates.

7. Evaluate your own professional status on the basis of the inventory by Miller and associates (1993) Use the Self-Asessment of Professionalism in Nursing format provided on the Intranet site.

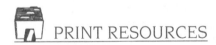
PRINT RESOURCES

References

American Nurses Association. (2004). *Nursing: Scope and standards of practice* (Publication No. 03SSNP). Washington, DC: American Nurses Publishing.

American Nurses Association. (2003). *Nursing's social policy statement* (2nd ed.) (Publication No. 03NSPS 15M 09/03). Washington, DC: American Nurses Publishing.

American Nurses Association. (2001). *Code of ethics for nurses with interpretative statements* (Publication No. CEN21 10M 08/01). Washington, DC: American Nurses Publishing.

Benner, P. (1984). *From novice to expert: Excellence and power in clinical nursing practice.* Menlo Park, CA: Addison-Wesley.

Bevis, E. O. (1989). *Curriculum building in nursing: A process* (3rd ed.) (Publication No. 15–2277). New York: National League for Nursing.

Callin, M. (1996). From RN to BSN: Seeing familiar situations in different ways. *Journal of Continuing Education in Nursing*, 27, 28–33.

Corrigan, M. S., Donaldson, M. S., Kohn, L. T., Maguire, S. K., & Pike, K. C. (2001). *Crossing the quality chasm: A new health system for the 21st Century*. Washington, DC: National Academy Press.

Fawcett, J. (2000). *Analysis and evaluation of contemporary nursing knowledge: Nursing models and theories*. Philadelphia: F. A. Davis.

Fawcett, J. (1995). *Analysis and evaluation of conceptual models of nursing* (3rd ed.). Philadelphia: F. A. Davis.

Greenwood, E. (1957). Attributes of a profession. *Social Work*, 2(3), 45–55.

Greiner, A. C., & Knebel, E. (eds.). (2003). *Health professions education: A bridge to quality*. Washington, DC: Institute of Medicine.

Henderson, V. (1966). *The nature of nursing: A definition and its implications for practice, education, and research*. New York: Macmillan.

Kerlinger, F. N. (1986). *Foundations of behavioral research* (3rd ed.). New York: Holt, Rinehart and Winston.

Kuhn, T. S. (1970). *The structure of scientific revolutions* (2nd ed.). Chicago: University of Chicago Press.

Mezirow, J. (1991). *Transformative dimensions of adult learning*. San Francisco: Jossey-Bass.

Miller, B. K., Adams, D., & Beck, L. (1993). A behavioral inventory for professionalism in nursing. *Journal of Professional Nursing*, 9, 290–295.

Pew Health Professions Commission. (1995). *Critical challenges: Revitalizing the health professions for the twenty-first century*. San Francisco: USCF Center for the Health Professions.

Wade, G. H. (1999). Professional nurse autonomy: Concept analysis and application to nursing education. *Journal of Advanced Nursing*, 30, 310–318.

Bibliography

American Nurses Association. (2003). *Scope and standards of diabetes nursing* (2nd ed.) (Publication No. 9808ST). Washington, DC: American Nurses Publishing.

American Nurses Association. (2003). *Scope and standards of pediatric nursing practice* (Publication No. PNP23). Washington, DC: American Nurses Publishing.

American Nurses Association. (2002). *Scope and standards of hospice and palliative nursing practice* (Publication No. HPN22). Washington, DC: American Nurses Publishing.

American Nurses Association. (2002). *Scope and standards of neuroscience nursing practice* (Publication No. NNS22). Washington, DC: American Nurses Publishing.

American Nurses Association. (2001). *Scope and standards of gerontological nursing practice* (2nd ed.) (Publication No. GNP21). Washington, DC: American Nurses Publishing.

American Nurses Association. (2001). *Scope and standards of nursing informatics practice* (Publication No. NIP21). Washington, DC: American Nurses Publishing.

American Nurses Association. (2001). *Scope and standards of professional school nursing practice* (Publication No. SHNP21). Washington, DC: American Nurses Publishing.

American Nurses Association. (2000). *Scope and standards of pediatric oncology nursing* (Publication No. PONP20). Washington, DC: American Nurses Publishing.

American Nurses Association. (2000). *Scope and standards of practice for nursing professional development* (Publication No. NPD-20). Washington, DC: American Nurses Publishing.

American Nurses Association. (2000). *Scope and standards of psychiatric–mental health nursing practice* (Publication No. PMH-20CM7). Washington, DC: American Nurses Publishing.

American Nurses Association. (1999). *Scope and standards of public health nursing practice* (Publication No. 9910PH). Washington, DC: American Nurses Publishing.

American Nurses Association. (1999). *Scope and standards of home health nursing practice* (Publication No. 9905HH). Washington, DC: American Nurses Publishing.

American Nurses Association. (1998). *Scope and standards of parish nursing practice* (Publication No. 9806ST). Washington, DC: American Nurses Publishing.

American Nurses Association. (1997). *Scope and standards of college health nursing practice* (Publication No. ST-1). Washington, DC: American Nurses Publishing.

American Nurses Association. (1997). *Scope and standards of forensic nursing practice* (Publication No. ST-4). Washington, DC: American Nurses Publishing.

American Nurses Association. (1998). *Statement on the scope and standards for the nurse who specializes in developmental disabilities and/or mental retardation* (Publication No. 9802ST). Washington, DC: American Nurses Publishing.

American Nurses Association. (1998). *Statement on the scope and standards of genetics clinical nursing practice* (Publication No. 9807ST). Washington, DC: American Nurses Publishing.

American Nurses Association. (1996). *Statement on the scope and standards of oncology nursing practice* (Publication No. MS-23). Washington, DC: American Nurses Publishing.

American Nurses Association. (1995). *Scope and standards of nursing practice in correctional facilities* (Publication No. NP-104). Washington, DC: American Nurses Publishing.

American Nurses Association. (1995). *Standards of clinical practice and scope of practice for the acute care nurse practitioner* (Publication No. MS-22). Washington, DC: American Nurses Publishing.

Kohn, L. T., Corrigan, M. S., & Donaldson, M. S. (1999). *To err is human: Building a safer health system*. Washington, DC: National Academy Press.

O'Neil, E. H. (1998). *Recreating health professional practice for a new century*. San Francisco: Pew Health Professions Commission.

Whall. A. L., & Hicks, F. D. (2002). The unrecognized paradigm shift in nursing: Implications, problems, and possibilities. *Nursing Outlook*, 50, 72–76.

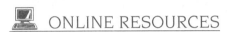 ONLINE RESOURCES

References

American Association of Colleges of Nursing.(2003). *Mission.* http://www.aacn.nche.edu/ContactUs/aboutaacn.htm

American Association of Critical Care Nurses. (2002). *Mission.* http://www.aacn.org

American Nurses Association. (2003). ANA's *statement of purpose.* http://nursingworld.org/about/mission.htm

American Nurses Association. (2002). N*ursing's agenda for the future*: A *call to the nation.* http://www.nursingworld.org/naf

National League for Nursing. (2003). A*bout* NLN: NLN *mission statement.* http://nln.org/aboutnln/ourmission.htm

Sigma Theta Tau. (2003). The society's vision and mission. http://www.nursingsociety.org/about/overview.html

Bernadette Dorsch Curry

2
chapter

Coping with Returning to School

> *Change is an opportunity—an opportunity to grow, to discover, to risk, to thrive, to make a difference.*

Chapter Objectives

On completion of this chapter, the reader will be able to:

1. Evaluate personal and professional goals.
2. Identify personal and professional role conflicts and stressors.
3. Develop time management strategies for family, work, and educational demands.
4. Assemble resources to help meet family, work, and educational demands.
5. Develop a personalized study environment and study strategies.

Key Terms

Goals	Resources	Streamlining
Role Transition		

Returning to school for an advanced degree in nursing may begin as an academic and professional goal. As the fullness of the experience unfolds, however, you will come to realize that education is more than academic exercises and credits. It is an intellectual pursuit that leads to personal growth in many areas. You have chosen the challenge and made the personal and professional commitment to goals. By adopting a positive attitude and using a variety of available resources, you can experience the exhilaration of success and the satisfaction of accomplishment.

 ## WHAT TO EXPECT

Expectations can set the tone and influence behaviors. When you are returning to school, it is important to have valid and realistic expectations of the experience and of yourself—to be informed, committed, and confident in your desire and ability to succeed. On the basis of experiences with registered nurse (RN) students in a baccalaureate nursing program, Donea Shane (1980) described observations and set forth what is known as the *returning to school syndrome*. She characterized emotional responses and captured the essence of the process. In addition to identifying and documenting the behaviors, she wanted to alert RN students to prepare for the challenges.

Returning to School Syndrome

The syndrome has three phases. In the first phase, called the "honeymoon," fascination with the new and different activities associated with academe casts a positive glow on the experience, and a strong sense of satisfaction can be derived from embarking on the journey.

In phase two, called "conflict," new and different perspectives of nursing are presented, and students experience a growing discomfort with previous knowledge and familiar concepts, often accompanied by waning confidence. Insecurity and self-doubt can cause students to question their capabilities or blame others for perceived unsatisfactory achievement in the program. RN students may have had minimal or no experience with nursing theory (Fawcett, 1995), for instance, and the abstract nature of theory may elicit anxiety in students who previously learned in concrete and structured educational modes and functioned professionally with technical expertise.

"Biculturalism," the third phase, is described as the "ability to be as comfortable and effective in one culture (school) as in another (work)." This is the phase in which students learn that growth does not require destroying strong foundations, but does require building on them. They realize that their past education and professional experiences serve as rich resources for professional development.

 ## SETTING PERSONAL GOALS

Deciding to return to school is a major lifetime decision and the beginning of a new phase of goal setting. **Goals** are powerful entities. They can provide a focus, sustain commitment, reinforce priorities, and provide a framework for current and future decisions. Goals help keep the decision-maker focused by addressing both the time needed and the scope of the task. It is easy to overlook the power of goals if they are considered simply an endpoint of a process.

Remember the following points when setting your goals:

- You alone are the goal-maker and in command of your personal quest.
- You alone create the goal, establish the plan, and accomplish the task.
- You can expect to invest considerable time and attention in developing your goals and their accompanying plans.
- Forethought, motivation, and creativity transform goals from ideas into reality.
- Personal goals are born of individual values,

ambition, and abilities and are the result of introspective and selective processes.

- Genuine personal goals are holistic and help you maintain perspective and respect priorities.

The planning associated with goals cannot be underestimated. Chenevert (1993) said that the "difference between a goal and a dream is a workable plan" (p. 135). Both long- and short-term goals, and the means to achieve them, must be realistic and must acknowledge individual strengths and limitations, available resources, and personal flexibility. Capitalize on your strengths, and use available resources to overcome your limitations.

Flexibility is particularly important. Change is to be expected and may require adjustments to your original plans. Consider revising your goals or readjusting your plans as a positive response to the new developments. Think of change as an opportunity, a possibility for improvement (Murphy,1999). When establishing your goals and plans, be sure to develop a "plan B," to increase your ability to adapt quickly to the new situation.

Consider achieving an advanced degree as a long-term goal. It requires patience, time, and energy to succeed. Building in short-term goals helps keep your achievements and remaining goals in perspective. Achieving these short-term goals provides a sense of satisfaction, which can energize and increase motivation. View each educational phase as a milestone and each course or semester completed as an accomplishment and progress toward the ultimate goal.

No matter how well you have set your goals, made realistic plans, or chosen appropriate actions, you will face occasional stress, frustration, discouragement, and low motivation. Achievement rarely occurs without challenge. During these times, it helps to recall your reasons for setting the goal and to review the potential benefits. Achieving a goal is fulfilling a commitment to yourself. It is by working through challenges and succeeding that you grow. Being true to yourself when setting and living out goals is vital and may be accomplished by heeding the words of Goethe, "things which matter most should never be at the mercy of things which matter least."

REFINING PROFESSIONAL IDENTITY

"Metamorphosis does not happen without our artful participation" (Moore, 1992, p. 76). Neither personal nor professional growth occurs without individual energy and creativity. The purposeful decision to return to school begins an ongoing series of transitions leading to the goal. Each of those transitions requires the thought, attention, and action of the individual and contributes to professional change and personal growth.

Change can be an uncomfortable and negative experience. However, it can also be invigorating and challenging and can have many positive results. Returning to the student role requires self-redefinition accompanied by motivation (Redman & Cassells, 1990). Curry (1994) found that the opportunity for career and educational mobility was the most influential factor for RNs deciding to pursue a baccalaureate degree. Personal desire to possess a bachelor's degree was the second. Interestingly, students in traditional baccalaureate nursing programs most often reported the same factors as being very influential in their decision to enroll (Curry, 1994). These motivators play an important part in the active roles expected of the student.

From the outset, you will have the opportunity to chart your own course of action, resulting in a change in professional identity. Planning is important because it allows time to develop a mindset, a time frame, and methods for the journey. Participating in educational decisions is a prime example of engaging in active change (Grant, 1994), and it sets the tone for establishing a new professional identity. In **role transition**, you not only assume but develop the new role (Strader & Decker, 1995); it is the opportunity for you to individualize educational and professional experiences and to use education as a vehicle for true change in your professional role.

Nursing education is designed to develop

professionals who think critically and to provide the principles and guidelines for the myriad of diverse situations they encounter. The fullness of your nursing role is limited only by your own imagination, creativity, and ability. During this transitional period, remember that health care is also in transition. As a student, you can craft a professional identity in tune with contemporary nursing as well as with your personal interests and professional talents. As you progress, the change and personal growth in your professional persona will enrich your experience and serve as an impetus for lifelong learning.

CONFLICTS AND STRESSORS

Nurses returning to school may encounter a variety of new conflicts and stressors.

Role Conflicts and Stressors

Returning to school creates a new role for the nurse, and the time, attention, and energy it requires must be found from a finite supply. Rearranging an established lifestyle and pattern of daily activities to accommodate the additional workload is often a necessary and thought-provoking challenge. The overall balance of life activities and parts of life roles can be affected and must be addressed.

Most nurses who return to school are employed, balancing concurrent roles of parent, nurse, student, and homemaker (Lengacher, 1993). Though they may be challenging, multiple roles can yield a number of rewards and pleasures, providing a positive synergy the individual might not experience from only one role. Functioning in multiple roles can be instrumental in redefining your identity, goal setting, and personal achievement. Negative consequences, however, can also occur, particularly, role conflict in women (Lengacher, 1993).

What are the sources of role conflict, or stressors, a returning student might experience? Any facet of the student's life has the potential for conflict or stress, varying with the individual. However, adequate planning and flexibility can minimize difficulties.

Educational Conflicts and Stressors

Being an adult learner may present your first challenge. For some, the label itself elicits a sense of not belonging, of not "fitting in," or of lagging behind the traditional education schedule. In most disciplines, however, adult learners currently constitute a significant percentage of college students. You will not be the lone adult in nursing courses, on campus, or in an online chat room.

Initial selection of courses presents a maze of choices and possibilities, which may seem overwhelming and strange. Keep in mind that the goal of the institution is to promote the success of each student. Faculty members are available to help and advise you. Be prepared to seek out your faculty advisor and to participate actively in your education. You have both a right and a responsibility to ask for guidance (Bruner & Donahue, 1992, p. 143). Effective education includes two-way communication, and you will be both encouraged and expected to be an active student.

Grades

Most educational endeavors involve criteria and some form of evaluation, and grades are the most common format. Although grades are usually important to all students, the mature student may place undue emphasis on them. Some students may assume that previous professional experience or age requires them to excel in their courses. This assumption is both unrealistic and an unnecessary burden. Concern for grades can lead to a mental battle for self-esteem that focuses more on getting good grades than on assimilating information. A grade less than an "A" should not be perceived as a threat to your identity. Grades do not automatically equal the time and money invested. Academic achievement evolves from effort and understanding. Communication with professors about course objectives, policies, and specifics of assignments can facilitate achievement.

Contracting for a grade is an alternative that allows the student to select a grade and an accompanying level of performance criteria. The selected grade ("A" through "C") is agreed upon by student and professor via a contract at the beginning of the course and is awarded upon successful completion of the required elements for the specific grade level. Contracting permits the student to be independent and take ownership of planning and implementing objectives for the assignment (Knowles, 1988).

Test Anxiety

Test anxiety is common among all learners and can be a major problem. Remember that some degree of anxiety is expected. However, excessive anxiety before and during examinations can interfere with thinking. Adequate preparation and understanding of the material and a positive, self-confident attitude can control test anxiety. Keep in mind that "tests measure performance not personal value," and that "your grade does not reflect the kind of person you are or your ability to succeed" (Katz, 2004, p. 246).

Some basic tips to reduce test anxiety are as follows:

- Plan and use adequate time for study.
- Do not cram.
- Study with others after you have studied alone.
- Take control.
- Think positively.
- Keep your normal, reasonable routine.
- Use stress-reducing tapes.
- Pace your time to answer the questions.
- Do not be afraid to ask the professor for clarification.

Writing Papers

Assembling the material and thoughts to write a paper may seem overwhelming at first. However, every college uses a format that can guide you through the process. Your course professor will provide direction and will be available to explain expectations. Plan

sufficient time to research and develop the topic. Ask the professor for feedback as you proceed, and use the library staff to help acquire the appropriate references. Make sure you have a copy of the writing format (American Psychological Assocation [APA], Modern Language Association [MLA], etc.) at home. Computer software for the APA format is available and can save a lot of time and effort. Once you have the first draft written, put it aside; review it with an objective eye the next day. Pay attention to grammar and flow to convey thoughts accurately.

Active Classroom-Active Learner

Today's classroom may vary significantly from your previous experiences. Note-taking and passive learning have been replaced by group work, presentations, simulations, distance learning, and many other creative educational strategies, producing a dynamic environment that addresses many learning styles and promotes critical thinking (Boyer, 1987). Be an active listener—learn to sense the entire message, then interpret, evaluate, and react (Katz, 2004). Be active and vocal, and realize that your point of view is respected. Often there are many answers and no wrong answers. Multiple views can enliven the discussion and expand perspectives. Active participation can be a distinct advantage in learning.

> *Tell me and I'll forget.*
> *Show me and I may remember.*
> *Involve me and I'll understand.*
> Chinese Proverb

Computer Anxiety

If you have little or no experience with computers, you may have doubts about computer-assisted exercises, submitting an assignment on disk, or participating in chat rooms. Developing computer skills while taking courses can be time-consuming and is not necessarily a confidence booster at the start. However, computers can produce a high-quality, finished document and generate multiple copies. They allow you to edit and duplicate readily. The computer is also an excellent tool for searching for and printing material for papers, saving time and trips to campus. Introductory courses to develop basic computer skills are usually available, and computer lab staff can assist you with problems. Books explaining computer programs in simple terms (e.g., *Word for Dummies*) are available at a reasonable price.

Work-Related Problems

Working while attending school presents a host of stressors. Although scheduling classes around professional responsibilities may create some problems, it can also provide wonderful opportunities to implement new concepts learned. Speak with your immediate supervisor and the human resources department about your decision, and emphasize that you intend to honor your responsibilities at work but want to explore time flexibility and any possibility for funding of courses. Some coworkers may be interested in sharing flexible time schedules.

At times, academic responsibilities may be more time-consuming than anticipated, and you may be tempted to adjust work schedules as a solution. However, this approach may cause additional complications with finances, colleagues, or supervisors. Try to develop support, understanding, and alternate plans in the workplace before complications arise.

Family Complications

The biggest conflicts or stressors may arise from situations involving those people closest to the student, especially family. Reorganizing responsibilities during school sessions can help, but continuing an education should never require the student to choose sides against family. In fact, family support and understanding of the experience are essential from both practical and emotional standpoints and have been recognized as such for many years (Campaniello, 1988).

A supportive partner can be the most important asset in your education experience. However, do not expect a partner to understand immediately the expectations and pressures of the process. You will need to talk about the pressures of your new role if you expect your partner to understand and support your endeavor. Accurate and adequate communication is essential to formulating new expectations within the family. When time with your family is curtailed to accommodate the demands of a course, you may experience considerable role strain and question the decisions and compromises you must make to pursue the degree.

The characteristically nurturing roles of wife and mother in American society have been compatible with nursing, a traditionally gendered profession, for many decades. However, these roles can be significant stressors for nurses returning to school (Lengacher, 1993). Certainly, the parental role should not be taken lightly, and the addition of school-related activities to an already busy schedule can prompt feelings of guilt and anxiety. These feelings may be more intense for a single parent. In addition, the need for competent child care frequently extends beyond day care to evening care. Reliable supervision for school-age and teenage children is an equally important issue that may require much more coordination than the care of younger, less mobile children. It can be extremely difficult for a student to concentrate in class knowing that a teenage son with a new driver's license is driving home from school.

Students who are part of the "sandwich generation" may bear responsibility for both parents and children. Even though the parents do not live in the student's home, they may require additional time, attention, and emotional support.

Single students without children may have fewer family responsibilities but also fewer resources and support to draw on while still being responsible for the multiple functions of a single-person household. Few people experience a totally uncomplicated return to school.

The number of men in nursing schools is growing. Besides the increasing percentage of young men who enter nursing programs, there is a noticeable increase in the number of men choosing nursing as a second career (Curry, 1994). Men can be subjected to societal stressors and experience role conflict when they enter a primarily female profession. Returning to school may cause similar stressors when the male student is questioned about his continuing education or his career choice. The conventional roles of husband, father, and breadwinner are not often linked with nursing. Exposure to such narrow thinking can affect the many dedicated men striving to advance both themselves and the profession of nursing. The situation can be compounded when male mentors, role models, and peer support are not readily accessible. However, the numbers of men are increasing, and they have shown they can successfully fufill the role and distinguish themselves in the profession (Billings & Halstead,1998).

Multiple family roles added to the roles of nurse and student create a challenging combination. Yet multiple roles can have positive aspects, such as improvements in confidence, satisfaction, and perspective. Adding or modifying roles does not necessarily have negative consequences. In fact, a study of RN students employed during their coursework showed that they did not experience "burnout" more frequently than other nurses (Dick & Anderson, 1993).

Nontraditional students come to the educational arena with a repertoire of life events that can ease adapting to new situations. In addition, those mature students who perceive themselves as "hardy" tend to experience less anxiety adjusting to school (Patton & Goldenberg, 1999). Stress can result from almost any type of change, even positive change. The happiest and most desirable things in life can take a physical and mental toll on the individual. Holmes and Rahe (1967) showed that both positive and negative life events can have a negative effect on health. It would be unrealistic to expect balance and harmony among all life roles during coursework (Table 2–1)

TABLE 2–1
Social Readjustment Rating Scale

Life Event	Mean Value
Death of spouse	100
Divorce	73
Marital separation	65
Jail term	63
Death of close family member	63
Personal illness or injury	53
Marriage	50
Fired from work	50
Marital reconciliation	47
Retirement	45
Change in family member's health	44
Pregnancy	40
Sex difficulties	39
Addition to family	39
Business readjustment	39
Change in financial status	38
Death of close friend	37

(continued)

TABLE 2–1
Social Readjustment Rating Scale *(continued)*

Life Event	Mean Value
Change to different line of work	36
Change in number of marital arguments	35
Mortgage or loan more than $10,000	31
Foreclosure of mortgage or loan	30
Change in work responsibilities	29
Son or daughter leaving home	29
Trouble with in-laws	29
Outstanding personal achievement	28
Spouse begins or stops work	26
Starting or finishing school	26
Change in living conditions	25
Revision of personal habits	24
Trouble with boss	23
Change in work hours, conditions	20
Change in residence	20
Change in schools	20
Change in recreational habits	19
Change in church activities	19
Change in social activities	18
Mortgage or loan less than $10,000	17
Change in sleeping habits	16
Change in number of family gatherings	15
Change in eating habits	15
Vacation	13
Christmas season	12
Minor violation of the law	11

Source: Holmes, T., & Rahe, R. (1967). The social readjustment rating scale.
Journal of Psychosomatic Research, 2(4), 213–218.

Personal Stressors

The most intense stress or conflicts students experience may be the pressures that come from within. Doubt, insecurity, and discouragement can become overwhelming enemies. Strive to be faithful to the commitment to yourself, and have trust in yourself, faith in your decisions, and courage to continue. To ensure success, embark on a plan of organization that will streamline activities, use resources, delegate tasks, and maximize results of efforts, and will not create unnecessary stress.

 ## TIME MANAGEMENT

Time is a precious, intangible commodity that cannot be stored, stopped, or renewed. It is invisible yet constantly makes its presence known, and it can hang heavily on the hands of some and quickly fly by for others.

Contemporary society is fascinated by time and ways to save it. *Time management* is a popular but inappropriate term. People do not manage the clock but, rather, organize their activities within the framework of time. The returning student has considerable experience with time from both personal and professional perspectives, but the student role can present new and different challenges. Time management can be effective for returning students, especially if they approach with a positive attitude rather than a stopwatch mentality and view it as an opportunity to plan and use time to their advantage.

Time is one of the most elusive entities an individual encounters. As people progress through the decades of life, they can experience a true sense of the days, weeks, and months passing at an ever-increasing pace. The student's perception of time, the accuracy of that perception, and how the individual functions in relation to time are extremely important to the educational experience. Achievement of academic objectives requires time—to read, write, review, and assimilate, among many other things.

Creativity does not necessarily flow on demand. If this "block" happens when you are facing a deadline, do not panic. Seasoned adult learners usually know to expect academic tasks to take twice as long as the time originally allotted. Learning to allot sufficient time allows the opportunity to concentrate, develop and nurture thoughts, and provide for critical review. Allowing adequate time for an activity is especially crucial when other people are involved. Ironically, the word "holiday" may take on a totally new and different meaning to the student; any opportunity for additional time may be viewed as a gift.

Practical Planning and Organization

Students benefit greatly when they take inventory of daily activities and develop a time plan that realistically addresses personal needs, family and professional responsibilities, and academic goals and expectations. The value of a schedule cannot be overrated. However, to be effective, it must be realistic and consider the time frame and the importance of other people and things involved. When you develop and use your plan for time management, you should keep in mind some key elements:

- The plan is simply a blueprint and can be modified.
- Its purpose is to assist in, not hinder, the use of time.
- Periodic reassessment and necessary modification are wise.
- The semester system provides an automatic time frame for reassessment in educational matters.
- Feasibility of the plan is essential.

Neither the most worthy goal nor unbounded motivation can turn an unrealistic plan into reality. A poignant example of realistic timing, given by Covey, Merrill, and and associates (1994), is referred to as the "law of the farm." They observe that to have a crop in the fall, the farmer must plant seeds in the spring. You cannot "cram" on the farm. They also note that shortcuts and cramming in education are not effective. The knowledge acquired by these means is often temporary and does not serve the student well.

Time Plans

Realistic, individualized time plans cannot be purchased at the campus bookstore. However, many time management methods and aids are available and can be used to meet individual student needs. Various forms of calendars and schedules can help you arrange activities into a reasonable time frame. Recording your schedule or list in writing is an important part of the time management process; it can serve as a point of direction, a reminder, and a visual commitment to the task. The written schedule tends to carry more importance and to improve organization.

It is important to organize from both short- and long-term perspectives. Within the framework of an academic year or semester, the student can plan according to monthly, weekly, and daily calendars. Meltzer and Palau (1993) state that these three time planning segments have slightly different functions: Monthly calendars assist students in arranging activities for long-term projects, weekly calendars help with developing consistency, and daily calendars aid in prioritizing (p. 5).

To implement effective daily planning, you should set aside a few minutes each night to determine and list things to do the next day. Priorities can then be identified by ranking each item from 1 to 10 or by assigning items a level of importance (A, B, or C). The list should be very specific regarding the activity and the time allotted. Crossing off accomplished items can give the student satisfaction and motivation to continue. When items are still on the list at the end of the day, there are three choices: Do the task then and be done with it; plan it for the next day; or eliminate it because it was not important. Covey and associates (1994) suggest that organizing on a weekly rather than daily plan helps reduce the problem of operating on a crisis basis. It allows the individual more flexibility without the pressure of a fixed daily schedule.

It is advisable to "frontload" whenever possible, accomplishing partial or complete assignments at the earliest opportunity. This eliminates working under increasing pressure when unanticipated complications arise. All too often, students take time, health, and necessary people and things for granted. Try to leave a buffer zone in time plans. Your mind might be ready to work when your body needs to rest, or your child is ill, or an elderly relative asks for help. You should always plan to complete assignments before their due dates. Although some people claim to work better under pressure, working up to the last minute of a deadline on a regular basis is physically and emotionally exhausting, and the possibility always exists that circumstances will arise to prevent you from completing the task.

Barriers to Time Management

Watch out for the following barriers, any of which can be the downfall of an effective time management plan.

Procrastination

Delaying the inevitable can increase the emotional pressure attached to accomplishing a task or meeting a deadline. Procrastination creates a domino effect, pushing the task into a time slotted for other activities. Guilt often accompanies the delays, adding even more pressure, which interferes with your concentration when you finally address the task. Procrastinating in family responsibilities in order to meet academic requirements can elicit enormous self-imposed guilt when families are understanding and cooperative.

If you find you are procrastinating, look for the core reason for the delaying tactic, and act on it. If the task seems overwhelming, seek advice, break it down into smaller parts, and get started with a simple aspect. Simply thinking about a project does not accomplish the work, and perfection is not expected on the first attempt. Getting started can easily consume the most time and energy of a project, especially when the people involved allow themselves to be controlled by the situation rather than controlling it.

Interruptions

Interruptions can easily derail the most well-planned schedule. The lost time can range from minutes to months, and the impact can be monumental. Some interruptions are caused by other people or the environment, and others come from within. When you are attempting to meet responsibilities of multiple roles, the saying "timing can be everything in life" can be brutally true. One of the most common forms of interruption was invented by Alexander Graham Bell. The ring of the telephone arrives without permission and often at inopportune times. A well-intentioned friend or relative who calls to say hello not only takes precious time but disrupts a line of thought that can never be retrieved again. At times you can feel victimized by the telephone because it seems impolite to keep the call brief. Conversely, the telephone may seem like a welcome distraction when you are involved in a difficult or unpleasant task. In either case, it takes time from the original plan. Either arrange for other family members to answer the telephone, field the questions, and take messages or turn on the answering machine. The most endearing interruption can be from a child who wants to spend time with a parent. Those times are important and cannot be replaced.

Time Savers

There are many ways to manage time and activities successfully. As you use time more effectively, you may develop new and different strategies specific to your individual situation. Follow these time management methods to experience more productive and enjoyable days:

- *Assess yourself*: When are you best able to concentrate? When are you most energetic? Many people are most productive in the early morning, when the world is very quiet, the mind clear, and the body refreshed.
- *Avoid the marathon approach:* Eight consecutive hours is a long time to focus on any one task, whether it is writing a paper or washing floors. The productivity level increases if activities are varied and performed in smaller blocks of time.
- *Allow for time spillovers:* Try to plan time with leeway between activities, to accommodate meetings that run late, unexpected appointments, or simply losing track of time.
- *Plan adequate travel time:* Not all trips from work to campus to home have to resemble an Indianapolis 500 race. Checking the most time-efficient routes, and having a backup plan for heavy traffic or inclement weather, can save valuable time and anxiety. Familiarize yourself with school policy regarding communication of closings due to weather conditions. Allow sufficient time to find a parking space and walk to buildings.
- *Use 5-minute fillers:* While waiting for a meeting or class to start, use the 5- or 10-minute time slot to make a telephone call, photocopy an article, or review a study question with another student.

- *Make a "waiting room" portfolio:* Keep a portfolio of portable tasks that can be accomplished in the 20 or 30 minutes you spend in a dentist's or doctor's waiting room, or in the car during practice before a youngster's soccer game, or when a class or meeting is canceled. Keep a supply of notepads and pencils to make "to do" lists, outline projects, or write overdue letters. Thirty minutes can make a visible difference on a piece of needlework planned as a gift.
- *Keep a pocket calendar*: Combine family, work, school, and social events on the calendar to give yourself an overview and enable you to arrange appointments or meetings on the spot. Save time by writing the telephone number with a name in the time slot in case of change. Keep a list of frequently used numbers on the calendar.
- *Do "double work" activities:* Always have some type of task ready to be done during telephone conversations. While conversing with a colleague about work or school, you can perform simple tasks, such as folding the laundry, washing dishes, polishing furniture, and sorting papers.
- *Use travel time:* Public transportation is a waiting room in motion and provides hands-free time for reading texts, reviewing policies for work, or keeping current with professional journals. Travel time in a car can be valuable time with yourself. It can be used to mentally gear up for, or wind down from, a busy day. Newscasts and informational talk shows capsulize current issues. Listening to audiotapes for course review, relaxation, or motivation is an especially good way to pass this time.
- *Consider a cellular connection:* If you have a cellular telephone, you can save time by calling ahead to confirm meetings or notify of delays. Telephone calls made "on the go" can open time slots in a busy schedule and accomplish personal business calls in privacy.
- *Time your time:* Keep track of time to stay on task without becoming obsessive. Be mindful of the positive or negative results in relation to the time being invested. If time escapes you easily, use a watch or pocket timer to time intervals. At home, the timer

on the stove can alert you to keep on pace or move to the next task.

- *Leave open time:* Schedule times for nothing. An occasional blank space in a busy week can be a welcome event, to be used as you choose.

Time management involves developing a respect for the clock, because time continues even when your energy and ideas are diminishing or depleted.

Setting Limits and Achieving Balance

Setting limits is not intended to create a restrictive environment or mindset. In fact, it encourages you to focus on goals and to be proactive rather than reactive. Setting limits involves responsible assessment and recognition of boundaries. It requires being aware of capabilities and acknowledging limitations. Self-management is an important strategy leading to taking control of the direction of your life (Case, 1997). Setting limits puts you in control. It allows you to be the decision-maker and determine what is realistic and beneficial. The words *realistic* and *beneficial* are key elements in limits, and students can become painfully aware that things that could be helpful or desirable are not always possible.

Setting limits is not confined to time. Many aspects of daily life, including energy, money, and activities of all types, can be subject to limits. Effective limit-setting involves balancing the various facets of life as well as the demands within each facet (social, professional, intellectual, physical, etc.). *Balancing* does not mean designating a time slot for everything each day but addressing your needs and goals weekly and monthly.

Balance requires firsthand knowledge of priorities and respect for individual needs, abilities, and interests. It means that you identify the minimum and maximum efforts required to meet your goals. Contemporary society often seems committed to the concept of maximum, sometimes to the point of excess. However, less is sometimes better; and you must use your judgment to determine

these circumstances. Remember the adage "Work expands to fill the allotted time." Learn to set limits.

> *Setting limits involves responsible assessment and recognition of boundaries. It requires being aware of capabilities and acknowledging limitations.*

A prime principle of limit setting is learning to say "No." This two-letter, one-syllable word is often the most difficult word to articulate. The desire to participate, to please, and to be viewed as cooperative and competent is very human. The altruistic nature common among nurses adds to their difficulty in limiting time and efforts, resulting in time binds and exhaustion. Responsibility to oneself is an important part of setting limits. It takes considerable self-discipline to leave a social gathering early to study for an examination or write a paper. It takes even more self-control to say "No" and stay on task when no one else is present or will know of your efforts or infractions. In reality, you are responsible for determining the appropriate balance and limitations, regardless of the presence or pressure of others. You will be the prime beneficiary of thoughtfully constructed limitations. You can, however, become a victim if limits are ill conceived or not honored.

Pace

A positive attitude, motivation, and zeal for knowledge enhance learning; however, unbridled enthusiasm can also lead you to push yourself beyond reasonable expectations. Overextending yourself at school can seriously limit the time and attention you have to devote to other responsibilities and can also lead to academic burnout. Remember that achieving a degree is a growth process— not a race, but a process of completion. Pace yourself so that you devote adequate time to all your work activities.

Lack of pacing can result in frustration, diminished quality of effort and work, depletion of physical and mental resources, or abandonment of your goal. Set and abide by speed limits. Take advantage of opportunities and address unanticipated events, but always keep your setpoint at a realistic level. Reasonable pacing allows you to complete academic assignments, courses, and curricula and to participate in other life activities.

ASSEMBLING RESOURCES

Before embarking on a new venture, thoroughly assess the situation and take inventory of your available **resources**. They usually fall into three basic categories—educational, professional, and family. Each category offers a variety of opportunities for assistance, and students are encouraged to take advantage of all types (Table 2–2)

Assess all aspects of life to develop a comprehensive picture, and identify resources that are currently accessible. Resources can come in many forms, including human, inanimate, and intangible. They serve varied purposes and can provide information, support, motivation, and physical convenience, among many other benefits. Take advantage of readily available assistance. Create a plan to determine how to use existing resources to meet your goal. Then be on the alert for new and additional sources of help. Just as new and different needs can emerge, so can resources. A proactive approach is necessary because resources do not necessarily come neatly packaged, labeled, and delivered. It is your responsibility to seek out and negotiate for resources and to know when and how to use them appropriately. Although it can be comforting to know that something is accessible, the true value of a resource lies in its use rather than its potential: "A little knowledge

TABLE 2–2	
Examples of Where to Find Resources	
Educational	Department chair
	Faculty
	Academic advisor
	Course professor
	Student orientation programs
	Adult and continuing education department
	Learning centers
	Library
	Financial aid office
	Bulletin boards
	Special-interest student groups
	Other students
Professional	Professional organizations
	Employer
Family/Friends	Available babysitters
	Family or friends with special talents, such as a computer whiz
	Neighbor willing to carpool
	Someone with library privileges at a nearby university
	Local groups that offer educational funding
	Access to computer or photocopying

that acts is worth infinitely more than knowledge that is idle," said Kahlil Gibran.

Educational Resources

The college campus, the very setting that facilitates achievement of the desired degree, is often the resource students are least familiar with. You should make an all-out effort to become aware of all the services and opportunities that are connected with the institution, both physically and online. Some resources may be apparent or mentioned in the application and admission process. Once you are enrolled, however, become familiar with the academic expectations and the people, methods, and activities to help meet those expectations. College offers many forms of assistance, but you must spend time and energy to become knowledgeable, and you must be a proactive student.

Campus Communication

A number of college resources are designed to distribute information. A brief review of your college's literature, such as the catalog, view book, and department brochures, can provide an overview of its program, policies, and services. A campus map is extremely helpful to orient you to the physical layout and enable you to identify key locations and services quickly. Semester schedules and an array of weekly announcements are posted to inform students of current curricular and extracurricular activities. Routine review of bulletin boards informs you of upcoming events that are beneficial or required.

Student orientation programs, especially those designed for mature students, are extremely helpful. These sessions capsulize the information in the institution's literature and focus on the practical aspects of the college experience. Orientation usually provides answers to commonly asked questions and alleviates some anxiety. Besides imparting information, the programs provide opportunity for interaction with key college personnel. Department chairs, faculty, and students are usually present and interested in talking with incoming students. An added benefit of attending orientation is meeting other incoming students—your academic peers.

Academic Advisor

One key resource in the educational setting is the faculty member who serves as your academic advisor. The importance of an advisor cannot be overestimated. Plan to meet with him or her at the beginning of the first semester and regularly throughout the experience. The advisor will assist you with course selection and will monitor your academic progress, but the role entails much more. You can expect your advisor to help you assess strengths and weaknesses and maintain focus and to serve as a source of encouragement and information. By serving as a sounding board, the advisor can help you develop independence and critical thinking. An advisor guides each student through the education process in an individualized manner, to meet his or her specific learning needs and the criteria of the program. You must be a willing and active participant, however, and understand that the advisor's role is to guide and facilitate, not to handle your responsibilities or errands. The advisor can serve as a role model and an ongoing source of guidance and information for the process of socialization into academe.

Campus Services and Personnel

An advisor may direct the student to a variety of resources on the campus. Many institutions have a specific department or office that works with adult learners. This unit is often known as the Lifelong Learning, Adult Education, or Nontraditional division. It provides information on issues relevant to mature students, including transfer and life-experience credit and financial opportunities for older students.

Every college also has a division that focuses on improving specific learning skills. Personnel with varied educational backgrounds work with students individually or in small groups to enhance abilities. Services can range from remediation in a specific learning area, such as mathematics, to supplemental instruction in sciences, to assistance in developing and writing papers. A variety of technological devices and methods may be available for educational goals such as increasing reading rate. These learning centers are designed for students who desire to improve their methods and abilities. Study groups in subject areas and tutors can be arranged through the center. Students can be referred by a professor or an advisor or can seek assistance on their own. International or culturally diverse students can expect to find an office on campus dedicated to bridging cultural variation in the educational setting. Courses in English as a second language may come under the direction of this office.

One of the most traditional educational resources is the campus library. Students benefit from a formal orientation to the facility or an individual appointment with a librarian to learn about the reference services available and the computerized catalog and information search operations. Libraries often have individual study carrels and typing and photocopy equipment for the convenience of students. Some college libraries provide free photocopying service. Looking through copies of daily newspapers, weekly journals, and past issues bound in the stacks can help students develop current and historical perspectives for various courses. Also be aware of other libraries, public or university affiliated, that offer different or additional holdings. Some health-care institutions have libraries and librarians at the worksite. Collections in these libraries often reflect the focus of the hospital or agency. The library can also be a very convenient, quiet, and efficient place to work.

Financial aid is available for all students, not just those coming directly from high school. The nursing department and financial aid office can apprise students of their eligibility for public funding. Employee benefit programs are another possible source of funding. A variety of state and federal assistance programs exist in addition to Veterans Administration benefits for students associated with the military. RNs can also benefit from scholarships and stipends offered by pro-

fessional and civic groups exclusively for adult students. Sometimes students have received funding from community organizations. Diligent monitoring of announcements can be financially advantageous.

The course professor is an often overlooked resource. He or she is your first point of communication and usually welcomes the opportunity to clarify or expand topics. The professor can provide the course perspective, develop criteria, and evaluate progress as well as refer students to other valuable resources as needed. Faculty members maintain office hours designated exclusively for interacting with students. Meetings with the course professor can correct assumptions, dispel rumors, and assist you in understanding the material. Students whose work and family schedules prevent them from meeting with professors during office hours can arrange a telephone discussion or e-mail contact.

Student Peers

One of the most valuable educational resources for the student is the student peer. Sharing the common educational experience can forge an intellectual and emotional bond. Student peers offer information, understanding, and support. Fellow students have similar goals and circumstances. They can comprehend the pressures of your return to school in a way that no family member does, and they can offer creative solutions that have worked for them.

Study groups also can be helpful for reviewing course content, preparing for examinations, or developing projects. Discussion and exchange of ideas in a group can energize individuals and the whole. Group interaction creates a network of additional eyes and ears to garner information for a course assignment. The interplay of common goals and varied experiences can expand perspectives, broaden understanding, and make the task more enjoyable.

The student peer group can also provide immeasurable personal support. The camaraderie can help keep motivation at a productive level or assist in overcoming disappointment. Some students act as role models and serve as sources of encouragement, whereas others provide information or support. Each student brings unique characteristics, talents, and abilities that can be shared. Interaction as brief as a conversation during a class break may still be supportive. Instructors often promote such support groups (Dick & Anderson, 1993).

Students who choose not to belong to a student group should make a point of interacting with some students individually. Exchanging telephone numbers helps, especially when students are on campus only one or two days a week. Occasional student social gatherings add pleasure and balance to a goal-oriented schedule. Incorporate a lunch or dinner with other students into your campus or study regimen.

Academic Items and Technology

Educational pursuits cannot take place in a vacuum, and certain items can be helpful in accomplishing academic tasks. Besides the required textbooks for each course, the student should have a current-edition dictionary, a thesaurus, and a copy of the format for writing papers (e.g., American Psychological Association [APA], Modern Language Association [MLA]) preferred by the college.

A computer—either at home or conveniently available for use—is an efficient tool for developing, storing, and retrieving information. Depending on the capability of the computer and the student, information can be accessed from libraries and many other locations. As Catalano (2003) notes, a myriad of Web sites can provide a wealth of information about nursing. A sample of popular Web sites is listed in Table 2–3 Students who do not have computers at home will find that most colleges have a computer facility for student use. If the campus location and times are not convenient, you can buy computer time and photocopy services at one of several franchise businesses located throughout the country. Such businesses are usually open 24 hours a day, which is helpful to students with full schedules and erratic hours. Owning a computer and acquiring computer skills can be an integral part of the college experience. A knowledgeable friend, computer laboratory personnel, and instruction books are valuable resources.

TABLE 2–3
Popular Nursing Web Sites

American Association of Colleges of Nursing	http://www.aacn.nche.edu/
American Association of Nurse Attorneys	http://www.taana.org
American College of Nurse Practitioners	http://www.nurse.org/acnp/
American Nurses Association	http://www.ana.org/
	http://www.nursingworld.org/
Association of Perioperative Registered Nurses	http://www.aorn.org
Association of Women's Health, Obstetric, and Neonatal Nurses	http://www.awhonn.org
Australian Electronic Journal of Nursing Education	http://www.scu.edu.au/schools/ nhcp/nejne/aejne/aejnehp.htm
National Association of Orthopedic Nurses	http://naon.inurse.com
National Association of Pediatric Nurses Associates & Practitioners	http://www.napnap.org
National Association of School Nurses	http://www.nasn.org
National Institute of Nursing Research	http://www.nih.gov/ninr
National League for Nursing	http://www.nln.org/
Sigma Theta Tau International Nursing Society	http://www.nursingsociety.org

Professional Resources

The professional arena holds many resources. The cooperation of your immediate superior in the workplace is pivotal in facilitating the integration of professional responsibilities and educational goals. When you decide to return to school, you should schedule a meeting to notify your superior of your decision. Be prepared to present a well-defined plan, including how it will benefit the nurse, the unit, and the institution. It is important for the superior who is responsible for assignments, schedules, and evaluations to understand your circumstances and potential. The meeting may be an appropriate time to ask about adjusting your workload and schedule in the future and to note any precedent. It is primarily your role to devise viable possibilities and options compatible with the function of the unit. Supervising personnel can provide additional input and insight into constraints for schemes presented. Enlist the cooperation of clinical colleagues to serve as interim backups or resources.

Many health-care agencies recognize the value of continued education and subsidize personnel for a portion of or the full cost of a course. Some institutions require that a specific grade be achieved for reimbursement. Such policies provide both financial and academic motivation for education.

Professional nursing organizations are resources in many ways. The continual dissemination of materials through such associations provides students with a current supply of professional information and issues. Conferences and workshops sponsored by nursing organizations give students the opportunity to listen to and possibly interact with leaders in the profession. Organization workshops or panels allow students to participate as presenters. Local and state chapters of many groups may have funds available for student education. Sigma Theta Tau, the international nursing honor society, fosters student achievement and rewards it with induction into the membership. State nurse and student nurse associations provide a stream of information and give members an opportunity to speak on contemporary issues of the profession.

Within the professional milieu, you may discover a person to serve as your mentor. Developing a relationship with a mentor is especially beneficial. A mentor is more than a role model and can offer much more than intellectual substance. You can expect to receive support and guidance from a person attuned to the politics, power, and processes of career paths. Mentors characteristically assist in the development of personal and professional growth. Although adult learners are self-directed, seeking a mentor is tied to the desire to obtain the expertise and resources to actively meet practical needs (Knowles, 1988). Having a mentor is not essential, but it can be a positive experience and often improves your success potential, leading to your service as a mentor in the future. This chain of mentoring constitutes an ongoing form of repayment to the profession.

Participating in a professional position concurrently with college studies places the student in regular touch with contemporary care. The clinical experiences put real faces on the pages of textbooks and make the lessons relevant. Involvement in the workplace maintains access to an interdisciplinary network, which is necessary given the changes of a health-care system in transition.

Family Resources

Even your most devoted family and friends can never share your perspective about returning to school. However, most families are eager to encourage and support you, despite a limited understanding of the total picture. The encouragement and admiration of your family can help sustain your motivation throughout the semesters. Likewise, you can readily serve as a role model for both children and adults and can gain self-esteem and confidence from the experience. Additionally, the family can provide assistance in practical ways that save you time and energy. Some family and household responsibilities can be adjusted to accommodate your schedule or workload without overlooking the responsibilities and interests of other family members. The experience can benefit individual members in many practical ways, perhaps enhancing the sense of family for the group.

Negotiate and delegate with partner, children, or parents according to the needs of the family. Develop each individual's talents and abilities so there is opportunity for others to share or take on new responsibilities. Appreciate their help, no matter how small, and be sure to show your appreciation. Ease your standards. For instance, do not redo a task because the outcome does not meet your standards. It does not matter whether the towels are not folded and stacked the way you would do it. Students who are parents should keep in mind that they can learn from how a child approaches a project. A child who is computer literate can help you learn to use the computer, and you can both benefit from the shared experience.

Do not eliminate the support you might get from a telephone conversation with a relative or friend hundreds of miles away. Willing friends and neighbors can help by offering to assist with carpools, babysitting, or caring for an older parent. Interested, well-meaning people are not necessarily expecting for you to reciprocate in kind, and often are genuinely happy to help and be a part of the endeavor—a true resource.

Health: An Overlooked Resource

One very important resource frequently taken for granted is good health. Despite their professional knowledge and experience, even nurses can undervalue personal wellness until they have a problem. To maintain physical and mental stamina, students must attend to the basic premises of health promotion and wellness. Disregard for individual health can lead to illness and can negatively influence academic schedules and goals. Regular exercise, good nutrition, and plenty of rest can help you approach responsibilities with a sense of vitality; they help you balance your activities and lifestyle. Cultivate the art of relaxation; it brings a host of physical and mental benefits and influences coping skills (Leddy & Pepper, 1998). Humor can be a healthy coping mechanism that helps put your day in perspective. Laughter often results in a sense of relaxation and defuses stress (Schuster, 2000). With a positive atti-

tude toward personal health, you can achieve a higher level of wellness, feel better, enjoy the college experience, be more productive, and position yourself for academic success (Curry, 2001).

Summary

Assembling resources consists of lining up assets and opportunities. It involves drawing on or using the knowledge, service, and access to resources available. Resources can be found as far as the Internet reaches or as near as your personal collection of nursing journals. Interaction and exchange are important in identifying and developing resources. Talking about activities and projects to family, friends, coworkers, and fellow students can increase your "brain power" and extend your network of available assistance. Some resources are readily identified and available, and others may have to be created.

 STREAMLINING WORK

The *Random House Unabridged Dictionary defines* **streamlining** as designing or organizing to give maximum efficiency (Flexner, 1993, p. 1881); it connotes concepts such as "expertly assembled," "minimal resistance," "swiftness," "smooth progress," and "unencumbered." These are positive and desirable qualities for work. Try to streamline work in each of the various facets of life—family, social, professional, and educational. Streamlining work in one area of life can positively affect the other areas.

Streamlining involves carefully considering all your ideas and plans. It is the coordination of goals, limits, resources, and time management in an action-oriented process geared toward efficiency and saving energy. It requires much organization and fine tuning how things are usually done. Streamlining means eliminating the unnecessary and making work a pleasant and productive experience. Be careful not to eliminate everything, because functioning with only the absolute essentials can turn work into hard labor.

Simplify your life, but do not close down your world.

Educational Streamlining

The educational arena has many requirements and essential activities, yet you can simplify the process and still achieve your objectives. Life and your nursing career provide you with processes integral to streamlining educational activities. Educational streamlining does not focus on the study process per se but rather helps create life circumstances that foster conditions conducive to study.

Accruing Credit

One aspect of streamlining is using resources effectively. This is particularly important in looking at the overall curriculum and various courses involved. The mass of information and number of academic courses necessary may seem overwhelming. However, you may already possess some of the required knowledge, and there is no reason to "reinvent the wheel." Discuss your experience with an advisor and explore the variety of ways, besides taking courses, that you can demonstrate knowledge and receive credits. This can be done during the application and admission process.

Once you have a better understanding of the requirements, you may want to analyze how your experience can earn you credits. You may qualify for transfer credits for courses taken at another institution that are comparable in content to those in the curriculum. You may also become eligible for credits by taking the Credit for Life Learning Experience examinations or those designed by faculty. These tests are designed to demonstrate knowledge covered in the course. Be aware of fees associated with taking the challenge examination and receiving credit, and the university and department may stipulate a time for completion. In addition, some universities grant credit to adult learners toward elective courses for "life experience." This is usually granted through an adult learning office and entails documenting achievement of specific objectives by the student in settings outside the classroom. The criteria are set by and vary according to the university; however, this type of credit is not usually awarded for work associated with your academic major.

Course Timing

The time at which a course is offered, especially a required course, is crucial to busy adults within many roles. Always check a course's schedule carefully to note whether it has multiple sections, and possibly one at a more convenient time or place. When you have a time conflict for an essential course, talk with your advisor about taking the class at a satellite location or another school. Explore the availability of telecourses. Distance education programs, which send live video broadcasts to one or more remote classroom locations, are also options. Whenever possible, it is helpful to chain courses together. This minimizes the number of trips to campus and saves transportation time and expense. When there are intervals between classes, it is wise to plan to use the time for a specific task, such as library research, review of notes, or study groups.

Using the Library

Make trips to the campus library as productive as possible. If you did not receive a formal orientation to the library, ask a librarian to describe the policies and features. When using journal articles, it is best to photocopy the material for current and future use at home and highlight the important information. Students should make sure the photocopy shows the complete information for citation, including journal volume and edition. For books, note the ISBN number and citation information for quick retrieval in the future. It is helpful to keep a supply of index cards handy to write citations and any pertinent information. Honor due dates. Attach a note with the due date on the front of the book to remind yourself to return it on time. Review your books weekly the night before a campus day to avoid a needless return trip.

When you go to the library for one course, check the availability of materials for other courses. Assist other students by being alert for materials relevant to their topics of interest; they can do the same for you. A class list with selected project or paper topics can guide you. Carefully monitor your time in the library. It is easy to spend inordinate amounts of time in the library because it is usually quiet and serene, with no sense of the passing time.

Portfolio System

Organizing things is just as important as organizing your life. A portfolio system is extremely helpful for easy access to important materials. Devote one portfolio to your academic progress, including such items as letters of acceptance, catalogs, course schedules, an advisement or curriculum plan, and any correspondence with the college. Transcripts, paid receipts, and other relevant materials can be added each semester. Keep a personal copy of any information requested by the college, such as an annual health history and physical forms, immunization records, or documentation of cardiopulmonary resuscitation certification.

A second portfolio should pertain to course work, with pertinent materials for each course, such as course outline, schedule, reading list, completed assignments, and papers for future reference. Copies of relevant journal articles can be included with the respective course or maintained in a separate portfolio for articles.

Another portfolio can contain printed copies of any computer materials. When using a computer, be sure to store information on a floppy disk and the hard drive, appropriately catalogued. It is wise to have a "traveling disk" readily available in a briefcase or handbag, so you can access information when opportunities arise. Always check disks for viruses before using them in each machine, especially if you use a computer that has multiple users. A computer virus can easily destroy many hours of work.

A portfolio created for programs and brochures for conferences, workshops, and professional meetings is also useful. It can provide an overview of upcoming events for possible participation and a record of events attended, along with names and information. These events can expand your professional perspective and contribute to your coursework.

Communication

Efficient communication is part of streamlining. Using e-mail and "fax" communications can save considerable time in transmitting information. Most colleges have a system for student e-mail accounts. If you do not have access to a fax machine at home, work, or school, many commercial locations can be used. Carrying a list of school-related places and people, with their telephone and fax numbers and e-mail addresses, will also enhance communication. The names and numbers of other students, your advisor, the department secretary, and the library are a few frequently used items. Students who do not use business cards in their professional roles may consider having cards with home address and appropriate phone numbers.

Forming a carpool with another student offers several advantages, including the opportunity to discuss class projects and review material. Students who audiotape courses can use travel time for review. As you progress in your educational program, your academic networks will expand, and more people and information will be available for you to use in the process of streamlining.

Professional Streamlining

Even those employed on a part-time basis usually have to assess and reorganize their situations to accommodate school. Adjustments range from exchanging a few hours to taking a leave of absence.

Negotiation with superiors, and sometimes peers, is often a successful approach to resolving the situation. Cost-conscious employers and supervisors can be extremely receptive to innovative plans that maintain quality performance and increase cooperation and morale. If timing of the workday is an issue, "flex time" may be the answer. Condensing work hours to fewer days may help. Sometimes arriving early or adding an hour on specified days is all that is necessary to allow a student to leave the workplace in time to attend a class. Trading holiday coverage for class time and job sharing are other options. If you are a manager or supervisor, delegate functions and authority as appropriate. A leave of absence is sometimes the most appropriate method. Most reasonable requests to realign work schedules to gain an education will be considered, and many are granted.

Streamlining Domestic Functions

One of the first tasks of streamlining is to get all involved in your home life to realize that you cannot continually relegate schoolwork to the end of the night, after everything else is finished, or to an already crammed weekend. Most home tasks can be rearranged, reprioritized, or eliminated to improve your quality of life.

Have a family discussion and encourage new ideas for getting the work done, determining what can be eliminated, or obtaining volunteers. Use incentives and rewards for a job well done. New interests and unrecognized talents may be developed in the streamlining process.

Hiring household help to clean periodically can provide significant assistance at moderate expense. Neighborhood teenagers or college students may be available. Grandparents or other relatives may be pleased to provide child care for a few hours a week. Arrange with neighbors to exchange child care or carpooling responsibilities.

Thinking in quantities and doing two things at once can help. Buy and prepare food in quantity. One night a week, while you are cooking dinner, it is possible to prepare two dishes, with one to be served on another evening. On occasion, ask a family member to do the grocery shopping or to accompany you—to turn the task into a pleasant time to

be together. Schedule these activities early in the week, when your ambition and energy are usually high. Plan to eat out once a week, for family enjoyment and less work.

Some basic practices to increase efficiency in domestic responsibilities are as follows:

- Select and lay out clothes the night before each working day.
- Do a morning check to make sure all necessary family items for the day are ready.
- Know the daily schedule and telephone numbers for each family member.
- Plan a route for each day. Chain activities and errands together to avoid driving in circles.
- Handle mail only once—read and relegate.
- Post a list for needed household items, making an automatic grocery list.
- Make a monthly medicine cabinet check.
- Plan time for routine car maintenance so you can handle daily schedules without delay.

Reorganizing activities can result in better working conditions, greater productivity, more time for the important things and people, and an improved quality of life.

STUDY TIPS

You have already spent several years in a study mode and have an established learning style. However, a few years may have passed since then, and you need to focus on recapturing successful study strategies and possibly developing new techniques. By enrolling in college, you have voluntarily committed yourself to education. A positive attitude may be your most valuable tool, because it can facilitate the learning process and allow you to enjoy the experience.

Study Environment

Have a designated area at home that is conducive to studying and concentrating. The room should have functional furniture and should be capable of holding educational equipment and materials. Furniture that is too comfortable may defeat the purpose. Adequate lighting is imperative, and the room temperature and noise level should be considered to prevent distractions. A quiet atmosphere is needed for activities involving concentration, although some learners find that background music or sounds are helpful and may even accelerate the pace of activity. Ellis (1985) expressed the traditional belief that "silence is the best form of music for study" (p. 49). Individual differences exist, however, and not everyone or all academic activities require total silence or isolation. Whatever your personal preferences, the environment should be designed to signal your brain that it is entering a work zone

Preparation for Study

Just as you prepare the environment, you must prepare yourself for study. Your body and mindset have to be open to academic business. Hunger and fatigue are unwelcome distractions and should be addressed before work begins. Any necessary materials should be on hand and within reach, to allow an undisturbed flow of work. A positive attitude, a sense of control, and a concrete plan set the stage for a productive session. You will need to acknowledge the transition and allow time to enter into the task. To participate effectively, you must mentally shift gears and assume the appropriate level of concentration. When projects are ongoing, it can be difficult to regain the mental perspective of the previous work session immediately. A quick review of the last section completed helps focus your attention and reduces startup time. Ending each work session of a continuing project by attaching a note detailing specific directions and ideas for the start of the next session may be beneficial.

Be cautious about unnecessary delays. Activities may give the appearance of efficiency, organization, and productivity and a sense of attending to the task at hand but, in fact, may be time and energy demons. Spending excessive amounts of time on preparation or process does not produce substance or achieve goals. A neatly labeled, color-coded collection of folders is of little value if the time you took to acquire and assemble them was taken from the time you needed to create content. Procrastination in the guise of preparation is not productive.

Study Process

Although individual study preferences exist and styles emerge, some practices have been successful for many people and can benefit the returning student with a busy schedule. It is helpful to establish a routine time for study, if possible. A routine facilitates readiness for the work and helps the student stay on task during the allotted time. Short study sessions interspersed with breaks and alternated with some physical activity are usually more productive than one continuous daylong effort. A break to read the mail, have lunch, vacuum the carpet, or take a quick walk or run serves the student well.

Each textbook is a valuable resource, and you should know its layout to gain a comprehensive view of its content and features. Take advantage of all the information authors provide. Objectives, key words, headings, highlights, and summaries are not window dressing; they provide direction and facilitate understanding. Illustrations clarify concepts. Diagrams, pictures, graphs, listings, and tables expand and enhance the mental images constructed by the written words. A glossary defines terms from the perspective of the subject area. An index assists students in quickly locating relevant information. Marking frequently used pages with a labeled tab or note can be helpful.

Reading the introduction and summary and paying attention to key words and headings before you read a chapter may help you identify the main points and understand the total concept. Visualizing while reading can create a mental picture and may help improve your comprehension. When questions arise, or you do not understand the material, tab the page, write the question on an index card, and speak with the professor. Many professors routinely interact with their students via e-mail.

Although initial study must be done individually, you can benefit from a study group.

To be effective, the group should have an agenda and a set time for each meeting. The gathering gives students an opportunity to compare notes from class, discuss content or questions from readings, and brainstorm about possible test questions. Group study works best when done on a regular, preferably weekly, basis.

Besides reading and discussion, you gain a significant amount of information through note-taking. It is important to be an active listener and to record pertinent information. Note-taking requires listening for and documenting key words and central thoughts and ideas. Verbatim notes are neither efficient nor realistic. Listen and understand first, and then summarize the information presented. Develop a consistent and efficient method of note-taking to ease the process and improve the content. Always date your notes and indicate the topic. Use paragraphs and headings to group and identify information. Record any reference your professor makes to pages in the text or names of other works and authors, and be alert to the importance of listings and definitions. Streamline notes to those points that are necessary and meaningful without being too brief or cryptic. Use common abbreviations and symbols, or develop an individual form of shorthand. Drawings and diagrams offer additional perspective on the words. Most important, handwriting must be legible for your notes to be of value.

The Cornell Notetaking Format is a useful tool. The format uses a lengthwise border on the left side of the paper, with notes written on the right side, the left portion is used for questions, comments, and additional information.

Taping lectures on an audiocassette reinforces the note-taking process. Tapes allow the student to add to notes already taken and to clarify details. The portable nature of tapes permits convenient repetition of the material in private settings, such as at home or in the car. Some international students may find tapes especially helpful in adapting to the English language and its nuances or to a professor who speaks rapidly. Any student who wishes to tape a lecture should have ample long-playing tapes available and should request permission of the presenter before taping. Some professors do not permit taping, and some students are reluctant to participate in discussion if it is being taped.

Cross-course activities help streamline and add depth to your education. The concept is to use information or processes from one course in another course or academic endeavor. It involves reprocessing information, reframing ideas, and implementing information or methods in new and creative ways. It does not mean submitting the same paper for two courses, but it can involve developing a new perspective on already researched material. For example, if appropriate to course objectives, a topic such as alcoholism could be used for papers in biology, sociology, psychology, and community nursing courses, among others. A different perspective directs the focus in each case. Students could merge aspects of work already produced to develop new perspectives and draw correlations. In the process, they deepen their knowledge, expand the scope of methods, and improve their critical thinking.

Bibliography cards are a simple, successful, and portable method of storing and transferring information. When researching any topic, you should write the citation in the correct form on an index card, along with notation of any pertinent information, quotes, or statistics. When the project or paper is completed, the bibliography will be complete, and merely rearranging the cards will produce the alphabetical order for typing. The cards can

 ONLINE CONSULT

To learn the Cornell Notetaking Format, consult the following Web sites. The first one offers the steps of the format, and the second contains an example:
www.ucc.vt.edu/stdysk/cornell.html
http://www.bucks.edu~specpop/Cornl.htm

then be filed according to a variety of categories (topic, course, alphabetically, etc.) to be retrieved for use later. You may also consider using a personal digital assistant to record information. With either procedure, the information can be transferred to computer at home, or the entire process can be adapted to a laptop computer.

A future use file can contain any materials with potential for use. Contents can include articles, quotes, cartoons, and brochures among many other things. Categories for filing can be established according to academic courses or topics, with a miscellaneous category. This file gives students a place to put information received or discovered that is pertinent to a specific area as well as a possible resource for any endeavor.

Advice on how to study could fill volumes, and many good publications on study strategies are available. Effective use of study methods can lead to cognitive energy and success.

However, you must accept the responsibility for determining and implementing the sound study practices most appropriate and realistic for you.

 CONCLUSION

If you honor the commitment to yourself, plan realistic strategies, use time and resources effectively, and maintain a balance in life activities, you can enjoy the challenge of the educational experience and achieve your goals. You are entitled to enjoy, not simply endure, the educational journey. Give yourself the opportunity to sense the growth, to measure the road you have traveled, and to determine future directions. The growth does not stop with conferral of the degree—it pervades your professional endeavors and guides your goals.

Key Points

- Personal goals involve commitment, require time and thought to formulate, and should be individualized and feasible. A series of short-term goals can help you accomplish long-term goals.
- Refining professional identity and role transition involves change that can be an uncomfortable but positive experience with personal and professional rewards.
- A mentor offers a role model, support, and assistance to avoid pitfalls.
- Responsibility to yourself can be both a key motivator and a monitor of actions.
- It is important to plan activities in realistic time frames to achieve goals and to focus on quality rather than be directed primarily by the clock.
- Recognition of your abilities, limitations, and resources is essential for realistic implementation of personalized strategies and success.
- Streamline work to direct time and attention to changing priority areas, maintain quality performance, and provide balance in a multiple-role lifestyle.
- Flexible thinking and change in perspective indicate growth related to the education experience.

 Thought and Discussion Questions

1. Review the quotation about change on the first page of the chapter in the context of the rest of the chapter, and be prepared to discuss it in class.

Interactive Exercises

1. Complete the Interactive Exercise on the Intranet site entitled "R & R," and be prepared to discuss your findings in class.
2. Complete the Interactive Exercise on the Intranet site entitled "Support Search," and be prepared to discuss your findings in class.
3. Complete the Interactive Exercise on the Intranet site entitled "Time Wasters," and be prepared to discuss your findings in class.
4. Complete the Interactive Exercise on the Intranet site entitled "Time Plan," and be prepared to discuss your findings in class.
5. List the things that you can delegate or eliminate to streamline your life while in school.
6. Start a collection of motivational sayings. Review and add to them each week; for example:
   - Live the life you've imagined.
   - Happiness is not the absence of problems, but the ability to deal with them.
   - It is more important to do your best than to be the best.

 PRINT RESOURCES

References

Boyer, E. L. (1987). College. *The undergraduate experience in America*. New York: Harper & Row.

Bruner, B., & Donahue, A. (1992). Marketing for the returning adult population. In *Symposium for the marketing of higher education*. Chicago: American Marketing Association.

Campaniello, J. (1988). When professional nurses return to school: A study of role conflict and well being in multiple role women. *Journal of Professional Nursing*, 4(2), 136–140.

Case, B. (1997). *Career planning for nurses*. Albany, NY: Delmar Publishers.

Catalano, J. (2003). *Nursing now: Today's issues, tomorrows trends*. Philadelphia: F.A. Davis.

Chenevert, M. (1993). *Pro nurse handbook*. St. Louis: Mosby.

Covey, S. R., Merrill, A., & Merrill, R. (1994). *First things first* [audiocassette]. New York: Simon & Schuster, Audio Division.

Curry, B. D. (1994). Societal and marketing influences on enrollment into baccalaureate nursing programs. In *Symposium for the marketing of higher education* (pp. 211–216). Chicago: American Marketing Association.

Curry, B. D. (2002). International inroads to wellness. Presentation, Vienna, Austria.

Dick, M., & Anderson, S. E. (1993). Job burnout in RN to BSN students: Time commitments, and support for returning to school. *Journal of Continuing Education in Nursing*, 24(3), 105–109.

Ellis, D. B. (1985). *Becoming a master student*. Rapid City, SD: College Survival Inc.

Fagin, C. (1994). Women and nursing: Today and tomorrow. In E. Friedman (Ed.), *An unfinished revolution: Women and health care in America*. New York: United Hospital Fund.

Fawcett, J. (1995). *Analysis and evaluation of conceptual models of nursing* (3rd ed.). Philadelphia: F.A. Davis.

Flexner, S. B. (Ed.). (1993). *Random House unabridged dictionary* (2nd ed.). New York: Random House.

Grant, A. B. (1994). *The professional nurse: Issues and actions*. Springhouse, PA: Springhouse Publishing.

Holmes, T. H., & Rahe, R. (1967). The social readjustment scale. *Journal of Psychosomatic Research*, 2(4), 213–218.

Katz, J. R. (with Carter, C., Bishop, J., & Kravits, S. L.) (2000). *Keys to science success*. Upper Saddle River, NJ: Prentice Hall.

Knowles, M. (1988). *The adult learner: A neglected species*. Houston, TX: Gulf Publishing.

Leddy, S., & Pepper, J. (1998). *Conceptual bases of professional nursing*. Philadelphia: Lippincott Williams and Wilkins.

Lengacher, C. (1993). Development of a predictive model for role strain in registered nurses returning to school. *Journal of Nursing Education*, 32(7), 301–308.

Meltzer, M., & Palau, S. M. (1993). *Reading and study strategies for nursing students*. Philadelphia: W. B. Saunders.

Moore, T. (1992). *Care of the soul*. New York: Harper Collins.

Murphy, J. (1999). *Think change*. USA: Successories Library

Patton, T., & Goldenberg, D. (1999). Hardiness and anxiety as predictors of academic success in first year, full time and part time RN students. *Journal of Continuing Education in Nursing, 30,* 158–167.

Redman, B. K., & Cassells, J. M. (Eds.). (1990). *Educating RN's for the baccalaureate.* New York: Springer.

Schuster, P. (2000). *Communication: The key to therapeutic relationships.* Philadelphia: F.A. Davis.

Shane, D. (1980, June.). The returning to school syndrome. *Nursing 80,* 86–88.

Strader, M. K., & Decker, P. J. (1995). *Role transition to patient care management.* Norwalk, CT: Appleton & Lange.

Bibliography

Burkhardt, M., & Nathaniel, A. (1998). *Ethics and issues in contemporary nursing.* Albany, NY: Delmar Publishers.

Covey, S. R. (1995). *Living the 7 habits* [audiocassette]. New York: Simon & Schuster, Audio Division.

Covey, S. R. (1990). *The 7 habits of highly effective people.* New York: Simon & Schuster.

Ellis, J. R., & Hartley, C. L. (1995). *Nursing in today's world* (5th ed.). Philadelphia: Lippincott.

Friedman, E. (Ed.). (1994). *An unfinished revolution: Women and health care in America.* New York: United Hospital Fund.

Hughes, E. C., Hughes, H., & Deutscher, I. (1958). *Twenty thousand nurses tell their story.* Philadelphia: Lippincott.

Khan, K., Schmidt, P. L., Schoville, R., & Williams, M. (1993, September). From expert to novice. *American Journal of Nursing,* September, 53–56.

Lancaster, J. (1999). *Nursing issues in leading and managing change.* St. Louis: Mosby.

Yoder-Wise, P. (1995). *Leading and managing in nursing.* St. Louis: Mosby.

Zerwekh, J., & Clabom, J. C. (1994). *Nursing today: Transitions and trends.* Philadelphia: W. B. Saunders.

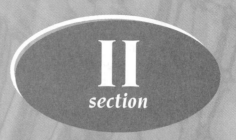

II
section

Theoretical Basis of Nursing Practice

Rose Kearney-Nunnery

3
chapter

What Is Theory?

> Theory and research are not solely the province of the academic, just as practice is not solely the field of the practitioner.
>
> *Glanz and associates (2002, p. 23)*

Chapter Objectives

On completion of this chapter, the reader will be able to:

1. Define key terms in theory development.
2. Discuss Maslow's theory of motivation with the hierarchy of basic needs.
3. Describe the components of developmental theories and their application to individuals across the life span.
4. Describe the components and application of systems theory.
5. Discuss the impact of theory on practice.

Key Terms

Theory	Construct	Hierarchy of Needs
Model	Variables	Developmental Theories
Framework	Propositions	General System Theory
Conceptual Model or	Theory Description	
Framework	and Evaluation	
Concept		

One characteristic of a profession is that it is built on a theoretical base. This base includes theoretical foundations unique to the profession as well as those borrowed or adapted from other scientific disciplines. Chapter 1 discussed paradigms and the metaparadigm concepts of nursing. Kuhn (1970) described a paradigm as "universally recognized scientific achievements that for a time provide model problems and solutions to a community of practitioners" (p. vii). When the paradigm is no longer useful in explaining phenomena, practice, and research in that particular scientific community, a paradigm shift occurs, and a new structure evolves.

In 1957, Merton used a paradigm to analyze sociological theory. He viewed the paradigm as a "field glass" to illuminate and view concepts and interrelationships and make assumptions clear on the body of knowledge for analysis and testing. Merton (1957) identified the purposes of a paradigm as providing for the following:

1. Parsimonious arrangement of concepts and propositions showing interrelationships.
2. A logical guide showing derivations and avoiding hidden assumptions and concepts.
3. Culmination in theory development as a building process.
4. Systematic arrangement and cross-tabulation of concepts for analysis.
5. Codification of qualitative research methods (pp. 13–16).

From a cultural perspective, Leininger (2002) defined a *worldview* as "the way an individual or group looks out on and understands their world about them as a value, stance, picture, or perspective about life or the world" (p. 83). In the professional culture of nursing, these are the values, attitudes, beliefs, and practices unique to the profession. Thus, a scientific community has the tools to create and test theory for knowledge development and use of this knowledge in practice. The worldview furnishes the philosophical assumptions that are considered "givens" by the theorist or the scientific community. In

nursing, this provides us with the process: the metaparadigm concepts to various paradigms, and the development of theory on which to base research, practice, administration, and education.

TERMINOLOGY IN THEORY DEVELOPMENT AND ANALYSIS

Professions such as nursing are based on unique theory. Kerlinger (1986) defined a **theory** as "a set of interrelated constructs (concepts), definitions, and propositions that present a systematic view of phenomena by specifying relations among variables, with the purpose of explaining and predicting the phenomena" (p. 9). This definition provides us with the components and aims of a theory, which must initially be described and then evaluated for potential use in practice, education, and research in a discipline. Some theorists, however, believe this definition is too narrow and excludes descriptive theories; descriptive theories, which focus on factor naming, are abundant in professional nursing and are often a first step for further research and development.

Before moving to the components of a theory, we need to address three similar terms frequently associated with theory: model, framework, and conceptual framework or model. A **model** is a graphic representation of some phenomenon. It may be a mathematical model (A + B = C) or a diagrammatic model, linking words with symbols and lines. A theoretical model provides a visual description of the theory using limited narrative and displaying components and relationships symbolically. A **framework** is another means of providing a structural view of the concepts and relationships proposed in a theory. Again, use of words and narrative is limited, but the structure of the theory is presented and allows translation, interpretation, and illumination of the narrative or text.

A **conceptual model or framework** is similar to a theory in that it represents some phenomenon of interest and contains concepts and propositions. However, with a conceptual model or framework, the concepts and especially the propositions are broader in scope, less defined, and less specific to the phenomenon of concern. As Fawcett (2000) noted, in professional nursing practice, conceptual models provide explicit and formal presentations of some nurses' images of nursing, but the concepts are "so abstract and general that they are not directly observed in the real world, nor are they limited to any particular individual, group, situation, or event" (p. 15).

A theory can evolve from a conceptual model or framework as concepts are further defined, specified, tested, and interrelated to represent some aspect of reality. Fawcett (1995, 2000) has described the structural hierarchy of contemporary nursing knowledge (Fig. 3–1) with its components, from the most abstract metaparadigm, influenced by different philosophies, to conceptual models that further evolve into theories and specific empirical indicators for testing. She applied this hierarchy to nursing practice, describing the role of conceptual models as "facilitating communication among nurses, reduc[ing] conflict among nurses who might have different implicit goals for practice, and provid[ing] a systematic approach to nursing research, education, administration, and practice" (Fawcett, 2000, p.17). Then, the function of a theory is "to narrow and more fully specify the phenomena contained in a conceptual model" (Fawcett, 2000, p. 19) Concepts become less abstract, and the population of interest is identified. This increase in specificity is evident in the examples proposed by Tomey and Alligood (2002) who, on the basis of Fawcett's structural hierarchy of nursing knowledge, correlated examples in theoretical structures as follows:

- Metaparadigm: Person, environment, health, and nursing
- Philosophy: Nightingale
- Conceptual Model: King's Systems Theory
- Grand Theory: King's Theory of Goal Attainment
- Theory: Goal Attainment in the hospital setting

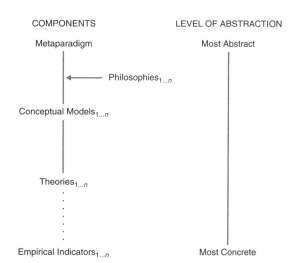

FIG. 3–1. The structural hierarchy of contemporary nursing knowledge: Components and levels of abstraction. (From Fawcett, J. [2005]. *Analysis and evaluation of contemporary nursing knowledge: Nursing models and theories.* [2nd. ed.] [p. 4.] Philadelphia: F.A. Davis, with permission.)

- Middle-range Theory: Use of goal attainment with adolescent diabetic clients in the community setting (p. 7)

As more is known about the phenomenon, more can be used in specific, meaningful client applications.

As knowledge about some phenomena increases, a theory is proposed to address phenomena or reality within the discipline. The components of a theory are the constructs (concepts), with their specific definitions, and the propositions that describe or link those constructs (concepts). At the simplest level, a **concept** is a view or idea that we hold about something. It can be something highly concrete, such as a pencil, or something highly abstract, such as quality. The more concrete the concept, the easier it is understood and consistently used. For instance, we are comfortable envisioning a pencil and can easily describe this to others. This ability to describe something directly in the concrete world shares the "concept." But the concept of quality is more abstract, and ensuring that all individual definitions are the same is difficult, often requiring indirect measures.

We strive to define a concept in operational terms—that is, how we view a specific entity and how it can be measured so that others know exactly what we mean. To meet the criteria of a theory, we need to define the concepts. Consider the concept of a pencil. We think of a pencil as a writing implement. This is the theoretical or conceptual definition of a pencil we read in a dictionary. But what do we truly mean by *pencil*? It is a yellow-painted, wooden-covered graphite instrument that we use to make marks on a paper. Does it have an eraser? Does a mechanical pencil fit into this definition? An operational definition narrows the definition to precisely what we view and how it can be measured for use in practice or research as a measurable, empirical indicator. In addition, concepts are broadened to constructs, such as with quality or identity, which can be multidimensional and difficult, if not impossible, to break down into component parts.

A **construct** is a more complex idea package of some phenomenon that contains many factors but cannot be truly isolated or confined to a more concrete concept. The construct of *identity*, for example, contains many pieces, such as personal perception, role expectations, and status. However, we must still provide an operational definition of a construct by specifying certain elements it contains (as indirect measures), such as self-image, ideal image, group image, role expectations, and status. The same multidimensionality occurs when we assess quality of health care.

In research, we often see the term **variables**, referring to some concept in the theory under study. Variables are concepts that can change and contain a set of values that can be measured in a practice or research situation. For example, a client's cholesterol reading is a variable. The concept of blood cholesterol has been operationally defined within certain parameters, and the level of the reading is the value for the variable.

Whether concepts, constructs, or a combination of the two are included in a specific theory, these concepts/constructs are the building blocks of the theory. Definitions are provided to help us understand the nature and characteristics of each block in the construction. We then need to relate these building blocks to each other. Describing and stating the relationships between or among the constructs (or concepts) provides the **propositions** of a theory. These are also called the *relational statements,* showing how the concepts are linked in the theory and relate to one another and to the total theoretical structure. They define how the structure is held together. In nursing theory, propositions refer to how the individual is characterized with specific abilities, knowledge, values, and traits and how these interrelate with the characteristics of health, the environment, and nursing.

Research is a means of supporting the concepts and relationships proposed in a theory. It provides supportive evidence and suggests further study and possible gaps or revisions needed in the theoretical structure. We can see this in the next chapters covering refinement of nursing and other health models, such as the health belief model revision. Research can be qualitative and inductive, for generating theory, or more quantitative, for deductively testing hypotheses as theoretical propositions.

As stated previously, Kerlinger defined the aims or purpose of theory as describing or explaining some phenomena of interest. In nursing, theory is further differentiated into levels that describe, explain, predict, and control. Dickoff and James (1968) developed a classic position paper proposing four levels of nursing theory (Box 3–1). All levels may be present as a practice theory evolves (factor-

---

BOX 3–1
DICKOFF AND JAMES (1968): FOUR LEVELS OF NURSING THEORY

1. Factor-isolating (naming) theories
2. Factor-relating (situation-depicting) theories
3. Situation-relating (predictive or promoting/inhibiting theories)
4. Situation-producing (prescriptive) theories

isolating and then relating), is subjected to further research, and is refined, becoming predictive and prescriptive. In application, testing, and refinement, theory is a continuum as long as the content meets the intent of the discipline and metaparadigm.

In addition, theories are classified according to their scope as grand, middle-range, or limited in scope or practice. This is the breadth of coverage of some phenomenon. General system theory is an example of a *grand theory*, or one with a broad scope. This theory, discussed later in the chapter, has been used in development, testing, and application in many scientific disciplines.

Merton (1957) was the first theorist to suggest "theories of the middle range: theories intermediate to the minor working hypotheses evolved in abundance during the day-by-day routines of research, and the all inclusive speculations comprising a master conceptual scheme from which it is hoped to derive it very large number of empirically observed uniformities of ... behavior" (pp. 5–6). As you will see in the next chapter, *middle-range theories* are narrower in scope, with a limited view of a phenomenon, and contain concepts and propositions that are measurable and can be empirically tested. Some of our traditional nursing theories meet the characteristics of a middle-range theory, as described in Chapter 4. Other middle-range theories are some of the developmental theories reviewed later in this chapter. Although these theories address psychosocial, cognitive, and moral development, they apply across disciplines as continual, incremental knowledge and skills developed by individuals. More limited nursing practice theories are evolving as hypotheses derived from middle-range theories are tested, clarified, and made specific to certain practice areas or types of health-care client. Chapter 5 shows examples of limited nursing practice models that are being tested and refined into theoretical frameworks, including Pender's health promotion model, the chronic illness trajectory framework, and Campinha-Bacote's model of cultural competence. Even more narrow in scope are *limited practice theories*, which focus on measurable variables and propositions that are based on

empirical research and now may be refined further, perhaps to a specific population or group of individuals with a common characteristic.

THEORY DESCRIPTION AND EVALUATION

To understand theories for use and application in practice, we use certain criteria to describe and evaluate them. Theory development is both an inductive and a deductive process. An inductive process is used to generate concepts and make inferences by stating interrelationships (propositions) within a framework to view phenomena. From observations of phenomena, we can name concepts and enumerate proposed relationships. Once the theory is generated, it is applied, in whole or part, for testing as a deductive process. For nursing **theory description and evaluation**, we consider the following three sets of criteria.

Chinn and Kramer (1999) differentiate between theory description and critical reflection of empiric theory. The theory is described by answering questions in the following five areas: purpose, concepts, definitions, relationships and structure, and assumptions. This process provides an understanding of the components and aims of the theory. Once the theory has been described, five issues are addressed in critical reflection:

- Clarity and consistency in presentation
- Simplicity and meaningfulness of relationships
- Generality or scope
- Accessibility as potential for use with empirically identifiable and applicable concepts
- Significance as leading to the values in practice, education, and research

This differentiation allows us to discriminate between understanding the theoretical structure and evaluating the theory's soundness and usefulness in practice, education, or research. These five areas for evaluation are used by Tomey and Alligood (2003) as clarity, simplicity, generality, empirical percision, and deriviable consequences (pp. 9–10).

Barbara Stevens Barnum (1998) proposes two categories of theory: descriptive theory and explanatory theory. *Descriptive theory* is factor-naming and factor-relating theory developed initially to characterize some phenomena. *Explanatory theory* brings us to the situating-relating and situation-producing levels of theory, looking at the "how," the "why," and the interrelationships in the theory (Barnum, 1998). Theory description is delineated as theory interpretation, with questions addressing the following areas:

- Major elements of the theory and their definitions
- Relationships among the elements
- Differentiating between descriptive and explanatory theory
- How the theory addresses, defines, and differentiates nursing
- The focus on the client, nurse, action, or relationship
- Unique language used and defined by the theorist (Barnum, 1990, 1994, 1998).

For critical analysis, internal criticism and external criticism are differentiated. *Internal criticism* is used to evaluate how the theory components fit together: the clarity, consistency, adequacy, logical development, and, sometimes, level of theory development (Barnum, 1998). *External criticism* deals with real-world issues such as reality convergence, usefulness, significance, and discrimination from other health-care disciplines (Barnum, 1998). This process allows us to discriminate between understanding the theoretical structure (internal criticism) and evaluating the soundness and usefulness of the theory for application in practice, education, or research (external criticism).

Fawcett (1993, 2000) has proposed criteria for theory analysis and evaluation that have undergone several revisions. *Analysis* refers to the description of the theory. Fawcett (2000) describes it as "a nonjudgmental description of the nursing model" while "analysis requires judgments to be made about the extent to which a nursing model satisfies certain criteria" (p. 63) Theory analysis is followed by theory evaluation, which requires thoughtful interpretation of the theory. Fawcett (2000) identifies a series of questions for analysis and evaluation of nursing models that stem from the components of the structural hierarchy. In this revision, Fawcett (2000) has proposed the three steps in a framework for the analysis of the nursing model and six steps for the evaluation of the model, as follows:

Analysis	Evaluation
Step 1: Origins of the Model	*Step 1:* Explication of Origins
Step 2: Unique Focus of the Model	*Step 2:* Comprehensiveness of Content
Step 3: Content of the Model	*Step 3:* Logical Congruence
	Step 4: Generation of Theory
	Step 5: Credibility: Social Utility, Social Congruence, Social Significance
	Step 6: Contributions to the Discipline

Application of this framework for theory analysis and evaluation will be evident in Chapter 4, which deals with specific nursing conceptual models and theories.

THEORIES FROM OUTSIDE OF NURSING, APPLIED TO NURSING

Nursing and other health-care disciplines have long used a variety of theories to guide practice. Some are discipline-specific, such as the nursing theories reviewed in Chapter 4. Other theoretical structures have been applied from other disciplines. Barnum (1990) describes early nursing theories as follows:

> As an applied science, much of nursing's theory is "borrowed" from other disciplines. Every discipline has similar boundary ambiguities, where the

inquiry and answers in one field overlap those in another. … Nursing's uniqueness in this respect does not lie in boundary overlap but in the number of boundary overlaps with which it must contend. A high number of overlaps occur in the discipline of nursing because it often attempts to deal holistically with a phenomenon (man) that has previously been dealt with in compartmentalized ways by other disciplines. (p. 218)

Chinn and Kramer (1999) agree on the usefulness of theories borrowed from other disciplines in some cases, but they recommend caution because some borrowed theories "do not take into consideration significant factors that influence a nursing situation" (p. 32). Recall the metaparadigm concepts. Borrowed theories may address the person, health, and the environment, but what of nursing? With collaborative practice, however, these theories provide a common ground and the opportunity for the application and sharing of middle-range theories. They also enable us to understand human nature, motivation, and development.

Several classic theories have been applied in nursing to view the person, family, community, and group. We use Maslow's hierarchy of needs to view the person and basic human needs. Developmental theories have been applied across the human life span as we seek to understand the complexity of human behavior. In looking at the person or group, we have applied systems theory to understand the interaction of person and environment. The following section briefly describes selected theories that are applied to the nursing discipline and are often used in the evolution of nursing models more specific to our metaparadigm concepts.

Maslow's Theory of Human Motivation and Hierarchy of Basic Needs

A theory widely used among disciplines is Maslow's theory of human motivation. In his original 1954 book, *Motivation and Personality*, Maslow described how his work emerged, and the work was published in segments in various journals and books. The book begins by presenting Maslow's philosophy as an approach to science. Human values are prevalent in the philosophy, and his worldview is described as holistic, functional, dynamic, and purposive. In his 1970 revised edition, Maslow reinforced his worldviews and described his theory as holistic-dynamic. He supported his original 16 propositions on motivation, on which his theory was based (see Chapter 10, on motivation in the teaching-learning process). This is a grand theory that views the complexity of human behavior, especially in relation to motivation of behavior. The theory of motivation is based on clinical and experimental data from psychology, psychiatry, education, and philosophy. It does not address specific nursing concerns except as they relate to human behavior with environmental influences.

Maslow's theory includes a hierarchical structure for human needs. This **hierarchy of needs** can be visualized as a pyramid (Fig. 3–2). At the base of the pyramid are the physiologic drives. Higher needs progress upward as safety, love and belonging, esteem, and self-actualization needs. Maslow (1954, 1970) described this as a "hierarchy of prepotency" to explain that the individual concentrates on the physiologic drives. The physiologic drives are considered the most powerful, but as physiologic needs are satisfied, higher needs emerge on which the individual focuses. This is the general structure for the hierarchy.

Individual differences are provided for in this theory. Some individuals have altered placement of needs in the hierarchy. Maslow (1970) described differences among individuals in placement of some of the higher needs such as a reversal of esteem and love/belonging needs. In addition, individuals may have different levels of need satisfaction. For example, one person might meet the physiologic drives at a 75 percent level, whereas another person's level for satisfaction is 85 percent. Individual differences also apply to the emergence of higher needs. Maslow (1970) regarded this as a gradual process; one person's safety needs may begin to emerge when his or her physiologic needs are being met at 25 percent, whereas another person may not begin to satisfy his or her safety needs until 30 percent of her physiologic needs are met. Levels of satisfaction and emergence of higher needs

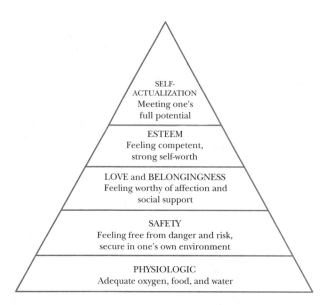

FIG. 3–2. Maslow's hierarchy of human needs.

therefore occur at different points in different people, as do pain thresholds in different people.

Looking again at the theoretical hierarchy, we see at the bottom level of the pyramid the physiologic drives, including the need to maintain homeostasis and the needs of hunger and thirst, sleep and rest, activity and exercise, sexual gratification and sensory pleasure, and maternal responses (Maslow, 1970). Meeting the physiologic hunger drive is very different from meeting one's nutritional requirements or treating anxiety or depression with a chocolate bar. When the individual is truly hungry or thirsty, not merely satisfying an appetite for food or drink, all energies and thoughts are directed to satisfying that drive for food or water. Consider the physiologic need of an individual with a chemical dependency. The person will focus all efforts on attaining the drug or addictive substance at the required level of satisfaction — while ignoring other needs, including the physiologic need for food or the next level of safey needs. When the physiologic drives and needs are relatively satisfied, higher-level needs emerge.

Safety needs are the next level of the hier-archy. Safety, both physical and emotional, must be achieved. Threats to a person's safety can become all-consuming. Think of an isolated person in an inner-city apartment whose fear for his safety motivates him to place bars on his windows and multiple chains and dead-bolt locks on his door. This person fears for his physical safety from a threat, real or imagined, of bodily harm. This is the main concern, not whether access is impeded in the case of a fire or accident. He places all focus on the quest for freedom from perceived danger.

Perceived safety can also be related to health, as with the fear of the client with chronic obstructive lung disease (COPD) to be near anyone who is coughing or sneezing. This person's safety need is to avoid a respiratory infection that could lead to pneumonia or even diminished oxygenation in an already compromised respiratory system. Even if the other person in the room is experiencing symptoms of a seasonal allergy, the individual with COPD seeks immediate escape from that environment because of the perceived danger of infection. Maslow (1954, 1970) also viewed safety needs more broadly in the need for the familiar and spiritual, religious, or philosophical meaning in life. He describes the use of rituals and ceremonial behaviors in children and individuals with psychological disorders as examples of focusing on safety needs.

Once the person satisfies these safety needs, the focus turns to the need for love and belonging. Inclusion and affection are important needs, not the isolated sex act, which is a physiologic drive. Maslow (1970) described the normal person as having a hunger and striving for affectionate relations and a place in a group, as opposed to the maladjusted person (pp. 43–44). Love and affection are manifested in many ways and are individually defined.

Satisfying the need for belonging and love brings us to the next level, esteem needs. Esteem needs involve a sense of dignity, worth, and usefulness in life. Maslow (1970) described two sets of esteem needs: (1) the sense of self-worth, including perceptions of strength, achievement, competence, and confidence; and (2) the esteem of others, including perceptions of deserved respect, status, recognition, importance, and dignity (p. 45). Satisfying the sense of self-worth and respect allows the next, and highest, level of basic needs to emerge.

The need for self-actualization at the top of the pyramid is the desire for self-fulfillment. This is the sense of being able to do all that a person can to answer the "why" of his or her existence. Maslow (1970) defined self-actualization as "the full use and exploitation of talents, capacities, potentialities, etc., such [that] people seem to be fulfilling themselves and ... developing to the full stature of which they are capable" (p. 150). Originally, Maslow (1954) proposed that self-actualized people included both older people and college students and children. But when he further examined the concept of self-actualization, he separated psychological health from self-actualization, which he limited to older people whose human potentialities have been realized and actualized (Maslow, 1970).

Maslow then developed support for his theory of basic needs and human actions using case studies and other research. Through observation of people, he proposed specific phenomena that are determined by basic gratification of cognitive-affective, cognitive,

character traits, interpersonal, and miscellaneous needs. He cited characteristics of people in relation to the hierarchy. For example, the following characteristics of self-actualized people emerged from Maslow's (1970) research and analysis of historical figures, public people, selected college students, and children:

1. More efficient and comfortable perceptions of reality
2. Acceptance of self, others, and nature
3. Spontaneity, simplicity, and naturalness in thoughts and behaviors
4. Problem-centered rather than ego-centered
5. Desire for detachment, solitude, and privacy
6. Autonomy with independence of culture and environment
7. Continued freshness of appreciation
8. Mystic and oceanic feelings with limitless horizons
9. Genuine desire to help people
10. Deeper and more profound interpersonal relationships
11. Democratic character structure
12. Strong ethical sense that discriminates means/ends and good/evil
13. Philosophical and unhostile sense of humor
14. Creativeness
15. Resistance to enculturation with an inner detachment (pp. 203–228)

Maslow created further hypotheses for testing. He described cases that diverged from his theory, such as the martyr who ignores survival needs for a principle. He called for further research, hypothesizing that satisfying basic needs earlier in life allows the individual to weather deprivation easier in later life (Maslow, 1954, p. 99). Maslow's work continued until his death in 1970. His hierarchy of needs has endured, and its applications have been extended in health care, education, industry, and marketing to understand people and their motivators. Needs related to individual, environmental, and health concerns are applicable to the nursing discipline. However, this theory is still a grand theory and does not address the specific domain of nursing.

	AGES	STRENGTHS & VIRTUES	DEVELOPMENTAL STAGE
8.	Ego Integrity vs. Despair	Renunciation & Wisdom	Older Adulthood
7.	Generativity vs. Stagnation	Production & Care	Middle Adulthood
6.	Intimacy vs. Isolation	Affiliation & Love	Young Adulthood
5.	Identity vs. Role Confusion	Devotion & Fidelity	Adolescence
4.	Industry vs. Inferiority	Method & Competence	School Age
3.	Initiative vs. Guilt	Direction & Purpose	Preschool
2.	Autonomy vs. Shame & Doubt	Self-control & Will Power	Toddler
1.	Trust vs. Mistrust	Drive & Hope	Infancy

FIG. 3–3. Erikson's (1963) eight ages of man.

Developmental Theories

A group of theories widely used in health care and education are the **developmental theories**. These middle-range theories address personality (Erikson and Havighurst), cognitive (Piaget), and moral (Kohlberg) development using a life span perspective. This perspective is based on progression and complexity in motor, personal-social, cognitive, or moral behavior. A brief review of each of the theories demonstrates how the theorist moved from a philosophy or worldview to identify concepts, propositions, and a model or theory based on observations, existing research, or case study presentations. Common to the developmental theories are predictable steps or stages through which the individual progresses during the life cycle. This is a building process. These theories are based largely on research through observation or case studies. Subsequent applications and research have been guided by the use of these theories to explain more specific phenomena or test hypotheses.

Personality Development

Erikson's (1963) eight ages of man represents a theory of psychosocial personality development in which the individual proceeds through critical periods in a step-by-step or epigenetic process (Fig. 3–3). This theory has been and continues to be used widely in health care and psychology. In offering the theory, Erikson presented his philosophy and case studies with Freudian and neo-Freudian applications. Each stage has positive and negative aspects that are defined and described. The basic goal is for the individual to develop a favorable ratio of the positive aspects for a healthy ego. Erikson (1963) further described basic virtues and essential strengths for each of his "ages" or stages of development. These strengths and basic virtues define the positive aspects of ego development required in each stage. Propositions are developed for each of the stages. This theory is supported mainly by case study, with suggestions and encouragement of further hypotheses for research and testing. Erikson's theory has been used widely in nursing to foster positive ego development and empowerment in individuals. Although this theory does not specifically address the domain of nursing, common concerns include the person, the environment, and psychosocial health.

Havighurst's developmental tasks and education represent another theory of personality development that includes principles of cognitive and moral development as well. In this perspective, the individual proceeds through six stages, accomplishing critical tasks.

Havighurst (1972) described his philosophy, including the origins of the concept, and proposed a method for analyzing individual developmental tasks based on the following five criteria: (1) nature or definition, (2) biological basis, (3) psychological basis, (4) cultural basis, and (5) educational implications (pp. 17–18). Table 3–1 illustrates the tasks for each of the six age groups.

Although descriptions of the tasks represent some gender bias and cultural limitations, the concept's biologic and psychological bases are applicable to health care. The tasks represent major milestones in biologic, psychological, emotional, and cognitive functioning or development that individuals must negotiate as they progress through life. Person, environmental, and health promotion concerns are

TABLE 3–1
Havighurst's Developmental Tasks

Stages	Tasks
I. Infancy and Early childhood	1. Learning to walk 2. Learning to take solid foods 3. Learning to talk 4. Learning to control the elimination of body wastes 5. Learning sex differences and sexual modesty 6. Forming concepts and learning language to describe social and physical reality 7. Getting ready to read 8. Learning to distinguish right and wrong and beginning to develop a conscience
II. Middle childhood	1. Learning physical skills necessary for ordinary games 2. Building wholesome attitudes toward oneself as a growing organism 3. Learning to get along with age-mates 4. Learning an appropriate masculine/feminine social role 5. Developing fundamental skills in reading, writing, and calculating 6. Developing concepts necessary for everyday living 7. Developing conscience, morality, and a scale of values 8. Achieving personal independence 9. Developing attitudes toward social groups and institutions
III. Adolescence	1. Achieving new and more mature relations with age-mates of both sexes 2. Achieving a masculine or feminine social role 3. Accepting one's physique and using the body effectively 4. Achieving emotional independence of parents and other adults 5. Preparing for marriage and family life 6. Preparing for an economic career 7. Acquiring a set of values and an ethical system as a guide to behavior 8. Desiring and achieving socially responsible behavior

(continued)

TABLE 3–1 Havighurst's Developmental Tasks *(continued)*	
Stages	**Tasks**
IV. Early adulthood	1. Selecting a mate 2. Learning to live with a marriage partner 3. Starting a family 4. Rearing children 5. Managing a home 6. Getting started in an occupation 7. Taking on civic responsibility 8. Finding a congenial social group
V. Middle adulthood	1. Assisting teenage children age to become responsible and happy adults 2. Achieving adult social and civic responsibility 3. Reaching and maintaining satisfactory performance in one's occupational career 4. Developing adult leisure-time activities 5. Relating oneself to one's spouse as a person 6. Adjusting and accepting the physiologic changes of middle age 7. Adjusting to aging parents
VI. Later maturity	1. Adjusting to decreasing physical strength and health 2. Adjusting to retirement and reduced income 3. Adjusting to death of a spouse 4. Establishing an explicit association with one's age group 5. Adopting and adapting social roles in a flexible way 6. Establishing satisfactory physical living arrangements

Source: *Developmental Tasks and Education* by Robert J. Havighusrt. Copyright © 1948 by the University of Chicago. Copyright ©) 1950 by Robert J. Havighurst. Copyright © (1952) by David McKay Company, Inc. Copyright © 1972 by David McKay Company. Reprinted by permission of Addison-Wesley Education Publishers, Inc.

apparent in the life-span perspective. Age-specific tasks relate well to activities of daily living during specific life stages and can easily be incorporated in care planning.

Cognitive Development

Piaget's theory of cognitive development focuses on the development of the intellect. Piaget was an example of a self-actualized person. Moving from the publication of his first monograph on birds at age 10 years, he detailed the development of the intellect in children through observations. His techniques were sometimes criticized by the scientific community. But his theory has since been accepted and used in practice and research by many students and professionals. Piaget's theory looks at the innate and environmental influences on the development of the intellect. This theory has four major periods of cognitive development: sensorimotor, preoperational thought, concrete operations, and formal operations (Table 3–2).

Within his theory, Piaget provided us with the concepts of schema, object permanence, assimilation, and accommodation. *Schema* are patterns of thought or behavior that evolve into more complexity as more information is obtained through assimilation and accommodation. *Object permanence*, the knowledge

TABLE 3–2
Piaget's Theory of Cognitive Development

Period of Cognitive Development	Age	Stage Description
Sensorimotor Stages		
• Reflexive	Birth–1 month	Use of primitive reflexes, such as sucking and rooting
• Primary circular reactions	1–4 months	Repeating an event for the result, such as thumb in mouth
• Secondary circular reactions	4–10 months	Combining events for a result, such as kicking a mobile over crib
• Coordination of secondary schema	10–12 months	Creating a behavior for some result, such as standing in crib to reach mobile
• Tertiary circular reactions	12–18 months	Looking for similar results from varying behaviors, such as shaking crib and jumping to observe movements of mobile
• Representational thought begins	18–24 months	Symbolic representation in thought such as hanging objects to create mobile
Preoperational	2–7 years	Making overgeneralizations, such as all cats are named Tiger; egocentric Focuses only on one concrete attribute Magical thought and symbolic play present
Concrete operations	7–11 years	Logical and reversible thought appears; conservation of matter and numbers
Formal operations	After 11 years	Theoretical and hypothetical thinking now possible; higher-order mathematics and reasoning

that something still exists when it is out of sight, develops when the child is between 9 and 10 months of age. *Assimilation* is the acquisition and incorporation of new information into the individual's existing cognitive and behavioral structures. *Accommodation* is the change in the individual's cognitive and behavioral patterns based on the new information acquired. Piaget's theory has been translated and applied worldwide and across disciplines. His work continued until his death in 1980, and further research and theory is still evolving from his contributions.

Piaget's work concentrated on cognitive development in children, including views on moral development. As such, it is more limited but has provided major insight into working with children. Applications are

seen in health teaching, especially in chronic or terminal illness situations. But with these limitations on cognitive development for some environmental influences, it can address only a portion of the domain of concern to nursing.

Moral Development

Kohlberg's theory of moral development was an outgrowth of Piaget's work on moral development in children. Kohlberg's extensive work on moral development (Kohlberg, 1984; Kohlberg et al., 1987) is based on research with children given scenarios to describe reactions and make judgments. He initially studied boys 10 to 16 years old

TABLE 3–3
Kohlberg's Theory of Moral Development

Level	Stage	Stage Description
Level I: Preconventional morality	1. Heteronomous morality	Egocentrically applies a fixed set of rules from authorities, e.g., parents, to avoid punishment.
	2. Individualism, purpose, and exchange	Sees that different individuals have different rules, e.g., parents and teachers, but selection based on individual interests with some fair exchange.
Level II: Conventional morality	3. Interpersonal expectations, relationships, and conformity	Motives of other person now emerge when considering right and wrong; use of the Golden Rule in considerations.
	4. Social system and conscience	The good of society as a whole now emerges with the individual having certain roles and rules in the system.
Level III: Postconventional morality	5. Social contract and individual rights	Believes in upholding laws and legal contracts looking at the greatest good for greatest number; sees but cannot deal well with ethical-legal conflicts.
	6. Universal ethical principles	Principles of justice and human rights are followed and upheld as a personal and universal ethical system.

Source: Adapted from Kohlberg, L. (1984) *Essays in moral development: Vol. II. The psychology of moral development* (pp. 174–176). San Francisco: Harper & Row, with permission.

from Chicago, later adding research with children of both genders and different backgrounds. Kohlberg's theory consists of six stages grouped into three major levels: preconventional, conventional, and postconventional (Kohlberg, 1984), illustrated in Table 3–3.

Kohlberg's theory confers major insight into moral development. He provided the theoretical structure, the supportive research, and applications in educational practice. The individual progresses through the levels and stages, not as a natural process, but through intellectual stimulation with a central focus on moral justice. This requires thinking about moral problems and issues. Further research and practices have been based on this theory and are ongoing. Consider the usefulness of this theory when you are working with a child or adolescent whose parent was recently diagnosed with a terminal illness.

As with Piagetian theory, Kohlberg's theory is limited to a specific area of development. The focus is on the person, such as the child, with ramifications for adult life. Environmental (e.g., social and cultural) factors provide insight for social and psychological health. The limitation to moral development addresses only a portion of the domain of concern to nursing.

Many developmental models are used and applied in nursing. Examine the conceptual models and theories presented in Chapter 4 for their application of developmental concepts. Several nursing theories have a decidedly developmental focus, whether as a main component, as in Watson's theory, or with specific concepts included, defined, and built on, as in King's model.

A life span, developmental, or life processes focus has major relevance for nursing, because we view the person in the context of environment and effects on health status.

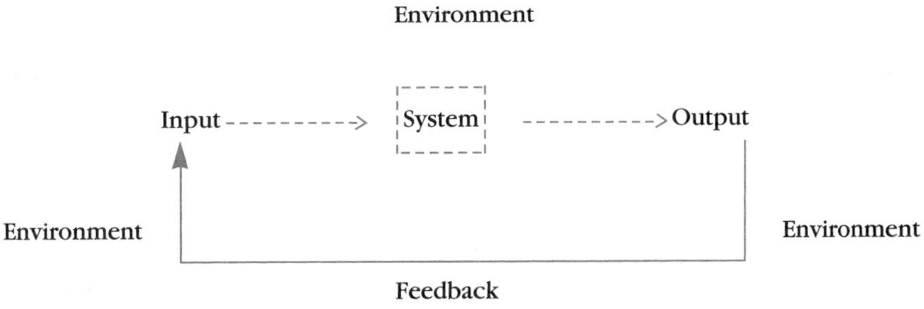

Environment

Input - - - - - - - - - > ┆System┆ - - - - - - - - -> Output

Environment   Environment

Feedback

FIG. 3–4. General systems model: A simple open system.

Systems Theory

The interrelationships with health and nursing are complex and must be specified for their applicability to the domain of nursing.

Perhaps the most widely used theory in multiple disciplines is systems theory. Systems have been in existence for ages, but in the late 1930s, Bertalanffy introduced systems theory to represent an aspect of reality. Thus, **general system theory** was incorporated in the paradigms of many scientific communities. This is a grand theory, wide in scope, that has generated numerous theories in many disciplines. Bertalanffy (1968) explained the wide applicability in many scientific communities as the various disciplines became concerned with "wholeness," not just focusing on isolated parts, but dealing with the interrelationships among them and between the parts and the whole. A system generally contains the following basic components: input, output, boundary, environment, and feedback. Figure 3–4 illustrates a basic view of a simple system.

The initial step in understanding and applying systems theory is to view the grand theory. Bertalanffy (1968) defined a *system* as a complex of interacting elements and proposed that every living organism is essentially an open system. The general system theory applies the following principles to human and organizational systems:

1. *Wholeness:* This indicates that the whole is more than merely the sum of the parts. To understand the whole, one must understand the components and their interactions with each other and the environment.
2. *Hierarchical order:* Some form of hierarchy exists in the system's components, structure, and functions.
3. *Exchange of information and matter (openness):* In an open system, there is an exchange and flow of information and matter with the environment through some boundary that surrounds the system. Inputs come through the boundary from the environment, are transformed through system processes (throughputs), and are sent as outputs through the boundary back into the environment. This exchange of information and matter is goal-oriented, whether to maintain the steady state or to fulfill the functions of the system. An important component of this process is feedback from the environment.
4. *Progressive differentiation:* Differentiation within the system leads to self-organization. Applying the laws of thermodynamics, entropy is a measure of order or organization in the system in the process of seeking equilibrium or some final goal. In an open system, entropy is decreased or negative, allowing for differentiation and self-organization.
5. *Equifinality:* In open systems, the final state can be reached from different initial conditions and in different ways. Initial conditions do not necessarily determine the final state or outcome of the system.
6. *Teleology:* Behavior in the system is directed toward some purpose or goal, as a human characteristic.

Environmental influences are a major consideration in health care. Systems theory provides a useful framework with which to visualize some phenomenon (the system), focusing on the components, structure, and functions as the internal environment (throughputs), and influenced by (inputs and feedback) and influencing (outputs) the environment. It is important to analyze the system carefully for all component parts, structures, and functions. Recall that the basis for general system theory is that "the whole is greater than the sum of the parts." This brings us to the need for a precise analysis of interrelationships among components and between the parts and the entire system. In addition, an open system has permeable boundaries receiving input and feedback from the environment. Problems occur when environmental factors are unknown, unclear, or ignored. Consider the broad health-service system. Since Institute of Medicine reports beginning in 1998, we have been greatly concerned about safety in health care. Systems issues have been a major focus, but moving from a culture of blaming individual practitioners, the challenge became one of improving components in the system, input, feedback, and outputs. In addition, the broader health-care environment and societal influences are included and visualized as crossing the system boundaries of an individual hospital setting.

In nursing, systems theory and various applications have been used to explain organizations, nursing and health-care delivery, and groups of people. Several nursing models are based on systems theory. Johnson's behavioral systems conceptual model views the person as a behavioral system and nursing as an external force. It exemplifies how a grand theory (general system theory) from another scientific community provided a basis for developing the conceptual model of nursing (Johnson's behavioral systems). Specificity to the metaparadigm concepts and interrelationships unique to nursing have provided the basis for the nursing conceptual framework. Further delineation of concepts and propositions leads to more specific nursing theory. Neuman's health-care model,

Roy's adaptation model, and King's conceptual framework and theory of goal attainment are examples of nursing conceptual models and theories based on systems models. Other nursing models use various components of general systems theory. Further applications of systems theory are evident in subsequent sections on management in organizations and change.

THE IMPACT OF THEORY ON PRACTICE

As Barnum (1998) states, "nursing knowledge, arising from practice, should shape our theories, and theories, reciprocally, should direct our practice" (p. 45). We use theory every day in our personal and professional lives, from the basic principles of asepsis in hygiene and standard precautions to understanding the complex communication channels of the organizational system in which we practice.

Theory, practice, and research are interrelated and interdependent. We need theory to guide practice predictably and effectively. We need research to support the significance and usefulness of the theory, because the dynamic nature of our metaparadigm concepts of person, environment, health, and nursing makes theories tentative and subject to refinement and revision. Professional practice must provide the questions for study based on problems and phenomena relevant to the discipline. As Chinn and Kramer (1999) have described, deliberate application of theory places theory within the context of practice to ensure that it serves the goals of the profession (pp. 141–142).

Again, recall that nursing is a profession and a scientific community. We practice using principles provided by our metaparadigm and theoretical bases. This furnishes us with the tools for critical thinking, provision of care, education, administration, research, and interdisciplinary collaboration. We have a paradigm that provides the models for problems and solutions in our knowledge base and practice community in line with Kuhn's (1970) descriptions of a paradigm. Our paradigms and theories are designed to address problems and solutions in practice, or we need to shift to a new structure with different theories and paradigms to explain our concerns for people, environments, health, and nursing.

The theory on which we base practice must be compatible with and must correspond to the phenomena of professional nursing practice. To ensure that the goals of theory and practice are consistent, Chinn and Kramer (1999) recommend considering the following questions:

1. Are the theory goals congruous with practice goals?
2. Is the intended context of the theory congruous with the situation in which the theory will be applied?
3. Is there, or might there be, similarity between theory variables and practice variables?
4. Are the explanations of the theory sufficient to be a basis for nursing action?
5. Does research evidence support the theory?
6. How will this new approach influence the practical function of the nursing unit? (pp. 142–146)

In the next chapter, conceptual models and theories unique to nursing are discussed. These models are the guides to practice in our highly complex profession. Implementing models for practice, whether unique to nursing or adapted, is a necessary but arduous and time-consuming task. The process is worth the effort to ensure quality care for recipients, but requires many of the skills addressed in subsequent chapters.

Key Points

- Kerlinger (1986) defined a theory as "a set of interrelated constructs (concepts), definitions, and propositions that present a systematic view of phenomena by specifying relations among variables, with the purpose of explaining and predicting the phenomena" (p. 9).

- A model is a graphic representation of some phenomena. A theoretical model provides a visual description of the theory using limited narrative but displays components and relationships symbolically. A framework is another means of providing a structural view of the concepts and relationships proposed in a theory. A conceptual model or framework represents phenomena of interest and contains concepts and propositions that are broader in scope, less defined, and less specific to the phenomena of concern than those in a theory.

- A concept is a view or idea we hold about something, ranging from something highly concrete to something highly abstract. A construct is a more complex idea package of some phenomena, containing many factors that cannot be isolated or confined into a more concrete concept. Definitions of concepts and constructs are theoretical or conceptual, such as those in dictionaries, or operational. An operational definition states precisely what we view as phenomena and how they can be measured. Variables are concepts that contain a set of values that can be measured in a practice or research situation.

- Propositions in a theory are the descriptions and relationships among the constructs (or concepts) that propose how the concepts are linked and relate to each other and to the total theoretical structure.

- Dickoff and James (1968) developed a classic position paper proposing four levels of nursing theory: factor-isolating, factor-relating, situation-relating, and situation-producing theories. *(continued)*

(continued)

- Theories are classified as grand, middle-range, or limited (practice) on the basis of their scope or breadth of coverage of phenomena.
- Theory description is a careful, nonjudgmental analysis of the component parts of a theory—its assumptions, concepts, definitions, propositions, context, and scope.
- Theory evaluation requires thoughtful interpretation relative to the clarity, significance, consistency, empirical support, and usefulness in explaining a phenomenon of concern.
- Maslow's theory of human motivation and hierarchy of basic needs proposes a hierarchical structure for human needs, from physiologic drives at the bottom, to needs for safety, belonging, love, esteem, and self-actualization at the top of the pyramid.
- Developmental theories are widely used in nursing and other health-care disciplines.
- Erikson's (1963) eight ages of man represents a theory of psychosocial personality development in which the individual proceeds through critical periods in a step-by-step or epigenetic process.
- Havighurst's developmental tasks and education represents another theory of personality development that involves principles of cognitive and moral development within six stages containing critical tasks for maturation.
- Piaget's theory of cognitive development focuses on the development of the intellect within four major periods of cognitive development: sensorimotor, preoperational thought, concrete operations, and formal operations.
- Kohlberg's theory of moral development was developed as an outgrowth of Piaget's six stages, grouped into three major levels: preconventional, conventional, and postconventional.
- A system generally contains the following basic component parts: input, output, boundary, environment, and feedback. General system theory is a grand theory applied to many disciplines. Bertalanffy (1968) defined a system as a complex of interacting elements with the following principles: wholeness, hierarchical order, open exchange of information and matter, progressive differentiation, equifinality, and teleology.
- Theory, practice, and research are interrelated and interdependent. When we are selecting a theory on which to base practice, the theory must be compatible and correspond to the phenomena of professional nursing practice.

Thought and Discussion Questions

1. Consider the following statement by Barnum (1990) describing early nursing theories: "A high number of [boundary] overlaps occur in the discipline of nursing because it often attempts to deal holistically with a phenomenon (man) that has previously been dealt with in compartmentalized ways by other disciplines" (p. 218). What does she mean by "holistically"? How do you think other disciplines may deal with the human being in a comparmentalized way?
2. Identify individuals who you think are self-actualized, and explain why.

3. Identify a theory used in your practice setting. Identify the concepts (constructs), how the component concepts are defined, the propositions that link the concepts, and the aims of this theory.

4. Describe how theory is used in your practice setting, and propose how it could be used further.

5. Review the Chapter Thought located on the first page of the chapter, and discuss it in the context of the contents of the chapter.

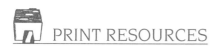

Interactive Exercises

1. Complete the exercise on the Intranet site on application of Maslow's theory of motivation, with its hierarchy of basic needs, to clients with the specified nursing diagnoses. Incorporate additional nursing diagnoses for clients specific to your practice areas in this table.

2. Read the case studies provided on the Intranet site. Apply a developmental theory to the situation, and give examples of how they are progressing according to the selected theory. Be prepared to discuss in class or online, as scheduled by your instructor.

3. Using the format on the Intranet site, apply systems theory to a work group of which you are a member. Describe examples applicable to general systems theory principles of wholeness, hierarchical order, open exchange of information and matter, progressive differentiation, equifinality, and teleology.

PRINT RESOURCES

References

Barnum, B. S. (1998). *Nursing theory: Analysis, application, evaluation* (5th ed.). Philadelphia: Lippincott Williams & Wilkins.

Barnum, B. J. S. (1994). *Nursing theory: Analysis, application, evaluation* (4th ed.). Philadelphia: J.B. Lippincott.

Barnum, B. J. S. (1990). *Nursing theory: Analysis, application, evaluation* (3rd ed.). Glenview, IL: Scott, Foresman/Little, Brown Higher Education.

Bertalanffy, L. V. (1968). *General system theory: Foundations, development, applications.* New York: George Braziller.

Chinn, P. L., & Kramer, M. K. (1999). *Theory and nursing: Integrated knowledge development* (5th ed.). St. Louis: Mosby.

Dickoff, J., & James, P. (1968). A theory of theories: A position paper. *Nursing Research, 17,* 197–203.

Erikson, E. H. (1963). *Childhood and society* (2nd ed.). New York: W. W. Norton.

Fawcett, J. (2005). *Analysis and evaluation of contemporary nursing knowledge: Nursing models and theories.* (2nd ed.). Philadelphia: F.A. Davis.

Fawcett, J. (2000). *Analysis and evaluation of contemporary nursing knowledge: Nursing models and theories.* Philadelphia: F.A. Davis.

Fawcett, J. (1995). *Analysis and evaluation of conceptual models of nursing* (3rd ed.). Philadelphia: F.A. Davis.

Fawcett, J. (1993). *Analysis and evaluation of nursing theories.* Philadelphia: F.A. Davis.

Glanz, K., Rimer, B.K., Lewis, F.M. (Eds.) (2002). *Health behavior and health education: Theory, research, and practice* (3rd. ed) San Francisco: Jossey-Bass.

Havighurst, R. J. (1972). *Developmental tasks and education* (3rd ed.). New York: David McKay.

Kerlinger, F. N. (1986). *Foundations of behavioral research* (3rd ed.). New York: Holt, Rinehart and Winston.

Kohlberg, L. (1984). *Essays in moral development: Vol. II. The psychology of moral development.* San Francisco: Harper & Row.

Kohlberg, L., DeVries, R., Fein, G., Hart, D., Mayer, R., Noam, G., Snarey, J., & Wertsch, J. (1987). *Child psychology and childhood education: A cognitive-developmental view.* New York: Longman.

Kuhn, T. S. (1970). *The structure of scientific revolutions* (2nd ed.). Chicago: University of Chicago Press.

Leininger, M. M. (2002). The theory of culture care and ethnonursing research method. In M. Leininger & M. R. McFarland, *Transcultural nursing: Concepts, theories, research, and practice* (3rd ed.) (pp. 71–980). New York: McGraw-Hill.

Maslow, A. H. (1970). *Motivation and personality* (2nd ed.). New York: Harper & Row.

Maslow, A. H. (1954). *Motivation and personality.* New York: Harper & Brothers.

Merton, R. K. (1957). *Social theory and social structure* (Rev. ed.). Glencoe, IL: Free Press.

Tomey, A. M., & Alligood, M. R. (2002). *Nursing theorists and their work* (5th ed.). St. Louis: Mosby.

Leininger, M. M. (1991). The theory of culture care diversity and universality. In M. M. Leininger (Ed.), *Culture care diversity and universality: A theory of nursing* (Pub. No. 15–2402) (pp. 5–68). New York: National League for Nursing.

Polan, E., & Taylor, D. (1998). *Journey across the life span: Human development and health promotion.* Philadelphia: F.A. Davis.

Power, F. C., Higgins, A., & Kohlberg, L. (1989). *Lawrence Kohlberg's approach to moral education.* New York: Columbia University.

Singer, D. G., & Revenson, T. A. (1998). *A Piaget primer: How a child thinks* (Rev. ed.). Madison, CT: International Universities Press.

Wadsworth, B. J. (1996). *Piaget's theory of cognitive and affective development: Foundations of constructivism* (5th ed.). New York: Addison Wesley Longman.

Bibliography

Erikson, E. H. (1980). *Identity and the life cycle.* New York: W. W. Norton.

Ginsburg, H. P., & Opper, S. (1988). *Piaget's theory of intellectual development* (3rd ed.). New York: Prentice-Hall.

Hardy, M. E. (1974). Theories: Components, development, evaluation. *Nursing Research, 23,* 100–107.

Johnson, B. M., & Webber, P. B. (2001). *An introduction to theory and reasoning in nursing.* Philadelphia: Lippincott Williams & Wilkins.

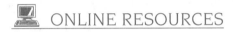 ONLINE RESOURCES

http://allnurses.com
http://www.enursescribe.com
http://www.tcns.org
http://www.maslow.com
http://www.nursing.gr/theory/theory.html

Jacqueline Fawcett
Barbara Swoyer

4
chapter

Evolution and Use of Formal Nursing Knowledge

"[A]rticulation of what nursing is and what nursing can be has never been more critical"
(Fawcett, 2000, p. iii).

Chapter Objectives

On completion of this chapter, the reader will be able to:

1. Describe the meaning of formal nursing knowledge as the basis for professional nursing practice.
2. Identify the different functions of conceptual models and theories.
3. Discuss the advantages of using explicit conceptual models of nursing and nursing theories to guide professional nursing practice.
4. Apply a conceptual model of nursing or nursing theory to a particular clinical situation.

Key Terms

Formal Nursing
  Knowledge
Nursing Knowledge
Conceptual Models of
  Nursing
Behavioral Systems Model
General Systems
  Framework
Conservation Model

Systems Model
Self-Care Framework
Science of Unitary
  Human Beings
Adaptation Model
Grand Theories of
  Nursing
Culture Care and
  Universality

Health as Expanding
  Consciousness
Human Becoming
Middle-Range Nursing
  Theories
Deliberative Nursing
  Process
Interpersonal Relations
Human Caring

This chapter describes the evolution of nursing knowledge—as it has been formalized—in conceptual models of nursing and nursing theories, and identifies the impact of that knowledge on professional nursing practice.

FORMAL NURSING KNOWLEDGE

Conceptual models of nursing and nursing theories represent **formal nursing knowledge**. That knowledge was organized by several nurse scholars who devoted a great deal of time to observing clinical situations, thinking about what is important to nursing in those situations, and then testing their thoughts by conducting nursing research (Fawcett, 1999). Nursing knowledge continues to evolve as nurse researchers and clinicians use conceptual models and theories to guide their research and clinical practice and then report the results at conferences and in publications. Consequently, all nurses can contribute to the evolution of nursing knowledge.

What Is Nursing?

Nightingale's (1859) book, *Notes on Nursing: What It Is, and What It Is Not*, contains the first ideas that can be considered formal nursing knowledge. More than 100 years later, Henderson (1966) published her definition of nursing, continuing the evolution of formal nursing knowledge. Although the intervening years were filled with many ideas about nursing, most of those ideas unfortunately were not presented as formal conceptual models and theories.

Florence Nightingale's Notes on Nursing

Nightingale's ideas about nursing, first published in 1859, represent the beginning of formal nursing knowledge. Nightingale maintained that every woman is a nurse because every woman, at some time in her life, has charge of the personal health of someone. Nightingale equated knowledge of nursing with knowledge of sanitation. The focus of nursing knowledge was how to keep the body free from disease or in such a condition that it could recover from disease. According to Nightingale, *nursing* ought to signify the proper use of fresh air, light, warmth, cleanliness, and quiet and the proper selection and administration of diet—all at the least expense of vital power to the patient; that is, she maintained that the purpose of nursing was to put the patient in the best condition for nature to act on him or her. She also asserted that nursing practice encompasses care of both well and sick people, and that nursing actions focus on both patients and their environments. Her 13 "hints" provided the boundaries of nursing practice (Box 4–1).

Virginia Henderson's Definition of Nursing

Henderson contributed to the evolution of nursing knowledge by providing a definition that has been accepted around the world. According to Henderson, the unique function of the nurse is to help individuals, sick or well, to perform those activities contributing to health or its recovery (or to peaceful death) that they would perform unaided if they had the necessary strength, will, or knowledge, and to do so in such a way as to help them gain independence as soon as possible. The practice of nursing requires nurses to know and understand patients by putting themselves in the place of the patients. Nurses should not take at face value everything that patients say, but rather should interact with patients to ascertain their true feelings. Basic nursing care involves helping the patient perform certain activities unaided (Box 4–2).

BOX 4–1
NIGHTINGALE'S 13 HINTS

1. *Ventilation and warming:* The nurse must be concerned first with keeping the air that patients breathe as pure as the external air, without chilling them.

2. *Health of Houses:* Attention to pure air, pure water, efficient drainage, cleanliness, and light will secure the health of houses.

3. *Petty Management:* All the results of good nursing may be negated by not knowing how to manage what you do when you are there and what shall be done when you are not there.

4. *Noise:* Unnecessary noise, or noise that creates an expectation in the mind, is that which hurts patients. Anything that wakes patients suddenly out of their sleep will invariably put them into a state of greater excitement, do them more serious and lasting mischief, than any continuous noise, however loud.

5. *Variety:* The nerves of the sick suffer from seeing the same walls, the same ceiling, the same surroundings during a long confinement to one or two rooms. The majority of cheerful cases are to be found among those patients who are not confined to one room, whatever their suffering, and the majority of depressed cases are seen among those subjected to a long monotony of objects about them.

6. *Taking Food:* The nurse should be conscious of patients' diets and remember how much food each patient has had and ought to have each day.

7. *What Food?:* To watch for the opinions the patient's stomach gives, rather than to read "analyses of foods," is the business of all those who have to decide what the patient should eat.

8. *Bed and Bedding:* The patient should have a clean bed every 12 hours. The bed should be narrow, so that the patient does not feel "out of humanity's reach." The bed should not be so high that the patient cannot easily get in and out of it. The bed should be in the lightest spot in the room, preferably near a window. Pillows should be used to support the back below the breathing apparatus, to allow shoulders room to fall back, and to support the head without throwing it forward.

9. *Light:* With the sick, second only to their need of fresh air is their need of light. Light, especially direct sunlight, has a purifying effect on the air of a room.

10. *Cleanliness of Rooms and Walls:* The greater part of nursing consists in preserving cleanliness. The inside air can be kept clean only by excessive care to rid rooms and their furnishings of the organic matter and dust with which they become saturated. Without cleanliness, you cannot have all the effects of ventilation; without ventilation, you can have no thorough cleanliness.

11. *Personal Cleanliness:* Nurses should always remember that if they allow patients to remain unwashed or to remain in clothing saturated with perspiration or other excretion, they are interfering injuriously with the natural processes of health just as much as if they were to give their patients a dose of slow poison.

12. *Chattering Hopes and Advices:* There is scarcely a greater worry that invalids have to endure than the incurable hopes of their friends. All friends, visitors, and attendants of the sick should avoid the practice of attempting to cheer the sick by making light of their danger and by exaggerating their probabilities of recovery.

13. *Observation of the Sick:* The most important practical lesson nurses can learn is what to observe, how to observe, which symptoms indicate improvement, which indicate the reverse, which are important, which are not, and which are the evidence of neglect and what kind of neglect.

Source: Nightingale, F. (1859). *Notes on nursing: What it is, and what it is not.* London: Harrison and Sons. [Commemorative edition printed 1992, Philadelphia: J. B. Lippincott]

BOX 4–2
VIRGINIA HENDERSON'S ACTIVITIES OF NURSING

- Breathe normally.
- Eat and drink adequately.
- Eliminate body wastes.
- Move and maintain desirable postures.
- Sleep and rest.
- Select suitable clothes, and dress and undress.
- Maintain body temperature within normal range by adjusting clothing and modifying the environment.
- Keep the body clean and well groomed and protect the integument.
- Avoid dangers in the environment and avoid injuring others.
- Communicate with others in expressing emotions, needs, fears, or opinions.
- Worship according to one's faith.
- Work in such a way that there is a sense of accomplishment.
- Play or participate in various forms of recreation.
- Learn, discover, or satisfy the curiosity that leads to normal development and health, and use the available health facilities.

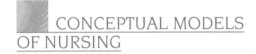

CONCEPTUAL MODELS OF NURSING

The terms *conceptual model, conceptual framework, conceptual system, paradigm,* and *disciplinary matrix* are frequently used interchangeably and have the same definition: a set of relatively abstract and general concepts that address the phenomena of central interest to a discipline, the statements that broadly describe those concepts, and the statements that assert relatively abstract and general relations between two or more of the concepts (Fawcett, 2000).

Definition

Each conceptual model presents a particular perspective about the phenomena of interest to a particular discipline, such as nursing. **Conceptual models of nursing** present diverse perspectives of the individuals, families, and communities who are participants in nursing; the environment of the nursing participant, and the environment in which nursing practice occurs; the health condition of

the nursing participant; and the definition and goals of nursing as well as the nursing process or practice methodology used to assess, label, plan, intervene, and evaluate.

Functions

One function of any conceptual model is to provide a distinctive frame of reference, or "a horizon of expectations" (Popper, 1965, p. 47), and "a coherent, internally unified way of thinking about ... events and processes" (Frank, 1968, p. 45) that tells nurses what to observe and how to interpret what they observe in practice. Each conceptual model, then, presents a unique focus that has a profound influence on nurses' ways of thinking about nursing participants and their environments in matters of health.

Another function of each conceptual model is the identification of a particular "philosophical and pragmatic orientation to the service nurses provide patients—a service which only nurses can provide—a service which provides a dimension to total care different from that provided by any other health professional" (Johnson, 1987, p. 195). Conceptual models of nursing provide explicit orientations not only for nurses but also for the general public. They identify the purpose and scope of nursing and provide frameworks for objective records of the effects of nursing assessments and interventions. As Johnson (1987) explains, "Conceptual models specify for nurses and society the mission and boundaries of the profession. They clarify the realm of nursing responsibility and accountability, and they allow the practitioner and/or the profession to document services and outcomes" (pp. 196–197). An overview of each of these nursing models is presented in the following section, along with the implications of each one for professional nursing practice.

Conceptual Models of Nursing

Currently, the works of several nurse scholars are recognized as conceptual models. Among the best known are Johnson's (1990) Behavioral Systems Model, King's (1990) General Systems Framework, Levine's (1991) Conservation Model, Neuman's Systems Model (Neuman and Fawcett, 2002), Orem's (2001) Self-Care Framework, Rogers's (1990) Science of Unitary Human Beings, and Roy's Adaptation Model (Roy & Andrews, 1999).

Dorothy Johnson's Behavioral Systems Model

Johnson's conceptual model of nursing, the **Behavioral Systems Model**, focuses on the person as a behavioral system, made up of all the patterned, repetitive, and purposeful ways of behavior that characterize life. The following seven subsystems carry out specialized tasks or functions needed to maintain the integrity of the whole behavioral system and to manage its relationship to the environment:

1. *Attachment or affiliative:* Function is the security needed for survival as well as social inclusion, intimacy, and formation and maintenance of social bonds.
2. *Dependency:* Function is the succoring behavior that calls for a response of nurtu-

rance as well as approval, attention or recognition, and physical assistance.
3. *Ingestive:* Function is appetite satisfaction in terms of when, how, what, how much, and under what conditions the individual eats, all of which is governed by social and psychological considerations as well as biologic requirements for food and fluids.
4. *Eliminative:* Function is elimination in terms of when, how, and under what conditions the individual eliminates wastes.
5. *Sexual:* Functions are procreation and gratification, with regard to behaviors dependent on the individual's biologic sex and gender role identity, including but not limited to courting and mating.
6. *Aggressive:* Function is protection and preservation of self and society.
7. *Achievement:* Function is mastery or control of some aspect of self or environment, with regard to intellectual, physical, creative, mechanical, social, and care-taking (of children, partner, home) skills.

The structure of each subsystem involves four elements:

- *Drive or goal*: The motivation for behavior.
- *Set*: The individual's predisposition to act in certain ways to fulfill the function of the subsystem.
- *Choice*: The individual's total behavioral repertoire for fulfilling subsystem functions, which encompasses the scope of action alternatives from which the person can choose.
- *Action*: The individual's actual behavior in a situation. Action is the only structural element that can be observed directly; all other elements must be inferred from the individual's actual behavior and from the consequences of that behavior.

The following three functional requirements are needed by each subsystem to fulfill its functions:

- Protection from noxious influences with which the system cannot cope
- Nurturance through the input of appropriate supplies from the environment
- Stimulation to enhance growth and prevent stagnation

Implications for Nursing Practice

Nursing practice is directed toward the restoration, maintenance, or attainment of behavioral system balance and dynamic stability at the highest possible level for the individual. Johnson's practice methodology, which is called the Nursing Diagnostic and Treatment Process, encompasses four steps (Box 4–3):

Step 1: Determination of the Existence of a Problem

The nurse obtains:

- Past and present family and individual behavioral system histories via interviews, structured and unstructured observations, and objective methodologies
- Data about the nature of behavioral system functioning in terms of the efficiency and effectiveness with which the client's goals are obtained
- Information to determine the degree to which the behavior is purposeful, orderly, and predictable
- Information on the condition of the subsystem structural components to draw inferences about: (1) drive strength, direction, and value; (2) the solidity and specificity of the set; (3) the range of behavior patterns available to the client; and (4) the usual behavior in a given situation

The client's behavior is compared with the

BOX 4–3
BEHAVIORAL SYSTEMS MODEL: DIAGNOSTIC AND TREATMENT PROCESS

- Determination of the Existence of a Problem
- Diagnostic Classification of Problems
- Management of Nursing Problems
- Evaluation of Behavioral System Balance and Stability

---

following indices for behavioral system balance and stability, as well as the reorganization and integration of the subsystems:

- The behavior is succeeding to achieve the consequences sought.
- Effective motor, expressive, or social skills are evident.
- The behavior is purposeful—actions are goal directed, reveal a plan and cease at an identifiable point, and are economical in sequence.
- The behavior is orderly—actions are methodical and systematic, build sequentially toward a goal, and form a recognizable pattern.
- The behavior is predictable—actions are repetitive under particular circumstances.
- The amount of energy expended to achieve desired goals is acceptable.
- The behavior reflects appropriate choices—actions are compatible with survival imperatives and the social situation.
- The client is sufficiently satisfied with the behavior.

Step 2: Diagnostic Classification of Problems

Classification occurs in two areas:

- *Internal subsystem problems*: Functional requirements are not met, inconsistency or disharmony among the structural components of subsystems is evident, and/or the behavior is inappropriate in the ambient culture
- *Intersystem problems*: The entire behavioral system is dominated by one or two subsystems, or a conflict exists between two or more subsystems

Step 3: Management of Nursing Problems

The general goals of action are to restore, maintain, or attain the client's behavioral system balance and stability and to help the client achieve an optimum level of balance and functioning when this goal is possible and desired. The nurse determines what nursing is to accomplish on behalf of the behavioral system by determining who makes the judgment regarding the acceptable level of behavioral system balance and stability. Nursing actions may occur in three areas:

- Temporary external regulatory or control mechanisms by setting limits for behavior by either permissive or inhibitory means, inhibiting ineffective behavioral response, helping the client acquire new responses, and reinforcing appropriate behaviors
- Repair of damaged structural components by reducing drive strength by changing attitudes, redirecting goal by changing attitudes, altering set by instruction or counseling, and adding choices by teaching new skills
- Fulfillment of functional requirements of subsystems by protecting the client from overwhelming noxious influences, supplying adequate nurturance, and providing stimulation to enhance growth and inhibit stagnation

The nurse negotiates the treatment modality with the client by establishing a contract with the client and helping him or her to understand the meaning of the nursing diagnosis and the proposed treatment.

Step 4: Evaluation of Behavioral System Balance and Stability

The nurse compares the client's behavior after treatment with indices of behavioral system balance and stability.

Imogene King's General Systems Framework

King's conceptual model of nursing, the **General Systems Framework,** focuses on the continuing ability of individuals to meet their basic needs so that they may function in their socially defined roles. It also concentrates on individuals' interactions within three open, dynamic, interacting systems.

Personal Systems

Personal systems are individuals who are regarded as rational, sentient, social beings. Concepts related to the personal system are:

- *Perception*: A process of organizing, interpreting, and transforming information from sense data and memory that gives meaning to one's experience, represents one's image of reality, and influences one's behavior
- *Self*: A composite of thoughts and feelings that constitute a person's awareness of individual existence, of who and what he or she is
- *Growth and development*: Cellular, molecular, and behavioral changes in human beings that are a function of genetic endowment, meaningful and satisfying experiences, and an environment conducive to helping individuals move toward maturity
- *Body image*: A person's perceptions of his or her body
- *Time*: The duration between the occurrence of one event and the occurrence of another event
- *Space:* The physical area called territory that exists in all directions
- *Learning:* Gaining knowledge

Interpersonal Systems

Interpersonal systems are defined as two, three, or more individuals interacting in a given situation. The concepts associated with this system are:

- *Interactions:* The acts of two or more persons in mutual presence; a sequence of verbal and nonverbal behaviors that are goal directed
- *Communication:* The vehicle by which human relations are developed and maintained; it encompasses intrapersonal, interpersonal, verbal, and nonverbal communications
- *Transaction:* A process of interaction in which human beings communicate with the environment to achieve goals that are valued

- *Role:* A set of behaviors expected of a person occupying a position in a social system
- *Stress:* A dynamic state whereby a human being interacts with the environment to maintain balance for growth, development, and performance, which involves an exchange of energy and information between the person and the environment for regulation and control of stressors
- *Coping:* A way of dealing with stress

Social Systems

Social systems are organized boundary systems of social roles, behaviors, and practices developed to maintain values, and the mechanisms to regulate the practices and rules. The concepts related to social systems are:

- *Organization:* Composed of human beings with prescribed roles and positions who use resources to accomplish personal and organizational goals
- *Authority:* A transactional process characterized by active, reciprocal relations in which members' values, backgrounds, and perceptions play a role in defining, validating, and accepting the authority of individuals within an organization
- *Power:* The process whereby one or more persons influence other persons in a situation
- *Status:* The position of an individual in a group or a group in relation to other groups in an organization
- *Decision-making:* A dynamic and systematic process by which goal-directed choice of perceived alternatives is made and acted on by individuals or groups to answer a question and attain a goal
- *Control:* Being in charge

Implications for Nursing Practice

Nursing practice is directed toward helping individuals maintain their health so they can function in their roles. King's practice methodology, which is the essence of the Theory of Goal Attainment, is called the Interaction-Transaction Process (Box 4–4).

Myra Levine's Conservation Model

Levine's conceptual model of nursing, the **Conservation Model**, focuses on conservation of the person's wholeness. *Adaptation* is the process by which people maintain their wholeness or integrity as they respond to environmental challenges and become congruent with the environment. Sources of challenges are:

- *Perceptual environment:* Encompasses that part of the environment to which individuals respond with their sense organs
- *Operational environment:* Includes those aspects of the environment that are not directly perceived, such as radiation, odorless and colorless pollutants, and microorganisms
- *Conceptual environment:* The environment of language, ideas, symbols, concepts, and invention

Individuals respond to the environment by means of four integrated processes that constitute the organismic response:

- Flight-or-flight mechanism
- Inflammatory-immune response
- Stress response
- Perceptual awareness: includes the basic orienting, haptic, auditory, visual, and taste-smell systems

Implications for Nursing Practice

Nursing practice is directed toward promoting wholeness for all people, well or sick. Patients are partners or participants in nursing care and are temporarily dependent on the nurse. The nurse's goal is to end the dependence as quickly as possible. Levine's practice methodology is a nursing process directed toward conservation (Box 4–5), which is defined as "keeping together," and which consists of three steps:

STEP 1: TROPHICOGNOSIS

Trophicognosis is formulation of a nursing care judgment arrived at by the scientific method.

BOX 4–4
KING'S PRACTICE METHODOLOGY: INTERACTION-TRANSACTION PROCESS

Assessment Phase:

1. *Perception:* The nurse and the client meet in a nursing situation and perceive each other. The nurse uses the goal-oriented nursing record (GONR) to record perceptions.

2. *Judgment:* The nurse and the client make mental judgments about each other; the nurse can use the GONR to record judgments.

3. *Action:* The nurse and the client take some mental action; the nurse can use the GONR to record mental actions.

4. *Reaction:* The nurse and the client mentally react to each one's perceptions of the other; the nurse can use the GONR to record mental reactions.

Diagnosis Phase:

Disturbance is the diagnosis phase, in which the nurse and the client communicate and interact, and the nurse identifies the client's concerns, problems, and disturbances in health. The nurse conducts a nursing history to determine the client's activities of daily living, using the Criterion-Referenced Measure of Goal Attainment Tool (CRMGAT). Also included with the nursing history are roles, environmental stressors, perceptions, values, learning needs, and goals. Data from the nursing history, the medical history and physical examination data, results of laboratory tests and x-ray examinations, information gathered from other health professionals and the client's family members, and the diagnoses are included on the GONR.

Planning Phase:

The planning phase includes mutual goal setting, exploration, and agreement. The nurse and the client set mutually agreed on goals.

• *Goal Setting:* If the client cannot verbally participate in goal setting, it is based on the nurse's assessment of the client's concerns, problems, and disturbance in health; the nurse's and client's perceptions of the interference; and the nurse's sharing of information with the client and his or her family to help the client attain the goals identified. The nurse records the goals on the GONR.

• *Exploration of Means to Achieve Goals:* The nurse and the client interact purposefully to explore the means to achieve the mutually set goals.

• *Agreement on Means to Achieve Goals:* The nurse and the client interact purposefully to agree on the means to achieve the mutually set goals, and these are recorded as nursing orders on the GONR.

Implementation Phase:

Transaction is the implementation phase of the process and refers to the valuational components of the interaction. The nurse and the client carry out the measures agreed on to achieve the mutually set goals. GONR flow sheet and progress notes are used to record the implementation of measures used to achieve goals.

Evaluation Phase:

Attainment of goals is the evaluation phase, in which the nurse and the client identify the outcome of the interaction-transaction process expressed in terms of the client's state of health or ability to function in social roles. The nurse and the client determine whether or not the goal was attained; and if not, why. CRMGAT is used to record the outcome, and the GONR to record the discharge summary.

The nurse observes and collects data that will influence nursing practice using appropriate assessment to establish an objective and scientific rationale for nursing practice. The nurse understands the basis for the prescribed medical regimen, including the medical diagnosis, the medical history, and the laboratory and x-ray examination reports, with specific reference to areas influencing the nursing care plan.

BOX 4–5
LEVINE'S PRACTICE METHODOLOGY:
CONSERVATION PRINCIPLES

- Conservation of Energy
- Conservation of Structural Integrity
- Conservation of Personal Integrity
- Conservation of Social Integrity

Assessment skills are directed at four conservation principles:

- *Conservation of energy* determines the ability to perform necessary activities without producing excessive fatigue. Relevant observations include vital signs, the patient's general condition, the patient's behavior, the patient's tolerance of nursing activities required by his or her condition, and allowable activity for the patient based on his or her energy resources.
- *Conservation of structural integrity* determines physical functioning. Relevant observations include status of any pathophysiologic processes, status of healing processes, and effects of surgical procedures.
- *Conservation of personal integrity* determines moral and ethical values and life experiences. Relevant observations include the client's life story, interest in participating in decision-making, and identifying sense of self.
- *Conservation of social integrity* takes the client's family members, friends, and conceptual environment into account. Relevant observations include identification of the client's significant others, participation in workplace and/or school activities, religion, and cultural and ethnic history.

The basis for implementation of the nursing care plan includes principles of nursing science and adaptation of nursing techniques to the unique cluster of needs demonstrated in the individual patient. The nurse identifies the provocative facts—that is, the data that provoke attention on the basis of knowledge of the situation—to provide the basis for a hypothesis, or trophicognosis. Observations are then recorded and transmitted.

STEP 2: INTERVENTION/ACTION

Intervention/action is a test of the hypothesis. The nursing care plan is implemented and evaluated within the structure of administrative policy, availability of equipment, and established standards of nursing. The general types of nursing intervention required are therapeutic nursing intervention, which influences adaptation favorably, or toward renewed social well-being, and supportive nursing interventions, which cannot alter the course of the adaptation and can only maintain the status quo or fail to halt a downward course. Nursing interventions are structured according to the four conservation principles as follows:

- Conservation of energy, based on the conservation of the individual patient's energy through an adequate deposit of energy resource and regulation of the expenditure of energy
- Conservation of structural integrity, which is conservation of the individual patient's structural integrity through maintenance or restoration of the structure of the body
- Conservation of personal integrity, based on the conservation of the patient's personal integrity through maintenance or restoration of the patient's sense of identity, self-worth, and acknowledgment of uniqueness
- Conservation of social integrity, which is conservation of the individual's social integrity through acknowledging the patient as a social being

STEP 3: EVALUATION OF INTERVENTION/ACTION

Evaluation of the intervention/action is the nurse's evaluation of the effects of the intervention/action and is used to revise the trophicognosis as necessary. An indicator of the success of nursing interventions is the patient's organismic response.

Betty Neuman's Systems Model

Neuman's conceptual model of nursing, the Systems Model, focuses on the wellness of the client system in relation to environmental stress and reactions to stress. The client system, which can be an individual, a family or other group, or a community, is a composite of five interrelated variables:

1. *Physiologic:* Bodily structure and function
2. *Psychological:* Mental processes and relationships
3. *Sociocultural:* Social and cultural functions
4. *Developmental:* Developmental processes of life
5. *Spiritual:* Aspects of spirituality on a continuum from complete unawareness or denial to a consciously developed, high level of spiritual understanding

The client system is depicted as a central core, which is a basic structure of survival factors common to the species, surrounded by three types of concentric rings:

- *Flexible line of defense:* The outermost ring is a protective buffer for the client's normal or stable state that prevents invasion of stressors and keeps the client system free from stressor reactions or symptomatology.
- *Normal line of defense:* Lies between the flexible line of defense and the lines of resistance and represents the client system's normal or usual wellness state.
- *Lines of resistance:* The innermost concentric rings are involuntarily activated when a stressor invades the normal line of defense. They attempt to stabilize the client system and foster a return to the normal line of defense. If these rings are effective, the system can reconstitute; if they are ineffective, death may ensue.

Environment represents all internal and external factors or influences surrounding the client system:

- *Internal environment:* All forces or interactive influences internal to or contained solely within the boundaries of the defined client system; the source of intrapersonal stressors

- *External environment:* All forces or interaction influences external to or existing outside the defined client system, the source of interpersonal and extrapersonal stressors
- *Created environment:* Is subconsciously developed by the client as a symbolic expression of system wholeness, and supersedes and encompasses the internal and external environments; functions as a subjective safety mechanism that may block the true reality of the environment and the health experience

Implications for Nursing Practice

Nursing practice is directed toward facilitating optimal wellness through retention, attainment, or maintenance of client system stability. The nurse uses the Neuman Systems Model Assessment and Intervention Tool, the Systems Model Nursing Diagnosis Taxonomy, and any other relevant clinical tools to guide collection of data and facilitate documentation of nursing diagnoses, nursing goals, and nursing outcomes. Neuman's practice methodology is the Neuman Systems Model Nursing Process Format (Box 4–6), which encompasses three steps:

STEP 1: NURSING DIAGNOSIS

The nurse establishes the database, which involves simultaneous consideration of the dynamic interactions of physiologic, psychological, sociocultural, developmental, and spiritual variables. The nurse identifies the client/client system's perceptions and his or her own perceptions, including basic structure factors and energy resources; flexible and

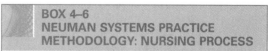

BOX 4–6
NEUMAN SYSTEMS PRACTICE
METHODOLOGY: NURSING PROCESS

- Nursing Diagnosis
- Nursing Goals
- Nursing Outcomes

normal lines of defense, lines of resistance, degree of potential or actual reaction, and potential for reconstitution following a reaction; and the internal and external environmental stressors that threaten the stability of the client/client system.

The nurse compares the client/client system's and the nurse's perceptions by identifying similarities and differences in perceptions. A comprehensive nursing diagnosis is presented that encompasses the client/client system's general condition or circumstances, including identification of actual or potential variances from wellness and available resources.

STEP 2: NURSING GOALS

The nurse prioritizes goals by considering the client/client system's wellness level, the meaning of the experience to the client/client system, system stability needs, and total available resources. Outcome goals and interventions are proposed that will facilitate the highest possible level of client/client system stability or wellness, maintain the normal line of defense, and retain the flexible line of defense. Desired prescriptive change or outcome goals are developed to correct variances from wellness with the client/client system, taking client/client system needs and resources into account. Specific prevention as intervention modalities are negotiated with the client/client system.

STEP 3: NURSING OUTCOMES

The nurse implements nursing interventions through the use of one or more of the three "prevention as intervention" modalities:

- *Primary prevention*: Nursing actions to retain system stability are implemented through such measures as preventing stressor invasion, providing resources to retain or strengthen existing client/client system strengths, and supporting positive coping and functioning.
- *Secondary prevention*: Nursing actions to attain system stability are implemented through such measures as protecting the

client/client system's basic structure, mobilizing and optimizing the client/client system's internal and external resources to attain stability and energy conservation, and facilitating purposeful manipulation of stressors and reactions to stressors.
- *Tertiary prevention*: Nursing actions to maintain system stability are implemented through such measures as attaining and maintaining the highest possible level of client/client system wellness and stability during reconstitution; educating, reeducating, and/or reorienting the client/client system as needed; and supporting the client/client system toward appropriate goals.

The nurse evaluates the outcome goals by confirming (with the client/client system) their attainment, and reformulating goals as necessary. The nurse and client/client system set intermediate and long-range goals for subsequent nursing action.

Dorothea Orem's Self-Care Framework

Orem's conceptual model of nursing focuses on patients' deliberate actions to meet their own and dependent others' therapeutic self-care demands. **The Self-Care Framework** also focuses on nurses' deliberate actions to implement nursing systems designed to assist individuals and multiperson units who have limitations in their abilities to provide continuing and therapeutic self-care or care of dependent others. The concepts of Orem's conceptual model are:

Self-Care

Self-care is behavior directed by individuals to themselves or their environments to regulate factors that affect their own development and functioning in the interests of life, health, or well-being.

Self-Care Agency

A self-care agency is the complex capability of maturing and mature individuals to determine the presence and characteristics of specific requirements for regulating their own functioning and development, make judgments and decisions about what to do, and perform care measures to meet specific self-care requisites. The person's ability to perform self-care is influenced by *ten power components:*

1. Ability to maintain attention and exercise requisite vigilance with respect to self as self-care agent and internal and external conditions and factors significant for self-care
2. Controlled use of available physical energy that is sufficient for the initiation and continuation of self-care operations
3. Ability to control the position of the body and its parts in the execution of the movements required for the initiation and completion of self-care operations
4. Ability to reason within a self-care frame of reference
5. Motivation (i.e., goal orientations for self-care that are in accord with its characteristics and its meaning for life, health, and well-being)
6. Ability to make decisions about care of self and to operationalize these decisions
7. Ability to acquire technical knowledge about self-care from authoritative sources, to retain it, and to operationalize it
8. A repertoire of cognitive, perceptual, manipulative, communication, and interpersonal skills adapted to the performance of self-care operations
9. Ability to order discrete self-care actions or action systems into relationships with prior and subsequent actions toward the final achievement of regulatory goals of self-care
10. Ability to consistently perform self-care operations, integrating them with relevant aspects of personal, family, and community living

The person's ability to perform self-care is also influenced by ten internal and external factors called *basic conditioning factors:*

- Age
- Gender
- Developmental state
- Health state
- Sociocultural orientation
- Health care system factors, for example, medical diagnostic and treatment modalities
- Family system factors
- Patterns of living, including activities regularly engaged in
- Environmental factors
- Resource availability and adequacy

Therapeutic–Self-Care Demand

The therapeutic–self-care demand is the action demand on individuals to meet three types of self-care requisites:

- *Universal self-care requisites*: Actions that need to be performed to maintain life processes, the integrity of human structure and function, and general well-being
- *Developmental self-care requisites*: Actions that need to be performed in relation to human developmental processes, conditions, and events and in relation to events that may adversely affect development
- *Health deviation self-care requisites:* Actions that need to be performed in relation to genetic and constitutional defects, human structural and functional deviations and their effects, and medical diagnostic and treatment measures prescribed or performed by physicians

Self-Care Deficit

The self-care deficit is the relationship of inadequacy between self-care agency and the therapeutic self-care demand.

Nursing Agency

Nursing agency is a complex property or attribute that enables nurses to know and help others to know their therapeutic self-care demands, meet their therapeutic self-care demands, and regulate the exercise or development of their self-care agency.

Nursing System

A nursing system is a series of coordinated deliberate practical actions performed by nurses and patients directed toward meeting the patient's therapeutic self-care demand and protecting and regulating the exercise or development of the patient's self-care agency.

Implications for Nursing Practice

Nursing practice is directed toward helping people meet their own and their dependent others' therapeutic self-care demands. Orem's practice methodology encompasses the Professional-Technologic Operations of Nursing Practice (Box 4–7). The operations are as follows:

CASE MANAGEMENT OPERATIONS

The nurse:

- Uses a case management approach to direct each of the nursing diagnostic, prescriptive, regulatory, and control operations.
- Maintains an overview of the interrelationships between the social, interpersonal, and professional-technological systems of nursing.
- Uses the nursing history and other appropriate tools for collection of information, documentation of information, and measurement of the quality of nursing.

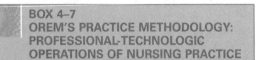

BOX 4–7
OREM'S PRACTICE METHODOLOGY: PROFESSIONAL-TECHNOLOGIC OPERATIONS OF NURSING PRACTICE

- Case Management Operations
- Diagnostic Operations
- Prescriptive Operations
- Design of Nursing Systems for Performance of Regulatory Operations
- Planning for Regulatory Operations
- Production of Regulatory Care
- Control Operations

DIAGNOSTIC OPERATIONS

The nurse:

- Identifies the unit of service for nursing practice as an individual, an individual member of a multiperson unit, or a multiperson unit.
- Determines why the individual needs nursing.
- Collects demographic data about the patient and information about the nature and boundaries of the patient's health care situation and nursing's jurisdiction within those boundaries.

PRESCRIPTIVE OPERATIONS

In collaboration with the patient or family, the nurse specifies:

- All care measures needed to meet the entire therapeutic self-care demand.
- The roles to be played by the nurse(s), patient, and dependent-care agent(s) in meeting the therapeutic self-care demand.
- The roles to be played by the nurse(s), patient, and dependent-care agent(s) in regulating the patient's exercise or development or self-care agency or dependent-care agency.

DESIGN OF NURSING SYSTEMS FOR PERFORMANCE OF REGULATORY OPERATIONS

The nurse designs a nursing system, a series of coordinated deliberate practical actions performed by the nurse and the patient. The actions are directed toward meeting the patient's therapeutic self-care demand and protecting and regulating the exercise or development of the patient's self-care agency or dependent-care agency.

PLANNING FOR REGULATORY OPERATIONS

The nurse specifies what is needed to produce the nursing system(s) selected for the patient, including:

- The time during which the nursing system will be produced
- The place where the nursing system will be produced
- The environmental conditions necessary for the production of the nursing system, as well as the equipment and supplies required
- The number and qualifications of nurses and other health care providers necessary to produce the nursing system and to evaluate its effects
- The organization and timing of tasks to be performed
- The designation of who (nurse or patient) is to perform the tasks

PRODUCTION OF REGULATORY CARE

Nursing systems are produced by means of the actions of nurses and patients during nurse-patient encounters; the nurse produces and manages the designated nursing system(s) and method(s) of helping for as long as the patient's self-care deficit or dependent-care deficit exists. The nurse:

- Performs and regulates the self-care or dependent-care tasks for patients or assists patients with their performance of self-care or dependent-care tasks.
- Coordinates self-care or dependent care task performance so that a unified system of care is produced and coordinated with other components of health care.
- Helps patients, their families, and others bring about systems of daily living for patients that support the accomplishment of self-care or dependent-care and are, at the same time, satisfying in relation to patients' interests, talents, and goals.
- Guides, directs, and supports patients in their exercise of, or in the withholding of the exercise of, their self-care agency or dependent-care agency.
- Stimulates patients' interests in self-care or dependent-care by raising questions and promoting discussions of care problems and issues when conditions permit
- Is available to patients at times when questions are likely to arise.

- Supports and guides patients in learning activities and provides cues for learning as well as instructional sessions.
- Supports and guides patients as they experience illness or disability and the effects of medical care measures and as they experience the need to engage in new measures of self-care or change their ways of meeting ongoing self-care requisites.

CONTROL OPERATIONS

The nurse performs control operations concurrently or separately from the production of regulatory care. The nurse makes observations and evaluates the nursing system to determine whether: (1) the nursing system that was designed is actually produced; (2) there is a fit between the current prescription for nursing and the nursing system that is being produced; (3) regulation of the patient's functioning is being achieved through performance of care measures to meet the patient's therapeutic self-care demand; (4) exercise of the patient's self-care agency or dependent-care agency is being properly regulated; (5) developmental change is in process and is adequate; and (6) the patient is adjusting to any decline in powers to engage in self-care or dependent care.

Martha Rogers' Science of Unitary Human Beings

Rogers' conceptual model of nursing, called the **Science of Unitary Human Beings,** focuses on unitary, irreducible human beings and their environments. The four basic concepts are:

- *Energy fields:* Irreducible, indivisible, pandimensional unitary human beings and environments that are identified by pattern and manifesting characteristics that are specific to the whole and that cannot be predicted from knowledge of the parts. Human and environmental energy fields are integral with each other.
- *Openness*: A characteristic of human and environmental energy fields; energy fields are continuously and completely open.

- *Pattern:* The distinguishing characteristic of an energy field. Pattern is perceived as a single wave that gives identity to the field. Each human field pattern is unique and is integral with its own unique environmental field pattern. Pattern is an abstraction that cannot be seen; what is seen or experienced are manifestations of field patterns.
- *Pandimensionality:* A nonlinear domain without spatial or temporal attributes.

The three principles of homeodynamics, which describe the nature of human and environmental energy fields, are as follows:

1. *Resonancy* asserts that human and environmental fields are identified by wave patterns that manifest continuous change from lower to higher frequencies.
2. *Helicy* asserts that human and environmental field patterns are continuous, innovative, and unpredictable, and are characterized by increasing diversity.
3. *Integrality* emphasizes the continuous mutual human field and environmental field process.

Implications for Nursing Practice

Nursing practice is directed toward promoting the health and well-being of all persons, wherever they are. Rogers' practice methodology is called the health patterning practice method (Box 4–8).

Pattern Manifestation Knowing— Assessment

The continuous process of apprehending and identifying manifestations of the human energy field and environmental energy field patterns that relate to current health events. The nurse uses one or more research instruments or clinical tools based on the Science of Unitary Human Beings to guide application and documentation of the practice methodology. The nurse acts with pandimensional authenticity—that is, with a demeanor of genuineness, trustworthiness, and knowledgeable caring. The nurse focuses on the client as a unified whole, a unitary human being.

Voluntary Mutual Patterning

The continuous process whereby the nurse, with the client, patterns the environmental energy field to promote harmony related to the health events. The nurse facilitates the client's actualization of potentials for health and well-being. The nurse has no investment in the client's changing in a particular way. The nurse does not attempt to change anyone to conform to arbitrary health ideals. Rather, the nurse enhances the client's efforts to actualize health potentials from the client's point of view.

Pattern Manifestation Knowing— Evaluation

The nurse evaluates voluntary mutual patterning by means of pattern manifestation knowing. Additional pattern information is monitored and collected as it unfolds during voluntary mutual patterning. The nurse considers the pattern information within the context of continually emerging health patterning goals affirmed by the client.

Callista Roy's Adaptation Model

Roy's conceptual model of nursing, the **Adaptation Model**, focuses on the responses of the human adaptive system, which can be an individual or a group, to a constantly changing environment. Adaptation is the central feature of the model. Problems in adaptation arise when the adaptive system is unable to cope with or respond to constantly changing stimuli from the internal and external environments in a manner that maintains the

---

BOX 4–8
ROGERS' HEALTH PATTERNING PRACTICE METHODOLOGY

- Pattern Manifestation Knowing— Assessment
- Voluntary Mutual Patterning
- Pattern Manifestation Knowing— Evaluation

integrity of the system. Environmental stimuli are categorized as:

- *Focal:* The stimuli most immediately confronting the person.
- *Contextual:* The contributing factors in the situation.
- *Residual:* Other unknown factors that may influence the situation. When the factors making up residual stimuli become known, they are considered focal or contextual stimuli.

Adaptation occurs through innate or acquired coping mechanisms used to respond to changing environmental stimuli:

- *Regulator coping subsystem (for individuals)* receives input from the external environment and from changes in the individual's internal state and processes the changes through neural-chemical-endocrine channels to produce responses.
- *Cognator coping subsystem (for individuals)* also receives input from external and internal stimuli that involve psychological, social, physical, and physiologic factors, including regulator subsystem outputs. These stimuli then are processed through cognitive/emotive pathways, including perceptual/information processing, learning, judgment, and emotion.
- *Stabilizer subsystem control process (for groups)* involves the established structures, values, and daily activities used by a group to accomplish its primary purpose and contribute to common purposes of society.
- *Innovator subsystem control process (for humans in groups)* involves the structures and processes necessary for change and growth in human social systems.

Responses take place in four modes for individuals and groups:

- *Physiologic/physical mode:*
  - *Physiologic mode (for individuals)* is concerned with basic needs requisite to maintaining the physical and physiologic integrity of the individual human system. It encompasses oxygenation; nutrition; elimination; activity and rest; protection; senses; fluid, electrolyte, and acid-base balance; neurologic function;

and endocrine function. The basic underlying need is physiologic integrity.
  - *Physical mode (for groups)* pertains to the manner in which the collective human adaptive system manifests adaptation relative to basic operating resources, that is, participants, physical facilities, and fiscal resources. The basic underlying need is resource adequacy, or wholeness achieved by adapting to change in physical resource needs.
- *Self-concept/group identity mode:*
  - *Self-concept mode (for individuals)* addresses the composite of beliefs and feelings that a person holds about himself or herself at a given time. The basic underlying need is psychic and spiritual integrity, the need to know who one is so that one can be or exist with a sense of unity, meaning, and purposefulness in the universe. The *physical self* refers to the individual's appraisal of his or her own physical being, including physical attributes, functioning, sexuality, health and illness states, and appearance. It includes the components of body sensation and body image. The *personal self* refers to the individual's appraisal of his or her own characteristics, expectations, values, and worth, including self-consistency, self-ideal, and the moral-ethical-spiritual self.
  - *Group identity mode (for groups)* addresses shared relations, goals, and values, which create a social milieu and culture, a group self-image, and coresponsibility for goal achievement. Identity integrity is the underlying need, which implies the honesty, soundness, and completeness of the group members' identification with the group and involves the process of sharing identity and goals. This mode encompasses interpersonal relationships, group self-image, social milieu, and group culture.
- *Role function mode (for individuals)* focuses on the roles that the individual occupies in society. The basic underlying need is social integrity, the need to know who one is in relation to others so that one can act. For the group, this mode focuses on the action components associated with group infrastructure that are designed to contribute to the accomplishment of the group's mission

or the tasks or functions associated with the group. The basic underlying need is role clarity, the need to understand and commit to fulfill expected tasks, so that the group can achieve common goals.

- *Interdependence mode (behavior pertaining to interdependent relationships of individuals and groups):* The basic underlying need is relational integrity, the feeling of security in nurturing relationships. For the individual, the mode focuses on interactions related to the giving and receiving of love, respect, and value, and encompasses affectional adequacy, developmental adequacy, resource adequacy, significant others, and support systems. For the group, it pertains to the social context in which the group operates, including both private and public contacts both within the group and with those outside the group, and encompasses affectional adequacy, developmental adequacy, resource adequacy, context, infrastructure, and resources.

The four modes are interrelated. Responses in any one mode may have an effect on or act as a stimulus in one or all of the other modes. Responses in each mode are judged as either adaptive or ineffective. A judgment of "adaptive modes" indicates promotion of the goals of the human adaptive system, including survival, growth, reproduction, and mastery. A judgment of "ineffective modes" does not contribute to the goals of the human adaptive system.

Implications for Nursing Practice

Nursing practice is directed toward promoting adaptation in each of the four response modes, thereby contributing to the person's health, quality of life, and dying with dignity. Roy's practice methodology is the Roy Adaptation Model Nursing Process, which encompasses six steps (Box 4–9).

Step 1: Assessment of Behavior

The nurse systematically gathers data about the behavior of the human adaptive system and judges the current state of adaptation in

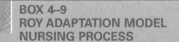

> **BOX 4–9**
> **ROY ADAPTATION MODEL NURSING PROCESS**
>
> - Assessment of Behavior
> - Assessment of Stimuli
> - Nursing Diagnosis
> - Goal Setting
> - Intervention
> - Evaluation

each adaptive mode. The nurse uses one or more of the Roy Adaptation Model–based research instruments or clinical tools to guide application and documentation of the practice methodology.

Step 2: Assessment of Stimuli

The nurse recognizes that stimuli must be amenable to independent nurse functions. Consequently, factors such as medical diagnoses and medical treatments are not considered stimuli, because those factors cannot be independently managed by nurses. The nurse identifies the internal and external focal and contextual stimuli that are influencing the behaviors of particular interest, in the order of priority established at the end of the Assessment of Behavior component of the Roy Adaptation Model Nursing Process.

Step 3: Nursing Diagnosis

The nurse uses a process of judgment to make a statement conveying the adaptation status of the human adaptive system of interest. The nursing diagnosis is a statement that identifies the behaviors of interest together with the most relevant influencing stimuli. The nurse uses one of the following three different approaches to state the nursing diagnosis:

- Behaviors are stated within each adaptive mode and with their most relevant influencing stimuli.
- A summary label for behaviors in each

ONLINE CONSULT

North American Nursing Diagnosis Association (NANDA) at
www.nanda.org

adaptive mode with relevant stimuli is used.
- A label that summarizes a behavioral pattern across adaptive modes that is affected by the same stimuli is used.

The nurse may link the Roy Adaptation Model–based nursing diagnosis with a relevant diagnosis from the taxonomy of the North American Nursing Diagnosis Association (NANDA).

Step 4: Goal Setting

The nurse articulates a clear statement of the behavioral outcomes in response to nursing provided to the human adaptive system. Goals are stated as specific short-term and long-term behavioral outcomes of nursing intervention. The goal statement designates the behavior of interest, the way in which the behavior will change, and the time frame for attainment of the goal. Goals may be stated for ineffective behaviors that are to be changed to adaptive behaviors and also for adaptive behaviors that should be maintained or enhanced.

Step 5: Intervention

The nurse selects and implements nursing approaches that have a high probability of changing stimuli or strengthening adaptive processes. Nursing intervention is the management of stimuli. The nurse may alter, increase, decrease, remove, or maintain stimuli.

Step 6: Evaluation

The nurse judges the effectiveness of nursing interventions in relation to the behaviors of the human adaptive system. The nurse systematically reassesses observable and nonob-

servable behaviors for each aspect of the four adaptive modes.

NURSING THEORIES DEFINED

The terms *theory, theoretical framework, theoretical model,* and *theoretical rationale* frequently are used interchangeably and have the same definition: one or more relatively concrete and specific concepts that are derived from a conceptual model, the statements that describe those concepts, and the statements that assert relatively concrete and specific relations between two or more concepts (Fawcett, 2000). Each theory presents a unique perspective about a particular phenomenon, such as a nursing participant, the environment, health, or a step of the nursing process or practice methodology.

Functions of Nursing Theories

The function of a nursing theory is to provide considerable specificity in the description, explanation, or prediction of some phenomenon. Theories are more concrete and specific than conceptual models. A *conceptual model* is an abstract and general system of concepts and statements, whereas a *theory* deals with one or more relatively concrete and specific concepts and statements. In addition, conceptual models are general guides that must be specified further by relevant and logically congruent theories before action can occur.

Grand Theories

Theories vary in scope—that is, they vary in the relative level of concreteness and specificity of their concepts and statements. Theories that are broadest in scope are called **grand theories**. These theories are made up of rather abstract and general concepts and statements that cannot be generated or tested empirically. Indeed, grand theories are developed through thoughtful and insightful appraisal of existing ideas or creative intellectual leaps beyond existing knowledge. Examples of grand theories of nursing are Leininger's (1991) Theory of Culture Care Diversity and Universality, Newman's (1994) Theory of Health as Expanding Consciousness, and Parse's (1998) Theory of Human Becoming.

The less abstract nature of grand theories compared with conceptual models is illustrated by Parse's (1998) theory, which was derived in part from Rogers's (1970, 1990) conceptual model. Rogers's conceptual model is a frame of reference for all of nursing, whereas Parse's theory limits the domain of interest to the unitary human's experience of becoming.

Madeleine Leininger's Theory of Culture Care Diversity and Universality

Leininger's grand nursing theory focuses on the discovery of human care diversities and universalities and ways to provide culturally congruent care to people. The 11 concepts of the **Theory of Culture Care Diversity and Universality** are described as follows:

- *Care:* Abstract and concrete phenomena related to assisting, supporting, or enabling experiences or behaviors toward or for others with evident or anticipated needs to ameliorate or improve a human condition or lifeway
- *Caring:* The actions and activities directed toward assisting, supporting, or enabling another individual or group with evident or anticipated needs to ameliorate or improve a human condition or lifeway or to face death
- *Culture:* The learned, shared, and transmitted values, beliefs, norms, and lifeways of a particular group that guides thinking, decisions, and actions in patterned ways; encompasses several cultural and social structure dimensions: technologic factors, religious and philosophical factors, kinship

and social factors, political and legal factors, economic factors, educational and cultural values, and lifeways
- *Language:* Word usages, symbols, and meanings about care
- *Ethnohistory:* Past facts, events, instances, experiences of individuals, groups, cultures, and institutions that are primarily people-centered (ethno) and that describe, explain, and interpret human lifeways within particular cultural contexts and over short or long periods of time
- *Environmental context:* The totality of an event, situation, or particular experiences that gives meaning to human expressions, interpretations, and social interactions in particular physical, ecological, sociopolitical, and/or cultural settings
- *Health:* A state of well-being that is culturally defined, valued, and practiced and that reflects the ability of individuals (or groups) to perform their daily role activities in culturally expressed, beneficial, and patterned lifeways
- *Worldview:* The way people tend to look out on the world or their universe to form a picture of or a value stance about their life or the world around them
- *Cultural care:* The subjectively and objectively transmitted values, beliefs, and patterned lifeways that assist, support, or enable another individual or group to maintain their well-being and health, to improve their human condition and lifeway, and to deal with illness, handicaps, or death; the two dimensions of cultural care are:
  - *Cultural care diversity:* The variabilities and/or differences in meanings, patterns, values, lifeways, or symbols of care within or between collectivities that are related to assistive, supportive, or enabling human care expressions
  - *Cultural care universality:* The common, similar, or dominant uniform care meanings, patterns, values, lifeways, or symbols that are manifest among many cultures and reflect assistive, supportive, facilitative, or enabling ways to help people
- *Care systems:* The values, norms, and structural features of an organization designed for serving people's health needs, concerns,

or conditions; the two types of care systems are:
- *Generic lay care systems:* Traditional or local indigenous health care or cure practices that have special meanings and uses to heal or assist people, which are generally offered in familiar home or community environmental contexts with their local practitioners
- *Professional health care system:* Professional care or cure services offered by diverse health personnel who have been prepared through formal professional programs of study in special educational institutions
- *Cultural-congruent nursing care:* Cognitively based assistive, supportive, facilitative, or enabling acts or decisions that are tailor-made to fit with individual, group, or institutional cultural values, beliefs, and lifeways in order to provide or support meaningful, beneficial, and satisfying health-care or well-being services; the three modes of cultural-congruent nursing care are:
  - *Cultural care preservation or maintenance:* Assistive, supportive, facilitative, or enabling professional actions and decisions that help people of a particular culture retain and/or preserve relevant care values so that they can maintain their well-being, recover from illness, or face handicaps and/or death
  - *Cultural care accommodation or negotiation:* Assistive, supportive, facilitative, or enabling creative professional actions and decisions that help people of a designated culture adapt to, or negotiate with, others for a beneficial or satisfying health outcome with professional care providers
  - *Cultural care repatterning or restructuring:* Assistive, supportive, facilitative, or enabling professional actions and decisions that help clients reorder, change, or greatly modify their lifeways for a new, different, and beneficial health care pattern while respecting the clients' cultural values and beliefs and still providing a beneficial or healthier lifeway than before the changes were coestablished with the clients

> **BOX 4–10**
> **THEORY OF CULTURE CARE DIVERSITY AND UNIVERSALITY: PRACTICE METHODOLOGY**
>
> - Goals of nursing practice are (1) to improve and to provide culturally congruent care to people that is beneficial, appropriate, and useful to the client, family, or culture group healthy lifeways; and (2) to provide culturally congruent nursing care in order to improve or offer a different kind of nursing care service to people of diverse or similar cultures.
> - Clients include individuals, families, subcultures, groups, communities, and institutions.

Implications for Nursing Practice

Nursing practice is directed toward improving and providing culturally congruent care to people. A practice methodology for the Theory of Culture Care Diversity and Universality is shown in Box 4–10.

Margaret Newman's Theory of Health as Expanding Consciousness

Newman's grand nursing theory, of **Health as Expanding Consciousness**, focuses on health as the expansion of consciousness, with emphasis on the idea that every person in every situation, no matter how disordered and hopeless the situation may seem, is part of the universal process of expanding consciousness. The concepts of the theory are consciousness and pattern.

Consciousness is the informational capacity of human beings, that is, the ability of humans to interact with their environments. Consciousness encompasses interconnected cognitive and affective awareness; physiochemical maintenance, including the nervous and endocrine systems; growth processes; the immune system; and the genetic code. Consciousness can be seen in the quantity and quality of the interaction between human beings and their environments. The process of life moves toward higher levels of consciousness. Sometimes this process is smooth, pleasant, harmonious; other times it is difficult and disharmonious, as in disease.

Pattern is information that depicts the whole, relatedness. People are identified by their pattern. The evolution of expanding consciousness is seen in the pattern of movement-space-time. Pattern is manifested as exchanging, communicating, relating, valuing, choosing, moving, perceiving, feeling, and knowing. Pattern encompasses three dimensions—movement-space-time, rhythm, and diversity:

- *Movement:* An essential property of matter; a means of communicating; the means whereby one perceives reality and becomes aware of self; the natural condition of life
- *Space*: Encompasses personal space, inner space, and life space as dimensions of space relevant to the individual, and territoriality, shared space, and distancing as dimensions relevant to the family
- *Time:* The amount of time perceived to be passing (subjective time); clock time (objective time)
- *Rhythm:* Basic to movement; the rhythm of movement is an integrating experience
- *Diversity:* Seen in the parts

Nursing practice is directed toward facilitating pattern recognition by connecting with the client in an authentic way and assisting him or her to discover new rules for a higher level of organization or consciousness. Newman's Research as Praxis Protocol is a research/practice methodology (Box 4–11). The phenomenon of interest is the process of expanding consciousness. The sequential patterns represent relationships. Any similarities of pattern among a group of study participants/clients having a similar experience may be designated by themes and stated in propositional form.

Rosemarie Parse's Theory of Human Becoming

Parse's grand nursing theory of **Human Becoming** focuses on human experiences of participation with the universe in the cocre-

> **BOX 4–11**
> **APPLICATION OF THE THEORY OF HEALTH AS EXPANDING CONSCIOUSNESS**
>
> The nurse:
> - Undertakes more intense analysis of the data in light of the Theory of Health as Expanding Consciousness after the interviews are completed.
> - Evaluates the nature of the sequential patterns of interaction in terms of quality and complexity and interprets the patterns according to the study participant/client's position on Young's spectrum of consciousness.

ation of health. The concepts of the theory are:

- *Human becoming:* A unitary construct referring to the human being's living health
- *Meaning:* The linguistic and imagined content of something and the interpretation that one gives to something
- *Rhythmicity:* The cadent, paradoxical patterning of the human-universe mutual process
- *Transcendence:* Reaching beyond with possibles—the hopes and dreams envisioned in multidimensional experiences and powering the originating of Transforming
- *Imaging:* Reflective-prereflective coming to know the explicit-tacit all-at-once
- *Valuing:* Confirming–not confirming cherished beliefs in light of a personal worldview
- *Languaging:* Signifying valued images through speaking–being silent and moving–being still
- *Revealing-concealing:* Disclosing–not disclosing all-at-once
- *Enabling-limiting:* Living the opportunities-restrictions present in all choosings all-at-once
- *Connecting-separating:* Being with and apart from others, ideas, objects, and situations all-at-once
- *Powering:* The pushing-resisting process of affirming–not affirming being in light of nonbeing

- *Originating:* Inventing new ways of conforming-nonconforming in the certainty-uncertainty of living
- *Transforming:* Shifting the view of the familiar-unfamiliar, the changing of change in coconstituting anew in a deliberate way

The three major principles of the theory of human becoming are:

1. *Structuring meaning multidimensionally* is cocreating reality through the languaging of valuing and imaging; means that humans construct what is real for them from choices made at many realms of the universe
2. *Cocreating rhythmical patterns of relating* is living the paradoxical unity of revealing-concealing and enabling-limiting while connecting-separating; means that humans live in rhythm with the universe coconstituting patterns of relating
3. *Cotranscending with the possibles* is powering unique ways of originating in the process of transforming; means that humans forge unique paths with shifting perspectives as a different light is cast on the familiar

Implications for Nursing Practice

Nursing practice is directed toward respecting the quality of life as perceived by the person and the family. The practice methodology is illustrated in Table 4–1 and Box 4–12.

Middle-Range Theories

Middle-range theories are narrower in scope than grand theories, encompassing a smaller number of concepts and a limited aspect of the real world. Middle-range theories are, therefore, made up of concepts that are empirically measurable and statements that are empirically testable. Examples of middle-range nursing theories are Orlando's (1961) Theory of the Deliberative Nursing Process, Peplau's (1952, 1992) Theory of Interpersonal Relations, and Watson's (1985, 1997) Theory of Human Caring.

The specificity of middle-range theory concepts and statements is illustrated by Orlando's (1961) theory. This theory predicts that using a particular communication technique is effective in identifying the patient's immediate need for help. The technique requires the nurse, using a personal pronoun, to share with the patient his or her perceptions, thoughts, or feelings about the patient's behavior and to ask the patient whether those perceptions, thoughts, or feelings are correct. An example is, "I think you do not want to do any exercises today? Am I correct?"

Ida Jean Orlando's Theory of the Deliberative Nursing Process

Orlando's middle-range predictive nursing theory, of the **Deliberative Nursing Process,** focuses on an interpersonal process between people. It helps identify the nature of the patient's distress and his or her immediate needs for help. The concepts of the theory are:

Patient's Behavior

The patient's behavior is behavior observed by the nurse in an immediate nursing-patient situation. The two dimensions are:

- *Need for help:* A requirement of the patient that, if supplied, relieves or diminishes immediate distress or improves immediate sense of adequacy or well-being
- *Improvement:* An increase in patients' mental and physical health, their well-being, and their sense of adequacy

The need for help and improvement can be expressed in both nonverbal and verbal forms. Visual manifestations of nonverbal behavior include such motor activities as eating, walking, twitching, and trembling as well as such physiologic forms as urinating, defecating, temperature and blood pressure readings, respiratory rate, and skin color. Vocal forms of nonverbal behavior—nonverbal behavior that is heard—include crying, moaning, laughing, coughing, sneezing, sighing, yelling, screaming, groaning, and singing. *Verbal behavior* refers to what a patient says,

TABLE 4–1
PRACTICE METHODOLOGY OF PARSE'S THEORY OF HUMAN BECOMING (SEE ALSO BOX 4–12)

Principle	Dimension	Process (Empirical Activities)
Practice Methodology		
1: Structuring meaning mutidimensionally	*Illuminating meaning:* Explicating what was, is, and will be	*Explicating:* Making clear what is appearing now through languaging
2: Cocreating rhythmical patterns	*Synchronizing rhythms:* Dwelling with the pitch, yaw, and roll of the human-universe process	*Dwelling with:* Immersing with the flow of connecting-separating
3: Mobilizing transcendence	*Mobilizing transcendence:* Moving beyond the meaning moment with what is not yet	*Moving beyond:* Propelling with envisioned possibles of transforming

BOX 4–12
PRACTICE METHODOLOGY OF PARSE'S THEORY OF HUMAN BECOMING (SEE ALSO TABLE 4–1)

Contexts for nursing:
• Nurse-person situations and nurse-group situations
• Participants include children and adults
• Locations include homes, shelters, health care centers, parish halls, all departments of hospitals and clinics, rehabilitation centers, offices, and other milieus where nurses are with people

   Goal of the discipline of nursing is quality of life from the person's, family's, and community's perspective.
   Goal of the human becoming nurse is to be truly present with people as they enhance their quality of lives.
   True presence is a special way of "being with" in which the nurse is attentive to moment-to-moment changes in meaning as she or he bears witness to the person's or group's own living of value priorities.
   Coming-to-be-present is an all-at-once gentling down and lifting up. True presence begins in the coming-to-be-present moments of preparation and attention.

including complaints, requests, questions, refusals, demands, and comments or statements.

Nurse's Reaction

The nurse's reaction is the nonobservable response to the patient's behavior. The three dimensions are:

• *Perception:* Physical stimulation of any one of the five senses by the patient's behavior
• *Thought:* An idea that occurs in the nurse's mind
• *Feeling:* A state of mind inclining the person toward or against a perception, thought, or action; it occurs in response to the nurse's perceptions and thoughts

Nurse's Activity

Nurse's activity is the observable actions taken by the nurse, including instructions, suggestions, directions, explanations, information, requests, and questions directed toward the patient; making decisions for the patient; handling the patient's body; administering medications or treatments; and changing the patient's immediate environment. The two dimensions of nurse's activity are:

- *Automatic nursing process:* Actions decided on by the nurse for reasons other than the patient's immediate need
- *Deliberative nursing process (process discipline):* A specific set of nurse behaviors or actions directed toward the patient's behavior that ascertain or meet the patient's immediate needs for help

Implications for Nursing Practice

Nursing practice is directed toward identifying and meeting the patient's immediate needs for help through use of Orlando's practice methodology (Box 4–13).

Hildegard Peplau's Theory of Interpersonal Relations

Peplau's middle-range descriptive nursing theory focuses on the phases of the interpersonal process that occur when an ill person and a nurse come together to resolve a health difficulty. The one concept of the **Theory of Interpersonal Relations** is the nurse-patient relationship, which is an interpersonal process made up of four components—two persons, the professional expertise of the

BOX 4–13
ORLANDO'S PRACTICE METHODOLOGY

Observations:
Encompass any and all information pertaining to a patient that the nurse acquires while on duty; form the raw material with which the nurse makes and implements plans for the patient's care

- *Direct Observations:* Nurse's Reaction to Patient's Behavior: Consists of any perception, thought, or feeling the nurse has from her own experience of the patient's behavior at any or several moments in time
- *Indirect Observations:* Other Information About the Patient's Behavior: Consists of any information that is derived from a source other than the patient; this information pertains to, but is not directly derived from, the patient

Actions:
Carried out with or for the patient

- *Nurse's Activity:* Deliberative Nursing Process: The process used to share and validate the nurse's direct and indirect observations. Clinical protocols contain the specific requirements for the deliberative nursing process.
- *Direct Help:* The nurse meets the patient's need directly when the patient is unable to meet his or her own need and when the activity is confined to the nurse-patient contact.
- *Indirect Help:* The nurse meets the patient's need indirectly when the activity extends to arranging the services of a person, agency, or resource that the patient cannot contact by himself or herself.
- *Reporting:* The nurse receives reports about the patient's behavior from other nurses and from other health professionals and reports observations.
- *Recording:* The nurse records the nursing process, including (1) the nurse's perception of or about the patient; (2) the nurse's thought and/or feeling about the perception; and (3) what the nurse said and/or did to, with, or for the patient.

nurse, and the client's problem, or need for which expert nursing services are sought—and which has three discernible phases:

- *Orientation phase:* The phase in which the nurse first identifies herself or himself by name and professional status and states the purpose, nature, and time available for the patient. This is the phase during which the nurse conveys professional interest and receptivity to the patient, begins to know the patient as a person, obtains essential information about the patient's health condition, and sets the tone for further interactions.
- *Working phase:* The phase in which the major work occurs. The two subphases are:
  - *Identification:* The subphase during which the patient learns how to make use of the nurse-patient relationship
  - *Exploitation:* The subphase during which the patient makes full use of available professional services (Peplau, 1952)
- *Termination phase:* The phase in which the work accomplished is summarized and closure occurs.

Implications for Nursing Practice

Nursing practice is directed toward promoting favorable changes in patients, which is accomplished through the nurse-patient relationship. Within that relationship, the nurse's major function is to study the interpersonal relations between the patient/client and others. Peplau's clinical methodology, which can be used for both nursing practice and research, is described in Box 4–14.

Jean Watson's Theory of Human Caring

Watson's middle-range explanatory nursing theory focuses on the human component of caring and the moment-to-moment encounters between the one who is caring and the one who is being cared for, especially the caring activities performed by nurses as they interact with others. The concepts of the **Theory of Human Caring** are:

- *Transpersonal caring relationahip:* Human-to-human connectedness, whereby each person is touched by the human center of the other. This is a special kind of relationship involving a high regard for the whole person and his or her being-in-the-world. The concept of transpersonal caring relationship encompasses three dimensions:
  - *Self:* Transpersonal-mind-body-spirit oneness, an embodied self, and an embodied spirit.
  - *Phenomenal field:* The totality of human experience, one's being-in-the-world.
  - *Intersubjectivity:* "Transpersonal" refers to an intersubjective human-to-human relationship in which the person of the nurse affects and is affected by the person of the other, both of whom are fully present in the moment and feel a union with the other.
- *Caring occasion/caring moment:* The coming together of nurse and other(s), which involves action and choice both by the nurse and the other. The moment of coming together in a caring occasion presents them with the opportunity to decide how to be in the relationship—what to do with the moment.
- *Caring (healing) consciousness:* A holographic dynamic that is manifest within a field of consciousness and that exists through time and space and is dominant over physical illness.
- *Carative factors:* Those aspects of nursing that actually potentiate therapeutic healing processes for both the one caring and the one being cared for. The ten carative factors are:
  - Forming a humanistic-altruistic system of values
  - Enabling and sustaining faith-hope
  - Being sensitive to self and others
  - Developing a helping-trusting, caring relationship
  - Promoting and accepting the expression of positive and negative feelings and emotions
  - Engaging in creative, individualized, problem-solving caring processes
  - Promoting transpersonal teaching-learning

BOX 4–14
PEPLAU'S CLINICAL METHODOLOGY

- *Observation:* Identification, clarification, and verification of impressions about the interactive drama, of the pushes and pulls in the relationship between nurse and patient, as they occur.
- *Nurse's Behavior:* Observation of the nurse's words, voice tones, body language, and other gestural messages.
- *Patient's Behavior:* Observation of the patient's words, voice tones, body language, and other gestural messages.
- *Interpersonal Phenomena:* Observation of what goes on between the patient and the nurse.
- *Reframing Empathic Linkages:* Occurs when the nurse's and/or the patient's ability to feel in self the emotions experienced by the other person in the same situation is converted to verbal communications by the nurse asking, "What are you feeling right now?"
- *Communication:* Aims are the selection of symbols or concepts that convey both the reference, or meaning in the mind of the individual, and referent, the object or actions symbolized in the concept; and the wish to struggle toward the development of common understanding for words between two or more people.
- *Interpersonal Techniques:* Verbal interventions used by nurses during nurse-patient relationships aimed at accomplishing problem resolution and competence development in patients.
- *Principle of Clarity:* Comments and questions to force the patient to think, to respond, and to use those capacities that will produce the necessary data.
- *Principle of Continuity:* Occurs when language is used as a tool for the promotion of coherence or connections of ideas expressed and leads to discrimination of relationships or connections among ideas and the feelings, events, or themes conveyed in those ideas. Continuity is promoted when the nurse is able to pick up threads of conversation that the patient offers in the course of a conversation and over a longer period, such as a week, and when she aids the patient to focus and to expand these threads.
- *Recording:* The written record of the communication between nurse and patient, that is, the data collected through participant observation and reframing of empathic linkages. The aim is to capture the exact wording of the interaction between the nurse and the patient.
- *Data Analysis:* Focuses on testing the nurse's hypotheses, which are formulated from first impressions or hunches about the patient.
- *Phases of the Nurse-Patient Relationship:* Identify the phase of nurse-patient relationship in which communication occurred: orientation phase; working phase, identification subphase, exploitation subphase; termination phase
- *Roles:* Identify the roles taken by the nurse and the patient in each phase of the nurse-patient relationship.
- *Relations:* Identify the connections, linkages, ties, and bonds that go on or went on between a patient and others, including family, friends, staff, and the nurse.
- *Pattern Integrations:* Identify the patterns of the interpersonal relation between two or more people that together link or bind them and that enable the people to transform energy into patterns of action that bring satisfaction or security in the face of a recurring problem.

- Attending to supportive, protective, and/or corrective mental, physical, societal, and spiritual environments
- Assisting with gratification of basic human needs while preserving human dignity and wholeness
- Allowing for, and being open to, existential-phenomenologic-spiritual dimensions of caring and healing that cannot be fully explained scientifically through modern Western medicine

Implications for Nursing Practice

Nursing practice is directed toward helping persons gain a higher degree of harmony within the mind, body, and soul, which generates self-knowledge, self-reverence, self-healing, and self-care processes while increasing diversity, which is pursued through use of the 10 carative factors. Watson's practice methodology is described in Box 4–15.

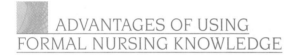

ADVANTAGES OF USING FORMAL NURSING KNOWLEDGE

Recognition of nursing as a profession confers a certain status on nurses. The status conferred by being a member of a profession, rather than having an occupation or a trade, carries with it the responsibility to use formal nursing knowledge. Anderson (1995) explained that, as members of a profession, nurses "must ensure that we have a solid scholarly and scientific foundation upon which to base our practice" (p. 247). Conceptual models of nursing and nursing theories are that foundation; they provide explicit frames of reference for professional nursing practice by delineating the scope of nursing practice. Furthermore, conceptual models of nursing and nursing theories (1) specify innovative goals for nursing practice, (2) introduce ideas that are designed to improve practice (Lindsay, 1990), and (3) enhance the quality of people's lives by facilitating the identification of relevant information, reducing the fragmentation of health care, and improving the coordination of all aspects of health care (Chalmers, as cited in Chalmers, Kershaw, Melia, & Kendrich, 1990).

> *The use of conceptual models of nursing and nursing theories moves the practice of nursing away from that driven by a medical or institutional model and, therefore, fosters autonomy from medicine and a coherent purpose of practice (Bélanger, 1991; Bridges, 1991; Ingram, 1991; Parse, 1995).*

BOX 4–15
WATSON'S PRACTICE METHODOLOGY

Requirements for a Transpersonal Caring Relationship:
The nurse considers the person to be valid and whole, regardless of illness or disease. The nurse makes a moral commitment and directs intentionality and consciousness to the protection, enhancement, and potentiation of human dignity, wholeness, and healing, such that a person creates or cocreates his or her own meaning for existence, healing, wholeness, and caring.

Authentic Presencing:
The nurse:
- Is authentically present as self and other in a reflective mutuality of being and becoming.
- Centers consciousness and intentionality on caring, healing, and wholeness, rather than on disease, problems, illness, complications, and technocures.
- Attempts to (1) stay within the other's frame of reference; (2) join in a mutual search for meaning and wholeness of being; and (3) potentiate comfort measures, pain control, a sense of well-being, or spiritual transcendence of suffering.

More specifically, the use of formal nursing knowledge to guide nursing practice "represents nursing's unique contribution to the health care system" (Parse, 1995, p. 128). It is the hallmark of professional nursing practice. As Chalmers pointed out, "Nursing models [and theories] have provided what many would argue is a much needed alternative knowledge base from which nurses can practice in an informed way. An alternative, that is, to the medical model which for so many years has dominated many aspects of health care" (Chalmers et al., 1990, p. 34).

Formal nursing knowledge also provides an alternative to the institutional model of practice, in which "the most salient values [are] efficiency, standardized care, rules, and regulations" (Rogers, 1989, p. 113). The institutional model, moreover, typically upholds, reinforces, and supports the medical model (Grossman & Hooton, 1993). Thus, the use of conceptual models of nursing and nursing theories moves the practice of nursing away from that driven by a medical or institutional model and, therefore, fosters autonomy from medicine and a coherent purpose of practice (Bélanger, 1991; Bridges, 1991; Ingram, 1991; Parse, 1995).

The major practical advantage of using a conceptual model of nursing is the identification of a comprehensive nursing process format or practice methodology that encompasses particular parameters for assessment, labels for problems, a strategy for planning nursing interventions, a typology of nursing interventions, and criteria for evaluation of the outcomes of nursing practice. More specifically, whereas the generic nursing process tells the nurse only to assess, label, plan, intervene, and evaluate, the nursing process associated with a particular conceptual model tells the nurse what to assess, what labels are possible, how to plan, what interventions are appropriate, and what outcomes to evaluate.

The major practical advantage a nursing theory provides is greater specificity in one or more phases of the nursing process. For example, Orlando's (1961) Theory of the Deliberative Nursing Process tells the nurse exactly how to identify the patient's immediate need for help. Orlando's theory can be used very effectively in combination with Roy's Adaptation Model (Roy & Andrews, 1999).

It should be obvious by now that formal nursing knowledge identifies the distinctive nursing territory within the vast arena of multidisciplinary health care (Feeg, 1989). Each conceptual model of nursing and nursing theory provides a holistic orientation for nursing practice and reinforces the view that nursing practice ultimately is "for our patients' sake" (Dabbs, 1994, p. 220). In addition, the use of formal nursing knowledge "help[s] nurses better communicate what they do" (Neff, 1991, p. 534) and why they do it. The importance of communicating what nursing is and what nurses do was underscored by Feeg (1989), who identified the following three reasons for implementing conceptual model-based or theory-based nursing practice:

1. In this time of information saturation and rapid change, we know it is not valuable to focus on every detail and, therefore, we need [conceptual models and theories] to help guide our judgments in new situations.
2. In this time of technologic overdrive, we need a holistic orientation to remind us of our caring perspective.
3. In this time of professional territoriality, it has become even more important to understand our identity in nursing and operationalize our practice from a [formal nursing] knowledge base. (p. 450)

The number of nurses throughout the world who recognize the advantages of using formal nursing knowledge is rapidly increasing. Indeed, although some clinicians hold the "unfortunate view [that nursing models and theories] are the inventions and predictions only of scholars and academics [that have] little significance for their own practice environments," many other clinicians recognize the beneficial effects of formal nursing knowledge on practice (Hayne, 1992, p. 105). Moreover, Cash's (1990) claim that "there is no central core that can distinguish nursing theoretically from a number of other occupational activities" (p. 255) is readily offset by many claims to the contrary. In particular, Cash's claim clearly fails to take into account the contributions made by formal nursing knowledge to the development of practices that enable all nurses to talk nursing (Chalmers et al., 1990), to think nursing (Nightingale, 1993; Perry, 1985), and to engage in thinking nursing (Allison & Renpenning, 1999), rather than just doing tasks and carrying out physicians' orders (Le Storti et al., 1999).

Nurses are able to think nursing and talk nursing because the conceptual models and theories that constitute formal nursing knowledge provide a distinctive nursing language. The lack of a nursing language in the past, and in the present when conceptual models of nursing and nursing theories are not used, "has been a handicap in nurses' communications about nursing to the public as well as to persons with whom they work in the health field" (Orem, 1997, p. 29). Thus, the content of each conceptual model of nursing and nursing theory, which is stated in a distinctive vocabulary, should not be considered jargon. Rather, the terminology used by the author of each conceptual model or theory should be recognized as the result of considerable thought about how to convey the meaning of that particular perspective to others (Biley, 1990). "The attention to language," Watson (1997) maintained, "is especially critical to an evolving [profession], in that during this postmodern era, one's survival depends on having language; writers in this area remind us 'if you do not have your own language you don't exist'" (p. 50). Elaborating, Akinsanya (1989) explained, "Every science has its own peculiar terms, concepts and principles which are essential for the development of its knowledge base. In nursing, as in other sciences, an understanding of these is a prerequisite to a critical examination of their contribution to the development of knowledge and its application to practice" (p. ii). Indeed, the differences in the vocabularies of the various conceptual models and theories are the same as the differences in the vocabularies of diverse medical specialties, such as obstetrics, gynecology, cardiology, neurology, psychiatry, and geriatrics.

Thinking nursing within the context of formal nursing knowledge helps nurses to "clarify their thinking on their role, especially at a time when the roles of many health professionals are becoming blurred" (Nightingale, 1993, p. 2). Moreover, thinking nursing within the context of formal nursing knowledge may shape the way in which specialized nursing practice is viewed. Indeed, nurses may elect to specialize in the use of a particular conceptual model of nursing or nursing theory, or they may elect to specialize in a particular concept of a particular conceptual model of nursing or nursing theory. A nurse could, for example, specialize in one behavioral subsystem of Johnson's Behavioral System Model (Rogers, 1973).

Risks and Rewards of Using Formal Nursing Knowledge

Johnson (1990) noted that although individual clinicians and nursing departments take risks when the decision is made to implement conceptual model- or theory-based nursing practice, the rewards far outweigh the risks. She stated:

> To openly use a nursing model [or theory] is risk-taking behavior for the individual nurse. For a nursing department to adopt one of these models [or theories] for unit or institution use is risk-taking behavior of an even higher order. The reward for such risk-taking for the individual practitioner lies in the great satisfaction gained from being able to specify explicit concrete nursing goals in the care of patients and from documenting the actual achievement of the desired outcomes. The reward for the nursing department is having a rational, cohesive, and comprehensive basis for the development of standards of nursing practice, for the evaluation of practitioners, and for the documentation of the contribution of nursing to patient welfare. (Johnson, 1990, p. 32)

Accumulating anecdotal and empirical evidence indicates that additional rewards of using formal nursing knowledge to guide nursing practice include reduced staff nurse turnover, more rapid movement from novice to expert nurse, greater patient and family satisfaction with nursing, increased nurse job satisfaction, and considerable cost savings (Fawcett, 2000). Furthermore, as the use of formal nursing knowledge grows, both nurses and participants in nursing are empowered. Indeed, "[nursing] knowledge is power" (Orr, 1991, p. 218), and it can be used to empower individuals, families, and communities to fully participate in decisions about their health care (Lister, 1991; Malin & Teasdale, 1991). The challenge, then, is to help each nurse select an explicit nursing model or theory to guide his or her nursing practice.

SELECTING A CONCEPTUAL MODEL OR NURSING THEORY FOR PROFESSIONAL NURSING PRACTICE

Although formal nursing knowledge is made up of many conceptual models and theories, using more than one model or theory at the same time will create much confusion. Therefore, each nurse should select just one as a guide for professional practice. The following six steps can help you select an appropriate conceptual model of nursing or nursing theory:

1. Identify your own beliefs and values related to the phenomena of interest to all nurses. State your beliefs about the participants in nursing, the relevant environment, health, and the goals of professional nursing practice.
2. Identify the patient population with which you would like to work. The population may be based on a specific medical diagnosis, such as cancer or renal failure; an age group, such as children and adolescents or the elderly; a type of illness, such as an acute crisis or chronic illness; or a particular symptom, such as chest pain or an elevated temperature.
3. Systematically analyze and evaluate the content of several conceptual models of nursing and nursing theories. Review the summaries of the conceptual models and theories presented in the chapter as well as the primary source material for each conceptual model and theory. This review will

provide a firm foundation for your selection of the conceptual model or theory.
4. Compare your own beliefs and values with the philosophical claims undergirding the selected conceptual model.
5. Identify the conceptual models and nursing theories that are appropriate guides for nursing with the patient population in which you are interested.
6. Choose the conceptual model or theory that most closely matches your beliefs and values and the patient population with which you want to work. Then use the model or theory to guide your practice with several nursing participants so that you can determine its utility. If you find that the conceptual model or theory you have chosen is not useful, select another model or theory and test its utility.

USING CONCEPTUAL MODELS TO GUIDE PROFESSIONAL NURSING PRACTICE

The use of an explicit conceptual model of nursing to guide professional nursing practice is exemplified in the following two case studies

Research findings indicate that nurses feel vulnerable and experience a great deal of stress when they attempt to achieve professional aspirations within a rapidly changing, medically dominated, bureaucratic health care delivery system (Graham, 1994). As structures for critical thinking within a distinctively nursing context, formal nursing knowledge provides the intellectual skills and points to the practical skills that nurses need to survive at a time when cost containment through reduction of professional nursing staff is the modus operandi of managed care and the administrators of health care delivery systems, including hospitals, home-health care agencies, and health maintenance organizations.

As a novice user of a conceptual model of nursing or nursing theory, you should not

Case Study

OREM'S SELF-CARE FRAMEWORK

Gerry Smith is a 64-year-old, well-nourished man with long-standing non–insulin-dependent diabetes mellitus (NIDDM). He underwent emergency open-heart bypass graft surgery 7 weeks ago and remains hospitalized with a serious leg wound. Mr. Smith had an uneventful cardiac recovery after his surgery, but the graft site on his left leg became infected and failed to heal properly. Two weeks after the open-heart surgery, Mr. Smith underwent emergency arterial bypass surgery to improve circulation to his left lower limb.

He currently is a patient on the rehabilitation unit for management of the leg wound. Sterile dressing changes are required three times daily. Mr. Smith transfers with moderate assistance, and ambulates using a walker and minimal to moderate assistance, depending on his pain and fatigue level. He requires moderate assistance for dressing, toileting-hygiene, and bathing, and minimal assistance for meal set-up. Mr. Smith has urinary and bowel control with occasional urgency of bowel secondary to diarrhea caused by multiple antibiotics. Mr. Smith has the support of his wife of 42 years and four grown sons.

Mrs. Smith is currently learning the skin care dressing techniques. She will be the primary caregiver when Mr. Smith is discharged in approximately 2 weeks. Mr. Smith has been experiencing periods of moodiness and depression since his operations. He admits that the long hospitalization has left him feeling overwhelmed at times, but he is hopeful for the future. He expresses gratitude that his leg was saved. More than anything else, Mr. Smith wants to regain enough ability to enjoy a hunting trip.

Initial assessment of Mr. Smith's self-care agency—that is, his ability to perform self-care—reveals that he currently is unable to meet what Orem calls his therapeutic self-care demand. Therapeutic self-care demand is defined as "the known self-care requisites [that are] particular for individuals in relation to their conditions and circumstances." (Orem, 1995, pp. 65, 123). Three types of self-care requisites make up the therapeutic self-care demand: universal, developmental, and health deviation. Comparing the therapeutic self-care demand with Mr. Smith's current self-care agency reveals several self-care deficits.

Mr. and Mrs. Smith, along with his nurse, agree that the goal is to enhance Mr. Smith's self-care agency and Mrs. Smith's dependent care agency through the use of all three types of nursing systems. The wholly compensatory nursing system is needed to provide both blood glucose monitoring and sterile dressing changes three times daily. The partly compensatory nursing system is needed to assist Mr. Smith with dressing, toilet transfers, bathing, and ambulation. The supportive-educative nursing system is needed to teach Mr. and Mrs. Smith about his personal care and to provide psychological support to facilitate coping with a chronic illness. Consequently, the nursing staff will initially provide wound care to Mr. Smith's leg, but will teach Mrs. Smith how to perform sterile dressing care when Mr. Smith goes home. In summary, the nursing staff will give Mr. and Mrs. Smith the necessary guidance and teaching to allow them to meet his therapeutic self-care demand once he is discharged from the hospital.

become discouraged if your initial experiences with the model or theory seem forced or awkward. Adopting an explicit nursing model or theory does require using a new vocabulary and a new way of thinking about nursing situations. Repeatedly using the conceptual model or theory should, however, lead to more systematic and organized applications. Broncatello's (1980) words, written more than 20 years ago, continue to provide the encouragement needed to start using a conceptual model of nursing or nursing theory to guide professional nursing practice.

Case Study

ROY'S ADAPTATION MODEL

Sue Jones is a 28-year-old, thin, single mother of three young children who has recently been hospitalized and diagnosed with hepatitis C. Ms. Jones is a recovering heroin addict, having been free of illegal drug use for 2 years. She currently is maintained on methadone 80 mg daily, which she receives at a methadone clinic located approximately 20 minutes from her home. Ms. Jones is currently experiencing severe fatigue, nausea, and abdominal pain. Today her physician advised her to begin interferon treatments in an attempt to slow down the virus's assault on her body. Ms. Jones appears withdrawn and depressed, expressing remorse because, "I caused my own illness. If only I had never gotten so wrapped up in drugs. I was so stupid." Ms. Jones lives with her divorced mother, Jane Brown. Mrs. Brown is supportive of her daughter and devoted to her grandchildren, but admits feeling overwhelmed and angry that Sue's past drug use is causing yet more turmoil in their lives.

The initial nursing assessment based on Roy's Adaptation Model indicates that Ms. Jones is exhibiting ineffective behaviors in all four response modes. More specifically:

- Assessment of physiologic mode responses reveals that Ms. Jones has a very poor appetite and is below average weight. Ms. Jones is also experiencing abdominal pain, fatigue, and difficulty sleeping.
- Assessment of self-concept mode responses indicates that Ms. Jones is struggling with the shame she feels about her previous lifestyle and drug use, the powerlessness she feels about her current situation, and the guilt she feels about causing her mother more trouble.
- Assessment of role function mode responses reveals that Ms. Jones feels like a failure as a mother and provider for her children. She expresses concern about her children's future and their opinion of her as a mother.
- Assessment of the interdependence mode responses indicates that Ms. Jones is fearful she may have finally pushed her relationship with her mother to the edge and is distraught about the prospect of losing her mother's love. Ms. Jones also expresses sadness about the lack of a significant other and states that she is lonely.

When Ms. Jones meets with the nurse case manager assigned to her, they agree that Ms. Jones's primary goal is to convert ineffective responses to adaptive ones, thereby contributing to her personal health and quality of life. Learning how to manage her hepatitis C and improving her parenting skills are goals made by Ms. Jones. Together, the case manager and Ms. Jones begin to identify specific behaviors that need to be modified or developed. They work to develop a timetable of short- and long-term goals for behavioral changes. Nursing intervention for Ms. Jones focuses on increasing the focal stimulus of social support through individual counseling, participation in a support group for hepatitis C patients and their families, and weekly Narcotics Anonymous meetings.

The nurse's consistent use of any model [or theory] for the interpretation of observable [patient] data is most definitely not an easy task. Much like the development of any habitual behavior, it initially requires thought, discipline and the gradual evolvement of a mind set of what is important to observe within the guidelines of the model [or theory]. As is true of most habits, however, it makes decision making less complicated. (p. 23)

Clearly, using formal nursing knowledge allows the nursing profession to be clear about its mission in the constantly changing health care arena. Now, perhaps more than ever before, it is crucial that nurses explicate what they know and why they do what they do. In other words, it is crucial that all nurses communicate distinctive nursing knowledge and explain how that knowledge governs the actions performed on behalf of or in conjunction with people who require nursing. Thus, it is incumbent on all nurses to use formal nursing knowledge. Only if they do so can nurses continue to claim a place on the multidisciplinary health care team.

Key Points

- Conceptual models of nursing present diverse perspectives of the participant in nursing, who can be an individual, a family, or a community; the environment of the nursing participant and the environment in which professional nursing practice occurs; the participant's health state; and the definition and goals of nursing as well as nursing actions or interventions.

- The most practical function of a conceptual model is its delineation of goals for nursing practice and a nursing process format or practice methodology that encompasses parameters for assessment, labels for problems, a strategy for planning nursing interventions, a typology of nursing interventions, and criteria for evaluation of the outcomes of nursing practice. A conceptual model of nursing provides a structure for documentation of all aspects of the nursing process, from patient assessment to evaluation of outcomes. A conceptual model also helps identify standards of nursing practice and criteria for quality assurance reviews.

- The function of a nursing theory is to provide considerable specificity in the description, explanation, or prediction of some phenomenon. Theories are more concrete and specific than conceptual models. A conceptual model is an abstract and general system of concepts and statements, whereas a theory deals with one or more relatively concrete and specific concepts and statements. In addition, conceptual models are general guides that must be specified further by relevant and logically congruent theories before action can occur.

- Conceptual models of nursing and nursing theories move the professional practice of nursing away from that driven by a medical or institutional model and, therefore, foster autonomy from medicine and a coherent purpose for professional nursing practice.

- Six steps are used to select a conceptual model or nursing theory to guide professional nursing practice: (1) state your philosophy of nursing, in the form of beliefs and values about the nursing participant, the environment, health, and nursing goals; (2) identify the particular patient population with which you wish to practice; (3) thoroughly analyze and evaluate several conceptual models of nursing and nursing theories; (4) compare the philosophical claims on which each conceptual model and nursing theory is based with your own philosophy of nursing; (5) determine which conceptual models or nursing theories are appropriate for use with the patient population you are interested in; and (6) select the conceptual model or nursing theory that most closely matches your philosophy of nursing and the patient population of interest.

Thought and Discussion Questions

1. List two ways in which a conceptual model differs from a grand theory or a middle-range theory.
2. List two criteria to use in the selection of a middle-range theory to flesh out a conceptual model more fully.

3. Many people select nursing as a career because they enjoy "taking care of" other people. Orem's conceptual model of nursing focuses on individuals with limited abilities to provide continuing self-care or care of dependent others. Describe the difference between "taking care of people" as a general term and professional nursing practice directed toward helping people meet their own and their dependent others' therapeutic self-care demands.

4. Describe the focus of Orem's self-care framework in relation to chronically ill patients and their families as they struggle to adjust to changes in the patients' ability to meet self-care demands.

5. Think about your personal feelings when dealing with patients similar to Ms. Jones (see Roy's Adaptation Model Case Study):

    *   Do you let your own beliefs interfere with how you interact with these patients? Explain your answer.
    *   Is your practice standard for all patients? Explain your answer.

6. Explain how conceptual models of nursing provide a framework for objective measurement of the effects of your nursing assessments and interventions.

7. Review the Chapter Thought located on the first page of the chapter, and discuss it in the context of the contents of the chapter.

Interactive Exercises

1. Complete the exercise on the Intranet site using the six steps to select a conceptual model or nursing theory to guide professional nursing practice.

2. Analyze the applicability of a nursing model in a community setting. First, attend a Narcotics Anonymous or Alcoholics Anonymous meeting in your area. After the meeting, answer the questions located on the Intranet site. Be prepared to participate in an online discussion, to be scheduled by your instructor.

PRINT RESOURCES

References

Akinsanya, J. A. (1989). Introduction. *Recent Advances in Nursing, 24,* i–ii.

Allison, S. E., & Renpenning, K. (1999). *Nursing administration in the 21st century.* Thousand Oaks, CA: Sage.

Anderson, C. A. (1995). Scholarship: How important is it? *Nursing Outlook, 43,* 247–248.

Bélanger, P. (1991). Nursing models—A major step towards professional autonomy. AARN *Newsletter, 48*(8), 13.

Biley, F. (1990). Wordly wise. *Nursing* (*London*), 4(24), 37.

Bridges, J. (1991). Working with doctors: Distinct from medicine. *Nursing Times,* 87(27), 42–43.

Broncatello, K. F. (1980). Auger in action: Application of the model. *Advances in Nursing Science,* 2(2), 13–23.

Cash, K. (1990). Nursing models and the idea of nursing. *International Journal of Nursing Studies,* 27, 249–256.

Chalmers, H., Kershaw, B., Melia, K., & Kendrich, M. (1990). Nursing models: Enhancing or inhibiting practice? *Nursing Standard,* 5(11), 34–40.

Dabbs, A. D. V. (1994). Theory-based nursing practice: For our patients' sake. *Clinical Nurse Specialist,* 8, 214, 220.

Fawcett, J. (2000). *Analysis and evaluation of contemporary nursing knowledge: Nursing models and theories.* Philadelphia: F.A. Davis.

Fawcett, J. (1999). *The relationship of theory and research* (3rd ed.). Philadelphia: F.A. Davis.

Feeg, V. (1989). From the editor: Is theory application merely an intellectual exercise? *Pediatric Nursing,* 15, 450.

Frank, L. K. (1968). Science as a communication process. *Main Currents in Modern Thought,* 25, 45–50.

Graham, I. (1994). How do registered nurses think and experience nursing: A phenomenological investigation. *Journal of Clinical Nursing,* 3, 235–242.

Grossman, M., & Hooton, M. (1993). The significance of the

relationship between a discipline and its practice. *Journal of Advanced Nursing,* 18, 866–872.

Hayne, Y. (1992). The current status and future significance of nursing as a discipline. *Journal of Advanced Nursing,* 17, 104–107.

Henderson, V. (1966). *The nature of nursing. A definition and its implications for practice, research, and education.* New York: Macmillan.

Ingram, R. (1991). Why does nursing need theory? *Journal of Advanced Nursing,* 16, 350–353.

Johnson, D. E. (1990). The behavioral system model for nursing. In M. E. Parker (Ed.), *Nursing theories in practice* (pp. 23–32). New York: National League for Nursing.

Johnson, D. E. (1987). Evaluating conceptual models for use in critical care nursing practice [Guest editorial]. *Dimensions of Critical Care Nursing,* 6, 195–197.

King, I. M. (1990). King's conceptual framework and theory of goal attainment. In M. E. Parker (Ed.), *Nursing theories in practice* (pp. 73–84). New York: National League for Nursing.

Leininger, M. M. (Ed.). (1991). *Culture care diversity and universality: A theory of nursing.* New York: National League for Nursing.

Le Storti, L. J., Cullen, P. A., Hanzlik, E. M., Michiels, J. M., Piano, L. A., Ryan, P. L., & Johnson, W. (1999). Creative thinking in nursing education: Preparing for tomorrow's challenges. *Nursing Outlook,* 47, 62–66.

Levine, M. E. (1991). The conservation principles: A model for health. In K. M. Schaefer & J. B. Pond (Eds.), *Levine's conservation model: A framework for nursing practice* (pp. 1–11). Philadelphia: F.A. Davis.

Lindsay, B. (1990). The gap between theory and practice. *Nursing Standard,* 5(4), 34–35.

Lister, P. (1991). Approaching models of nursing from a postmodernist perspective. *Journal of Advanced Nursing,* 16, 206–212.

Malin, N., & Teasdale, K. (1991). Caring versus empowerment: Considerations for nursing practice. *Journal of Advanced Nursing,* 16, 657–662.

Neff, M. (1991). President's message: The future of our profession from the eyes of today. *American Nephrology Nurses Association Journal,* 18, 534.

Neuman, B., & Fawcett, J. (2002). *The Neuman systems model* (4th ed.). Upper Saddle River, NJ: Prentice Hall.

Newman, M. A. (1994). *Health as expanding consciousness* (2nd ed.). New York: National League for Nursing Press.

Nightingale, F. (1859). *Notes on nursing: What it is, and what it is not.* London: Harrison and Sons. [Commemorative edition printed 1992, Philadelphia: J. B. Lippincott]

Nightingale, K. (1993). Editorial. *British Journal of Theatre Nursing,* 3(5), 2.

Orem, D. E. (1997). Views of human beings specific to nursing. *Nursing Science Quarterly,* 10, 26–31.

Orem, D. E. (2001). *Nursing: Concepts of practice* (6th ed.). St. Louis: Mosby.

Orlando, I. J. (1961). *The dynamic nurse-patient relationship: Function, process and principles.* New York: G. P. Putnam's Sons. [Reprinted 1990, New York: National League for Nursing]

Orr, J. (1991). Knowledge is power. *Health Visitor,* 64, 218.

Parse, R. R. (1998). *The human becoming school of thought: A perspective for nurses and other health professionals.* Thousand Oaks, CA: Sage.

Parse, R. R. (1995). Commentary. Parse's theory of human becoming: An alternative guide to nursing practice for pediatric oncology nurses. *Journal of Pediatric Oncology Nursing,* 12, 128.

Peplau, H. E. (1992). Interpersonal relations: A theoretical framework for application in nursing practice. *Nursing Science Quarterly,* 5, 13–18.

Peplau, H. E. (1952). *Interpersonal relations in nursing.* New York: G. P. Putnam's Sons. [Reprinted 1991, New York: Springer]

Perry, J. (1985). Has the discipline of nursing developed to the stage where nurses do 'think nursing'? *Journal of Advanced Nursing,* 10, 31–37.

Popper, K. R. (1965). *Conjectures and refutations: The growth of scientific knowledge.* New York: Harper and Row.

Rogers, C. G. (1973). Conceptual models as guides to clinical nursing specialization. *Journal of Nursing Education,* 12(4), 2–6.

Rogers, M. E. (1990). Nursing: Science of unitary, irreducible, human beings: Update 1990. In E. A. M. Barrett (Ed.), *Visions of Rogers' science-based nursing* (pp. 5–11). New York: National League for Nursing.

Rogers, M. E. (1989). Creating a climate for the implementation of a nursing conceptual framework. *Journal of Continuing Education in Nursing,* 20, 112–116.

Rogers, M. E. (1970). *An introduction to the theoretical basis of nursing.* Philadelphia: F.A. Davis.

Roy, C., & Andrews, H. A. (1999). *The Roy adaptation model* (2nd ed.). Stamford, CT: Appleton and Lange.

Watson, J. (1997). The theory of human caring: Retrospective and prospective. *Nursing Science Quarterly,* 10, 49–52.

Watson, J. (1985). *Nursing: Human science and human care. A theory of nursing.* Norwalk, CT: Appleton-Century-Crofts. [Reprinted 1988, New York: National League for Nursing]

Bibliography

Alligood, M. R., & Marriner-Tomey, A. (2002). *Nursing theory: Utilization and application* (2nd ed.). St. Louis: Mosby.

Parker, M. E. (Ed.). (2001). *Nursing theory and nursing practice.* Philadelphia: F.A. Davis.

Parker, M. E. (Ed.). (1993). *Patterns of nursing theories in practice.* New York: National League for Nursing Press.

Parker, M. E. (Ed.). (1990). *Nursing theories in practice.* New York: National League for Nursing.

Rose Kearney-Nunnery

Models for Health and Illness

> I can enter your world, as one who invites your growth or as a strangler of your possibilities, a prophet of stasis.
>
> Sidney M. Jourard

Chapter Objectives

On completion of this chapter, the reader will be able to:

1. Differentiate among the various health and illness models for applicability to professional nursing practice.
2. Discuss the advantages and disadvantages of the various models.
3. Apply a health belief or health promotion model to a given nursing care situation.
4. Analyze differences in health beliefs held by members of various cultural groups.

Key Terms

Health
Health Promotion
Health Protection
Preventive Services
Primary Prevention

Secondary Prevention
Tertiary Prevention
High-level Wellness
Health Belief Model
Health Promotion Model

Chronic Illness Trajectory
   Framework
Functional Health
   Patterns
Cultural Competence

Health is a condition we seek, promote, and hope to maintain. Health is more than the absence of illness, or infirmity. A multidimensional construct of health is determined by the individual's worldview and philosophical assumptions. If we subscribe to our four metaparadigm concepts of nursing, health is specified in the nursing theory that guides our practice. Health as a part of the metaparadigm is interrelated with concepts of person, environment, and nursing. Considering your particular view of the world and your concept of health, we can now approach ways of promoting health using a sample of different models. This selection of model is, again, determined by one's worldview and theoretical guide.

In Chapter 4, health is illustrated within individual theoretical structures. For example, consider the three definitions of health provided by King, Roy, and Leininger. King (1981) defines health as "dynamic life experiences of a human being, which implies continuous adjustment to stressors in the internal and external environment through optimum use of one's resources to achieve maximum potential for daily living" (p. 5). Roy defines health as "a state and a process of being and becoming an integrated and whole person. ... Health as a state reflects the adaptation process and is demonstrated by adaptation in each of the four integrated adaptive modes. ... Health is a process whereby individuals are striving to achieve their maximum potential" (Lutjens, 1991, pp. 9–10). And Leininger (2002c) defines health as "a state of well-being or restorative state that is culturally constituted, defined, valued, and practiced by individuals or groups that

enables them to function in their daily lives" (p. 84).

In other nursing theories and models, the concept of health may not be well defined but is interpreted, as in Rogers's theory, as a "value term defined by the culture or individual" (Gunther, 2002, p. 229). Or, in Parse's (1981) theory, health is a process of becoming (p. 159). Still, health or well-being is represented in each framework on which practice is based. Before delving into the theories of health and illness—in the context of health promotion and illness prevention—and cultural perceptions of health, it is first important to understand the different levels and types of health promotion and illness prevention activities.

LEVELS OF PREVENTION

When considering health promotion activities, we frequently refer to illness and disability prevention. In 1990, national health promotion and disease prevention activities were developed under the auspices of the U.S. Department of Health and Human Services (USDHHS) and published as Healthy People 2000. Interestingly, the publication distinguished between health promotion and health protection strategies, with an individual versus a community focus, as follows:

> **Health promotion** strategies are those related to individual lifestyle–personal choices made in a social context—that can have a powerful influence over one's health prospects. These include physical activity and fitness, nutrition, tobacco,

alcohol and other drugs, family planning, mental health and mental disorders and violent and abusive behavior. ... **Health protection** strategies are those related to environmental or regulatory measures that confer protection on large population groups. These strategies address issues such as unintentional injuries, occupational safety and health, environmental health, food and drug safety, and oral health. **Preventive services** include counseling, screening, immunization, or chemoprophylactic interventions for individuals in clinical settings. (USDHHS, 1992, pp. 6–7)

These preventive activities and services address the three levels of prevention: primary, secondary, and tertiary. Health promotion activities are both protective and preventive, but they require consumers actively involved in all levels of prevention. And this focus on health promotion and health protection strategies became an important component of Healthy People 2010 (2000) with the national goals to increase the quality and years of healthy life and to eliminate health disparities.

Primary prevention refers to healthy actions taken to avoid illness or disease. Examples are healthy nutrition, smoking cessation, exercise programs, parenting classes, community awareness programs, and mental health programs and activities. *Primary prevention* refers to the individual lifestyle health promotion strategies recommended in Healthy People 2000 and Healthy People 2010. These are becoming more popular and prevalent as people take responsibility for their own health. Health columns have appeared more frequently in publications. We have also seen a growing number of health food and holistic health stores, "healthy" fast food options, Web sites, and educational programs for the general public. But consumers can still have difficulty acquiring sufficient information on a selected topic before they become frustrated.

Secondary prevention involves screening for early detection and treatment of health problems. With secondary prevention, the individual is seeking health care not for a specific problem but, rather, for early detection of a potential problem, to mobilize resources and reduce its intensity or severity if the problem is identified. Secondary prevention usually involves use of some procedure or measurement tool in addition to the health history and physical assessment. Examples of secondary prevention are screening procedures used by health-care consumers or health-care professionals for physiologic, developmental, or environmental problems. Physiologic procedures include screening for hypertension or specific forms of cancer. Mental health screening procedures range from simple tests for orientation to more elaborate instruments such as mental status questionnaires for aging clients. In young children, examples of secondary prevention activities are use of growth charts to assess growth along established percentiles and the Denver II developmental screening test to detect problems in the areas of personal-social skills, motor activities, and language. Note the difference between using parenting classes as primary prevention for developmental stimulation and screening for developmental problems with the Denver II test as secondary prevention. Environmental screening procedures include testing air and water quality and home safety assessments. If a problem is detected, a referral is made for a differential diagnosis and institution of early treatment.

Tertiary prevention occurs during the rehabilitative phase of an illness to prevent complications or further disability. The individual has already entered the health-care system and is recovering from or learning to cope with a health deficit. Tertiary prevention builds on this care to prevent further deficits. Examples of tertiary prevention are counseling and teaching after recovery from a cardiovascular event, an accident or injury, an abusive situation, or any other physical, psychosocial, mental, or environmental disruption from usual health and functioning. Support from self-help groups is a large component of tertiary prevention. Continuing with the example of preventive activities for children with parenting classes and the Denver II test, an example of tertiary prevention is family counseling after identification of a child in a physically abusive situation.

Professional nursing practice involves not only health promotion but also all three levels of preventive activities. Because the health of individuals, families, communities, and groups is a major concern in nursing, professional skill and expertise in the area of prevention activities are presumed in practice, education, research, and administrative functions.

THEORIES OF HEALTH AND ILLNESS

Aside from the nursing conceptual or theoretical frameworks, different models are available to guide assessment of health factors and promote and preserve health. Benner and Wrubel (1989) have described five theories of health as (1) an ideal, (2) the ability to fulfill social roles, (3) a commodity, (4) a human potential, and (5) a sense of coherence. Health is more than an ideal. We strive for the person, family, community, or group to reach a positive state of well-being. Defining health as the ability to perform one's role is limiting and fails to meet our holistic concern for the person. As Benner and Wrubel (1989) observe, "this view focuses on doing rather than being and ignores the person's sense of fulfillment and well-being" (p. 151). Health as a commodity implies that it can be bought, sold, traded, and withheld. This view fails to meet the intent of a caring professional practice discipline. Health as a commodity is described as a "medicalized view," promising instant cures without personal involvement (Benner & Wrubel, 1989, pp. 151–153).

Health defined as a human potential is consistent with the beliefs of many in nursing and other health-care disciplines and is the basis of the first three health models presented here. Health as a human potential includes physical, mental, and spiritual health. Benner and Wrubel (1989) based their model on the premise that all people have the potential for health, with the limitation that they are always pursuing but not attaining health. This definition depends on whether health is viewed as a defined goal or a dynamic state that we continue to strive toward. Dunn's high-level wellness model, the health belief model, and Pender's health promotion model are consistent with health viewed as human potential.

A fifth view of health takes a phenomenologic approach. *Phenomenology* is the lived experience of the individual, from his or her unique perspective. This view focuses on one's lived experience rather than an opinion derived from another person's observations of the experience. Benner and Wrubel's (1989) approach to health as a mind-body-spirit integration in a state of becoming is an example of health as a sense of coherence. A focus on the person's belonging to a sociocultural group makes this integration unique. Benner and Wrubel define the term *well-being* as a better indication of health with challenges and involvement in the following definition: "Well-being is defined as congruence between one's possibilities and one's actual practices and lived meanings and is based on caring and feeling cared for" (Benner & Wrubel, 1989, p. 160).

In this view, a model must be based on a qualitative approach to address individuals' well-being, because it depends on the lived experience of those persons in their context. As Benner and Wrubel (1989) state, "health as well-being comes when one engages in sound self-care, cares, and feels cared for—when one trusts the self, the body, and others. Breakdown occurs when that trust is broken. Well-being can be restored" (p. 165). The chronic illness trajectory framework is consistent with the view of health as coherence.

Model of High-Level Wellness

Dunn developed his model of **high-level wellness** starting with the 1947 definition of health from the World Health Organization that emphasized physical, mental, and social well-being. He stressed that well-being includes the positive, dynamic, and unique integration of mind, body, and spirit of the individual within his or her environment, including work, family, community, and society. Dunn (1973) defined high-level wellness for an individual as "an integrated method of functioning which is oriented toward maximizing the potential of which the individual is capable. It requires that the individual maintain a continuum of balance and purposeful direction within the environment where he is functioning" (pp. 4–5).

Dunn regarded high-level wellness as an ongoing challenge to the highest level possible, the individual's maximum potential. Meeting basic needs and striving for higher needs were components of his view of individual health and well-being. Dunn (1973) viewed high-level wellness as "an open-ended and ever-expanding tomorrow with its challenge to live at full potential" (p. 223). He also considered high-level wellness, with similar components, for the family, community, environment, and society.

Dunn's beliefs about high-level wellness evolved into a health grid (Fig. 5–1) that demonstrates a person or group at some point along a health continuum or horizontal axis, from death at the left side to peak wellness at the right. The person or group was further influenced by the environment (the vertical axis), from a very favorable environment at the top to a very unfavorable environment at the bottom. This grid illustrates the person or group in context, within one of the four quadrants ranging from poor health to protected poor health, high-level wellness, and emergent high-level wellness. The high-level wellness model provides an explanation of the person-environment relationship in health but gives no direction as to movement among quadrants, and it also compartmentalizes

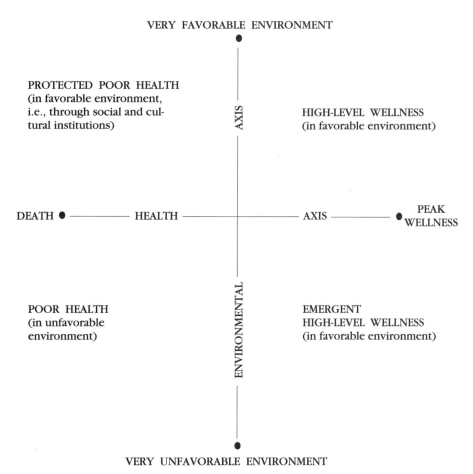

FIG. 5–1. Dunn's high-level wellness. (From U.S. Department of Health, Education, and Welfare. Public Health Service, National Office of Vital Statistics.)

wellness The model could be effectively used to address health disparities for the client who is currently in an unfavorable environment (poorly accepted services related to language) to a favorable environment where we strive to promote more culturally relevant, understandable, and acceptable services and health care.

Health Belief Model

The **health belief model** is a valuable tool for looking at both health promotion and actions directed at maintaining or restoring health. Originally, the model was based on the following hypothesis:

> Persons will not seek preventative care or health screening unless they possess minimal levels of relevant health motivation and knowledge, view themselves as potentially vulnerable and the condition as threatening, are convinced of the efficacy of intervention, and see few difficulties in undertaking the recommended action (Becker et al., 1977, p. 29).

The health belief model was designed as an organizing framework to advance health promotion activities by targeting interventions on certain individual variables. The three major concepts in the model were individual perceptions, modifying factors, and likelihood of action. Individual perceptions involve how the person considers the risk of susceptibility or the severity of the illness— in other words, how likely he or she believes it is that the disease or condition could happen to him or her. Modifying factors are a set of demographic, sociopsychological cues to action from family, friends, professionals, or the media relative to the perceived threat of the disease. Sociopsychological variables include personality, interpersonal influences, and socioeconomic status. The modifying factors, along with individual perceptions, lead to the likelihood of action in the direction of health. The concept of motivation is central to this model (Becker et al., 1977, p. 31).

An extensive review of research on variables in the health belief model led to a subsequent revision. The model was expanded from a diagram of health belief concepts and their relationships to a full explanation of and prediction about health-related behaviors (Fig. 5–2). The three major concepts were (1) readiness to undertake recommended compliance behavior, (2) modifying and enabling factors, and (3) compliant behaviors. On the basis of research, readiness to undertake recommended compliance behavior broadened individual perceptions from perception of susceptibility and severity to perceptions of motivations, values for threat reduction, and subjective risk/benefit considerations that the compliant behaviors would be safe and effective. Modifying factors were expanded to more inclusive modifying and enabling factors on the basis of research findings. A reciprocal relationship between readiness and modifying/enabling factors also became more apparent in the revised model. The outcome in the revised model was the likelihood of compliant behaviors with preventive recommendations or prescribed regimens.

The original version of the health belief model focused on health promotion or preventive behaviors. Since its inception, the model has been widely used in research and practice. In addition to use in understanding utilization of health-care services and health promotion behaviors, the model has guided research in client compliance to health care. An extensive body of research on patient compliance for the revised model demonstrated applicability in a wide range of health-care situations. Insights for use of the model in practice and education were offered. Concerning education, Becker and associates (1977) recommended that health-care providers understand the following principles:

1. Behavior is motivated.
2. Certain beliefs seem central to a client's decision to act.
3. Not all persons possess these beliefs and motives to equal degrees.
4. Intellectual information, although necessary, is often not sufficient to stimulate needed beliefs.
5. Health providers need to view the importance of client education and accept substantial responsibility in this activity (p. 42).

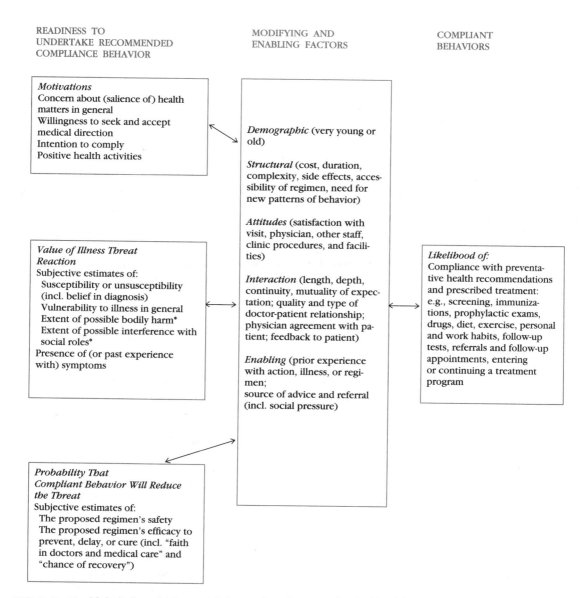

READINESS TO
UNDERTAKE RECOMMENDED
COMPLIANCE BEHAVIOR

MODIFYING AND
ENABLING FACTORS

COMPLIANT
BEHAVIORS

Motivations
Concern about (salience of) health
matters in general
Willingness to seek and accept
medical direction
Intention to comply
Positive health activities

*Value of Illness Threat
Reaction*
Subjective estimates of:
  Susceptibility or unsusceptibility
  (incl. belief in diagnosis)
  Vulnerability to illness in general
  Extent of possible bodily harm*
  Extent of possible interference with
  social roles*
Presence of (or past experience
with) symptoms

*Probability That
Compliant Behavior Will Reduce
the Threat*
Subjective estimates of:
  The proposed regimen's safety
  The proposed regimen's efficacy to
  prevent, delay, or cure (incl. "faith
  in doctors and medical care" and
  "chance of recovery")

Demographic (very young or
old)

Structural (cost, duration,
complexity, side effects, accessibility of regimen, need for
new patterns of behavior)

Attitudes (satisfaction with
visit, physician, other staff,
clinic procedures, and facilities)

Interaction (length, depth,
continuity, mutuality of expectation; quality and type of
doctor-patient relationship;
physician agreement with patient; feedback to patient)

Enabling (prior experience
with action, illness, or regimen;
source of advice and referral
(incl. social pressure)

Likelihood of:
Compliance with preventa-
tive health recommendations
and prescribed treatment:
e.g., screening, immunizations, prophylactic exams,
drugs, diet, exercise, personal
and work habits, follow-up
tests, referrals and follow-up
appointments, entering
or continuing a treatment
program

FIG. 5–2. Health belief model for explaining and predicting individual health-related behaviors. (From Becker, M. H., Haefner, D. P., Kasl, S. V., Kirscht, J. P., Maiman, L. A., & Rosenstock, I. M. [1977]. Selected psychosocial models and correlates of individual health-related behaviors. *Medical Care, 15*[5], 30. Reproduced with permission, Philadelphia: Lippincott-Raven Publishers.)

These principles are consistent with the discipline of professional nursing practice and are routinely incorporated into care plans and health teaching. Consideration of the belief systems of the individual, family, or group is essential in assessing a client and choosing interventions. The extent of detail and inclusion of this information is the challenge to the nurse, whose health teaching role is an integral component of professional practice.

As a part of the health history, readiness, as motivations in health behaviors, is easily included in the interview. Soliciting and understanding the client's "subjective estimates" of the threat, potential reduction, and care options are less commonly included in the assessment, depending on the professional's impressions of time restraints and knowledge of the client, or even on cultural or interpersonal differences between the professional and the client. In a nursing health assessment, we frequently acquire demographic information and some structural information that provides insight into modifying and enabling factors. The challenge is to acquire the additional structural information, such as cost and accessibility, and voluntarily to seek information from the client about quality, satisfaction, and social pressures for additional knowledge of attitudinal, interaction, and enabling factors. This information can be used to increase compliant behaviors.

Nevertheless, the model has limitations. First, the language is directed to physician-patient relationships, quite possibly a product of the roles and functions of other heath-care providers in 1977. More recently, the health belief model has been used in further research consistent with views of nursing. Ongoing research and applications of health behavior have been demonstrated at the level of the individual, dyad, group, organization, and community (Glantz, Rimer, & Lewis, 2002). Second, as Pender (1987, 1996; Pender et al., 2002) indicates, the health belief model is directed at preventive services or health protection behaviors in the context of a provider-consumer relationship rather than individual health promotion behaviors. To be empowered consumers in today's health-care system, individuals must take personal responsibility for their own health long before they seek care from a health professional. This concept is now beginning to be addressed in the health belief model, especially in application related to health education.

Health Promotion Model

Pender's **health promotion model**, an outgrowth of the health belief model, is based on research and information on health and health-protecting behaviors. It is primarily a

nursing model and has been revised with evolving knowledge. In the health promotion model, health promotion is motivated by the desire to increase the level of wellness and actualization of an individual or an aggregate group (Pender, 1996, p. 7). Pender states that the nine assumptions of the model "emphasize the *active role* of the client in shaping and maintaining health behaviors and in modifying the environmental context for health behaviors" (Pender et al., 2002, p. 63). She points out that "unlike the health belief model, the health promotion model does not include 'fear' or 'threat' as a source of motivation for the health behavior" (Pender et al., 2002, p. 61).

Structurally, the model had been designed as a schematic representation similar to the original health belief model. After extensive research, however, the model was revised, and significant variables were reorganized (Fig. 5–3). The knowledge obtained through research led to the later addition of three new variables in the health promotion model: activity-related affect, commitment to a plan of action, and immediate competing demands and preferences.

The revised health promotion model contains two principal components that interact for participation in health-promoting behaviors: (1) individual characteristics and experiences and (2) behavior-specific cognitions and affect. Individual characteristics and experiences are similar to the individual perceptions in the health belief model, in that they involve looking at health through past experiences (prior related behavior) and personal factors. Pender points out that "empirical studies indicate that often the best predictor of behavior is the frequency of the same or a similar behavior in the past" (Pender et al., 2002, p. 68). Personal factors include biologic variables (age, gender, body mass, etc.), psychological variables (such as self-esteem, self-motivation, perceived health status), and sociocultural variables (ethnicity, aculteration, educational level, socioeconomic status) (Pender et al., 2002, p. 69).

On the basis of research evidence, these biologic, psychological, and sociocultural personal factors were included in the model as further predictors of individual health percep-

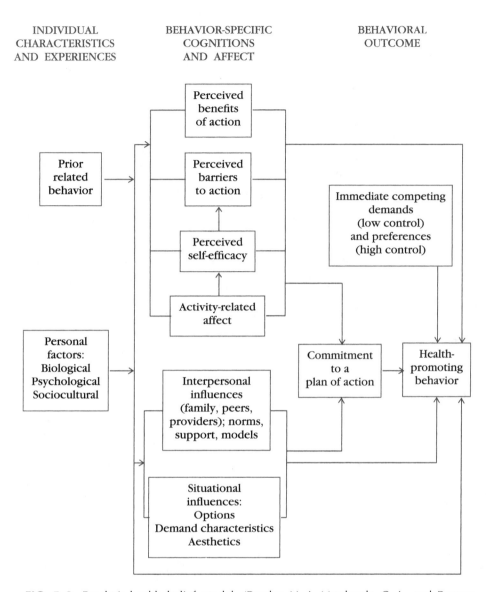

INDIVIDUAL
CHARACTERISTICS
AND EXPERIENCES

BEHAVIOR-SPECIFIC
COGNITIONS
AND AFFECT

BEHAVIORAL
OUTCOME

FIG. 5–3. Pender's health belief model. (Pender, N. J. Murdaugh, C. L. and Parsons, M. A. [2002]. *Health promotion in nursing practice* [4th ed.] Stamford, CT: Prentice Hall. Reprinted with permission.)

tions and behaviors. For example, consider the health-seeking behaviors demonstrated by clients of different socioeconomic groups, family backgrounds, and experiences in the health-care system. As stated in the first theoretical proposition of the model, prior behavior and individual characteristics influence beliefs, affect, and enactment of health-promoting behaviors (Pender et al., 2002, p.

63). A later section of this chapter addresses specific cultural differences in health beliefs that also influence health-seeking behaviors.

The behavior-specific cognitions and affect are similar to the health belief model's modifying or enabling factors but relate more to the nomenclature of nursing. As Pender has indicated, this category of variables is of "major motivational significance" and provides the critical "core," because they are subject to modification based on nursing interventions (Pender et al., 2002, p. 63). These behavior-specific cognitions and affects include perceived benefits, perceived barriers, perceived self-efficacy, activity-related affect (subjective feelings), interpersonal influences, and situational influences. Interpersonal and situational influences are identified as having both direct and indirect effects on health promotion behaviors. Consider the older adult walking through a shopping mall and noticing a free hypertension screening clinic. Indirect situational influences to obtain a screening test may include the perceived camaraderie of people in the clinic compared with a tedious wait for an office appointment. The direct influence is the availability of the screening during this older adult's routine exercise program at the mall.

The variables of perceived benefits, perceived barriers, self-efficacy, interpersonal influences, and situational influences have been supported in research studies as predictors of health promotion behaviors (Pender, 1996; Pender et al., 2002). Activity-related affect, a variable added in the revised health promotion model, addresses the individual's subjective feelings related to the health promotion behavior. Because of the recent inclusion of this variable in the model, limited support is available for it as a predictor of health promotion behaviors.

Behavioral outcome, the third component of the model, includes actions toward the healthy behavior. These actions lead to the attainment of a positive health outcome. Two variables (immediate competing demands and preferences; and commitment to a plan of action) were added to the revised health promotion model to further explain the behavioral outcome of the health-promoting behavior. Pender describes the commitment to the plan of action with two distinct cognitive processes: (1) the commitment to carry out a specific action at a given time and place and with specified persons or alone, irrespective of competing preferences, and (2) identification of definitive strategies for eliciting, carrying out, and reinforcing the behavior (Pender et al., 2002, p. 72).

The health-promoting behavior can be affected by the immediate competing demands and preferences the individual perceives. These are viewed as alternate behaviors. Competing demands are behaviors over which the person has little control because of environmental factors, like family commitments. Competing preferences are behaviors with powerful reinforcing properties—such as a sudden urge for a particular food—over which the person has a high level of control (Pender et al., 2002, pp. 73–74). This component is greatly influenced by nursing interventions related to values clarification, encouragement, and reinforcement of healthy behaviors.

In the earlier version of the health promotion model, Pender (1987) described the model as a flexible organizing framework, subject to revision after further testing. Fifteen theoretical propositions have now been derived from the model. Research has been ongoing for testing of the model. With the empirical support of variables, the revised model has greater potential to predict and intervene for health promotion activities. Health promotion settings are the social environment in which we live, work, and play, such as family, school, workplace, health-care agencies, and the community at large. Ongoing research studies have focused on a variety of client populations to target theory testing for this model and to further validate the utility of its theoretical structure in the discipline of nursing.

Comparison of the Two Models

Table 5–1 compares the health belief model and the health promotion model. Both models propose that the health professional must understand how the person perceives the world and makes personal decisions through identified readiness or individual characteristics and experiences. The modifying factors or behavior-specific cognitions and affect are the social, situational, and environmental influences related to the person's conception of healthy behavior. Both models include demographic variables, because research supports

TABLE 5–1
Comparing the Health Belief Model and the Health Promotion Model

Model	Individual Characteristics	Mediating Factors	Outcomes
Health Belief Model (Becker et al., 1977)	Readiness for Recommended Behavior: Motivations, including general health concerns, willingness and compliance behaviors, positive health attitudes Value of illness threat reduction, including subjective estimates and past experiences Probability that compliant behavior will reduce threat (subjectively)	Modifying/Enabling Factors: • Demographic • Structural • Attitudes • Interaction • Enabling	Compliant Behaviors: Likelihood of compliance with preventive health recommendations and prescribed regimens
Pender's Health Promotion Model (1996)	Individual Characteristics and Experiences: Prior related behavior Personal factors • Biological • Psychological • Sociocultural	Behavior-Specific Cognitions and Affect: • Perceived benefits • Perceived barriers • Perceived self-efficacy • Activity-related affect • Interpersonal influences • Situational influences	Behavioral Outcomes: • Commitment to a plan of action • Immediate competing demands and preferences • Health promoting behaviors

the importance of differences. For example, the choice between surgery and irradiation is very different for a 28-year-old patient and an 88-year-old patient, in terms not only of physiologic differences but also of past experiences. Attention to these differences turns the focus of health-care consumers to their specific outcomes and increases chances of success in the health promotion activity.

Chronic Illness Model

Although the health belief model has been used in research and practice settings with clients who have chronic illnesses, Corbin and

Strauss's chronic illness model is specific to chronicity. Despite its focus on chronic illness, it is still a health promotion model. As Corbin and Strauss (1992a) state:

> The focus of care in chronicity is not on cure but first of all on the prevention of chronic conditions, then on finding ways to help the ill manage and live with their illness should these occur. Interventions are aimed at fostering the prevention of, living with, and shaping the course of chronic illnesses, especially those requiring technologically complex management, while promoting and maintaining quality of life. (p. 20)

The **chronic illness trajectory framework** (Corbin & Strauss, 1992a), shown in Table 5–2, is a substantive theory that applies

TABLE 5–2 The Chronic Illness Trajectory Framework (Corbin & Strauss, 1992a)	
Trajectory phasing	Eight phases: pretrajectory, trajectory onset, crisis, acute, stable, unstable, downward, dying; sub-phasing within each phase for fluctuations as improvements, plateauing, reversals, or deterioration occurs during course of illness
Trajectory projection	Vision of the illness course
Trajectory scheme	Shaping the course, controlling symptoms, and handling disability
Conditions influencing management	Technology used, resources, past experience, motivation, setting of care, lifestyle/ beliefs, inter-actions/ relationships, type of chronic condition and physiologic involvement, symptoms, political and economic climate affecting legislation
Trajectory management	Management of symptoms, side effects, crises, and complications through the trajectory scheme
Biographical and everyday living impact	Identity adjustments and management of limitations
Reciprocal impact	Consequences with management and problems related to illness, biography and everyday activities

to individuals with a broad range of chronic conditions. Benner and Wrubel's (1989) concept of health as coherence applies to this model. Corbin and Strauss (1992a) describe the development of the framework as based on 30 years of qualitative, grounded theory research. The original framework was developed with the following concepts: key problems, basic strategies, organizational or family arrangements, and consequences (Strauss & Glaser, 1975; Strauss et al., 1984). It evolved into a nursing theory through its use and research base, but the developers maintain that potentially it applies to all health-care disciplines. The framework or model is based on the following assumptions:

1. The course of chronic conditions varies and changes over time.
2. The course of a chronic condition can be shaped and managed.
3. The technology involved is complex and can potentially create side effects.
4. The illness and technology pose potential consequences for the individual's physical well-being, biographical fulfillment (iden-

tify over time), and performance of daily activities.
5. Biographical needs and performance of daily activities can affect illness management choices and the course of the illness.
6. The course of illness is not inevitably downward.
7. Chronic illnesses do not necessarily end in death. (Corbin & Strauss, 1992a, p. 10; 1992b, p. 97)

Corbin and Strauss (1992a) describe the framework as a conceptual model organized under the central concept of trajectory. This central concept was proposed to indicate the management of the evolving course of the chronic condition, as "shaped" by the person, family members, and health-care providers. From this central organizing or umbrella concept flow the other major theoretical concepts.

These concepts are described as leading to the structure of the nursing process, with the following steps:

1. Locating the client and family, and setting goals

2. Assessing conditions influencing management
3. Defining the intervention focus, the target of intervention
4. Intervention
5. Evaluating the effectiveness of intervention.

This model focuses on the person to illustrate the management of an evolving course of a chronic condition the individual experiences that is influenced by that individual, the family, and health-care providers. It takes us a step further than the health belief model because this model is more grounded in the individual's unique, personal history and patterns of life. Chronic illness has been studied further by Mishel (1990), who focused on the concept of uncertainty in both chronic and acute illness situations. The chronic illness experience is distinctively different for an elderly, frail Anglo-American woman living in an urban high-rise apartment and for the African-American elder with a physical disability living in a rural farm area. The difference involves more than the issue of compliance; it focuses on quality. This model is extremely relevant to nursing care as we experience the rising numbers of chronic illnesses managed in contemporary practice and the growing population of aging adults who are living longer while dealing with a chronic illness. In addition, the importance of cultural relevance, the beliefs and values of individuals, families, communities, and groups, and environmental factors, are major considerations in health care.

Conclusions

All of these models require a thoughtful and thorough nursing assessment. Valid data are needed for their application. As part of the nursing assessment, the application of Gordon's **functional health patterns** could assist in this application (Box 5–1). Nursing assessment of each of these areas provides valuable data for application of a health or illness model to address health and illness focused on human potential or a sense of coherence.

> **BOX 5–1**
> **FUNCTIONAL HEALTH PATTERNS**
>
> Gordon (2002) has identified 11 functional health patterns for inclusion in the nursing assessment and diagnosis process:
> - Health perception and health management
> - Nutrition and metabolic
> - Elimination
> - Activity and exercise
> - Sleep and rest
> - Cognitive and perceptual
> - Self-perception and self-concept
> - Role and relationship
> - Sexuality and reproductive
> - Coping and stress tolerance
> - Values and beliefs

 CULTURAL INFLUENCE ON HEALTH PERCEPTIONS AND PROMOTION

Healthy People 2000 and Healthy People 2010 targeted selected groups of at-risk populations requiring special health promotion strategies. These reports illustrated significant health problems in some minority groups, but more importantly, they emphasized individuals within subgroups. As originally reported in Healthy People 2000, individual differences, beyond racial group, socioeconomic status, and educational level, affect health status and access to health care. These reports pointed out that "our health care programs are characterized by unacceptable disparities linked to membership in certain racial and ethnic groups"(USDHHS, 1992, p. 31). To address this issue, the Commonweath Foundation conducted a field study, reporting that "minorities have difficulty getting apropriate, timely, high-quality care because of language barriers and that they may have different perspectives on health, medical care, and expectations about diagnosis and treatment" (Betancourt et al., 2002, p. 3). The issue then goes beyond access to the need for the provi-

ONLINE CONSULT

Agency for Healthcare Research & Quality at
www.ahrq.gov
The Commonwealth Fund at
www.cmtw.org
Healthy People at
www.healthypeople.gov
U.S. Dept. of Health & Human Services at
www.hhs.gov

sion of acceptable of health care to address the existing disparaties.

These reports highlight the need for a concerted effort to understand and embrace diversity in our daily personal and professional lives. But much is implied within the construct of "diversity." When people speak of ethnicity and race, they generally refer to a group, tribe, or nation of people united by some common characteristics, whether biologic, environmental, or social. In the United States, we tend to classify people into five ethnic groups: African-Americans, Asian-Americans and Pacific Islanders, Hispanic-Americans, Native Americans, and white Americans. But this tendency does little to help us understand the health beliefs, practices, needs, or diversity represented within each of these population classifications. It may, in fact, encourage us to impose stereotypical judgments on persons within these groups.

This point leads us to the concept of culture as a way of life and the increasing focus on **cultural competence**. Betancourt and associates (2002) describe three components of cultural competence—organizational, systemic, and clinical—and propose recommendations to address racial and ethnic disparities in health care. The focus on clinical cultural competence is to enhance "health professionals' awareness of cultural issues and health beliefs while providing methods to elicit, negotiate, and manage the information once it is obtained" "(Betancourt et al., 2002, p. 17).

Our cultural inheritance has a powerful influence on our health beliefs, both con-

scious and unconscious. We bring into our personal and professional lives the influences from our ancestors, family, peers, and colleagues. We are affected by history, genetics, social customs, religion, language, politics, law, economics, education, and many other factors. We mutually influence and are influenced by others because of these endowments. When we talk about cultural diversity, we mean more than an inherited background. "Culture" implies social, familial, religious, national, and professional characteristics that affect the way we think and act; it is a combination of all these things.

Research demonstrating individual differences and perceptions provided valuable data for the revision of the health belief model. Educational, ethnic, and social class differences were identified for careful assessment of client beliefs and perceptions (Becker et al., 1977). These data are is significant whether one is dealing with individual clients or families with a specific health-care deficit or a larger population group with informational needs for health promotion activities. To address health disparities further, Baldwin (2003) proposes that in "promoting wellness a healthy lifestyle is key in eliminating unequal burdens in mortality and morbidity for ethnic and racial groups" (p. 4).

But it is important to consider the characteristics of both the client and the health professional. The values for cultural diversity and culturally sensitive care are clearly illustrated in position statesments of our nursing organizations. However, as Andrews (2003) indicates, "health professionals must have positive experiences with members of other cultures and learn to value genuinely the contributions all cultures make to our multicultural society" (p. 9).

> "as Mazanec and Tyler (2003) so aptly point out," cultural competence demands that nurses look at patients through both their own eyes and the eyes of patients and family members" (p. 52).

One's health beliefs are the result of cultural inheritance, educational information, reasoned opinions, and, often, unfounded impressions. The proportion of each of these factors is individually determined. Babcock and Miller (1994) describe three paradigms for cultural influence on health care: (1) magico-religious, (2) scientific or biomedical, and (3) holistic (Table 5–3). The three different views show us how individuals differ in their beliefs in the supernatural, the scientific community, or the holistic mind-body-spirit interrelationship. It is worth noting that the traditional health-care system operates from the scientific worldview, which diverges from that of many cultures and their subgroups. Spector (2000) describes this dominant health-care system in America—acute care, chronic care, rehabilitation, psychiatric/mental health, and community/public health—as "allopathic" and as a culture onto itself. Significant differences can exist in health beliefs and roles between the client with a health-care need and the health-care provider, considered the "expert."

In our health-care system, we generally view the roles of health-care providers and those of consumers in traditional ways. We consider the disease or illness, including all the pathophysiology and treatment modalities. We are aware of health-care and health promotion services in both the hospital and community setting. We usually present them through our words and behaviors as norms to which clients must adhere. Otherwise, they are termed "bad patients," "noncompliant," or even "problem cases." For example, the health-care community carefully conducts, evaluates, and uses research to identify biologic, chemical, structural, and physical factors to treat, manage, or cure a disease. Faced

with clients whose belief system includes the "hot/cold" theory of disease causation and treatment—which holds that imbalance of the four body humors of yellow and black bile, phlegm, and blood resulting in a "hot" infectious condition must be treated with appropriate foods or herbs—we may ignore or patronize the client. Many scientific minds reject this theory, creating conflict and failure to provide health care. As Benner and Wrubel (1989) observe, "changes in lifestyles and health habits work best when they are integrated into the person's own cultural patterns and traditions [for] it is hard to sustain new patterns if they go against the grain of one's normal social patterns" (p. 155).

Models of Cultural Care

Madeleine Leininger proposed a transcultural nursing theory entitled Culture Care Diversity and Universality. Leininger's (1970) early definition of *culture* referred to a way of "life belonging" to a designated group, through accumulated traditions, customs, and the ways the group solves problems that are learned and transmitted systematically, largely through socialization practices that are reinforced through social and cultural institutions (pp. 48–49). Within her culture care theory, Leininger (2002c) defined culture as "patterned lifeways, values, beliefs, norms, symbols, and practices of individuals, groups, or institutions that are learned, shared, and usually transmitted intergenerationally over time" (p. 83). Taking this one step further as a health belief, Leininger (2002c) defined *cultural care* as "the synthesized and culturally constituted assistive, supportive, and facilitative caring acts toward self or others focused on evident or anticipated needs for the client's health or well-being or to face disabilities, death or other human conditions" (p. 83).

On the basis of in-depth qualitative research, Leininger has identified dominant cultural values and culture care meanings and action modes for many different American subculture groups, showing differences with the Anglo-American health care value structure. She defines *subcultures* as "small or large

TABLE 5–3
Summary of Belief Systems about Health and Illness

	Magico-religious	Scientific/Biomedical	Holistic
Worldview	Fate of world is under control of supernatural forces God(s) or other supernatural forces for good and evil are in control, while humans are at the mercy of natural forces	Life is controlled by physical and biochemical processes that can be studied and manipulated by humans	Harmony, natural balance Human life is only one aspect of nature and part of the general order of the cosmos Everything in universe has a place and role according to laws that maintain order
Illness/disease	Initiated by supernatural agent with or without justification, via sorcery Cause of health or illness is not organic, but mystical Causes: possession by evil spirits, breaching a taboo, supernatural forces (sorcery, witchcraft)	Wear and tear, accident, injury, pathogens, and fluid and chemical imbalance Cause-effect relationship exists for natural events Life related to structure and functions like machines Life can be reduced or divided into smaller parts Mind and body two distinct entities Cause exists, if only it were known	Disease, imbalance, and chaos result when these laws are disturbed
Health	Gift or reward given as a sign of God's blessing and good will	Illness prevention activities, restoration through exercise, medication, treatments, and other means	Environment, behavior, and sociocultural factors are influential in maintaining health and prevention of disease Maintaining and restoring balance are important to health
Ethnic group	Hispanic-Americans, African-Americans; components found in other groups	White Americans	Native Americans, Asian-Americans; components found in other groups
Other concepts			Yin/yang Hot/cold Harmony/disharmony

Source: Babcock, D. E., & Miller, M. A. (1994). *Client education: Theory and practice.* St. Louis: Mosby. Modified from Albers, cited in Herberg, P. (1989). Theoretical foundations of transcultural nursing. In J. S. Boyle, M. M. Andrews (Eds.), *Transcultural concepts in nursing care.* Boston: Scott, Foresman, with permission.

groups living in a dominant culture that retain certain values and beliefs that are different from the dominant culture" (Leininger, 2002a, p. 122). The Anglo-American cultural values include individualism, independence and freedom, competition and achievement, materialism, technology, instant time and actions, youth and beauty, equal rights (gender), leisure time, scientific facts and numbers, and a sense of generosity in time of crisis; action modes include stress alleviation, personalized acts, self-reliance, and health instruction. These characteristics are consistent with the prevailing culture of the practitioners and organizations that make up the health-care system. In her book, *Culture, Care, Diversity, and Universality: A Theory of Nursing,* Leininger lists information on a sample of some American subgroups (Leininger, 1991a, p. 355). She has identified further special groups as subgroups, such as the homeless, drug users, homosexuals, the deaf, those infected with acquired immunodeficiency syndrome and human immunodeficiency virus, and nurses Leininger, M. M. (1991a).

Difficulties arise when significant values are unknown, in conflict, or poorly understood. The client's cultural values can be quite different from those of the health-care provider. As Leininger (1991a) details in her book, of the 15 sample subgroups presented, 10 share none of the dominant characteristics of health-care systems and Anglo-American clients, and few characteristics are shared by the remaining subgroups. In addition, consider the importance of religious or dominant spiritual influence in all but three of the cultural subgroups presented. Knowledge of the dominant values can assist in providing health promotion or health maintenance information, activities, and programs. An example was noted by Armmer and Humbles (1995), who considered the support from and linkages with church leaders crucial to the success of a health promotion program for African-Americans. We have since seen the increasing importance of the use of the faith communities in community health promotion activities. Leininger (1994) stresses that nurses as primary, secondary, and tertiary care providers, through their close and continuous

contact with culturally diverse clients, must move from unicultural personal and professional knowledge to provide meaningful culturally based nursing care (p. 255). Time, openness, and a growing understanding are critical components of a clinician's development of higher levels of cultural competence.

Campinha-Bacote (2003) has proposed a model specifically to address becoming culturally competent, *The Process of Cultural Competence in the Delivery of Healthcare Services Model.* She describes cultural competence as "the process in which the nurse continuously strives to achieve the ability and the availability to effectively work within the cultural context of a client (individual, family or community)"(Campinha-Bacote, 1998, p. 6). The model is illustrated as a volcano; as cultural desire erupts, it leads to "becoming culturally competent" rather than "being," to illustrate the process through cultural awareness, cultural knowledge, cultural encounters, and cultural skill (p. 3–4). Time, openness, and a growing level of understanding are required of the clinician to develop the cultural skills. This ongoing process of becoming culturally competent is similar to Maslow's Hierarchy of Needs and the quest for self-actualization at the top of the hierarchy. Cultural competence is the pursuit of a goal.

Consider the results of a research study by Froman and Owen (2003). The purpose of the research was to validate an instrument used with hospitalized clients on advanced directives. The researchers found that the instrument was valid, in both the English and Spanish versions. However, differences were also found in the preferences, in that the Hispanic adult participants had less knowledge of advanced directives and a higher preference for life-support interventions. Froman and Owen (2003) were able to support the validity of the instrument but did recommend further study to address the "great diversity among Hispanic regions and culture" (p. 36). Consider the following variables:

- Time with clients to become accepted and gain an understanding of their belief system

- Differences in belief systems among generations and geographic origin
- Religious influences
- Familial influences
- Understanding of advanced directives
- Acceptance of the health-care services, systems, and practitioners
- Linguistic issues.

Other individual values may not be initially apparent or may grow more dominant. Complementary and alternative medicine (CAM) and health-care practices, such as acupuncture, imagery, and herbal medicines, are being tried as people become dissatisfied with the biomedical view and move to holistic care. These practices may differ from a client's inherited cultural background but may be adopted or become more dominant. In addition, they may be used along with (complementary) or instead of (alternative) conventional medicine, and their use may or may not be reported by the client to the health-care provider. Spector (2000) reports the rapidly growing use of homeopathic health-care choices as alternative or complementary (e.g., aromatherapy, biofeedback, hypnotherapy, massage) and ethnocultural or traditional (e.g., herbals and holistic healing practices and rituals). And the research and body of knowledge on many of these practices is growing. This increase in use and acceptance of CAM also points to the need for a comprehensive cultural assessment with the client and may require of the clinician great openness, sensitivity, and time.

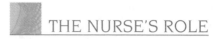 THE NURSE'S ROLE

Nurses have a primary responsibility in health promotion, health maintenance, and prevention activities; in fact, such activities represent the essence of professional nursing practice. The focus of nursing is on the health of the individual, family, community, and societal group. Health promotion roles are guided within the theoretical framework on which nursing practice is based, including how you, as the professional, view the client, the concept of health, the environment, and the practice of nursing as well as your accord with a model's definitions and relationships. This is the purpose of the middle-range theories discussed in Chapter 3, from which you can move to a practice model that is applicable to your specific function or practice setting. Before you decide on the best framework to guide your own professional practice, consider the following two examples.

Example 1

Suppose your practice is guided by King's theory of goal attainment. In this theory, nursing is defined as "a process of human interactions between nurse and client whereby each perceives the other and the situation, and through communications, they set goals, explore the means to achieve them, agree to the means, [and] their actions indicate movement toward goal achievement" (King, 1987, p. 113). Health promotion, health maintenance, and prevention activities are all implied in this definition of *health* as adjustment to stressors in the system environments and use of resources. Health is viewed as a potential and the goal of the process. Specific assessment and intervention activities must address the theory's theoretical concepts and propositions. Personal perceptions of the client are important components of the health belief model, Pender's Health Promotion Model, and the Chronic Illness Trajectory Framework. If your practice setting is a clinic with a large population that needs health promotion strategies addressing individual lifestyles and the preventive services identified in Healthy People 2010, you may find the health belief model or Pender's health promotion model quite useful with your clients. These same models can address health maintenance as secondary and tertiary prevention. On the other hand, if your practice setting is a hospice or you work primarily with patients with cancer and their families, you may find the chronic illness trajectory framework more useful for guiding your practice and use of the nursing process.

Example 2

If your practice is guided by Leininger's (1991b, 2002c) Culture Care Diversity and Universality model, three modes of cultural care guide your nursing judgment, decisions, and actions: preservation and maintenance, accommodation and negotiation, and repatterning or restructuring. In Leininger's concept of culturally congruent nursing care, these modes all focus on health promotion, health maintenance, and prevention activities within the context of the client's cultural belief system. She defines culturally *congruent nursing care* as "the specific use of culturally based care and health knowledge in sensitive, creative, and meaningful ways to fit the general lifeways and needs of individuals or groups for beneficial and meaningful health and well-being or to face illness, disabilities, or death" (Leininger, 2002c, p. 84). The practice models and assessment tools you select must be culturally sensitive and must include individual focus on each of the assessment factors in the sunrise model, which is used by Leininger (1991b, 2002c) to depict the dimensions of her theory visually.

Selecting a health model involves a deliberate and reflective process that takes into account your views, the theory that guides your professional practice, and the unique characteristics of the people and environment in which you work. You may practice under several similar models, depending on a changeable environment or client group interactions.

Key Points

- Health promotion and health protection strategies relate to individual lifestyle and environmental influences on health status and health prospects. Preventive activities and services address three areas of prevention. Primary prevention consists of healthy actions taken to avoid illness or disease. Secondary prevention involves screening for early detection and treatment of health problems. Tertiary prevention during the rehabilitative phase of an illness prevents complications and further disability.
- Health is more than the absence of illness, disease, or infirmity. A concept of health is determined by one's worldview and philosophical assumptions.
- Benner and Wrubel (1989) have described five theories of health as (1) an ideal, (2) the ability to fulfill social roles, (3) a commodity, (4) a human potential, and (5) a sense of coherence.

(continued)

(*continued*)

- Dunn's high-level wellness emphasizes well-being, including the positive, dynamic, and unique integration of mind, body, and spirit of the individual functioning within his or her environment and the individual's maximum potential.

- The health belief model was designed as an organizing framework to advance health promotion activities by targeting interventions to certain individual variables. Three major concepts explain and predict health-related behaviors: (1) readiness to undertake recommended compliance behavior, (2) modifying and enabling factors, and (3) compliant behaviors.

- Pender's health promotion model is a schematic representation with three components for health-promoting behaviors. Individual characteristics and experiences include prior related behavior and personal factors (biologic, psychological, and sociocultural factors). Behavior-specific cognitions and affect include perceived benefits, perceived barriers, perceived self-efficacy, activity-related affect interpersonal influences, and situational influences. The behavioral outcome is attainment of a positive health outcome through commitment to the plan of action and competing demands and preferences.

- The chronic illness trajectory framework (Corbin and Strauss, 1992a) is a conceptual model organized under the main concept of trajectory for managing an evolving course of a chronic condition.

- Gordon's (2002) 11 functional health patterns can be used as a valuable tool in the nursing assessment and diagnosis process and in the application of models to address health and illness focused on human potential or a sense of coherence.

- Culture involves a combination of social, familial, religious, national, and professional characteristics that affect the way we think, act, and interact with others. Differences among groups and subgroups produce diversity that can lead from uniculturalism to appreciation of a multicultural environment and health-care behaviors.

- "Cultural competence demands that nurses look at patients through both their own eyes and the eyes of patients and family members" (Mazanec & Tyler, 2003, p. 52).

- Leininger (2002c) defines cultural care as "the synthesized and culturally constituted assistive, supportive, and facilitative caring acts toward self or others focused on evident or anticipated needs for the client's health or well-being or to face disabilities, death or other human conditions" (p. 83).

- Campinha-Bacote (2003) has proposed the process of Cultural Competence in the Delivery of Healthcare Services Model to illustrate cultural desire leading to cultural awareness, cultural knowledge, cultural encounters, and cultural skill.

- Complementary and alternative medicine (CAM) and health-care practices, such as acupuncture, imagery, and herbal medicines, are being tried as people become dissatisfied with the biomedical view and move to holistic care.

- Nursing focuses on the health of the individual, family, community, and societal group. Health promotion roles are guided by the theoretical framework on which practice is based.

Thought and Discussion Questions

1. Select a definition provided for health from the nursing theories presented in Chapter 4. Discuss which of the five models of health they fit into, and suggest health promotion models for each.

2. Use Pender's health promotion model to plan a health promotion campaign for one of the following situations:
   - Immunization program in an urban apartment complex with a high density of families with young children
   - Home safety program at a senior citizens' center
   - Wellness program for employees in a manufacturing company
3. Recall a client with a chronic illness for whom you have provided nursing care in the past. Retrospectively apply the chronic illness trajectory framework to the client's experiences that you were able to observe.
4. Think of an example from your experience in which culture affected perception of health, illness, or treatment. How did you or could you alter your approach to the client?
5. Review the Chapter Thought located on the first page of the chapter, and discuss it in the context of the contents of the chapter.

 ## Interactive Exercises

1. Levels of prevention using the health belief model: Find an organization not mentioned in the chapter that has a mission of health promotion. Complete the online activity comparing the organizational activity on the Intranet with the Health Belief Model, and identify specific examples of activities directed at primary, secondary, and tertiary levels of prevention.
2. Comparisons of cultural beliefs and practices: Select a cultural subgroup other than your own. Interview several representatives from that subgroup and from your own extended family on the topics listed in the Intranet site. Summarize what is said about each topic in the online activity. Analyze the differences between the two groups. Choose an appropriate health promotion model for use with that group, and describe areas to which you will need to pay particular attention in assessment and intervention activities. Be prepared to discuss your comparisons and findings in an online chat or in class.
3. Conduct an online search using the keyword "cultural competence" for a health-care site and its mission. Compare the results with the position statements on cultural diversity for the following nursing organizations:
   - American Association of Colleges of Nursing at **http://www.aacn.nche.edu/Publications/positions/diverse.htm**
   - American Nurses Association (ANA) at **http://www.nursingworld.org/readroom/position/ethics/etcldv.htm.**
   - Cross Cultural Health Care at **http://www.xculture.org**

   Be prepared to participate in a class or online discussion on the topic, to be scheduled by your instructor.
4. Find an example of a specific magico-religious belief about health by conducting an online search. Be prepared to participate in a class or online discussion on the topic, to be scheduled by your instructor.
5. Complete an online search for complementary and alternative medicine (CAM) practice. Determine how it could fit with the traditional alliopathic view of health care. Be prepared to participate in a class or online discussion on the topic, to be scheduled by your instructor.

6. Complete an online search on COPD, childhood asthma, or fibromyalgia. Determine how practice could be guided by the chronic illness model. Be prepared to participate in a class or online discussion on the topic, to be scheduled by your instructor.

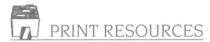

PRINT RESOURCES

References

Andrews, M. M. (2003). Theoretical foundations of transcultural nursing. In M. M. Andrews, & J. S. Boyle, *Transcultural Concepts in Nursing Care* (4th ed.). Philadelphia: Lippincott Williams & Wilkins.

Armmer, F. A., & Humbles, P. (1995). Parish nursing: Extending health care to urban African-Americans. *Nursing and Health Care: Perspectives on Community*, 16, 64–68.

Babcock, D. E., & Miller, M. A. (1994). *Client education: Theory and practice*. St. Louis: Mosby.

Becker, M. H., Haefner, D. P., Kasl, S. V., Kirscht, J. P., Maiman, L. A., & Rosenstock, I. M. (1977). Selected psychosocial models and correlates of individual health-related behaviors. *Medical Care*, 15(5, Supplement), 27–46.

Benner, P., & Wrubel, J. (1989). *The primacy of caring: Stress and coping in health and illness*. Menlo Park, CA: Addison-Wesley.

Betancourt, J. R., Green, A. R., & Carrillo, J. E. (2002, October). *Cultural competence in health care: Emerging frameworks and practical approaches* (Field Report, Publication No. 576). New York: The Commonwealth Fund.

Campinha-Bacote, J. (2003). *The process of cultural competence in the delivery of healthcare services: A culturally competent model of care* (4th. ed.). Cincinnati, OH: Transcultural C.A.R.E. Associates. Also *http://www.transculturalcare.net*.

Corbin, J. M., & Strauss, A. (1992a). A nursing model for chronic illness management based upon the trajectory framework. In P. Woog (Ed.), *The chronic illness trajectory framework: The Corbin and Strauss nursing model* (pp. 9–28). New York: Springer.

Corbin, J. M., & Strauss, A. (1992b). Commentary. In P. Woog (Ed.), *The chronic illness trajectory framework: The Corbin and Strauss nursing model* (pp. 97–102). New York: Springer.

Dunn, H. L. (1973). *High level wellness*. Arlington, VA: Beatty.

Froman, R. D., & Owen, S. V. (2003). Validation of the Spanish Life Support Preference Questionnaire (LSPQ). *Journal of Nursing Scholarship*, 35(1), pp. 33–36.

Glanz, K., Rimer, B. K., Lewis, F. M. (Eds.) (2002). *Health behavior and health education: Theory, research, and practice* (3rd. ed). San Francisco: Jossey-Bass.

Gordon, M. (2002). *Nursing diagnosis: Process and application* (10th ed.). St. Louis: Elsevier Science.

Gunther, M. E. (2002). Martha E. Rogers: Unitary human beings. In A. M. Tomey & M. R. Alligood (Eds.), *Nursing theorists and their work* (5th ed.) (pp. 226–249). St.Louis: Mosby.

Jourard, S. M. (1971). *The transparent self*. New York: Litton Educational.

King, I. M. (1987). King's theory of goal attainment. In R. R. Parse (Ed.), *Nursing science: Major paradigms, theories, and critiques* (pp. 107–113). Philadelphia: W. B. Saunders.

King, I. M. (1981). *A theory for nursing: Systems, concepts, process*. New York: John Wiley & Sons.

Leininger, M. (2002a). Culture care assessments for congruent competency practices. In M. Leininger & M. R. McFarland, *Transcultural nursing: Concepts, theories, research, and practice* (3rd ed.) (pp. 117–143). New York: McGraw-Hill.

Leininger, M. (2002b). Cultures and tribes of nursing, hospitals, and the medical culture. In M. Leininger & M. R. McFarland, *Transcultural nursing: Concepts, theories, research, and practice* (3rd ed.) (pp. 181–204). New York: McGraw-Hill.

Leininger, M. (2002c). The theory of culture care and ethnonursing research method. In M. Leininger & M. R. McFarland, *Transcultural nursing: Concepts, theories, research, and practice* (3rd ed.) (pp. 71–98).. New York: McGraw-Hill.

Leininger, M. M. (1994). Transcultural nursing education: A worldwide imperative. *Nursing and Health Care*, 15, 254–257.

Leininger, M. M. (1991a). Selected culture care findings of diverse cultures using culture care theory and ethnomethods. In M. M. Leininger (Ed.), *Culture care diversity and universality: A theory of nursing* (Pub. No. 15–2402) (pp. 345–371). New York: National League for Nursing.

Leininger, M. M. (1991b). The theory of culture care diversity and universality. In M. M. Leininger (Ed.), *Culture care diversity and universality: A theory of nursing* (Pub. No. 15–2402) (pp. 5–68). New York: National League for Nursing.

Leininger, M. (1970). *Nursing and anthropology: Two worlds to blend*. New York: John Wiley & Sons.

Lutjens, L. R. J. (1991). *Callista Roy: An adaptation model*. Newbury Park, CA: Sage.

Mazanec, P., & Tyler, M. K. (2003). Cultural considerations in end-of-life care. *American Journal of Nursing*, 103(3), 50–59.

Mishel, M. H. (1990). Reconceptualization of the uncertainty in illness theory. *Image: Journal of Nursing Scholarship*, 22, 256–262.

Parse, R. R. (1981). *Man-living-health: A theory of nursing*. New York: John Wiley & Sons.

Pender, N. J. (1996). *Health promotion in nursing practice* (3rd ed.). Stamford, CT: Appleton & Lange.

Pender, N. J. (1987). *Health promotion in nursing practice* (2nd ed.). Norwalk, CT: Appleton & Lange.

Pender, N. J., Murdaugh, C. L., and Parsons, M. A. (2002). *Health promotion in nursing practice* (4th ed.). Upper Saddle River, NJ: Prentice Hall.

Spector, R. E. (2000). *Cultural diversity in health & illness* (5th ed.). Upper Saddle River, NJ: Prestice Hall Health.

Strauss, A. L., Corbin, J., Fagerhaugh, S., Glaser, B. G., Maines, D., Suczek, B., & Wiener, C. L. (1984). *Chronic illness and the quality of life* (2nd ed.). St. Louis: C. V. Mosby.

Strauss, A. L., & Glaser, B. G. (1975). *Chronic illness and the quality of life*. St. Louis: C. V. Mosby.

U.S. Department of Health and Human Services, Public Health Service. (1992). *Healthy People 2000: Summary Report*. Boston: Jones & Bartlett.

Bibliography

Endelman, C. L., & Mandle, C. L. (2002). *Health promotion throughout the lifespan* (5th ed.). St. Louis: Mosby.

Clark, C. C. (2000). *Integrating complementary health procedures into practice*. New York: Springer.

Clark, C. C., Gordon, R. J., & Harris, B. (2000). *Encyclopedia of complementary health practice*. New York: Springer.

Frankenburg, W. K., Dodds, J. B., Fandal, A. W., Kazuk, E., & Cohrs, M. (1975). *Denver developmental screening test* (Rev. ed.). Denver: LADOCA Project & Publishing Foundation.

Kelley, M. L., & Fitzsimons, V. M. (1999). *Understanding cultural diversity: Culture, curriculum, and community in nursing*. Boston: Jones & Bartlett/NLN.

Munhall, P. L., & Boyd, C. O. (1999). *Nursing research: A qualitative perspective* (2nd ed.). New York: Appleton-Century-Crofts.

Munro, B. H. (2003). Caring for the Hispanic populations: The state of the science. *Journal of Transcultural Nursing, 14*, 174–176.

Purnell, L. D., & Paulanka, B. J. (1998). *Transcultural health care: A culturally competent approach*. Philadelphia: F.A. Davis.

Rundle, A. K., Carvalho, M., & Robinson, M. (1999). *Honoring patient preferences: A guide to complying with multicultural patient requirements*. San Francisco: Jossey-Bass.

Snyder, M., & Lindquist, R. (2002). *Complementary/alternative therapies in nursing* (4th ed.). New York: Springer.

Tate, D. M. (2003). Cultural awareness: Bridging the gap between caregivers and Hispanic patients. *Journal of Continuing Education in Nursing, 34*, 213–217.

Zahn, L. (1999). *Asian voices: Asian and Asian American health educators speak out*. Boston: Jones & Bartlett/NLN.

 ONLINE RESOURCES

References

Baldwin, D. M. (2003). Disparaties in health care: Focusing efforts to eliminate unequal burdens (Continuing Education). *http://www.nursingworld.org/mods/mod560/cebrdnfull.htm*

Campinha-Bacote, J. (January 31, 2003). Many faces: Addressing diversity in health care. *Online Journal of Issues in Nursing, 8* (1), Manuscript 2. *http://nursingworld.org/ojin/topic/tpc20_2.htm*.

Campinha-Bacote, J. (1998). The process of cultural competence in the delivery of healthcare services: A culturally competent model of care. Cincinnati, OH: Transcultural C.A.R.E. Associates. *http://www.transcultur-alcare.net*

U.S. Department of Health and Human Services. (2000). *Healthy People 2010: Understanding and improving health*. *http://www.healthypeople.gov/publications*.

U.S. Department of Health & Human Services, Public Health Service, (USDHHS, PHS). *Healthy People* 2010 (Conference Edition, in Two Volumes). Washington, DC: U.S. Government Printing Office. Available online: *http://www.health.gov/healthypeople*.

Resources

The Center for Cross-Cultural Health. *www.crosshealth.com*

Initiative to Eliminate Racial & Ethnic Disparities in Health. *http://racehealth.hhs.gov*

Office of Minority Health. *http://odphp.osophs.dhhs.gov*

National Center for CAM. *http://nccam.nih.gov*

National Center for Cultural Competence. *www.georgetown.edu/research/gucdc/nccc*

Transcultural C.A.R.E. Associates. *www.transculturalcare.net*

Agency for Healthcare Reseach & Quality. *www.ahrq.gov*

The Commonwealth Fund. *www.cmwf.org*

U.S. Dept. Of Health & Human Services. *www.hhs.gov*

Rose Kearney-Nunnery

Evidence-Based Practice

We may search for information, but once gained, how does it become wisdom?

Chapter Objectives

On completion of this chapter, the reader will be able to:

1. Explain the importance of evidence-based practice for the profession of nursing.
2. Define basic terminology used in research for application of findings in practice.
3. Describe legal and ethical considerations applicable to research with human subjects.
4. Describe different ways to participate in nursing research.
5. Analyze barriers to evidence-based practice.
6. Prepare a basic critique of a published research study.
7. Plan for the inclusion of a higher level of evidence-based care in his or her practice setting.

Key Terms

Evidence-Based Practice
Research
Ethical Codes
Basic Human Rights
Beneficence
Full Disclosure
Self-Determination
Privacy and
    Confidentiality

Minimal Risk
Empirical Research
Qualitative Research
Research Critique
Research Problem
Literature Review
Hypotheses
Research Design

Operational Definition
Variables
Sampling
Data Collection
    Procedures
Instruments
Descriptive Statistics
Inferential Statistics

Theory guides practice, but current knowledge and practice must be based on evidence of efficacy rather than intuition, tradition, or past practice. Out of a national concern for safety initiatives in 1999 and a focus on systems issues in 2001, the national call came for changes in the education and competencies of health professionals in all disciplines in 2003. The result was the identification of the five core competencies for health professionals identified in Chapter 1. The importance of employing evidence-based practice was described as follows:

> The committee feels that it is critical for interdisciplinary health teams and each of the disciplines to be able to tap this evidence base effectively at the point of patient care, determining whether an intervention, such as a preventive service, diagnostic test, or therapy, can be expected to produce better outcomes than alternatives—including the alternative of doing nothing. (Greiner & Knebel, 2003, p. 56)

Sigma Theta Tau (2003), the International Honor Society of Nursing, defines the use of **evidence-based practice** as "an integration of the best evidence available, nursing expertise, and the values and preferences of the individuals, families, and communities who are selected" (p. 2). This does not sound unique to our view of nursing and quality health care. The problem is that we are not consistently *using* the best evidence available to guide care to clients. And the next questions become: Do we have the best evidence available? Where is the information? And, are we applying appropriate knowledge in clinical situations? A paradigm shift occurred, with the call for evidence-based practice.

Research supports our knowledge base and answers questions of clinical concern. It provides sound information on which to base practice, as evidence-based nursing practice. Evidence can come from a number of sources, but as Mulhall (2001) observes, "evidence from research studies is crucially important to best practice" (p. 124). We need both seekers and users of the information in practice to develop knowledge. Clinicians in the practice setting have the questions. These questions must be refined and studied so that nurse researchers can find solutions to health-care practice problems. And we further need the validation from the consumer as to the appropriateness of the intervention. This is truly evidence-based practice.

 NURSING RESEARCH

Research has been defined as a "systematic, controlled, empirical and critical investigation of natural phenomena guided by theory and hypotheses about the presumed relations among such phenomena" (Kerlinger, 1986, p. 10). Given this definition, research is still viewed by some as an academic exercise. But it is much more in nursing. The purposes of research are to describe, explain, predict, and control phenomena and to provide information for future use in practice or for expansion of the knowledge base.

Nursing research began with Florence Nightingale and her identification of environmental influences on health and illness. In her classic *Notes on Nursing: What It Is, and What It Is Not* (1859), Nightingale identified factors that influence health and wellness, supporting them with observational accounts, statistics, and deductive reasoning. Following her landmark efforts, non-nurse researchers performed limited research on nurses and nursing education. Then in the mid-20th century, graduate nursing programs began to proliferate, as did nurses' involvement in research studies, often on nurses and delivery of nursing services. The introduction of the journal *Nursing Research* in 1952 provided a specific channel for disseminating research findings to other nurses.

During the second half of the 20th century, the number of graduate and baccalaureate nursing programs grew. Content on research became prevalent in baccalaureate nursing curricula during the 1970s and early 1980s. Graduate student enrollments increased with the growth in doctoral programs in the 1980s.

Research findings were used to develop and refine conceptual and theoretical models. More nurses were now doing research, and the American Nurses Association (ANA) Cabinet on Nursing Research identified research expectations by level of education in 1981. The primary focus of research changed during this time from educational programs and methods to the focus of nursing: people as patients, clients, and members of society. Support has grown for research as we see the needs to investigate the domain of nursing, test theories and interventions, and demonstrate efficacy and efficiency of nursing actions and client outcomes.

Nursing research is further supported in the position statement of the American Association of Colleges of Nursing (AACN, 1999a). This organization of member schools with baccalaureate and graduate programs believes that its membership facilitates the conduct of research and the utilization of research findings through the education of professional nurses and nurse scientists (AACN, 1999a, p. 1). This concept has implications for the baccalaureate-prepared nurse in the identification of research problems, the support of ongoing research, and the use of applicable findings in practice.

The establishment of the National Center for Nursing Research (NCNR) as part of the National Institutes of Health (NIH) in April 1986, under the Health Research Extension Act of 1985 (PL99-158), demonstrated the importance of research for and by the profession. In 1993, the National Institute of Nursing Research (NINR) was established, a change from the former divisional and center status, with fiscal year appropriations from Congress growing, thus further demonstrating the importance of generating knowledge in nursing. An important component of the mission of the NINR is to support "clinical and basic research to establish a scientific basis for the care of individuals across the life span—from management of patients during illness and recovery to the reduction of risks for disease and disability, the promotion of healthy lifestyles, promoting quality of life in those with chronic illness, and care for individuals at the end of life" (NINR, 2003). Extramural research programs for the NINR concern (1) health promotion and disease prevention, (2) acute and chronic illness, and (3) nursing systems.

Research proposals are highly competitive at NINR, more so than in many other areas of NIH. Research proposals are reviewed by a panel of experts and scored according to the consistency with the mission of NINR and the merit of the research project. During the initial phase of NINR initiatives, research priorities were specified for investigations. In 2004, the NINR issued research opportunities to focus on the following nursing initiatives:

Chronic Illnesses or Conditions

- Chronic Illness Self-Management and Quality of Life

Behavioral Changes and Interventions

- Decreasing Low Birth Weight Infants Among Minority Populations
- Enhancing Health Promotion Among Minority Men

Responding to Compelling Public Health Concerns

- End-of-Life: Bridging Life and Death
- Nursing Research Training and Centers

A vital issue is the need for reliable and valid research on questions of clinical concern for decision-making and change. In nursing, research must be directed at interventions over which nursing has control so that the

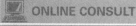

ONLINE CONSULT

National Institute of Nursing Research at
www.nih.gov.ninr
Federal Opportunities for Research Funding at
www.grants.gov

knowledge developed can lead to needed change. This is the essence of evidence-based professional nursing practice.

For some time, Sigma Theta Tau has recognized the importance of generating and using research. The purposes of this honor society include encouraging scholarly and creative work. This purpose is applicable to both the conduct and utilization of research. Scholarship involves discovery, integration, application, and teaching. Utilizing and communicating research in nursing practice projects and conferences have been focuses of Sigma Theta Tau International. The organization also supports research investigations that generate nursing knowledge through competitive extramural grants for researchers, as does the American Foundation of Nursing. Nurses have a major responsibility to identify research problems, support ongoing research, and use applicable findings in practice along with continuing to learn in this area of scholarly nursing practice.

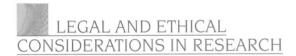

LEGAL AND ETHICAL CONSIDERATIONS IN RESEARCH

An additional responsibility in professional nursing practice is protecting the rights of research subjects.

Background

The rights of people in research have been of great concern to ethicists, legislators, and professionals, leading to ethical codes and guidelines for the protection of research subjects. History has provided much of the impetus for our professional codes and federal regula-

tions. During World War II, experiments noted for the unethical treatment of subjects included the Nazi medical experiments and the Japanese concentration camp experiments on human subjects. As a result, international **ethical codes** evolved. In 1949, the Nuremberg Code set standards for involving human subjects in research, with guidelines for consent, protections, risks and benefits, and qualifications of researchers. The Declaration of Helsinki (1990), made in 1964 and revised in 1975 and 1989, provided guidelines on therapeutic and nontherapeutic research along with the requirements for disclosing the risks and potential benefits of the research and obtaining written consent for participation from research subjects.

Safety, Health, and Welfare

In the United States, the Tuskegee syphilis study on sharecroppers, the Jewish Chronic Disease Hospital study of oncology patients, and the Willowbrook hepatitis study in children are further examples of unethical treatment of research subjects. In the quest for knowledge, researchers failed to consider the basic human rights of their subjects, especially the right of informed consent and considerations for vulnerable populations. Federal regulations evolved from the original guidelines of the former Department of Health, Education and Welfare, culminating in the National Research Act in 1974. This law specified the composition and authority of institutional review boards (IRBs). IRBs were now mandated as oversight bodies to ensure protection of research subjects, especially for research projects seeking federal funding.

The Belmont Report (1979) was the outcome of a National Commission for the

 ONLINE CONSULT

U.S. President's Commission for the Study of Ethical Problems in Medicine and Behavioral Research. (1982). *Compensating for research injuries: The ethical and legal implications of programs to redress injured subjects* (Vol. I). at http://www.gwu.edu/~nsarchiv/radiation/dir/mstreet/commeet/meet16/brief16/tab_b/br16b1a.txt

Protection of Human Subjects of Biomedical and Behavioral Research mandated by the National Research Act. This commission was charged with identifying principles and developing guidelines. The report specified boundaries between practice and research. Basic ethical principles were reinforced, highlighting respect for persons and defining the principles of beneficence (doing no harm, with maximum benefits and minimal risks) and justice (fairness relative to one's share, need, effort, contribution, and merit). Specific applications that resulted from the Belmont Report (1979) were: (1) guidelines on informed consent, including provision of information and ensuring comprehension and voluntariness; (2) assessment of risks and benefits; and (3) selection of subjects. The Belmont Report provided the basis for federal laws, including the federal codes on the Protection of Human Subjects.

All activities involving humans as subjects must provide for the safety, health, and welfare of every individual. Subjects do not abdicate rights with their participation in a research study. Four **basic human rights** must be ensured for research subjects. These principles speak to ethical considerations and human rights:

1. **Beneficence** (do no harm)
2. **Full Disclosure**
3. **Self-determination**
4. **Privacy and confidentiality**

The "do no harm" concept includes careful consideration of the risk-benefit ratio with any research project. One must keep in mind that **minimal risk** requires that "the probability and magnitude of harm or discomfort anticipated in the research are not greater in and of themselves than those encountered in daily life or during the performance of routine physical or psychological examinations or tests" (Protection of Human Subjects, 45 CFR 46, §42.102 [i]). Full disclosure of informa-

---

BOX 6–1
GENERAL PRINCIPLES/ETHICAL GUIDELINES FOR RESEARCH ON HUMAN SUBJECTS

- Risk to the subjects is minimized.
- Risks are reasonable in relation to anticipated benefits to subjects.
- Selection of subjects is equitable.
- Informed consent will be sought from each prospective subject or the legally authorized representative.
- Informed consent will be appropriately documented.
- The research plan makes adequate provision for monitoring the data collected to ensure the safety of subjects.
- Adequate provisions exist to protect the privacy of subjects and maintain the confidentiality of data.
- Special protections are in place for populations that are vulnerable, e.g., children, prisoners, the mentally disabled persons, pregnant women, or economically or educationally disadvantaged persons, because these subjects are vulnerable to coercion or undue influence.

Source: Title 45 Code of Federal Regulations Part 46 (45 CFR 46), §46.111

 ONLINE CONSULT

Federal Guidelines for the Rights of Human Subjects in Research at
http://ohrp.osophs.dhhs.gov/humansubjects/guidance/45cfr46.htm

ONLINE CONSULT

HIPAA. Office of Civil Rights at
http://hss.gov/ocr/hipaa

tion and self-determination by potential subjects are necessary conditions for informed consent. In addition, subjects' rights to privacy and confidentiality must be ensured throughout the process. As protections for these four rights, the guidelines must be considered by researchers and their respective IRBs (Box 6–1).

The issue of privacy of personal health information (PHI) was the focus of the Health Insurance Portability and Accountability Act (HIPAA) of 1996. The Act's Privacy Rule establishes:

[M]inimum Federal standards for protecting the privacy of individually identifiable health information. The Rule confers certain rights on individuals, including rights to access and amend their health information and to obtain a record of when and why their PHI has been shared with others for certain purposes (USDHHS, 2003, p. 2)

For researchers, informed consent is a necessary process. The Privacy Act requires further language in the consent process but does allow for the use of selected categories of PHI, as a *"Limited Data Set"* that may be used or disclosed, for purposes of research, public health, or health-care operations, without obtaining either an individual's authorization or a waiver for its use and disclosure, with a data use agreement (USDHHS, 2003, p. 26).

As with other areas of nursing practice, legal and ethical considerations are deliberated with any research activity. These issues occur in the planning, implementation, analysis, and reporting stages for a research endeavor. In the proposal or planning stage of any research study, the researcher must consider the rights of the subjects and the ethical nature of the study. When a researcher defines the problem and purpose of the research, the significance of the problem for the body of knowledge and the ethical issues associated with the proposed investigation are vital considerations.

The Institutional Review Board

Once the basic research plan is developed, an IRB must review and approve the start of the study. In the past, many IRBs were called "human subjects committees," but strict federal guidelines for review by an IRB must be adhered to, especially in agencies seeking funding for research. Human subjects' rights of full disclosure, self-determination (informed consent), privacy and confidentiality, and safety (not to be harmed) must be ensured. The research proposal, with statements of the problem and purpose or significance, literature support, theory and definitions, specific research questions or hypotheses, design, sampling plans, and data collection and analysis methods must be approved for use with human subjects. The researcher submits a proposal to an IRB for approval or exemption to proceed to the next step of data collection. During this stage of implementing the research project, the investigator must adhere to the procedures specified for data collection and analysis. Evaluation is done throughout the project to ensure that subjects are not placed at risk and that the integrity and confidentiality of the data are maintained during collection, analysis, and dissemination of the findings.

ANA Guidelines

In addition to basic ethical principles, federal, state, local, and institutional regulations, the ANA (1985) has specified human rights guidelines for nurses in research. These guidelines address the rights of both subjects and professionals. As with the federal rules, the nursing guidelines address the basic human rights of research subjects, including freedom from harm, informed consent, and preservation of privacy. Ten years later, and with the consideration of societal and professional practice changes that had occurred, new guidelines based on nine principles were published (Silva, 1995, p. 2). As shown in Box 6–2, these principles address beneficence, full disclosure, self-determination, privacy and confidentiality, and the skills of the researcher.

Each of the nine principles (see Box 6–2) charges the investigator with specific responsibilities. Explanatory commentary and specific research guidelines are presented for each of the nine principles. For example, with the protection of subjects against harm, vulnerable groups discussed specifically are pregnant women, children, persons with human immunodeficiency virus (HIV) or acquired immunodeficiency syndrome (AIDS), and the elderly. All of the principles require that professionals in a practice setting must be aware of any ongoing research and its associated risks to both subjects and participants. And nurses have both the right and the responsibility to participate in research. Participation

of nurses should be evident; for example, they should function as members of research teams and IRBs. Nurses can also actively participate by giving support and assistance to others involved in research for the advancement of knowledge and enhancement of professional practice. The process of research with human subjects must be diligent and must benefit subjects and participants through the acquisition and use of new knowledge.

Consult the government and institional Web sites for information on protections for human subjects in research.

 PROCESSES OF NURSING RESEARCH

The actual research process is generally thought of as the scientific method. However, this can be misleading when one considers the

---

BOX 6–2
ETHICAL PRINCIPLES IN THE CONDUCT, DISSEMINATION, AND IMPLEMENTATION OF NURSING RESEARCH

The Investigator:

1. Respects autonomous research participant's capacity to consent to participate in research and to determine the degree and duration of that participation without negative consequences.
2. Prevents harm, minimizes harm, and/or promotes good to all research participants, including vulnerable groups and others affected by the research.
3. Respects the personhood of research participants, their families, and significant others, valuing their diversity.
4. Ensures that the benefits and burdens of research are equitably distributed in the selection of research participants.
5. Protects the privacy of research participants to the maximum degree possible.
6. Ensures the ethical integrity of the research process by the use of appropriate checks and balances throughout the conduct, dissemination, and implementation of the research.
7. Reports suspected, alleged, or known incidents of scientific misconduct in research to appropriate institutional officials for investigation.
8. Maintains competency in the subject matter and methodologies of his or her research as well as in other professional and societal issues that affect nursing research and the public good.
9. If involved in animal research, maximizes the benefits of the research with the least possible harm or suffering to the animals.

Source: Silva, M. (1995). *Ethical guidelines in the conduct, dissemination, and implementation of nursing research* (p. 4). Washington, DC: American Nurses Association.

different types of research. To understand the basics of nursing research, first think about the scientific method as a systematic process for answering a question or testing a hypothesis. One problem emerges: This is easier done in a controlled laboratory setting, with variables such as chemicals, than in a natural setting in which the variables involve people, well or ill, who need nursing interventions. With this in mind, it is easiest to begin with empirical research using quantitative methods.

The Empirical Method

First, consider the steps of research. **Empirical research** is based on the strict rules of the scientific method and on the philosophical perspective of positivism. With this perspective, the focus is on an observable, measurable, and predictable world. It is guided by a controlled set of steps that one goes through to observe something or test a hypothesis. It is a deductive and linear method with the following steps:

1. Identification of the problem
2. Statement of the purpose
3. Review of the literature
4. Description of theoretical framework
5. Definition of terms
6. Statement of hypothesis(es)
7. Selection of the research design, population, and sample
8. IRB approval
9. Collection of data
10. Analysis and interpretation of data
11. Presentation of findings and recommendations

Using this empirical approach, the researcher may return to a prior step in the planning stage, for example, to refine the problem after the review of the literature, but will still go through all successive steps in a systematic and controlled manner to maintain the integrity of the process. Once the plans for the study are finalized, strict research protocols are adhered to with quantitative methods, to reduce threats to the validity of the study. Although some of the steps may be combined, nurse researchers using quantitative methods engage in the same process to describe, explain, predict, and control phenomena of concern to nursing. The following is a review of the research process.

In the initial step of *problem identification*, the researchers specify what they are interested in studying. This is the "what" that will be done as the study progresses. For example, a specific nursing intervention is compared with a traditional nursing intervention for a selected group of clients. Next, researchers specify the reason they are interested in this problem, or the *purpose of the research*. At this time, the significance of the problem for the body of knowledge and ethical issues associated with the proposed investigation are considerations. This is "why" the researchers want to investigate the new intervention, for example, to effectively improve the health awareness or healthy behaviors of the client group.

The researchers next search the *literature* to "discover" what is known on the topics: the interventions, the client group, cultural factors, useful theoretical bases (e.g., self-care), and what problems have been studied in the area. This provides the current information known on the topic. This is a time-intensive process that requires absorbing a great deal of information for the planning stage of the project. Researchers perform literature searches, followed by careful critique and assimilation of the information. Next, researchers specify the philosophical orientation that will guide the research, the *theoretical framework*. The *defining terms and variables* specific to the study emerge from the theoretical framework, as do specific research questions that will be addressed or the *hypotheses* (predictions) the study will test.

So far we have the basic idea for the investigation, but the researchers must select a design or plan for the study that is appropriate for the problem in light of the theoretical framework. Once the appropriate *design* has been selected, the researchers must *define the population*—those individuals or groups to whom the findings will be applicable or generalizable. Researchers know that not all the people to whom the research applies can be studied, so they must study a select group of the population: the *sample*. The researchers' decision about the type and the size of the sample is based on the research design, the theoretical framework, research purpose, and research problem. It all relates back in a linear manner, but the goals in sampling are to limit bias and statistical error and for the sample to be representative of the population.

The researchers now have the basic plan for their investigations, but no one has been studied yet. The rights of human subjects must be considered and protected. At this point the researcher submits a proposal to an IRB for approval or exemption to proceed to the next step of data collection. Once IRB approval has been secured, the researcher is ready to begin *collecting data*.

Plans for data collection and analysis have already been made in the research proposal and are strictly adhered to. Researchers must follow the proposed design when data are collected; for example, they cannot decide to replace interviews that were planned with a questionnaire. Data must be collected in an orderly and systematic manner and must be recorded before analysis and decision-making begin.

Measurement issues are of prime concern.

The type of data collected and the measurement instruments are, again, determined before the study is started, on the basis of the research problem, literature review, theoretical basis, research questions or hypotheses, research design, and sampling method. Issues of reliability (consistency of measurement) and validity (measuring the variable of interest properly) are considered by the researcher from prior methodologic studies, use in similar research, or a pilot study as a small-scale version or a formal trial to resolve any methodologic issues. Measurements may be self-reported, in writing, by the subjects in the sample (tests, questionnaires, diaries, etc.) or may require taping or note-taking by researchers in personal or telephone interviews.

Measurements can also be observations of behavior (ability to perform a skill, like a dressing change), responses by subjects on a scale (such as a Likert scale or a scale for pain perception from 0 to 10), physiologic measures (such as blood pressure, electrocardiogram, electroencephalogram, or oxygen saturation), review of records, or a number of other types of methods. Research protocols are strictly adhered to: the identical and detailed process is used with each research subject. Scripts are used to read instructions to subjects to ensure that each subject has been given the same information for the data collection process.

Once all subjects have been investigated and all data collected, the researcher moves into the *analysis stage*. The analysis provides information to answer the research questions or support or refute the hypotheses. The analysis stage seems to be the most threatening to the research novice. Keep in mind that the research depends on a good analysis of the data so that reliable, valid information is made available on the topic. The most important decisions for this stage were made before the study was started, with the selection of the correct statistical tests. In addition, computers or statisticians can easily perform calculations. Try to see this stage as one of discovery and understanding how the data provide answers to the research questions or hypotheses. The findings are reported objectively for each research question or hypothesis.

The results of the descriptive statistics (such

as frequencies, means, standard deviations, correlations) are reported to characterize the sample. Appropriate inferential statistics are used to generalize to the population (such as t-test, analysis of variance, correlations, and multivariate analysis), according to the type of measurement scale, the sample size, and the assumption of a normal distribution. From the point of reporting the statistics, the researcher then *interprets the meaning* and implications relative to the stated research questions or hypotheses. Recommendations for use of the findings and further research are then presented in the research report.

Disseminating the findings to others is the final responsibility of the researcher as part of the particular study. The findings can be disseminated locally, regionally, and nationally through presentations or publications. It is vital that the information be shared with others. If the findings are important and point to a need for change, practicing nurses must have the opportunity and responsibility to implement the information as appropriate to their practice settings. Further research is also needed. If the findings were not significant or were indifferent, then further research is needed, perhaps further specification of the problem, better measurement instruments, or a different environment or sample. If the research findings were negative, the new intervention was less effective than current ones. Still more research may be needed if there were problems with reliability and validity. If a safety issue emerged during the research, a subject would have been withdrawn from the study or the study halted. Still, it is necessary for others to know all situations to make use of good information or avoid problem areas.

Qualitative Research

The research process using qualitative research methods is somewhat different. These methods are inductive and theory-generating research. **Qualitative research** is used to generate theory to explore, describe, and illuminate phenomena. The basis of qualitative research focuses on the meaning and interpretation of experiences to understand some phenomena. Types of research classified as qualitative include ethnography, field studies, grounded theory, historical research, analytic induction, and phenomenology.

Major data collection methods are naturalistic observation (hence the term field studies) and on-site interviewing. Some researchers describe the data that emerge from this research as "information rich," because the researcher begins a study with a need to understand from the perspective of people in the environment. The researcher is not limiting the data collection to a few variables. Rather, he or she is trying to have the people in their environment describe the phenomena; the researcher then classifies concepts, identifies themes, and generates theory. This is why some also see qualitative research as a "humanistic" form of research that discovers people and their unique experiences.

In qualitative research, the linear steps of the process are not the procedure. The researcher must still complete the initial process of developing the project, with *identification of a "problem"* of a little-understood area or phenomena, and the *statement of purpose as an inquiry* for "discovery" of the phenomena. The *review of the literature* looks at what is known, which is often tangential, because little may be known before the research "uncovers" the phenomena. The *theory* will evolve from this research, rather than be driven by it, as are the *terminology* and *future study hypotheses* that use quantitative methods for theory testing. The process of IRB approval is still required prior to data collection, for the protection of human subjects.

Qualitative methods have different inquiry forms and processes. *Data collection* and *analysis* are driven by the particular qualitative method. Reliability and validity issues can be difficult with this form of research, and investigators frequently use triangulation of data to provide valid results. (*Triangulation* involves the use of multiple data sources, complementary investigations, or theoretical perspectives to improve the data's validity.) Dissemination of the findings through presentations and publication is the final step in the process, along with identification of future areas for inquiry.

Choice of Research Method

Whether quantitative or qualitative research methods are selected depends on the phenomena of interest and the purpose of the research. For example, the researcher may select or use qualitative methods to investigate health beliefs of a particular cultural group, but would use quantitative methods to test a new intervention designed to enhance the functional independence of older adults with a limitation in mobility. Comparisons of qualitative research to the empirical research process are illustrated in Table 6–1. Regardless of the methods selected to address the need for information on the problem, the research must respect the individual or group in the quest for knowledge.

THE ROAD TO EVIDENCE-BASED PRACTICE

We have a responsibility to base nursing practice on current knowledge. As Stone and associates (2002) have stated, "basing nursing practice on the best available evidence is now the expected standard of care" (p. 277). This consideration highlights an accountability issue for the profession and focuses the direction of nursing research on clinical issues for improved patient outcomes and effective care in a time when resources are stretched beyond limits. In 1985, Crane described research utilization as the use of research findings to define new practices and the use of research methods to assist in implementing new practices with accuracy and evaluating their impact on patients and staff (p. 262).

This development evolved from the landmark work for research-based nursing practice that began in the 1970s. The WICHE (Western Interstate Commission for Higher Education) Project was a 6-year project funded by the U.S. Department of Health, Education, and Welfare (HEW) between 1971 and 1975. It focused on both the conduct of research projects and the utilization of research findings. The initial thrust of the project was to support collaborative research endeavors followed by a focus on using research findings in practice (Lindeman & Krueger, 1977). The second federally funded activity was the CURN (Conduct and Utilization of Research in Nursing) Project, conducted in Michigan between 1975 and 1981. This project focused on use in the hospital setting of the knowledge from research already available. Finding the information and the applicability to the practice setting were the skills of concern. This led to the development of guidelines and specific protocols for research-based nursing interventions. Videotapes illustrating the process became available, to help nurses base their practice and interventions with clients on research evidence available in the literature.

We are now seeing a positive view of research. Since the 1970s, there has been a growing number of professional journals dedicated to publishing research findings. Specialty journals include special columns or research features. Professional conferences, both general and specialty, now provide more research presentations as special and concurrent offerings. These sessions are well attended, particularly as clinicians' comfort level with terminology and the thirst for the most current information increase. A focus on research has also emerged in certification examinations.

Then in 1981, the ANA Cabinet for Nursing Research developed guidelines for involvement in research based on level of nursing education. Subsequently, both the ANA (1997) and the AACN (1999b) have delineated expectations for nurses' involvement in research according to level of educational preparation. In these guidelines, the graduate with doctoral or postdoctoral preparation is seen as providing leadership on investigations, applying theory, and developing methods to generate knowledge for the discipline. With an expertise in specialty practice, the master's-prepared nurse is the facilitator for using research findings and conducting investigations.

Associate degree and baccalaureate nursing graduates are research consumers. Baccalaureate graduates are also responsible for identifying researchable problems and

TABLE 6–1
Empirical and Qualitative Research Methods

	Empirical Research	Qualitative Research
Identification of the problem	Narrow specification of what is to be studied	Identification of little understood area of phenomena
Statement of the purpose	The reason the problem is of interest; significance	Discovery of the phenomena
Review of Literature	Discover what is already known about the problem	Tangential subjects to demonstrate why little is known on the phenomena
Theoretical framework	Selection and application of a theory or model	To be generated
Definitions and terminology	Define terms as variables to be studied, consistent with the theoretical model	Terminology will emerge from the findings
Questions and hypothesis(es)	Specify questions or hypotheses to be tested, consistent with the theoretical model	Developing broad questions to be asked that will lead to others during the research as discovery
Selection of the research design, population, and sample	Selection of specific design and study instruments Specifying population of interest Identifying group and number of research subjects	Selection of a qualitative method and of a group to seek their descriptions of their human experience, and proposing methods to access the group
Approval of Internal Review Board	Approval of research proposal	Approval of research proposal
Collection of Data	Adherence to research protocol, controls, and steps specified with the study's measurement instruments; for example, the experimental group of subjects has one intervention while the control group received the usual treatment or intervention. Data is systematically recorded	Gaining entry to the group, proposing broad questions, receiving information, and seeking meaning. Further questions are emerging as the study progresses and are pursued in search of meaning and understanding. For example, using grounded theory to see the data falling into differing categories
Data analysis and interpretation	Application of the statistical tests on the specific study variables specified in the research proposal and drawing conclusions from these tests.	Creating meaning and themes from information in transcripts and documents that evolve into different areas and emerge into a theoretical framework.
Presentation of findings	Reporting the statistics on the questions or hypotheses as findings. Drawing conclusions based on the findings and proposing applications and futher investigation.	Proposing a theoretical framework to pursue further investigation of the categories of meaning discovered, thus adding to our theoretical bases described in Chapter 4.

findings from prior research on which to base practice. Nevertheless, there have been problems with disseminating findings and applying them in practice. National practice guidelines have been available since the 1990s, but studies have shown they have not been consistently incorporated in practice. Evidence-based practice is fundamental to contemporary nursing, providing a firm foundation for nursing interventions. It has been identified as one of the core competencies for health professionals in all disciplines. Proficiency in critiquing research is central to the ability to apply research findings to professional practice behavior.

 RESEARCH CRITIQUE

Consider both the objective process of critiquing a research study and the subjective process of evaluating its application to practice.

Objective Evaluation

A **research critique** is an objective analysis of a published research report. The reader must critically consider all components of the report—problem, purpose, supporting literature, theoretical framework, definitions, study questions or hypotheses, design, population and sample, data collection methods and procedures, analysis, and interpretation of findings (Box 6–3). The ultimate goal of a research critique is to evaluate applicability of appropriate scientific findings to one's own professional practice and knowledge base.

Thoughtful critique is based on critical thinking skills used to address the steps of the research process. When publishing research reports, researchers must provide the essential information gained from the study within the given space. This can create a challenge for the reader attempting to glean the vital information for a critique. A published research report is frequently organized into the following sections: abstract, introduction, review of literature, theoretical framework, methods, results, discussion, and references.

Preliminary information provides valuable information for the reader. First, the title of the study should clearly reflect the problem area and capture the reader's interest. Information provided about the researcher includes his or her background and qualifications in the practice area and for conducting the research study. The abstract briefly reviews the problem, purpose, methodology, findings, and conclusions, summarizing the

---

BOX 6–3
AREAS TO ADDRESS IN A RESEARCH CRITIQUE*

Areas to address while doing a thoughtful critique of a research study as a component of evidenced-based practice include:
- Title and abstract
- Introduction, problem, and purpose
- Literature review
- Theoretical framework
- Research questions or hypotheses
- Methods: design, ethics, sampling, data collection
- Results and analysis
- Discussion and recommendations

And now, are the findings applicable to your use in evidence-based practice?

*Further information on the areas to address in a research critique are located on the Intranet site.

content and also capturing the reader's attention.

Next comes the introduction to the research report. The opening paragraphs outline the background of the problem, including its purpose and significance to nursing and the care of clients. The **research problem** is the central question that the research has been designed to answer. It is the "what" that is being done in the study to describe, explain, predict, or control some phenomenon of concern to nursing. The research problem contains the major variables and the population of concern to the researcher. The author may also identify specific research aims in this introductory section.

Next, a **review of literature** pertinent to the research problem is provided. The literature review is a report and comparison of all pertinent prior investigations on the topic, variables of interest, theoretical models, and methods used. Unlike the library research done for a paper, a research literature review concentrates on primary references. A *primary* literature source is the actual report of an investigation or development of an instrument or theory written by the researcher or theorist. Using the primary source eliminates the chance of error in interpretation that could occur through analyses by others or loss of the context of the original work.

The literature review should provide a critical appraisal and synthesis of what is already known on the topic. Thus, the literature review supports the study and how the investigation proposes to contribute to the existing body of nursing knowledge. A review of literature may be conducted electronically with the availability of online databases, resources, and articles. However, caution is recommended on the use of research reports found in chat rooms or on personal Web pages versus a published report of research findings that has not been subjected to a thoughtful peer review process before it is accepted for publication in a referred (peer-reviewed) professional journal.

The theoretical framework may be described in a separate section or may be included with the literature review. As was discussed in Chapters 3 and 4, a theoretical framework or model is the way the researcher views the concepts and their interrelationships; it may be described in words or displayed symbolically. This underlying view drives the research in describing, explaining, predicting, or controlling the phenomena, as in the case of empirical research studies.

At this point, the researcher may present specific questions to address in the study or hypotheses to be tested. Specific research questions must flow from, and relate back to, the main research problem or purpose. **Hypotheses** are predictions about the variables that the investigation is testing with a subject group. Hypotheses may be null (statistical), predicting no relationship; conversely, the researcher may state research (alternative) hypotheses that do predict a difference and, in some cases, the direction of the difference (increase, decrease, greater, less). Both null and research hypotheses can be either simple (stating a prediction between two variables) or complex (stating a difference between more than two variables). Hypothesis testing uses inferential statistics, inferring from the sample to make generalizations about the population. Both research questions and hypotheses must be consistent with the framework that provides the theoretical guidance for the investigation. The variables to be investigated should be readily apparent in either the stated research questions or hypotheses.

The next major section in a published research report describes the methodology or methods. This section contains information on the research design, research subjects (including ethical considerations and sampling), and data collection and procedures used. The **research design** is the overall blueprint for the study. The design specifies the setting for the study, the subjects (sample group), the experimental or nonexperimental treatment or grouping methods, the data collection methods, and procedures or protocol. The research design is selected to address the variables of concern to answer the research questions or test the hypotheses. Study designs may be experimental or nonexperimental. Qualitative research studies are also useful in aiding the understanding of a phenomenon that is relevant to your practice area.

Experimental designs are classified as true experiments, quasi-experiments, and pre-experiments, with varying degrees of control, manipulation, and randomization. Nonexperimental study designs may be used to answer the research questions with less human subject involvement or intervention; such designs are ex post facto, correlational, survey, case study, needs assessment, secondary analysis, and evaluation studies. Additional designs you may see in the literature are methodologic (studies on research tools or instruments) and meta-analysis, which uses many previous studies to determine the overall effect. The design must "fit" the research problem, purpose, and theoretical framework.

The researcher provides definitions for all major variables included in the study. Both theoretical and operational definitions may be provided in the introduction or the review of the literature. Theoretical, or in some cases conceptual, definitions are the general description of a term, that is, the term as defined in a specific theoretical framework or the dictionary. Researchers must provide operational definitions of the major variables of interest, especially when quantitative research methods are used. An **operational definition** is the description specific to the use of the variable in the study. It is precisely what the researchers are looking at and how they are measuring it. For example, consider the term *stethoscope*. Every nurse knows it is an acoustical instrument used to measure heart rate apically or blood pressure peripherally. But the type of stethoscope must be specified in the operational definition, for example, bell-diaphragm combination, electronic, or pediatric. The specification ensures controls in quantitative methods, describing exactly what the researcher used and enabling others to reproduce the study results given a similar set of circumstances or apply to a specific practice setting.

Generally, the researcher provides operational definitions of the study variables in the section on methodology. **Variables** are concepts and constructs defined and manipulated, controlled, or measured in a research study. Independent variables are variables manipulated by the researcher, such as the cause, treatment, or difference between the groups (such as the type of dressing used). Dependent variables are the outcome variables that the researcher is measuring and analyzing. The researcher wishes to see whether the change in the independent variable (type of dressing) caused a difference in the dependent variable (healing time or bacterial colony count). Uncontrolled or confounding variables (such as nutritional status) must also be considered because they can have extraneous and unwanted effects on the dependent variable (healing time). The researcher often attempts to control the extraneous effects by selecting a population or study procedures that meet specific criteria, to reduce the chance of occurrence of the unwanted influences. In the methods section, special attention is given to the descriptions of the subjects. Ultimately, this allows the readers to determine the applicability of results to practice with their specific client group. Ethical considerations specific to the sample should also be described.

Sampling is the use of a subset (sample) of the population as a feasible group to study, ultimately generalizing the findings to the population. The population is the total group to which the researcher wishes the results of the research to be generalized. For example, not all cardiac patients in a rehabilitation program can be interviewed in person. Yet the researcher would like the study results to be applicable to all patients similar to the subjects interviewed in the study, so that the information will add to the body of nursing knowledge. Samples may be selected by probability (based on statistical chance of selection) or nonprobability sampling. Types of probability samples are random, systematic, stratified, and cluster. Nonprobability samples include convenience, purposive, snowball, quota, and expert samples. Each type of sample has advantages and disadvantages that must be considered. At this point, look for the sample size. Smaller sample sizes are associated with qualitative methods. On the other hand, minimum sample sizes are necessary with some statistical procedures in quantitative methods and analysis.

Specific research methods are described as **data collection procedures**. *Data* are the measures or responses obtained from the subjects in the study. Analyzed data become information. Research methods may be quantitative or qualitative. Quantitative methods focus on numerical data that can be obtained from subjects using any one or a combination of measurement instruments. Qualitative methods focus on information gathered from individuals and groups, often in their natural environment, to explore their unique qualities in depth and generate theory on a little-known topic or construct. The different research methods can use similar or different instruments to obtain or measure data.

Instruments are the measurement tools for collecting data. They include paper-and-pencil instruments (such as questionnaires, diaries, or scales), biophysiologic instruments (such as a stethoscope, sphygmomanometer, pulse oximetry, electrocardiograph, or electroencephalograph), interview guides, videotapes and audiotapes, and others, depending on the specific investigation and variables. Important considerations for use of any instrument, including an observer as data collector, are the reliability and validity of the measurement. Researchers report the reliability and validity tests before they discuss the findings of their study.

Instrument reliability describes whether the instrument provides consistent measurement. The reliable instrument measures the variable consistently over time. The need for instrument reliability is apparent in examples of a calibrated scale that dependably provides a reading of the client's weight or the test that consistently estimates the client's stress level. The types of instrument reliability that are reported in studies are test-retest (stability of the measure over time), internal consistency or alpha (statistical measure on items or parts of a test), equivalent forms of tests, and interrater (equivalence among data collectors).

Instrument validity considers whether the instrument measures what it is intended to measure, such as body surface area and not weight. Types of instrument validity include content, construct, and criterion-related. A panel of experts may assess the content validity of an instrument, ensuring that it adequately addresses the variable or area of interest. Construct validity is described with prior research on the instrument and may be reported as findings from a factor analysis or other statistical test. Criterion-related validity is important when the variable cannot be measured directly, such as family and visitor contacts, cards and gifts, and discussions (as another criterion) to discover social support for a study on the psychosocial stress of the hospitalized client.

Once the data collection methods have been described, the researcher describes methods used to analyze the data and reports the results in the findings or results section. Methods for analysis of the data are based on the specified research methods and the type of data involved. For numerical data, statistics are used in the analysis of quantitative research methods. **Descriptive statistics** are used to summarize and describe data through graphic displays of the information (percentages and frequency counts), measures of central tendency (means, medians, modes), and measures of dispersion (ranges, variances, and standard deviations). **Inferential statistics** are used to test hypotheses, make predictions, and infer from the sample (statistic) to the population (parameter). Depending on the variables, data, and sample size and distribution, inferential statistics used include nonparametric tests (chi square, Spearman rho, median test) and parametric tests (t test, analysis of variance [ANOVA], Pearson r). The results are reported for each research question or hypothesis in an objective manner.

Finally, the researcher presents his or her interpretation of the results in a discussion section. Conclusions should be consistent with the theoretical framework used to guide the study. The discussion also includes the researcher's identification of limitations and recommendations for using the findings in practice, teaching, administration, and further research.

Guidelines to assist with a thoughtful critique of a research study have been posted on the Intranet site.

Subjective Evaluation; Incorporating Evidence-Based Practice

At this point, the reader must determine the applicability of the results to the individual practice area. A research critique is an objective assessment of the information presented in the report against some criterion, such as the critique questions. The subjective evaluation for use of the findings in one's own practice area is made after the objective critique of the value of the study's process and results. If the critique is positive, you must decide whether the results are applicable in your practice area. If so, it is a professional responsibility to implement information found to be beneficial to clients, rather than to continue to practice on the basis of tradition instead of fact and efficacy—your competence in evidence-based practice.

Reading professional journals and keeping abreast of current knowledge are essential in contemporary nursing practice. Acquiring critique skills is an integral part of this aspect of nursing. Access to quality journals and the depth of reading must also be considered. Look carefully at the professional journals to which you subscribe and the journals that are available at your work site. Do they contain research reports? If so, are you reading research studies as well as the narrative and practice articles? Consider different levels of reading, from skimming the information to a careful analysis of the content or a comparison with other literature to synthesize the information known on the topic. At what level are you reading? Critiquing a research article is at the level of analytic reading rather than merely looking for articles of interest to your practice area. Make time, on a consistent basis, to look for and evaluate research in the professional literature. Effec-tive communication is a vital component of this process.

As an additional aid to the implementation of evidence-based practice, alternate sources beyond traditional research articles are available to assist the clinician. Pape (2003) identifies cognitive clustering for integration of findings on a specific research topic through sources such as published meta-analyses, systematic reviews, practice guidelines, online reviews, and Internet searches. Youngblut and Brooten (2001) state that the use of evidence-based practices developed by others saves the institutional and individual resources and list these sources as journals, specialty organizations, government organizations, and commercial organizations (p. 471).

As mentioned previously, national clinical guidelines have been available since the 1990s but are not consistently accessed or used. The National Guideline Clearinghouse provides archives of current practice guidelines that have been reviewed, revised, or deleted within the past 5 years, organized by health conditions and national organizations. The Agency for Healthcare Research and Quality also provides useful information for clinicians on current research and quality measures for application in evidence-based practice.

Once you have obtained the information from the professional literature or resources, the issue is implementation and sharing. Are you sharing the information with colleagues? This can be done informally among your colleagues or can be formally presented at a unit conference or during an interdisciplinary grand rounds session. Having access to "user-friendly" databases or a library is essential for acquiring information on a clinical issue. Investigate what is available in your environment. Attending "brown bag lunches" and participating in a journal club focused on research studies are ways of making this activity more enjoyable and rewarding.

ONLINE CONSULT

Agency for Healthcare Reseach & Quality at
http://www.ahrq.gov
National Guidelines Clearinghouse at
http://www.guideline.gov

Obtaining new information is the intended aim of attending a clinical conference, whether or not you need continuing education units for relicensure or recertification. Quality of programs and significance of the topics to your practice area must be considered for evidence-based practice. Selecting research-based concurrent sessions is a good way to hear current research information. Attendance at grand rounds in an institution committed to research is also a valuable experience. Research questions specific to nursing or interdisciplinary collaboration may become available. Your work setting may have a nursing or interdisciplinary research committee. Participating on a research committee can be a challenging and rewarding experience. Nurses can collaborate on different stages of the research process. In addition, the practice problems specific to your setting can emerge, be developed, and be investigated when professionals start the discussion and raise the issues. It can be quite a stimulating and fun experience.

ELIMINATING BARRIERS TO EVIDENCE-BASED NURSING PRACTICE

Barriers to evidence-based nursing practice should be diminished or removed to further professional practice. Such barriers are real and perceived lacks of educational preparation, administrative support, resources, and time. In this time of diminishing resources, the use of the most reliable and accurate information is crucial. Trial-and-error strategies as the basis for a client intervention waste valuable resources and are unconscionable if there is contrary evidence. We need an increasing sense of professional commitment to practice based on evidence of effective outcomes for our clients.

Negative attitudes toward research or researchers must be replaced with greater collaboration among clinicians, researchers, administrators, and educators. Barnsteiner and Prevost (2002) have prosposed the following strategies for facilitating evidence-based practice:

- Change viewpoints about research
- Increase knowledge about the evidence-based-practice process
- Harness new knowledge
- Consider potential consequences
- Institute system changes
- Collaborate locally and globally.

Clinicians have firsthand awareness of problem areas but must be assisted in accessing the current knowledge base, looking at problems in the domain of nursing that address the need for improved client outcomes, having the professional commitment to go the extra mile and take time to get involved with research activities, basing their nursing interventions on the current evidence of efficacy, and receiving some form of recognition for their efforts.

The support and encouragement of the chief nurse administrator or executive are a must to ensure that the organizational climate, resources, and philosophy of practice are present in the practice setting. Moving to evidence-based practice will not be an easy transition without a dynamic person spearheading the process. Clinicians must keep an open mind and make a professional commitment to identify research problems and search the current knowledge base for information. Researchers must collaborate with clinicians to address nursing questions and avoid speaking or talking in "researchese," thus providing clear practice implications in publications and presentations. Educators must also assist in the development of critique and research skills.

Commitment must be made to the ongoing nature of building knowledge and basing practice on evidence of efficacy. Our knowledge base has been evolving since the time of Nightingale and before. It will constantly evolve because of the nature of the information and our focus on people in a dynamic environment. The profession needs more extensive research that is generalizable to and supportive of nursing as a major player in health-care issues. We need more replications to add reliability and validity to instruments and information. Constant updating and modification of any protocol is needed as more information becomes available. Gaining critique skills and learning the language of research are components of this process.

Key Points

- Evidence-based practice, a core competency for health professionals, is defined as the use of clinical expertise and interventions that are based on evidence of efficacy for client outcomes and the preferences of the clients served.
- Research is a process for generating scientific knowledge and utilizing the knowledge on which to base practice. Using evidence of efficacy for practice is a vital professional attribute and a responsibility.
- Nursing research began with Florence Nightingale and has become vital to both professionals and consumers in investigating the domain of nursing, testing theories and interventions, and demonstrating the efficacy and efficiency of nursing actions.
- Highly evident in the research priorities of the National Institute of Nursing Research is testing of nursing interventions that promote health behaviors in individuals or population groups.
- Ethical considerations in research must include the four basic human rights:
  - Do no harm (beneficence)
  - Full disclosure
  - Self-determination
  - Privacy and confidentiality
- A professional nurse should be an active consumer of nursing research, promoting use of current and valid scientific knowledge and identifying the questions to be addressed in further research. Professional accountability demands that one read the literature, attend educational sessions, use critique skills, participate in investigations, and promote evidence-based interventions.
- Empirical research is based on the strict rules of the scientific method, with the following steps:
  - Identification of the problem
  - Statement of the purpose
  - Review of the literature
  - Description of theoretical framework
  - Definition of terms
  - Statement of hypothesis(es)
  - Selection of the research design, population, and sample
  - Approval by the IRB
  - Collection of data
  - Analysis and interpretation of data
  - Presentation of findings and recommendations
- A research critique is an objective analysis of a published research report. The reader must critically consider all components of the report, including problem, purpose, literature support, theoretical framework, definitions, study questions or hypotheses, design, population and sample, data collection methods and procedures, analysis, and interpretation of findings. The ultimate goal of a research critique is to consider applicability of appropriate scientific findings to one's own professional practice and knowledge base.
- A research problem is the main issue or central question that the researcher addresses in the investigation. Specific research questions or hypotheses flow from the main research problem.
- The literature review is a report and comparison of all pertinent prior investigations on the topic, variables of interest, theoretical models, and methods used. The researcher focuses on primary sources for a critical appraisal and synthesis of what is currently known. *(continued)*

(*continued*)

- Variables are concepts and constructs defined and manipulated, controlled, or measured in a research study. Independent variables are manipulated by the researcher, such as the cause, treatment, or difference between the groups. Dependent variables are the outcome variables that the researcher is measuring and analyzing.
- Hypotheses are predictions about the variables that the researcher is testing with a subject group. Hypothesis testing uses inferential statistics to infer from the sample and make generalizations about the population.
- The research design is the overall blueprint and methods for the study.
- Research methods may be quantitative or qualitative. Quantitative methods focus on numerical data that can be obtained from subjects through any one or a combination of measurement instruments. Qualitative methods focus on information gathered from individuals and groups, often in their natural environment, to explore in depth their unique qualities and generate theory on a little-known topic or construct.
- Sampling is the use of a subset (sample) of the population as a feasible group to study and ultimately generalize findings to the population.
- Instruments are the measurement tools for collecting data. Important considerations for use of any instrument are the reliability and validity of the measurement.
- Statistics are used in analyzing quantitative research methods. Descriptive statistics are used to summarize and describe data. Inferential statistics are used to test hypotheses, make predictions, and infer from the sample to the population.

Thought and Discussion Questions

1. Describe activities present in your practice setting that demonstrate the use of evidence-based practice.
2. Develop a plan to encourage or promote evidence-based practice in your nursing practice environment. Select a clinical protocol or problem. Use the following six phases of the research utilization process to organize your plan: (1) identification of clinical problems and access to research bases; (2) evaluation of the knowledge and the potential for application in the organization, along with policy and cost determinants; (3) planning for implementation and evaluation of the innovation; (4) clinical trial and evaluation; (5) decisions to adopt, modify, or reject innovations on the basis of evaluation; and (6) if the innovations are adopted, planning for their extension to other units (Horsley et al., 1978). Describe who will be involved in the process and how the new practice or protocol will be implemented. Finally, identify evaluation criteria.
3. Identify practice issues that can be developed into a nursing research problem for investigation.
4. Find the requirements for the IRB at your college or institution. Be prepared to participate in a discussion on the requirements for the preparation of a research proposal for consideration by the IRB.
5. Look further at PHI and current privacy issues. Be prepared to participate in a discussion as scheduled by your instructor.
6. Review the Chapter Thought located on the first page of the chapter and discuss it in the context of the contents of the chapter.

Interactive Exercises

1. Critique a nursing research article. First, locate a current research article that pertains to your clinical practice area. Try to select an article that has subheadings containing words such as theoretical framework or hypotheses, literature review, sample, findings, and discussion. Develop an objective critique of the study using the guidelines and format provided on the Intranet site. Discuss the applicability of this research to, and the potential for using the findings in, your practice setting.

2. Conduct an online search for information on the Tuskeegee Syphillis Study, the Jewish Chronic Disease Hospital Study, and the Willowbrook Hepatitis Study. Explain how these studies led to the need for additional human protections.

3. Conduct an online search on end-of-life issues, and locate an empirical study and a qualitative study on the topic. Identify the ethical issues and protections for the subjects included in each study. Be prepared to participate in an in-class or online discussion, to be scheduled by your instructor.

4. Go to the National Institute for Nursing Research (NINR) Web site **(http://nih.gov/ninr)**:
   - Identify the current priorities or research opportunities and future themes.
   - Take the online training for nurse scientists.
   - Be prepared to participate in an in-class or online discussion on the general profile of NINR, including its mission, strategic plan, research initiatives, and impact.

5. Investigate funding opportunities for clinical nursing research. Start with the information provided at the NINR, DHHS, and Sigma Theta Tau Web sites.

6. Go to the Web site of the National Guideline Clearinghouse **(http://www. guideline.gov)**. Identify a current guideline appropriate to your practice area that is not being implemented. Explain why it is not appropriate for the client population or propose how you will introduce this information to your colleagues for potential application.

PRINT RESOURCES

References

American Nurses Association. (1985). *Human rights guidelines for nurses in clinical and other research* (Pub. No. D-46 3M 9/87R). Kansas City, MO: American Nurses Association.

American Nurses Association Commission on Nursing Research. (1981). *Guidelines for the investigative function of nurses*. Kansas City, MO: American Nurses Association.

Barneteiner, J., & Prevost, S. (2002). How to implement evidence-based practice: Some tried and true pointers. *Reflections on Nursing Leadership, 28*(2), 18–21.

Belmont Report: Ethical principles and guidelines for the protection of human subjects of research, 79 Fed. Reg. 12065 (1979).

Crane, J. (1985). Research utilization: Theoretical perspectives. *Western Journal of Nursing Research, 7*, 261–268.

Declaration of Helsinki. (1990). Recommendations guiding physicians in biomedical research involving human subjects. *Bulletin of Pan American Health Organization, 24*(4), 606–609.

Greiner, A. C., & Knebel, E. (Eds.). (2003). *Health professions education: A bridge to quality*. Washington, DC: Institute of Medicine.

Horsley, J. A., Crane, J., & Bingle, J. D. (1978). Research utilization as an organizational process. *Journal of Nursing Administration, 8*(7), 4–6.

Kerlinger, F. N. (1986). *Foundations of behavioral research* (3rd ed.). New York: Holt, Rinehart & Winston.

Lindeman, C. A., & Krueger, J. C. (1977). Increasing the quality, quantity, and use of nursing research. *Nursing Outlook, 25*, 450–454.

Mulhall, A. (2001). Nursing research and nursing practice: An exploration of two different cultures. *European Journal of Oncology Nursing*, 5(2), 121–127.

Nightingale, F. (1859). *Notes on nursing: What it is, and what it is not.* London: Harrison and Sons. [Commemorative edition printed 1992, Philadelphia: J. B. Lippincott]

Pape, T. M. (2003). Evidence-based nursing practice: To infinity and beyond. *Journal of Continuing Education in Nursing*, 34, 154–161, 189–190.

Silva, M. (1995). *Ethical guidelines in the conduct, dissemination, and implementation of nursing research.* Washington, DC: American Nurses Association.

Stone, P. W., Curran, C. R., & Bakken, S. (2002). Economic evidence for evidence-based practice. *Journal of Nursing Scholarship*, 34, 277–281.

Youngblut, J. M., & Brooten, D. (2001). Evidence-based nursing practice: Why is it important? AACN *Clinical Issues*, 12, 468–476.

Bibliography

Barnard, S., Casella, P .J., Coffin, C., Hughes, T., Hurst, J. W., Rasey, J. S., Redding, D., Robillard, R. J., St James, D., & Ullery, S. C. (2001). *Writing, Speaking, and Communication Skills for Health Care Professionals.* New Haven, CT: Yale University.

Colling, J. (2003). Demystifying nursing research: Defining the problem to be studied. *Urologic Nursing*, 23, 225–226.

Edwards, N., & Valley, J. (2003). The research process: Using a "recipe" to increase successful outcomes. *Journal of Gerontological Nursing*, 29(9), 49–54.

Fain, J. A. (1999). *Reading, understanding, and applying nursing research: A text and workbook.* Philadelphia: F.A. Davis.

Fawcett, J. (1998). The relationship of theory and research (3rd ed.). Philadelphia: F.A. Davis.

Fullbrook, P. (2003). Developing best practice in critical care nursing: Knowledge, evidence and practice. *Nursing Critical Care*, 8, 96–102.

Larson, E. (1989). Using the CURN Project to teach research utilization in a baccalaureate program. *Western Journal of Nursing Research*, 11, 593–599.

Melnyk, B. M., & Fineout-Overholt, E. (2002). Putting research into practice. *Reflections on Nursing Leadership*, 28(2), 22–25, 45.

Polit, D. F., & Beck, C. T. (2003). *Nursing research: Principles and methods* (7th ed.). Philadelphia: Lippincott Williams & Wilkins.

Profetto-McGrath, J., Hesketh, K. L., Lang, S., & Estabrooks, C. A. (2003). A study of critical thinking and research utilization among nurses. *Western Journal of Nursing Research*, 25, 322–337.

Rizzuto, C., & Mitchell, M. (1970). Outcomes of a research consortium project. *Journal of Nursing Administration*, 20(4), 13–17.

Sandeloski, M, & Barroso, J. (2002). Finding the findings in qualitative research. *Journal of Nursing Scholarship*, 14, 213–219.

Schreiber, R. S., & Stern, P. N. (2001). *Using grounded theory in nursing.* New York: Springer.

Streubert Speziale., H. J., & Carpenter, D. R. (2002). *Qualitative nursing research: Advancing the humanistic perspective* (3rd. ed.). Philadelphia: Lippincott Williams & Wilkins.

Thomas, S. P., & Pollio, H. R. (2002). *Listening to patients: A phenomenological approach to nursing research and practice.* New York: Springer.

Titler, M. G., Cullen, L., & Ardery, A. G. (2002). Evidence-based practice: An administrative perspective. *Reflections on Nursing Leadership*, 28(2), 26–27, 46.

ONLINE REFERENCES

American Association of Colleges of Nursing (AACN). (1999a). Position statement on defining scholarship for the discipline of nursing. *http://www.nchu.edu/Publications/positions/scholar.htm.*

American Association of Colleges of Nursing (AACN). (1999b). Position statement on nursing research. *http://www.nchu.edu/Publications/positions/rscposst.htm.*

American Nurses Association. (1997). Position statement: Education for participation in nursing research. *http://www.nursingworld.org/readingroom/position/research/rseducat.htm.*

National Institute of Nursing Research. (2003). National Institute of Nursing Research mission statement. *http://www.nih.gov/ninr.*

National Institute of Nursing Research. (2004). National Institute of Nursing Research mission statement. *http://www.nih.gov/ninr.*

Protection of Human Subjects, 45 CFR S 46 (1991). Http://hhs.gov.-or Title 45 Code of Federal Regulations Part 46 (45CFR 46), §46.111. *http://ohrp.osophs.dhhs.gov/humansubjects.*

Sigma Theta Tau. (2003). Evidence-based nursing position statement. *http://www.nursingsociety.org*

United States Department of Health and Human Services (USDHHS). (2003). *Protecting personal health information in research: Understanding the HIPAA Privacy Rule* (NIH Pub. No. 03–5388). *http://privacyruleandresearch.nih.gov/pr_02.asp.*

U.S. President's Commission for the Study of Ethical Problems in Medicine and Behavioral Research. (1982). *Compensating for research injuries: The ethical and legal implications of programs to redress injured subjects* (Vol. 1). *http://www.gwu.edu/~nsarchiv/radiation/dir/mstreet/commeet/meet16/brief16/tab_b/br16b1a.txt.*

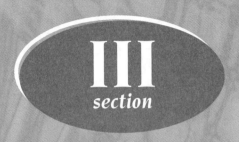

III
section

Critical Components
of Professional
Nursing Practice

Jacqueline Owers Favret

7
chapter

Effective Communication

Chapter Objectives

On completion of this chapter, the reader will be able to:

1. Describe and understand the various communication models.
2. Explain the various forms of communication, such as verbal and nonverbal communication.
3. Evaluate the use of therapeutic communication in the health-care setting.
4. Differentiate between ways the nurse receives information from the client.
5. Discuss the various types of barriers to communication.

Key Terms

Communication
Communication
    Models
Source
Encoder
Message
Channel
Receiver
Decoder
Noise

Relationships
Transactions
Contexts
Metacommunication
Verbal Communication
Nonverbal
    Communication
Proxemics
Cultural Variations
Kinesics

Facial Expressions
Physical Appearance
Therapeutic
    Communication
Active Listening
Silence
Questions
Barriers to
    Communication
Collaboration

Communication is a comprehensive and complex process. The word *communication* is similar to words like love, health, and freedom; intuitively, each of us thinks that we know what it means, but really people base their definitions on their own life experiences, cultures, and surroundings. For the nurse, communication is an essential element, not only in the relationship with the client but also in working effectively with the interdisciplinary health team. The process of interactions between humans can be verbal or nonverbal, written or unwritten, planned or spontaneous. It is therefore essential for communication to be defined within the context of nursing. **Communication** consists of "all the cognitive, affective, and behavioral responses used to convey a message to another person" (Watson, 1979, p. 33). Within this context there is no such thing as "no communication" between individuals. All behavior, whether verbal or nonverbal, has both meaning and a message value.

Effective communication within the client-nurse relationship is not necessarily a natural process; it is a learned skill. Clear and appropriate communication is essential for providing effective nursing care and presents a unique challenge to nurses today. Society is composed of many different cultures using many different languages. "Nearly 32 million people in the United States speak a language other than English at home" (Andrews & Boyle, 1999, p. 37). In the aftermath of the September 2001 terrorist attack in New York, one of the biggest challenges faced by the Red Cross workers was communicating with individuals who spoke so many different languages. When a nurse is giving care to a client, the nurse's message must be understandable to the client and the nurse should be adept at understanding whatever the communication is from the client. Nurses must be aware not only of what they are saying in their words but also what their body language is saying to their clients.

The 21st century poses an additional challenge to nurses in communicating via technology. Nurses are expected to be proficient in computer skills, using nursing documentation systems and e-mail. Nurses also use many different types of communication in their care of clients—in person, through the written word, over the telephone, through facsimile (fax) and electronic mail, and through the Internet. Finding effective ways to overcome communication barriers gives nurses the opportunity to bridge culture gaps within their community and provide care to a larger number of individuals.

COMMUNICATION MODELS

The chapter first presents an overview of basic **communication models** to help the reader understand the complex process of communication, especially in the health-care setting.

Basic Components

Whether or not sources of communication are effective depends on a combination of factors (Berlo, 1960). All types of communication require the following components:

- **Source:** The individual who decides what message is to be sent
- **Encoder:** The person who interprets the message
- **Message:** The content of meaning
- **Channel:** The medium or way chosen to convey the message
- **Receiver:** The one who receives the message
- **Decoder:** The one who interprets the message sent

In intrapersonal communication, the source and the encoder are the same person. The message is then communicated either by verbal or nonverbal language. The message may be sent to any or all of a person's five senses. The receiver is also the decoder. According to Berlo (1960), in effective communication, the receiver is the most important line in the communication process. If the source does not

reach the receiver with the intended message, the source might just as well have talked to himself or herself.

In written communication, the reader is most important. In spoken communication, the listener is most important. When the source chooses a "code" for his message, he must choose one that is familiar to his receiver. An example of poor communication in the health-care setting is when a nurse gives information to a client using only the jargon or terms known within the profession. The client can receive the information but does not have the knowledge to decode the message.

> *Human communication is a two-person process in which both individuals influence and are influenced by each other.*

Shannon-Weaver Model

Claude Shannon, a mathematician, and Warren Weaver, an electrical engineer, developed one of the early contemporary communications models in 1947. Both men were employed by Bell Telephone Laboratory and were referring to electronic communication, not human communication (Berlo, 1960). Yet behavioral scientists have found the linear Shannon-Weaver Model (FIG. 7–1) very useful in describing human communication.

They defined communication in a "very broad sense to include all of the procedures by which one mind may affect another" (Shannon & Weaver, 1949, p. 95). In this model, the *information source* selects a desired *message* out of a set of possible messages. The *transmitter* changes this *message* into the *signal* that is then transmitted to the *receiver*. The transmitter is the encoder of the message; the receiver is the decoder (Shannon & Weaver, 1949). Noise is a distinctive entity of this model. In the process of transmission of the message, certain things are added to the signal that were not intended by the information source. **Noise** refers to any disturbances, such as actual static, environmental noises, or the psychological or perceptual distortion of the receiver. In a nurse-client interaction, noise could represent an environment that is not conducive to receiving the message, such as a room that is too cold or a loud television playing in the background. This model does demonstrate a communication path but fails to show any type of reciprocal interaction on the part of the receiver.

Source-Message-Channel-Receiver Model

David Berlo (1960), a professor at Michigan State University, developed the source-message-channel-receiver (SMCR) model of the

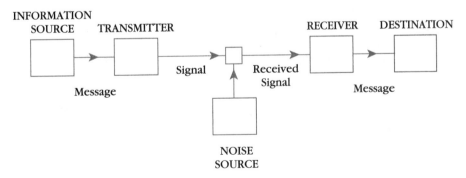

FIG. 7–1. Shannon-Weaver model. (From Shannon, C. E., & Weaver, W. [1949]. *The mathematical theory of communication*. [p. 720]. Champaign, IL: University of Illinois Press. Copyright 1949 by the Board of Trustees of the University of Illinois. Used with permission of the University of Illinois Press.)

communication process (FIG. 7–2). This paradigm emphasizes the importance of a thorough understanding of human behavior as a prerequisite to communication analysis. The SMCR model represents a communication process that occurs as a *source* formulates *messages* based on the source's communication skills, attitudes, knowledge, and sociocultural system. These messages, which have unique elements, structure, content, treatment, and codes, are then transmitted along channels. *Channels* are the various senses, such as seeing, hearing, touching, smelling, and tasting. The *receiver* interprets messages on the basis of his or her own communication skills, attitudes, knowledge, and sociocultural system.

The strength of the SMCR model is that it demonstrates the complex process of communication and shows that communication is not a static event. It incorporates the sociocultural context of both sender and receiver as a critical component in the communications process. The model comes up short, however, by omitting the feedback component of communication (Northouse & Northouse, 1992).

Leary Model

According to Timothy Leary (1955), interpersonal communication is the aspect of personality psychology that is concerned with the social effect that one human being has on another. Leary developed a model that is truly a transactional and multidimensional model, stressing the relationship aspect of interpersonal communication (FIG. 7–3). It demonstrates that human communication is a two-person process in which the two individuals influence and are influenced by each other (Leary, 1955).

As a psychotherapist, Leary noted that patients influenced the way he behaved toward them. He concluded that individuals actually "train" others to respond to them in ways that are pleasing for the individuals' own preferred interpersonal behaviors. From this perspective, according to the Leary model, every communication message can be viewed as occurring along two dimensions: dominance/submission and hate/love. Leary (1955) stated that two rules govern how these dimensions function in human interaction:

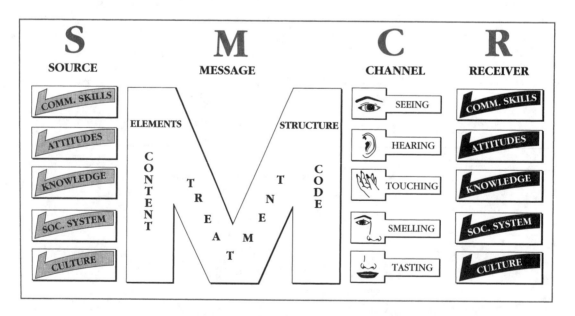

FIG. 7–2. Source-message-channel-receiver (SMCR) model of communication. (From Berlo, D.K. [1960]. The process of communication: An introduction to the theory and practice [p. 7]. New York: Holt, Rhinehart & Winston, with permission.)

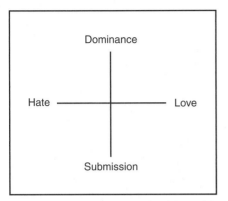

FIG. 7–3. Leary's reflexive model. (Adapted from Leary, T. [1955]. *The theory and measurement methodology of interpersonal communication.* Psychiatry, 18, 152. The William Alanson White Psychiatric Foundation, Inc.)

- *Rule 1:* Dominant or submissive behavior usually stimulates the *opposite* behavior in others. For example, if we prefer to be dominant, we condition others to behave submissively; conversely, if we like to be submissive, we condition others to behave in a way that is dominant towards us.
- *Rule 2:* Loving or hateful behavior usually stimulates the *same* behavior from others. Being kind to another individual usually encourages kindness from others, but if we display aggressive behavior, the other person will usually react in a hostile manner.

Leary says that these rules operate reflexively; our own responses toward one another are involuntary and immediate.

The Leary model of communication can be directly applied to the health-care arena. In the past, clients were generally passive about their health-care and needs, and often assumed a submissive role, allowing the health-care professionals to assume the dominant role. Amidst current trends of consumerism and the availability of information about health-care, however, clients are tending to take a more active role in their health care. When consumers become more assertive, the health-care providers have to relinquish some of their own control and authority. The strength of Leary's model is the transactional way in which he describes these power and affiliation issues in our everyday

interactions with others. It is important to be aware of what each person brings to interactions with others.

Health Communication Model

The models previously described provided the foundation for Northouse and Northouse (1992) to construct the health communication model (HCM) (FIG. 7–4), which specifically applies to transactions between participants in health care about health-related issues. The HCM's primary focus is on the health communication that occurs within the various kinds of relationships in health-care settings. This model also takes a broader systems view of communication and emphasizes the way in which a series of factors can affect the interactions in the health-care setting. Three major factors illustrate the health communication process: relationships, transactions, and contexts.

Relationships

From a systems perspective, the HCM illustrates four major types of **relationships** that exist in the health-care setting:

- Professional/professional
- Professional/client
- Professional/significant other
- Client/significant other

When an individual is involved in health communication, he or she is involved in one of these types of relationships. In this model, the term *health professional* is any individual who has the education, training, and experience to provide health services to others. Health professionals include nurses, health administrators, social workers, physicians, and occupational and physical therapists (Northouse & Northouse, 1992). Each of these professionals brings unique characteristics and beliefs to health-care settings that affect the way they interact with the client and with the other members of the interdisciplinary health-care team.

Clients are the people who are the focus of

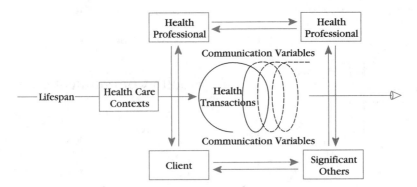

FIG. 7–4. Health Communication model. (From Northouse, P. G. & Northouse, L. L. [1992]. *Health Communication Strategies for the health professional* [p. 16]. Norwalk, CT: Appleton & Lange, with permission.)

the health-care services being provided. The term also encompasses the characteristics, values, and beliefs that these individuals bring to the health-care setting. Just as the personal characteristics of the nurse and other professionals influence their interactions, the characteristics of clients influence their interactions with others. Within the social network of the client, the client's *significant others* are family members and friends who have been found to be essential in supporting clients as they maneuver through the health-care system. Significant others are all the people who are significant in their lives but are not health professionals.

> *The client's self esteem, emotional stability, and sense of identity will define how the client relates to the health-care professionals as well as those significant individuals in his or her life.*

Northouse and Northouse (1992) realized that too often, health professionals overlook the important role played by family members and other significant individuals in enhancing the health of the person. Their model includes this aspect because as clients live longer with chronic health problems, significant others assume an even more central role as patient advocates and are more involved in the direct care of the client. This concept is also true when the nurse is visiting the client in the home. The dynamics within the family and the support of the significant others around

the client can help the client realize the full potential of a healthy lifestyle.

Transactions

Transactions, the second major element in the HCM, are the health-related interactions between the nurse or other health professional, the client, and the client's significant others. These transactions about health can include both verbal and nonverbal communication behaviors, which are equally important and are most effective when they are compatible with each other. Northouse and Northouse (1992) represent these health transactions with a circle from which an unending spiral emerges, signifying that communication is not static but is an interactive process that occurs at various points in a person's life. This continuous feedback allows the message to be changed in accordance with the situation.

Contexts

Contexts, the third major element in the model, is defined as the settings where the health communication takes place and includes the properties of these settings. At one level *context* can refer to the health-care setting, such as a hospital room or the client's home. For example, if the professional is communicating with the client in an ambulatory clinic, there may be many distractions and infringements of privacy. Each particular health-care setting affects the dynamics of the transactions that take place. However, at another level, health-care *contexts* can refer to the number of participants within the particular health-care setting. Communication can take place in a one-to-one situation or in small groups. The number of participants present influences the overall interactions in the setting.

The health communication model is based on the assumption that communication is ongoing, dynamic, and always changing. It is transactional, in that each participant affects the other participants, and it has both a content and relationship dimension that are inextricably bound together in the interactions. It is a model that incorporates the thoughts, feelings, attitudes, and current roles of the participants and demonstrates that all of these things can affect the accuracy of the communication.

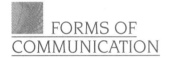

FORMS OF COMMUNICATION

In order to share information, people express messages in a complex composite of both verbal (spoken or written) and nonverbal behaviors. Individuals express themselves through language, gestures, voice inflection, facial expressions, and use of space. Within the nurse-client relationship, information exchanged between two individuals must be interpreted not only by the nurse but also by the client. The health-care provider should be aware of styles of communication and should have observational skills that enhance the encounter.

Metacommunication

Metacommunication is a broad term used to "describe all of the factors that influence how the message is perceived" (Arnold & Boggs, 2003, p. 217) and has long been recognized as being of enormous value in the nurse-client therapeutic relationship. Metacommunication includes all things taken into account when the receiver is interpreting

a message, such as the role of the communicator, the nonverbal messages sent, and the context in which the communication is taking place. These messages may be hidden within verbal messages or conveyed by nonverbal expressions or gestures. An example is the "play fighting" observed in children and animals. Bateson noted that for an organism to "play" at fighting, it must be able to both appear that it is fighting and simultaneously appear not to be fighting but merely simulating the act of fighting (Mitchell, 1991).

In the nurse-client relationship, metacommunication conveys messages about how to interpret both verbal and nonverbal communication clues. For example, a nurse can convey a message of caring by saying to the client, "That's important. Let's talk about it." If the nurse sits in a chair and uses nonverbal cues such as maintaining eye contact, smiling, having a relaxed posture, and listening intently, the verbal and nonverbal messages are congruent. If the same verbal message is delivered while the nurse fidgets and looks at a watch, the nurse may provide a nonverbal message that he or she does not have time or is not willing to listen. Metacommunication is the message conveyed when both verbal and nonverbal communication are perceived together.

Nurses must make sure that their verbal and nonverbal messages to clients are consistent and congruent in order to be sure that the clients interpret the messages clearly. Suppose you walk into a room and ask a client whether he is in pain and he answers no, but you observe that he is thrashing in bed, clutching his incision, and has deep grimaces on his face. How would you interpret this behavior? A nurse who is skilled in communication would realize that the verbal answer and the nonverbal cues are inconsistent and would clarify the situation. If the nurse points out the incongruent form of communication that he or she observed, the client may admit that he is in pain (Arnold & Boggs, 2003).

Verbal Communication

Verbal communication takes place when people use words to share experiences with others. Without the use of spoken language, individuals are severely limited in means of sharing with others what they are feeling. The choice of words that a person uses is based on language, educational background, age, race, and socioeconomic background as well as by the situation in which the communication takes place.

According to the individual's background and experience, interpretation of the words may also vary. One cannot assume that words have the same meaning to everyone who hears them. "Language is useful only to the extent that it actually reflects the experience it is designed to portray" (Arnold & Boggs, 2003, p.218). If a person speaks a different native language, consider the difficulty that person will have expressing his or her thoughts in English. This could also apply to a small child or a person who is afflicted with Alzheimer's disease.

Keep in mind that the intended meaning of the message may be represented in the emphasis placed on a particular word. The pitch and tone of a word can suggest mood and can either support or contradict the content of the verbal message. When a client is explaining something to the nurse, the nurse must consider that certain phrases and words may have entirely different meanings for the client and the nurse.

Potter and Perry (1999) state that the six most important aspects of verbal communication are (1) vocabulary, (2) denotative and connotative meanings, (3) intonation, (4) pacing, (5) clarity and brevity, and (6) timing and relevance.

Vocabulary

Vocabulary consists of the words or phrases that a person chooses and uses to communicate a message. Communication is unsuccessful if the receiver cannot translate or understand the sender's words and phrases. Nurses work with individuals of various ages, developmental stages, cultures, and educational backgrounds as well as individuals who have physical problems that distort their communication skills.

Nurses must be very aware of their use of nursing or medical jargon. Consider the nurse who is instructing a client before an operation. If the nurse says, "You are to be NPO after midnight and you are to void prior to the pre-op injection," what will the client be able to decipher from this instruction? At the same time, the nurse must not "talk down" or patronize the client. The nurse must respect the client and understand the best way to give him or her the information in a manner that can be understood readily.

Meaning

A single word may have several different meanings. The *denotative meaning* is the meaning that is shared by individuals who use a common language. The word *football* may be understood by all individuals who speak English but denotes a different meaning to individuals of different countries. The word *code* denotes a cardiac arrest to members of the health-care profession but has different meaning outside the health profession community. The *connotative meaning* is the interpretation or the way one's feelings, thoughts, experiences, or ideas about the word influence the meaning of the word. When a family is told that their loved one is in a "serious condition," they may interpret that phrase to mean that their loved one is near death. To the nurse, however, the term may merely describe the nature of the illness. Nurses should be extremely cautious to use words and phrases that will not be misinterpreted, especially when explaining a client's condition.

> When a nurse is giving instructions to a client, the nurse must use terms and phrases that the client understands. The best way to ensure that the client has understood the instructions is have the client repeat the instructions to the nurse. At that time, any questions can be answered, and the nurse can be assured that the client has the correct information.

Intonation

Intonation is the cadence and tone of the spoken word. The intonation of words in a message can readily change the meaning. Take the phrase "He is." If spoken one way it can be a sentence, but with a different tone it can be a question. Emphasizing the "he" or the "is" also changes the meaning of the phrase. The tone of voice can also dramatically affect the message's meaning, and emotions directly influence the tone of voice. Emotions such as anger, enthusiasm, and concern may be gleaned from the tone of voice that one uses. Nurses must be aware of this fact to avoid sending an unintended message. The nurse must also realize that the client's intonation may reflect the client's emotional state, even if the client's words do not.

Pacing

Pacing is the speed and rate of the spoken word. Communication is more successful when words are spoken at an appropriate speed or pace. Talking too rapidly or too slowly may express an inadvertent message. When the nurse is communicating important information to a client, the nurse must speak slowly and clearly and must pause at appropriate points to give emphasis. This approach allows the client time to absorb the message and to understand it more clearly. Pacing is improved if the message is thought out before it is delivered.

The nurse should also be aware of the pace of the client's spoken word. The speech may be slow and slurred if the client has some type of neurologic problem or is under the influence of drugs or alcohol. The client who is scared and nervous may speak very rapidly. Cultural variables may also influence the pace of the words; people from the southern part of the United States sometimes speak in a slow manner, and someone from the Northeast may speak very quickly. It is important for the nurse to be aware of these differences and be able to define the meanings attributed to a person's pace of speaking.

Clarity, Timing, and Relevance

The nurse should use words and phrases that express the idea simply and directly. Using examples tends to make the message clearer. *Timing* and *relevance* are likewise critical in communication. The client must be ready to hear what the nurse has to say. If a patient is distracted by pain, the nurse must realize that it is not the right time to give detailed instructions. Often the best time to communicate is when the client has expressed interest in a particular topic. Choosing this timing tends to make the client more attentive.

Nurses should also demonstrate *credibility*, which is defined as a sense of trustworthiness, sincerity, reliability, and integrity. The nurse must be dependable and believable. If the client asks the nurse a question that the nurse does not know the answer to, it is much better for the nurse to answer, "I do not know the answer to that but I will find out for you" than to give erroneous information. When a nurse establishes credibility in a nurse-client relationship, the communication is more reliable and reaches greater depths.

Nonverbal Communication

Nonverbal communication is communication without words; it includes messages that are created through body motions, facial expressions, use of space and sounds, and the use of touch. Birdwhistell (1970) studied the area of body movement and suggested that 65 to 70 percent of the social meaning of an interaction is transmitted by nonverbal communication. Although nonverbal communication does not include language, it can be either vocal or nonvocal. For example, if a client is moaning in pain, he or she can be giving a nonverbal cue that the nurse should ask more questions about the client's condition.

Nonverbal communication can be intentional or unintentional. If a nurse is giving important information to a client, the nurse should intentionally have a serious facial expression. A client who is giving the nurse information in an apparently relaxed and gleeful manner but whose face shows expressions of fear and uncertainty demonstrates unintentional nonverbal communication. A prime example of nonverbal communication is Holly Hunter's 1993 role in the movie "The

Piano." For the entire length of the movie, she does not speak one word of language, yet her nonverbal communication in the role is so effective that it earned her an Oscar for the best actress performance.

> *Monitoring subtle nonverbal communication clues accounts for the vast majority of communication between individuals.*

Most Americans are only dimly aware of their use of nonverbal language, although they use it every day. We are constantly communicating our real feelings in nonverbal ways (Hall, 1959). Arnold and Boggs (2003) categorize four areas in which nonverbal behaviors are used: (1) proxemics, (2) cultural variations, (3) kinesics, which include body language and facial expression, and (4) appearance.

Proxemics

Proxemics, the use of personal and cultural space, refers to how individuals use and interpret space in the communication process. Some areas of proxemics address questions of territoriality, personal space, and distance relevant to the health-care setting. Each culture has expectations for appropriate distance, depending on the context of communication. Personal space, or one's own territory, is important because it gives one a sense of identity, security, and control. A person may feel threatened or simply irritated when his or her personal space is invaded.

When people enter the health-care setting, they are required to give up their privacy and personal space. They are required to give personal and intimate information to strangers and may undergo procedures that further compromise their sense of privacy and personal space. Although nurses and other health professionals may not be able to eliminate these problems of personal space, the health-care professional should respect the client's territory, belongings, and right to privacy. The client should be given as much control over the situation as possible. For example, the client should be allowed to decide whether

the door to the room is left open and where personal items are placed. The client's body should be exposed as little as possible to minimize the discomfort involved with procedures that invade his or her privacy.

Cultural Variations

Cultural variations are learned unconsciously through the observations of behavior of significant individuals in the client's culture. Communication patterns vary in different cultures, even for such conventional social behaviors as smiling, a handshake, and direct eye contact. For many Hispanic clients, smiling and shaking hands are considered an integral part of sincere interaction and trust, whereas a Russian American client might perceive this behavior to be inappropriate. (Andrews & Bolye, 1999).

Sometimes a nonverbal *gesture*—a body movement usually with the hand—is totally acceptable in one culture and truly offensive in another one. For example, the nurse may mean to signal to a Brazilian client that things went well by making an "OK" circle with the thumb and index finger; in Brazil, however, this movement is considered an obscene gesture (Arnold & Boggs, 2003).

Cultural taboos can inhibit nonverbal behaviors. Different cultures have different rules about *eye contact*—looking directly into another person's eyes. In many Western cultures, making direct eye contact is interpreted as being interested and attentive. However, the use of eye contact is one of the most culturally variable nonverbal behaviors. Although most nurses have been taught to look directly at the client when speaking, individuals from other cultures may attribute other culturally based meanings to this behavior. Asian, Native American, Arab, and Appalachian clients may consider eye contact impolite or antagonistic, and they may divert their own eyes when talking to a nurse or physician. In some cultures, showing respect to the nurse dictates that the client should cast the eyes downward. Hispanic clients may expect eye contact from the nurse but will not necessarily reciprocate it (Andrews & Boyle, 1999).

In some cultures, *touching*—coming into physical contact with another person—is one of the most powerful means of nonverbal communication, but the nurse must give careful consideration to issues surrounding touch. Touch can take a variety of forms and can convey a range of meanings, but it is a powerful tool in health care when it communicates caring and respect. Touch can ease a client's sense of isolation and can make procedures seem less invasive. Care must be taken, however, to understand individual cultural customs about touching, which can vary dramatically. For example, the cultures of Muslim and Orthodox Jewish men dictate that they do not touch women outside their families. Such men may be very uncomfortable shaking the hand of a female health-care provider (Arnold & Boggs, 2003).

Unfortunately, there is no precise formula to determine when or when not to touch a client, and no universal meaning can be given to a touch. In order for clients to perceive touch positively in a therapeutic relationship, Northouse and Northouse (1992) suggest that nurses use the following guidelines:

- *Use a form of touch that is appropriate to the particular situation:* There are many types of touch that can be used in various ways. The nurse should use touch that seems compatible with the context of the way it is being used. For example, if a woman has just been told distressing information (e.g., that her child is diagnosed with leukemia), she may respond positively to the nurse's hand being placed on her arm. On the other hand, this type of touch may not be therapeutic or well received by a male adolescent who has just been told that he has diabetes and who is in the process of venting anger. It is better to let him get the anger out than to try to console him.
- *Do not use a touch gesture that imposes more intimacy on a client than he or she desires:* To some people, certain gestures may imply a level of intimacy or degree of closeness. When the touch suggests a degree of closeness that is not equally shared or agreed upon by both parties, distress may occur.
- *Observe the client's response to the touch:* Assessment of a touch is especially impor-

tant in the initial meeting with clients and when the nurse does not know how the client will respond. The nurse should observe the client's nonverbal behaviors. For example, if the client pulls away or displays a tense facial expression, he or she may be having a negative reaction or response to the touch. On the other hand, if a client appears relaxed and more comforted after the touch, it is likely that he or she is receiving the touch positively.

In health-care situations in which both the nurse and the client are comfortable with touch, and the use of touch is assessed for therapeutic effect, touch can be a very valuable mode of human communication.

Kinesics

Kinesics, commonly referred to as body language, is an important component of nonverbal communication (Arnold & Boggs, 2003). Kinesics is also defined as involving the conscious or unconscious body positioning and actions of the individual giving the message. Some dimensions of kinesics are posturing and gait, gestures, and facial expressions. Body stance can convey a message about the nurse or the client. If the client is in a slumped, head-down position, the nurse may assess that the client may have low self-esteem, whereas an erect posture and decisive movements may suggest confidence and self-control. Rapid, diffuse, or agitated body movements may indicate anxiety.

Facial expressions, the various movements in the face, provide emotional undertone and feeling whether or not they are accompanied by verbal communication. Throughout life, individuals respond to the expressive qualities of another face, often without realizing it. Mehrabian (1971), in studying the impact of words, vocalization, and facial expressions, noted that the power of the facial expression supporting the verbal content far outweighs the impact of the actual words. Research also suggests that individuals who make direct eye contact while talking or listening give a sense of confidence and credibility, whereas those people who look down or avert their eyes indicate submission, weakness, or shame (Arnold & Boggs, 2003). Remember, however, that eye contact varies with culture.

Facial expression is important in conveying a message; it either reinforces or changes the verbal message that the listener hears. When the verbal message is inconsistent or different from the individual's facial expression, the nonverbal expressions assume more prominence and meaning and are generally perceived as more trustworthy and meaningful than the spoken word (Mehrabian, 1971).

The face is the most expressive part of the body, adding obvious and subtle cues to the real focus of the message. Common facial expressions are surprise, sadness, anger, happiness and joy, disgust and contempt, and fear (Arnold & Boggs, 2003). A client's facial expression should be part of the nursing assessment. For example, if a client frowns after receiving information, he or she may be experiencing confusion or anger. The nurse can intervene by saying, "I see that you are frowning. Is something wrong?" The question would encourage the client to clarify his or her response.

In the health-care profession, it is very important for the nurse's facial expression to be congruent with the verbal message given to the client. When a nurse walks into a client's hospital room, the client will "search" the nurse's face for clues before the nurse can even speak. For example, if the client asks the nurse, "Do I have cancer?" the slightest change in the nurse's facial features can reveal the nurse's true feelings. Although it is difficult to control all facial expressions, the nurse should try to avoid showing overt shock, revulsion, dismay, and other distressing reactions in the client's presence. If the nurse comes into a client's room with an expression of anger, stress, or disgust, the client and his family may perceive the nurse to be uncaring.

Appearance

The nurse's **physical appearance,** including dress, grooming, posture, gestures, and ease of movements, makes an important impact on the client and conveys the nurse's attitudes

about himself or herself and others. Studies have shown that spoken words account for only 7% of the message; vocal quality accounts for 38%; and the way individuals look and act account for 55% or more of the message, depending on the culture (Hall, 1959).

The business world has been aware of the "dress for success" rule and has noted the role clothes play in projecting the image of the serious professional. Nursing is no different; the client reacts to the way a nurse is dressed. In the past, nurses wore white uniforms and caps that were designed from their various schools of nursing. In today's health-care environment there is no standard uniform for the professional nurse—a fact that does tend to confuse the layperson. What nurses wear is usually determined by the area of the hospital in which they work or the role they have in the community. Mangum and associates (1991) surveyed clients, nurses, and administrators to determine whether or not different styles of nursing uniforms are associated with the professional image of nursing. In their summary, they noted that the nurse is judged primarily by what is worn and presented at the bedside. The nurse should make a conscious effort to dress in a professional image.

THERAPEUTIC COMMUNICATION

Therapeutic communication, a term coined by Ruesch (1961), is defined as a purposeful form of communication between the health professional and the client that allows them to reach health-related goals through participation in a focused relationship. "Therapeutic communication differs from ordinary communication in that the intention of one or more of the participants is clearly directed at bringing about a change in the system and manner of communication" (Rusesch, 1961, p. 460). This type of communication differs from a social communication, because there is a specific purpose or planned direction to the communication. The nurse uses therapeutic communication to promote a psychological setting that allows positive change, growth, and healing for the client. As the professional caregiver, the nurse comes to know the client as an individual who has unique health needs, responses, and patterns of living. With this knowledge, the nurse uses a goal-directed approach when communicating with the client.

Therapeutic communication can take place in a variety of clinical settings, ranging from the acute care system to nursing homes. As health-care delivery moves to a community focus, therapeutic communication can take place in nontraditional health-care settings such as the client's home, schools, and ambulatory care settings. Therapeutic conversations in health-care settings are designed to help clients maintain healthy habits, learn about their illness, and learn ways of coping. The communication is goal-oriented and client-centered, has rules and boundaries, and uses individualized strategies (Arnold & Boggs, 2003).

Therapeutic Communication Techniques

A number of techniques are used in therapeutic communication (Box 7–1). Nurses should familiarize themselves with and make it a habit to use these techniques both in and outside of therapeutic situations.

Active Listening

Effective therapeutic communication between the nurse and client begins with **active listening** (Bush, 2001). Listening actively means that the listener is communicating interest and attention to the client. The goal of active listening is to comprehend and understand fully what the other person is trying to communicate.

Two important techniques used by the nurse in active listening are restatement and reflection (Craven & Hirnle, 1996). *Restatement* takes place when the nurse listens carefully to the client and then restates some or all of the content back to the client to ensure that the nurse has the correct under-

> **BOX 7–1**
> **THERAPEUTIC COMMUNICATION TECHNIQUES**
> - Active listening
> - Restatement
> - Reflection
> - Focusing
> - Encouraging elaboration
> - Looking at alternatives
> - Use of silence
> - Appropriate questions

standing of what the client has said. When the content is restated, the client has the opportunity to hear what he or she has said and therefore gains an understanding of how the nurse has perceived what he or she has communicated.

> *The nurse listens to the client for both content and emotions expressed through nonverbal facial expression, body posture, and emotional status.*

Reflection is the process of identifying the main emotional themes in the conversation and directing them back to the client (Box 7–2). The nurse listens for the underlying feeling that the client is conveying and then shares this with the client in a nonjudgmental, open manner. This process allows the

> **BOX 7–2**
> **REFLECTION AND RESTATEMENT**
> *Client:* I don't want to eat anything today. I can't even begin to think about food.
> *Nurse:* You don't want to eat and you can't think about food. (*Restatement*)
> *Client:* All I can think about is what the doctor will tell me about the biopsy. (*Client is wringing her hands and almost crying*)
> *Nurse:* The news about the biopsy result is worrying you and makes you unable to eat. (*Reflection*)
> *Client:* Yes, I'm very nervous that it will mean that I have to have more surgery. I'm really frightened.

client to explore his or her own ideas and gives the client a clearer understanding of the feelings being experienced.

Questions

Questions are an important part of all phases of therapeutic communication because they allow the nurse to obtain information from the client. The nurse needs to ask pertinent questions but not to the point that the client feels that he or she is being interrogated.

Arnold & Boggs (2003) suggest that questions can be divided into three categories: open-ended, close-ended, and circular. *Open-ended questions* are phrases stated in such a way that the client is able to elaborate beyond a simple yes or no answer. This gives the client a way to "tell a story." Think of such a question as an essay question on a test. It gives the client a chance to express thoughts about a problem or health need. Open-ended questions usually begin with words like "how," "what," "when," and "can you tell me about." Examples of open-ended questions are, "What brought you to the hospital?" and "Can you tell me about your being diagnosed with diabetes?" These questions are general, rather than specific, and are open to the client's interpretation.

Closed-ended questions require specific answers and limit a client's response. These types of questions are best used in emergency situations, and it may take more of them to get the desired response. In this situation, the nurse wants to obtain information quickly and the client's emotional reactions are secondary. Examples of closed-ended questions are "When did the pain start?" and "How long has it been since you saw the doctor?"

Circular questions focus on the impact of the illness or injury and how it will affect the family and significant others. The nurse uses circular questions as a type of family interviewing strategy. The nurse can use the information that the family or others provide as a basis for additional questions about the client or other family members. For example, the nurse asks family members about the care of a terminally ill client (the mother) in their home. From the family's response, the nurse may receive multidimensional information about the family that could not be learned by asking specific questions. This approach provides a basis for open discussion of the client and the family's circumstances.

Other Therapeutic Communication Techniques

Other techniques the nurse may use in therapeutic communication are focusing, encouraging elaboration, and looking at alternatives. *Focusing* means asking goal-directed questions that help keep the client focused on the subject at hand. The nurse is also conveying that she is helping the client discuss the main areas of concern. The nurse can also encourage *elaboration*. This technique allows the client to describe the concerns or problems under discussion in a more detailed manner. The nurse can look attentively at the client and use short responses like "I see" and "Go on" to allow the client to continue to explore feelings. *Looking at alternatives* allows the nurse to help the client increase the client's perceived choices. This technique should not be used until the client has a clear understanding of the current situation. Sometimes the client has to deal with emotions such as anger and denial before alternatives come into play.

Probably one of the hardest techniques the nurse must learn is the use of **silence**, that period when no words are being spoken between the nurse and the client. For Americans in particular, it takes experience to become comfortable with pauses in the conversation. Most people have a natural tendency to try to fill up the empty spaces with words. By contrast, many Native Americans consider silence essential to understanding and respecting what the nurse has said. In traditional Chinese and Japanese cultures, silence may mean that the speakers wants the listener to consider the importance of the content before continuing. British and Arab people may use silence as a sign of respect for the individual's privacy, whereas French, Spanish, and Russian individuals may consider silence a sign of agreement. Among some African Americans, silence is used to respond to what is perceived as an inappropriate statement (Andrews & Boyle, 1999).

In therapeutic relations, silent moments give the nurse and the client time to observe each other, digest what messages have been communicated, and think of things to say. Silence can be used deliberately and thoughtfully and can be a powerful listening tool. On the other hand, long silences may be very uncomfortable. By pausing briefly before continuing a conversation with a client, the nurse gives the client a chance to reflect and come up with questions of his or her own.

Barriers to Communication

In the therapeutic communication setting, the nurse must be aware of certain responses that may lower the client's self-esteem and limit full disclosure of client information. Several of these responses that tend to block communication, or **barriers to communication**, are as follows (Box 7–3):

False reassurance is the use of clichés or comforting phrases in order to attempt to reassure the client. These types of responses invalidate the client's feelings or fears. Expressions such as "Everything will be okay" and "Don't worry" send a message to the client that the nurse is not interested in the client's true feelings.

Giving advice is telling the client what to do or making a decision for the client. The nurse should avoid offering personal opinions to the client. Avoid phrases such as "should do" or "ought to do." These types of responses tend to center the interaction on the nurse's needs and perspective rather than on the client's. If a client asks a nurse for specific advice, the nurse can use a reflective statement and explore the various choices the client has in that situation.

Probing is asking questions out of curiosity rather than for information needed to assist the client. Many of these questions begin with the word "Why?" These types of questions from the nurse tend to put the client in a defensive mode and also violate the client's privacy.

> **BOX 7–3**
> **COMMUNICATION BARRIERS**
> - False reassurance
> - Giving advice
> - Probing
> - Stereotyping
> - Social comment
> - Changing the subject
> - Use of jargon

Stereotyping is the process of attributing characteristics to a group of people as though all people in that group possess those features. Stereotyping groups clients in a category and does not value or recognize their individuality. Stereotypes lead the nurse to false conclusions about the client, and if they are based on strong emotions, stereotypes can be identified as prejudices. It is important that the nurse convey an acceptance of the client as a unique individual.

Social comment is the use of polite, superficial comments that do not focus on what the client is feeling or trying to express to the nurse. The nurse can use social comments at the beginning of an interaction to make a connection with the patient. However, the nurse should focus on a therapeutic interaction with the client when talking about issues or concerns that affect the client's health. Socialization is inappropriate when a more serious approach to the client's situation is suitable.

Changing the subject when the client is trying to communicate about another topic is rude and shows lack of sensitivity. Changing the subject tends to block communication; the client may withhold information about important issues and fail to express his feelings openly. If the nurse does have to change the subject, the reason for this change should be given to the client.

The nurse should not use *nursing or medical jargon*—terminology that is used among nurses and other health professionals—when addressing the client. These unfamiliar words can cause confusion and anxiety for clients. They also may be frightening to some clients. Nurses should try to use common terms that the client is familiar with. And if nurses need to use jargon, they should make sure that they carefully explain what the terms mean.

CONCLUSION

Nurses should be aware of the various aspects of communication discussed and avoid common communication pitfalls with clients, their families and significant others, and other health professionals. Being a good communicator takes practice and may feel a bit unnatural at first. However, as nurses continue to integrate communication techniques into their communication pattern, the acquired skills become more natural. These acquired skills will be beneficial not only in communication with clients but also in communication with other health-care professionals. A valuable tool to evaluate communication patterns is a process recording where verbal and nonverbal behavior interactions are analyzed (see Table 7–1).

COMMUNICATION WITH COLLEAGUES

Nurses must also communicate effectively with a diverse group of professionals and unli-

censed personnel in caring for clients. When members of the health-care team communicate ineffectively with one another, delivery of health-care to the client suffers.

The nurse must use effective communication skills with all colleagues, regardless of their position, and must regard each individual with an attitude of respect. "Using clear, simple messages and clarifying the intent of others constitutes a positive goal in all personal and professional communication"(Chitty, 1997, p. 391). Just as a client must have trust in the health professional administering care, trust and respect must exist between colleagues for effective communication.

Collaboration, the collegial working relationship with other health-care providers, is intrinsic to nursing. Henneman and colleagues (1995) state that collaboration implies working in cooperation with other personnel and viewing them as a team. The relationship between individuals who are collaborating is nonhierarchical. The power is shared and is based on the knowledge and expertise that each individual brings to the setting, not on role or title (Henneman et al., 1995). In this team approach, each person recognizes the boundaries of each discipline and values the contribution that every person makes.

Because nurses are the managers of client

TABLE 7–1
Sample Process Recording for Evaluation of Communication

Client Response	Nurse Response	Nonverbal Behavior	Anaylsis of Content
	How are you feeling today?"		
"OK."		Client is grimacing and frowning.	The patient is exhibiting signs of postoperative pain by the look on the face.
	"You seem to be in pain. Can you tell me about how you feel?"		

care in acute care settings and are with the client for 24 hours, they obtain a lot of information that must be communicated to other health-care providers. Nurses must make a concerted effort to have a collaborative relationship with the team members, not just working in cooperation with others Silva & Ludwick, 2002). Collaboration allows the nurse to identify the contributions of the other disciplines and permits the integration of this information into the health-care plan for the client. It also helps enhance problem-solving skills by utilizing insights from other disciplines and health-care workers who deal with the client. Collaboration with other members of the health-care team is essential for the nursing profession to provide excellent health care to all clients.

 ONLINE CONSULT

http://carbon.cudenver.edu/~mryder/itc/comm_theory.html
http://cbpa.louisville.edu/bruce/mgmtwebs/commun_f98/Introduction.htm
http://www.acjournal.org/
http://stephan.dahl.at/nonverbal/

Key Points

- Effective communication within the client-nurse relationship is a learned skill and is essential for providing effective nursing care.
- Communication models illustrate the complex process of communication with the basic components: source/encoder, the message, the medium, and the receiver/decoder.
- The health communications model (Northouse & Northouse, 1992) uses a broad systems view of communication and emphasizes the way in which a series of factors (relationships, transactions, and contexts) can affect interactions in the health-care setting.
- When people share information, they express messages in a complex composite of both verbal (spoken or written) and nonverbal behaviors. Individuals express themselves through language, gestures, voice inflection, facial expressions, and use of space.
- Metacommunication is a broad term used to "describe all of the factors that influence how the message is perceived" (Arnold & Boggs, 2003, p. 217).
- Oral communication is the use of words by people to think about ideas, to share experiences with others, and to validate the perceptions of the world.
- Potter and Perry (1999) state that the six most important aspects of verbal communication are (1) vocabulary, (2) denotative and connotative meaning, (3) intonation, (4) pacing, (5) clarity and brevity, and (6) timing and relevance.
- Nonverbal communication is communication without words and includes messages that are created through body motions, facial expressions, use of space and sounds, and use of touch. Arnold and Boggs (2003) categorize four areas in which nonverbal behaviors are used: (1) proxemics, (2) cultural variations, (3) kinesics, which includes body language and facial expression, and (4) appearance.

(continued)

(*continued*)

- In order for clients to perceive touch in a positive therapeutic relationship, Northouse and Northouse (1992) suggests that nurses use the following guidelines: use touch that is appropriate to the particular situation, do not use a touch that imposes more intimacy on a client than he or she desires, and observe the client's response to the touch.
- Therapeutic communication is a purposeful form of communication that serves as a point of contact between the health professional and the client and allows them to reach health-related goals through participation in a focused relationship. Techniques include active listening, restatement, reflection, focusing, encouraging elaboration, looking at alternatives, use of silence, and use of appropriate questions.
- Barriers to communication are certain responses that may lower the client's self-esteem, limit full disclosure of client information, and block communication. These barriers include false reassurance, giving advice, probing, stereotyping, social comment, changing the subject, and use of jargon.
- Collaboration involves working in cooperation with other members of the health-care team. The power is shared and is based on the knowledge and expertise that each member brings to the setting; titles and roles do not matter.

Thought and Discussion Questions

1. Contrast the various communication models for use in the hospital versus the home setting.
2. Explain how nonverbal communication may be more "powerful" than spoken words.
3. Describe a collaborative relationship that you have experienced in your work setting.
4. Prepare a Process Recording of a 5-minute intervention with a client. Use the format shown in Table 7–1:
5. Review the Chapter Thought on the first page of the chapter and discuss it in the context of the contents of the chapter.

Interactive Exercises

1. Review the clinical scenarios provided on the Intranet site, and identify the communication techniques and barriers to therapeutic communication.
2. Conduct an interview with someone from a different culture, and identify the ways that this person perceives illness and/or hospitalization. Does the person's culture use any folk remedies or alternative health-care measures? You may conduct the interview via the Internet.
3. Complete the Interview Self-Assessment Questions located in the Interactive Exercises section of the Intranet in order to evaluate your own nonverbal communication.
4. Complete the Picture Taking Interactive Exercise located on the Intranet site in

order to see the nonverbal emotional cues that you are communicating with other people.

5. Perform the Setting Evaluation located in the Interactive Exercises on the Intranet site in order to identify the environmental factors in your facility that could frighten clients.

6. By completing the Barriers to Communication Interactive Exercise on the Intranet site, you will be able to understand better what you may be doing to create obstacles in communication with clients and colleagues.

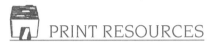

PRINT RESOURCES

References

Andrews, M., & Boyle, J. (1999) *Transcultural concepts in nursing care* (3rd ed.) Philadelphia: Lippincott.

Arnold, E., & Boggs, K. (2003). *Interpersonal relationships: Professional communication skills for nurses* (4th ed.) Philadelphia: W. B. Saunders.

Berlo, D. K. (1960). *The process of communication: An introduction to theory and practice.* New York: Holt, Rinehart & Winston.

Birdwhistell, R. L. (1970). *Kinesics and context.* Philadelphia: University of Pennsylvania Press.

Bush, K. (2001). Do you really listen to patients? RN 2001, 64 (3), 35–37.

Chitty, K. K. (1997). *Professional nursing concepts and challenges* (2nd ed.). Philadelphia: W. B. Saunders

Craven, R., & Hirnle, C. (1996). *Fundamentals of nursing human health and function* (2nd ed.). Philadelphia: Lippincott-Raven.

Hall, E. T. (1959). *The silent language.* Garden City, NY: Doubleday & Company.

Leary, T. (1955). The theory and measurement methodology of interpersonal communication. *Psychiatry,* 18, 147–161.

Mangum, S., Garrison, C., Lind, A., et al. (1991). Perceptions of nurses' uniforms. *Image,* 23, 127.

Mehrabian, A. (1971). *Silent messages.* Belmont, CA: Wadsworth Publishing.

Mitchell, R. W. (1991). Bateson's concept of meta-communication in play. *New Ideas in Psychology,* 9(1), 73–87.

Northouse, P. G., & Northouse, L. L. (1992). *Health communication strategies for health professionals* (2nd ed.). Norwalk, CT: Appleton & Lange.

Potter A., & Perry, G. (1999). *Basic nursing: A critical thinking approach* (4th ed.). St. Louis: Mosby.

Ruesch, J. (1961). *Therapeutic communication.* New York: W. W. Norton.

Shannon, C. E., & Weaver, W. (1949). *The mathematical theory of communication.* Urbana, IL: University of Illinois Press.

Watson, J., (1979). *Nursing the philosophy and science of caring.* Boston: Little, Brown.

Bibliography

Print Resources

Benson, A., & Latter, S. (1998). Implementing health promoting nursing: The integration of interpersonal skills and health promotion. *Journal of Advanced Nursing,* 27, 100–107.

Brown, G. (1995). Understanding barriers to basing nursing practice upon research: a communication model approach. *Journal of Advanced Nursing,* 21, 154–157.

Ceccio, J., & Ceccio, C. (1982). *Effective communication in nursing: Theory and practice.* Canada: John Wiley & Sons.

Craven, R., & Hirnle, C., (1996) *Fundamentals of nursing human health and function* (2nd ed.). Philadelphia: Lippincott–Raven.

Crowther, D. (1991). Metacommunication a missed opportunity? *Journal of Advanced Nursing,* 20, 703–706.

Davidhizar, R., & Giger, J. (1994). When your patient is silent. *Journal of Advanced Nursing,* 20, 703–706.

Edwards, B., & Brilhart, J. (1981). *Communication in nursing practice.* St. Louis: C. V. Mosby.

Leininger, M., & McFarland, M. (2002). *Transcultural nursing: Concepts, theories, research and practice* (3rd ed.). New York: McGraw-Hill.

Lindberg, J., Hunter, M., & Kruszewski, A. (1983). *Introduction to person-centered nursing.* Philadelphia: J. B. Lippincott.

Long, L. (1992). *Understanding/responding: A communication manual for nurses.* Boston: Jones and Bartlett.

Mehrabian, A. (1981) *Silent messages: Implicit communication of emotions and attitudes* (2nd ed.). Belmont, CA: Wadsworth Publishing

Mulaik, J., Megenity, J., Cannon, K., et al. (1997). Patient's perceptions of nurses' use of touch. *Western Journal of Nursing Research,* 13(3), 306–323.

Peplau, H. (1952). *Interpersonal relations in nursing.* New York: G. P. Putnam's Sons.

Peplau, H. (1960). Talking with patients. *American Journal of Nursing,* 60, 964 –966.

Salle, A. (1999). Effective communication. In B. Cherry & S. Jacob (Eds.), *Contemporary nursing issues, trends, & management* (pp. 378 – 402). St. Louis: Mosby.

Sieh, A., & Brentin, L. (1997). *The nurse communicates.* Philadelphia: W. B. Saunders.

Steel, Jean E. (1986). *Issue in collaborative practice* Orlando, FL: Grune & Stratton, Inc.

💻 ONLINE RESOURCES

http://carbon.cudenver.edu/~mryder/itc/comm_theory.html
http://cbpa.louisville.edu/bruce/mgmtwebs/commun_f98/ Introduction.htm
http://www.acjournal.org/
http://stephan.dahl.at/nonverbal/

References

Henneman, E. A., Lee, J. L., & Cohen, J. I. Collaboration: A concept analysis. Journal of advanced nursing, 21, 103–109.
Silva, M., and Ludwick, R. (August 30, 2002). Ethics Column: Ethical Grounding for Entry into Practice: Respect, Collaboration, and Accountability. *Online Journal of Issues in Nursing.* *http://www.nursingworld.org/ojin/ethicol/ ethics_9.htm*

Rose Kearney-Nunnery

8
chapter

Working with Groups

> We communicate in many ways, especially when working with others toward a common goal.

Chapter Objectives

On completion of this chapter, the reader will be able to:

1. Explain the techniques for effective communication in group settings.
2. Evaluate personal communication patterns used with clients and colleagues in a group.
3. Describe different types of groups, including their characteristics and roles of group members.
4. Differentiate between effective and ineffective groups and the characteristics of an effective group leader.
5. Evaluate communication patterns in a group for effective functioning in meeting the group's common goals.

Key Terms

Group	Effective groups	Ineffective groups
Group process	Goal attainment	Stages of group
Group structure	Member participation	development
Group composition	Cohesiveness	Functional task roles
Group roles	Decision-making	Functional group-building
Group focus	Communication patterns	roles
Professional groups	Attendance	Nonfunctional group roles
Work groups	Creativity	Organizational group
Educational groups	Power	Virtual meetings
Therapeutic groups		

Communication—verbal, nonverbal, and written—is integral to working with individuals and groups. DeWine and associates (2000) identify four contexts or environments in which communication takes place: interpersonal, group, organizational, and mass communication. Nurses must be skilled in each of these areas, from the interpersonal situation with a client or colleague, to small client or colleague groups, to larger organizational settings, and, finally, to mass communications with the public. Effective communication becomes more complex when multiple relationships and transactions are occurring while the purpose for and goals of a particular group are being addressed.

The concepts of effective group process are important components in professional nursing practice and require understanding of the types of groups, their composition and functions, and the roles played by the members. As nurses, we need to develop skills to use as both leaders and members of various work and professional groups as well as to apply group process to intervene therapeutically with clients. Examining the group's characteristics and evaluating the group's effectiveness provide the knowledge and skills needed to accomplish these goals. Note that understanding groups is an initial step in addressing the core competency for health professionals of working in interdisciplinary teams.

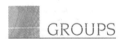 GROUPS

A **group** consists of three or more individuals with some commonality, such as shared goals or interests. Living in society, we are members of many groups—family, work, professional, and social. Each type of group has a specific goal and membership. As nurses, we are involved as participants in work groups and interact with groups of clients in their healthcare activities. We may also participate in therapy or support groups. We use the principles of group process in all these activities and in assisting our clients. Some of these groups

are structured loosely, with minimal rules, whereas others have clearly defined roles and limits. It is essential for the nurse to understand group processes to communicate and function effectively in the group as both an individual and a professional.

Group Process

Group process is the dynamic interplay of interactions within and between groups of humans. Interplay includes what is said and done in groups as well as how members interact with one another and the group leader. Wilson (1985) has vividly described the usefulness of systems theory as a framework for studying group process phenomena in terms of roles and behaviors, boundaries, and the communications within the group (p. 5). Recall from Chapter 3 that systems theory is concerned with holism as opposed to the isolated parts. The basic components of a system are the input, output, boundary, environment, and feedback. A group is a social system, composed of people with their unique characteristics and communication styles but focused on the group goals as the output from the system. And as Berol (1960) pointed out in his classic work on communication, "a knowledge of the composition and workings of a social system is useful in making predictions about how members of that system will behave in a given communication situation" (p. 135). This is particularly applicable to professional practice with the nurses' focus on the importance of working with groups in a variety of practice settings—client, family, self-help, self-awareness, peer, and task groups.

Group Characteristics

Groups can be classified according to structure, composition, roles, and focus. A particular group often fits more than one classification, especially in terms of its roles. For example, the initial purpose of developing a cancer support group might have been to provide the members with a sense of sharing and support. But this type of group often fills many other functions, such as education regarding medications, traditional and non-traditional treatment programs, and health-care providers; information sharing about benefits, wills, and finances; and strategy sharing on coping with symptoms and managing daily life.

Group Structure

Groups may be differentiated by **group structure**, such as whether a group is formal or informal. Formal groups are highly structured, with functions specified in job descriptions, contracts, policies, and procedures. Formal groups associated with nursing are the entire nursing staff and the professional standards committee. Each of these groups has particular requirements for membership and specific rules, procedures, and standards of practice. A professional group can also be viewed as a formal group, with requirements for membership, rules that govern meetings, and specific member expectations. An advantage of structured groups is their clear understanding of roles and expectations. This same benefit may become a disadvantage, if the group is not open to changing to meet the needs of the members. The leaders of more structured groups tend to have greater power. By contrast, informal groups are more loosely structured, at times disbanding or reconvening according to the needs of the membership. Examples of informal groups are special interest groups and support groups. Informal groups benefit from some degree of flexibility in roles, expectations, and leadership.

Composition of Groups

Groups can also be differentiated by the unique composition of the membership. **Group composition** may be homogeneous or heterogeneous, depending on the characteristics of the members. Members of homogenous groups are similar in some aspect, such as all adolescent male clients or female nurses

employed in the intensive care units. A benefit of working with a homogeneous group is the sense of shared connection that the members typically feel from the beginning. This sense may be expressed as "He has the same problem" or "She thinks the same way I do." Heterogeneous groups consist of a mix of individuals, such as clients with various diagnoses or ages, or a work group of both nurses and physicians working with patients in a cardiac intensive care unit. This type of group has a wider range of diversity and therefore usually a greater variety of opinions, beliefs, and needs. Facilitating a sense of connection among members is a key challenge for the heterogeneous group. With a heterogeneous group, however, group members have the advantage of learning from many different perspectives.

Group Roles

A third way to classify groups is in terms of the leader and participant **group roles.** Some groups are led by a professional who is responsible for instituting the rules, establishing the structure, and determining the membership. There are clear expectations for the leader and the participants. An example is an outpatient recovery group, in which a cardiac rehabilitation counselor leads the group, initiates themes for discussion, and often sets criteria for members' participation. Other groups have informal leadership as well as rules for members. Peer support groups are an example of this type. Traditionally, the leadership may be shared by members, who are usually working on a common issue. Members are free to attend or not, depending on their own needs and schedules. At times, the group may become engulfed in struggles for leadership, which can compromise the group's effectiveness.

Group Focus

Groups may also be classified according to their focus or approach. The **group focus** can be work-related, educational, therapeutic, or professional. Professional nursing groups were described in Chapter 1, along with their unique missions and membership requirements. These **professional groups** are generally formal and are directed at professional issues and at the objectives stated in their mission statements. **Work groups** are task oriented, focused on a particular work-related activity, as with a nursing department budget committee and the task of allocating resources.

Many of us are members of a variety of work groups. Nurses on a particular unit constitute one group, whereas the nursing department as a whole is another functioning work group. Committees that meet monthly are probably commonly viewed as work groups. They may be convened ad hoc (as needed), or they may be more or less a permanent standing group, such as the nursing standards committee, the safety committee, or the quality assurance committee. The membership changes over time, and the structure varies in level of formality. If the group is focusing on one specific issue or task, members may be expected to fulfill assigned roles. At other times there may be a more informal, shifting assignment of roles, as occurs in monthly staff meetings on a care unit. Attendance varies, depending on schedule, client load, and the issues involved.

Educational groups have a teaching focus, whether members are teaching clients about medications, treatments, parenting skills, or a variety of health promotion activities or educating their colleagues in areas of expertise. This type of group may actually convene only for an individual session, if held in a clinic or institutional setting, or it may have a series of sessions. An example is a stress reduction class for clients diagnosed with hypertension, which is scheduled on a weekly basis in a clinic or outpatient department. Membership and attendance vary depending on educational needs and appointment schedules. Although the group leader is a professional, the structure is typically less formal and directed at the learning needs of the audience. Teaching and learning principles, discussed in Chapter 10, are important considerations, along with the group process.

Therapeutic groups are varied in nature, depending on the specific treatment or client needs. This group is led by a professional and is a formally structured group that typically specifies when members can join and when they can leave the group. Examples of these groups are cognitive therapy groups for depressed clients, behavioral therapy groups for anger management, and therapeutic activity groups, such as a music therapy group for clients who have suffered cerebral vascular events. The group leader has special training in the different therapeutic approaches used. Advanced Practice Nurses (APRNs) can lead groups in specific therapies as defined in practice standards and as recognized by their State Practice Act.

Effective Groups

Effective groups have an identified purpose or need for the group and a commitment to the process. Once the decision is made to form a new group, several issues are involved in setting up or structuring the group. Arnold (2003) terms this the "pregroup phase," in which the following activities occur:

- Alignment of purpose and membership
- Determination of appropriate group size
- Creation of the appropriate environment

The first consideration is the purpose for forming the group. This purpose must be clearly stated for specification of the membership. Once the intended membership is determined, members can be recruited and goals set for the group. The size of the membership must be appropriate to addressing the group goals effectively. A professional group must be larger to effect change than a work group. A work or therapeutic group becomes less effective when it grows too large, becoming more heterogeneous and unable to focus on the task or treatment aims. For some groups, the leader also spends time interviewing potential members before the initial meeting. This step serves as an orientation to the group as well as a way to determine whether the individual will "fit in."

The room arrangement is another important factor for creating the appropriate environment. When the room is being set up, the goals of the group and interactions needed among members should be considered. A large conference table and chairs may be needed for a work group, whereas placing chairs in a circle to allow individuals to make eye contact without the barrier of a table is imperative in many therapeutic groups. Neither of these arrangements may be feasible or essential in an educational group.

Other factors to consider involve the basic setup issues are:

- The best meeting place and time for meetings
- Fees, dues, or cost factors
- Frequency and length of meetings
- Documentation needed for third-party payers or sponsoring organizations

> *Effective groups have an identified purpose or need for the group and a commitment to the process.*

An effective group will also determine whether there will be a single leader or coleaders. Those in favor of two-leader groups cite the enhanced ability to examine dynamics, provide feedback, and manage absences of the leader. Those against this style look at the possibility of problems arising between these two individuals in terms of power, equality, and accountability, with the potential for splitting of the group, creating factions, and ineffectiveness. The goal is to form a strong, viable group. Before initiating a group, a nurse should consider all of these concerns.

Evaluating Effectiveness of Groups

Effective groups are those that work toward the stated goals and whose members derive a sense of belonging and acceptance. How these outcomes can be accomplished requires a closer look at behaviors, strategies, and goals. In addition, organizations and third-party payers may determine their own criteria of effectiveness. General factors to consider in determining effectiveness of any group are identified in Box 8–1.

Goal attainment is the initial and most important criterion in determining the effectiveness of any group. It is an evaluation of

> **BOX 8–1**
> **FACTORS TO CONSIDER IN EVALUATING EFFECTIVENESS OF GROUPS**
>
> - Goal attainment
> - Member participation
> - Cohesiveness
> - Decision-making
> - Communication patterns
> - Attendance
> - Creativity
> - Power

whether the intended task or goal was accomplished, especially in a work group. In a professional association, goal attainment is focused on the activities related to the organization's mission. In a therapeutic group, goal attainment relates to the focus of the group, such as gaining insight, awareness, or skills.

Member participation is another important criterion for assessing the effectiveness of a group. Consider whether all members are included in the discussions and what roles they are playing as group members. On the other hand, think about a situation in which an autocratic leader limits the members' ability to participate in the group discussions. In an effective group, there is evidence of belonging, camaraderie, and acceptance. But participation does not imply that all members should be in agreement on all issues. "Group think" is the phenomenon by which all members are in constant agreement, which can limit creativity and lead to stagnation.

Cohesiveness among the group members indicates that they are working together toward the group's common purpose or goal. If all members are not focused on the purpose, the original goal for which the group was formed will be difficult to attain, and conflict may arise. To achieve cohesiveness, the group members must be refocused on the original intent for the group, with the leader and members supporting one another in their actions and demonstrating agreement on the common goal.

In an effective group, **decision-making** must occur at the group level, with all members being involved in decisions rather than unilateral actions being taken by the leader or a disruptive member. A democratic leader and involved, cohesive members directed toward the common goal usually signify effective group functioning as they actively work toward that goal.

The **communication patterns** among the members provide valuable information on whether there is a common focus, respect, and decision-making. Evaluate how the group's decisions are made. The group leader should facilitate effective communication patterns, thus allowing all members to be heard and involved in the group process. In an effective group, members are actively involved in a mutual communication process.

Attendance is regular and active in an effective group. Members are punctual and involved, energetically focused on the task or purpose of the group. When a group meeting is arranged in advance, members in an effective group honor their commitments to the meeting rather than making excuses for not attending or demonstrating routine tardiness.

A high level of **creativity** among the members is another sign of an effective group. The group members are spontaneously generating novel ideas for solutions on the common problem. Brainstorming sessions are focused on the goals, and communication is encouraged, with all ideas and contributions from members considered.

Typically, the leadership style in more effective groups is described as democratic, and the interactions among the members are interdependent and collaborative. **Power** is distributed, on the basis of the common purpose and abilities of the members to achieve their goal in an effective group. Power struggles disrupt group process, with members focusing inwardly rather than working collaboratively on the group's goals.

Ineffective groups have low levels of productivity. These groups contain much unrest and stagnation, and members feel that they do not belong or that it is not safe for them to share their thoughts, ideas, and feelings. The group members demonstrate an uncaring attitude toward one another, have little spontaneous involvement, or are reluctant participants. The members do not appear to trust one another, seem unwilling to take risks and, in work groups, rarely volunteer for or willingly accept assignments. The attendance may be uneven, with a high rate of dropout and tardiness. The leadership style in less effective groups is often described as autocratic or laissez-faire, and the group interactions as independent and competitive.

THE BASICS OF GROUP PROCESSES

The Stages of Group Development

Understanding the expected **stages of group development** and how to facilitate groups during these stages is essential to nursing practice, when the nurse is a group member or a leader. As with the developmental stages of individuals, groups go through predictable stages. An effective group leader must be aware of these stages and must motivate members and modify approaches accordingly. Consider the descriptions of the stages of group development in Table 8–1.

TABLE 8–1 Stages of Group Development	
Tuckman (1965)	• Forming • Storming • Norming • Performing • Mourning or termination
Yalom (1995)	• Orientation • Conflict • Cohesion • Working • Termination
Arnold (2003)	• Forming • Storming • Norming • Performing • Adjourning

We can use the traditional stages of the nurse-client relationship (initial, working, and termination), with the addition of the conflict and norming stages before the working phase, to understand the process of group development better. The stages of group development, along with expected goals and examples of appropriate nursing approaches, are illustrated in Table 8–2. Now, consider the five stages of group development: initial or forming, conflict or storming, norming, working or performing, and termination or adjourning.

Forming

In the initial or forming stage, the group is being formed. The members are becoming acquainted with one another, the group, and the purpose and outcomes. Arnold (2003) identifies the major group tasks during this forming stage as establishing the group contract, developing trust, and identification. The leader focuses on orienting the members and determining the structure in terms of time, duration, and frequency of meetings as well as the goals for the group. Cohesiveness of the group is enhanced by clearly stated goals and group norms. Work groups require an introduction, identification of goals and expectations, and orientation to the structure. Client groups also require this introduction and orientation information, but issues of confidentiality and personal disclosure are important considerations in their forming stage.

Storming and Norming

The next phase is the conflict or storming stage. This is the time when members become

TABLE 8–2
Group Stages, Expected Goals, and Nursing Techniques

Stage	Expected Goals	Nursing Techniques
Initial/forming	Sense of trust	Making introductions Structuring group Defining parameters and goals Encouraging the sense of group
Conflict/storming	Sense of commitment	Encouraging verbalizations Allowing interactions and role development Handling confrontations and setting limits
Norming	Sense of purpose	Setting limits, rules, and expectations Encouraging group cohesion
Working/performing	Sense of hope	Facilitating discussion Identifying themes and progress Refocusing as needed Identifying processes
Termination/adjourning	Sense of accomplishment	Summarizing and evaluating goals Facilitating transfer of knowledge and skills Supporting closure

more comfortable with the group but may be ambivalent about the need for the group and its intended goals. This ambivalence can be demonstrated by "testing" the authority of the leader through questioning, skipping sessions, or coming late. These issues must be dealt with openly and clearly so that the group can settle into its work. This becomes the time of norming, with the identification of standards and expectations of behavior. Some level of discomfort or conflict is often expressed overtly or covertly, until the group becomes functional. All groups need this time to set norms such as roles, rules, and structure.

Performing

The working or performance stage involves exactly that—performance of the work of the group. In this stage, the leader becomes less involved in running the group. The members themselves decide what to discuss and how to address the goals and, to some degree, manage the group themselves. Cohesiveness and creativity should be apparent and encouraged. The leader's role is to refocus and clarify as needed, handle problems and conflicts if they arise, and identify the process as it develops. In this process, members may avoid issues or tasks and engage in disruptive reactions and behaviors. By bringing problems and conflict out in the open, the participants can examine these issues and make changes. Some groups have established dates for each stage; others depend on the tasks and type of group. Another factor that depends on the particular group is whether members can join or leave at different times or whether all members must begin and terminate together.

Adjourning

Termination or adjourning is the formal ending of the group. How long this stage lasts depends on the purpose of the group and its duration. As in the orientation stage, the group leader assumes an active role at this stage. The goals are to assist the members in expressing what has been accomplished and preparing for closure. This can be an emotional stage, with some members striving for continual closeness in some therapeutic groups or the continued comradarie that is not experienced in the work setting. On the other hand, some work group members are relieved at having accomplished the intended goals.

The Role of the Group Leader

Leadership is an essential consideration for the viability of many groups. One consideration is whether the leader has been selected externally or whether has been determined internally through group consensus. This appointment status may affect both the leader and member behaviors within the group. Other factors that may influence the particular leadership style adopted by an individual are the person's personality and skills, the purpose of the group, the characteristics of group, and the participants or members.

Traditional group leadership styles have been described as democratic, autocratic, or laissez-faire. Group leaders often use a combination of styles or modify their style, depending on the group membership or the topic being discussed. With a democratic leadership style, the leader shares the authority and decision-making tasks with members. A democratic leader seeks greater participation by and feedback from group members. One of the benefits of this style is that it typically produces a greater sense of satisfaction among members. On the other hand, the need to have consensus or agreement may impede the progress of the group by monopolizing the discussion.

An autocratic leadership style is one in which the leader makes all pertinent decisions, informs members of the rules, and structures the sessions. This style can facilitate the group effectiveness and goal achievement because the expectations have been clearly delineated and actions controlled. However, it may limit group interaction and lead some members to feel that they are disenfranchised and that their opinions are not valued.

The laissez-faire leadership style is unstructured, allowing members a great deal of freedom and the ability to come and go at will. This style might also involve a change of leader from session to session, which can be effective with a highly functional, goal-directed population but will not work well with poorly focused or unmotivated groups.

Regardless of the leadership style, characteristics of an effective group leader include the ability to understand the dynamics of the group, listen attentively, focus on the goals, and facilitate the progress of the group. Again, effective communication and interpersonal skills are vital attributes of an effective leader. Interestingly, McKay and associates (1995) have proposed that every meeting have two purposes, (1) the group goal and (2) maintenance of the group morale. The maintenance of group morale is a major role of the group leader.

Leadership Skills

Consider the leadership skills necessary to successfully manage a group by analyzing the group's purpose, structure, member participation, communication, and goal attainment. One of the first tasks for the group leader is to establish a structure that will promote an effective working relationship. The leader is also responsible for securing a meeting place, deciding the length and frequency of meetings, and determining the goals for the group. These goals must be clearly communicated to the members so that they can assume their roles. At times, goal determination may be delayed to allow members to participate in goal development. The leader must also physically set up the room. As discussed earlier, the arrangement of the physical environment is crucial in some groups.

Another critical task for the group leader at this point is to orient the members to the group and its expectations and to allot sufficient time for the group to form before initiating work. The leader can accomplish this by ensuring that the interactions among the members during the initial period of forming remain on a superficial level while the members become acquainted. The stages of

forming, storming, and norming may be much briefer in a work group, but the leader must ensure that there is some time for the members to settle in. This may be accomplished in one meeting, but some allowance for introductions and getting to know one another is important, regardless of the group's focus.

Leadership skills are essential to facilitate the group in its deliberation and discussion for decision-making. Ensuring participation by all members, avoiding premature closure on the topic, and recognizing the recurring themes are important activities for an effective group leader. The leader can set the tone for the level of communication, whether superficial or personal, as well as set limits on appropriate and unacceptable communication styles. The leader uses techniques such as restatement, reflection, clarification, collaboration, and problem-solving while always attempting to promote open communication among the members. Another useful technique for the leader is role modeling for the group members on how to provide constructive feedback. In this way, the group leader is actually teaching the members effective communication skills.

Striving for group cohesiveness is another goal of the group leader. Coming together as a group and focusing on the common goal or purpose are reinforced by the effective group leader. This cooperative and cohesive group esprit de corps can occur and endure when the group leader provides the positive, supportive, and encouraging lead or model for the group. Conflict can arise in any type of group and must be managed. The best resolution entails a "win-win" situation with a solution satisfying to both sides. This is a challenge for the group leader in directing the members in creative problem-solving for both effective and satisfying group process. Nurses commonly face conflict situations in work group settings and need to keep in mind the four functional problems that Turniansky and Hare (1998) have identified—meaning, resources, integration, and goal attainment—as well as the four "must" activities to address these problems with groups in organizations. There must be:

- An overall meaning of the activity that sets both a direction and boundaries for the group
- Resources adequate for the task
- Integration in the form of role differentiation and level of morale for the group members to work together
- Enough coordination of the resources and the integration functions to provide for goal attainment (Turniansky and Hare, 1998, p. 111).

The Conflict Resolution Network (CRN) also further identifies 12 skills useful in a conflict situation (Box 8–2). The CRN (2003) is an international organization whose purpose is to research, develop, teach and implement the theory and practice of conflict resolution through a national and international network. Other techniques to use when dealing with difficult people are discussed later in this chapter. Try to identify conflict situations and use effective techniques for resolution in your next work or group session.

BOX 8–2
CONFLICT RESOLUTION NETWORK'S 12 USEFUL SKILLS

The Conflict Resolution Network recommends the following 12 skills for dealing with conflict situations:
- The win-win approach
- Creative response
- Empathy
- Appropriate assertiveness
- Cooperative power
- Managing emotions
- Willingness to resolve
- Mapping the conflict
- Developing options
- Negotiation
- Mediation
- Broadening perspectives

Leaders should avoid using the following ineffective communication techniques: giving advice, giving approval, blaming, and scapegoating. Giving advice and blaming are considered nontherapeutic. Group leaders must be vigilant not to inadvertently scapegoat a member or allow other group members to do so, especially a disruptive member. The leader needs to recognize these dynamics and intervene appropriately, creating a safe, open, and productive environment for the group. Giving approval is, perhaps surprisingly, not helpful. Giving approval can interfere with the group process and goal accomplishment by focusing on one individual. Rather than express approval for an individual's efforts or successes, the leader can reflect back the accomplishment to the person or other members, allowing them to express their feelings. The leader can use the group format as a means of teaching effective communication skills such as how to listen, give and receive feedback, and express feelings or opinions.

Goal accomplishment has already been identified as a benchmark of success for groups. Giving assignments, such as recording the group's discussion or trying out a particular suggestion from the group, is one helpful measure. The use of assignments communicates the belief that members are capable and that change involves work on the part of group members. In a work group, members are given specific areas to work on or research, with the expectation that the group will reconvene to put these pieces together. Ultimately, the leader is responsible for ensuring that activities in the group remain focused on the common goals that were set for the group.

Another leadership activity is facilitating closure. To provide for group closure, the leader must summarize progress at the end of each session as well as at the official termination of the group. If the members enter and leave the group at various individual points, the leader may actually summarize at

---

 ONLINE CONSULT

Visit the CRN at
http://www.crnhq.org/twelveskills.html

the start of each session to orient newer and continuing members to current status, goals, and tasks. This approach is also highly effective in educational groups as it serves to reorient learners to prior content. Regardless of the focus of the group, periodic summaries and closure can be essential for the successful functioning of both the group and its members. Group members need an opportunity to acknowledge their accomplishments.

Roles of Group Members

Group members demonstrate a variety of roles during particular meetings. These roles may be either functional or nonfunctional for the group process. They may remain similar or constant over the life of the group, or individuals may alter their role from meeting to meeting. It is vital for nurses to recognize the roles assumed in groups and to interact purposefully when necessary. Consider the last unit meeting you attended. Who led the

group? Did anyone stall or disrupt the discussion? Were the topics discussed major issues for the unit or "pet peeves" of one individual? Did all members participate in the discussion? How could you, if you had been the group leader, have changed this meeting?

Functional Group Roles

Functional group roles facilitate the group process and determine the ultimate effectiveness of the group, especially in accomplishing a task or attaining a goal. In any type of group, members may play both functional and nonfunctional roles for various periods. For the effectiveness of the group process, the goal is for members to demonstrate predominantly functional group roles. For nursing work groups, Tappen (2001, p. 125) differentiates between **functional task roles** (Table 8–3), which contribute to completion of the task, and **functional group-building roles** (Table 8–4), which support development and meet relational needs.

TABLE 8–3
Functional Task Roles

Initiator/ contributor	Makes suggestions and proposes new ideas, methods, or problem-solving approaches
Information giver	Offers pertinent information from personal knowledge appropriate to the group topic or task
Information seeker	Requests information or suggestions from other members appropriate to the group topic or task
Opinion giver/seeker	Offers or requests views, judgments, or feelings about the topic or suggestions under consideration by the group. Provides the opportunity for values clarification by the group members
Disagreer	Identifies errors in statements made or proposes a different viewpoint
Coordinator	Suggests relationships between the different suggestions or comments made by the group members
Elaborator	Elaborates or expands on suggestions already made
Energizer	Stimulates the group into action toward the goals either by introducing certain issues or topics or by behavior
Summarizer	Summarizes suggestions, actions, and accomplishments that have occurred in the group
Procedural technician	Provides the technical tasks needed for the group functions, such as arrangement of the group, including media, equipment and work supplies
Recorder	Takes notes to record the progress, suggestions, and decisions of the group

Adapted from Tappen, R. M. (2001). *Nursing leadership and management: Concepts and practice* (4th ed.). Philadelphia: F.A. Davis. Reprinted with permission.

TABLE 8–4 Functional Group-Building Roles	
Encourager	Accepts and praises contributions of the group and other group members
Standard setter	Reinforces the standards or processes for effective group functioning
Gatekeeper	Ensures that all members have contributed to the discussion and that the group is not being monopolized by the views of more verbal members
Consensus taker	Seeks the weighting of group sentiments or consensus on the issues
Diagnoser	Identifies barriers or blocks to group progress that are occurring
Expresser	Restates or identifies and expresses the feelings of the group
Tension reliever	Uses humor and mediation when group tensions rise and interfere with the group process and accomplishment of tasks
Follower	Consents to whatever is proposed by others in the group. Demonstrates no active participation without great encouragement

Adapted from Tappen, R. M. (2001). *Nursing leadership and management: Concepts and practice* (4th ed.). Philadelphia: F.A. Davis. Reprinted with permission.

Observe these roles in any work group setting, such as a committee or unit meeting. Many functional task and group-building roles are demonstrated by the group leader. The leader may start out as the information giver and standard setter during the forming stage, but then function as an information seeker, gatekeeper, and encourager as the group process evolves in the working stage. The leader may also demonstrate the functional roles of coordinator, energizer, summarizer, and consensus taker to facilitate group process and attainment of the group goals. Effective communication techniques will be apparent when the leader serves in the roles of diagnoser or expresser. However, other group members will also serve in these functional roles as they become more active and progress toward the achievement of the group's goals. Observe who acts as the procedural technician, helping the leader organize the group and supplying needed equipment and materials. Examine who appears to be the more passive follower in the group, who cracks jokes as the tension reliever, and who records the actions and progress of the group.

Although these roles have been discussed mainly for the work setting, they also apply to professional, educational, and therapeutic group settings. In a professional group, observe the leadership roles shared by the officers, procedural technician roles performed by the aides or room monitors, and the standard setter role taken by the parliamentarian. In an educational group, consider the specific content and the size of the audience. Observe the roles taken by the teacher or facilitator, the people who are seated close to the teacher, the people in the back of the room, and the people who are asking most of the questions or who may be cracking jokes. In a therapeutic group, observe the particular role of the leader and how he or she facilitates sharing of the members' feelings and beliefs. Observe the members who verbalize supportive comments versus those who disagree or give further information about similar feelings.

Nonfunctional Group Roles

At times, group members demonstrate nonfunctional roles when they interrupt the group process. An example is the individual who provides negative comments on whatever other group members propose. **Nonfunctional group roles** generally are disruptive to group-building, task accomplishment, and progress toward goal attainment. However, a group can actually be mobilized to act in response to the unacceptable actions of one member, such as the individual who repeatedly comes late and then insists on being updated on what already occurred. Tappen (2001) has identified the following nonfunctional roles: dominator, monopolizer, blocker, aggressor, recognition seeker, zipper-mouth, and playboy. Smith (2001) lists similar disruptive roles in a meeting as latecomers/early leavers, silent/shy persons, whisperers/side conversationalists, and talk-a-lots, including loudmouths, know-it-alls, and hostiles.

- The *dominator*, or *know-it-all*, controls conversations, determines what will be discussed, and may control or intimidate other members. The dominator is often focused on his or her own needs. An example of the dominator in a work group is a unit coordinator at a quality assurance meeting who suggests that the group focus on the number of requests for schedule changes. An example in a therapeutic group is a client who opens the group by suggesting that members discuss the upcoming holidays.
- The *monopolizer*, or *loudmouth*, seeks attention and demands that the group focus on him or her. He or she may repeatedly interrupt others and perceive his or her issues and problems as the most important. A work group example is the nurse who goes on and on about how she always has to work overtime. In a therapeutic group, an example is a client who repeatedly inter-

rupts and insists the group listen to his problem.

- The *blocker* interrupts the discussion, often focusing on another topic or personal concerns. The blocker can do this overtly or through side conversations, which can be highly disruptive to the group.
- The *aggressor*, or *hostile*, attacks during the discussion, making comments that may or may not be relevant to it. Often this individual is focused inwardly on personal needs and demands to be heard, regardless of relevance to the discussion. This member criticizes other group members because they do not have the same insights or experiences as the aggressor. This individual is readily signified in professional, work, educational, and therapeutic groups by his or her expression of hostile comments. Signs of discomfort or counterattacks may be apparent among other group members.
- The *recognition seeker* consistently attempts to draw the group's attention to his or her personal beliefs, values, and concerns. This individual has a need to stand out among the group members and be heard, respected, and perhaps admired. This member sometimes sounds like the leader but is usually working on personal issues. In our work group example, this is the nurse who declares, "It's not all shifts that are short-staffed. Mine is the one that's always short-staffed with temps, but I am able to orient them successfully after all."
- The *zipper-mouth* is a nonparticipant (Tappen, 2001, p. 126). In either a work or a therapeutic group, this is the silent individual who sits quietly and sulks, feeling unlucky to be in the group. This is not the *shy person*, who is tracking on the meeting content and perhaps needs more time in the group to develop trust, reflection, and opportunity.
- The *playboy* makes irrelevant remarks and does not take the group seriously (Tappen, 2001, p. 126). Unfortunately, we have all experienced these jokers in a group setting and can easily recognize the disruption they make in the group process. These individuals may also be consistently late without notice or may frequently leave early.

Dealing with Difficult People

The group setting is no different from routine interpersonal interactions. You will inevitably encounter people who are difficult to work with. Lundin and Lundin (1995) propose that there is no "one-size-fits-all" answer to dealing with the many categories of difficult people (Box 8–3). Being aware, however, of your own reactions, identification of the real problem, preparation, experimentation, and problem-solving are the steps toward resolution (p. 87). And in the group setting, this can make all the difference between stagnation or dissolution and meeting group goals.

As with interpersonal communication skills, there are effective ways to deal with difficult and disruptive group members. Consider the suggestions in Box 8–4. The

---

BOX 8–4
COMMUNICATION TECHNIQUES IN A GROUP WHEN DEALING WITH DIFFICULT MEMBERS

- Make observations and acknowledge contributions.
- Use the communication techniques of reflection and restatement.
- Refocus the discussion if it is getting off track.
- Set limits and adhere to the ground rules agreed upon by the group.
- Focus on potential solutions raised.
- Provide constructive feedback, not corrective feedback, which should be done privately.
- Promote balanced participation from members.
- Assign functional group roles to members displaying nonfunctional behaviors.
- Plan ahead and anticipate for the next group session.

BOX 8–3
CATEGORIES OF DIFFICULT PEOPLE

- Mean and angry
- Cynic
- Pessimist
- Unresponsive
- Suspicious
- Negativist
- Know-it-all
- Indecisive
- Complainer
- Sneak
- Whiner
- Politician
- Manipulator
- Procrastinator
- Staller
- Exploder
- Sniper
- Sarcastic
- Thin-skinned
- Shy and quiet

From Lundin, W., & Lundin, K. (1995). *Working with difficult people.* New York: American Management Association.

---

skillful and effective group leader or member can use a variety of these techniques, depending on the group structure, composition, roles, focus, and situational factors. In addition, Streibel (2003) suggests the inclusion of a "timeout" rule set at the first group meeting with periodic reminders of this rule at subsequent meetings, so "that any member of the group who feels at any time that the situation is getting out of control can call for a timeout" (p. 154). Having this rule empowers any member of the group to intervene in a conflict situation.

Effective communication techniques and interpersonal skills are critical to success in group process, whether a small working group to a larger organizational setting.

 ORGANIZATIONAL GROUPS

Communication issues among the larger **organizational group** and less tangible groups are also worth exploring.

Interorganizational versus Intraorganizational Groups

Interorganizational groups are those that occur between systems or organizations. Communication is a vital activity to reach out to these other groups or systems. The interorganizational groups may consist of the hospital and the community mental health center, the home health agency, or the various subgroups of a health department. Outpatient hospital groups and inpatient unit groups also fit this category. These groups are often highly structured, with functions specified in job descriptions, policies, and procedures.

Nurses are involved with and provide leadership for effective functioning between or among systems in interorganizational groups. Communication and interpersonal skills are valuable attributes of professional nurses in this process. Along with these skills, a full awareness of each system or organization and their interrelationships is needed. This awareness involves an understanding of each organization's subsystems, as illustrated in Chapter 12. Consistent goals and values, complementary technical subsystems, and compatible psychosocial, structural, and managerial subsystems promote effective functioning. In addition, consider the environment in which the different organizations or systems exist. Nursing involvement in interorganizational groups is growing as the complexity of health care and professional practice expand.

> *Collaboration in this process is vital for the client and for effective use of resources.*

Intraorganizational groups are those that exist within a single, overall system or organization. The nursing, housekeeping, and physical therapy departments are intraorganizational groups within a hospital system. These groups are somewhat similar in terms of their structure, with specified roles, policies, and procedures. It is imperative for nurses to learn how to interact and negotiate effectively with these intraorganizational groups. An example

is how to obtain needed supplies and services from the housekeeping department. Accomplishing this task often depends on the ability of members of each department to collaborate with the others. Activity for clients is a major consideration and incentive to work effectively together. For example, the client is the focus for physical therapy and nursing departments. A physical therapist has certain scheduling needs based on individual client progress. The nurse manager has different needs in scheduling staff for treatments, which may be predetermined by client census, staffing, and care needs. Collaboration in this process is vital for the client and effective use of resources.

Communication in Organizational Groups

In addition to the verbal and nonverbal interpersonal communication techniques, additional methods of communication are routinely used in large groups and organizations. The information we compile and the method we use to transmit it vary. Considering the purpose of communication in an organization is indispensable. Whether we are involved in health teaching or the transmission of physiologic findings, the method and receiver of the information are important. Clear, concise, and timely transmission of information is necessary for an effective process. The time frame and ongoing evaluation are also factors in the initial communication phase as well as in the feedback phase of the process.

Specifically, information can be sent or received by telephone, facsimile (fax), electronic mail, or messaging, depending on sender's and receiver's access to and skill with the available technology. A classic problem in some organizational settings is fear of technology. Consider the use of e-mail in organizations. The intent is to deliver information efficiently and rapidly to other individuals or groups of individuals in the sender's network while reducing paper and administrative costs. But some people avoid this form of mail, whereas others regularly check for messages. If the information is not sent correctly or received appropriately, the message is not communicated and the process is ineffective.

Personal skills in verbal and written communication must be continually developed and refined through specific techniques or technologies. For example, keep in mind that e-mail can be forwarded easily to others, thus communicating with a larger group. The original sender's message will be evaluated by others on the appropriateness of content, format, and presentation (including grammar and appearance). Evaluating the appropriate channels and preparing the information in the correct format are vital for effective communication in the organizational setting.

In essence, organizational communication can be thought of as being similar to the five rights of administering medications. In organizational communications, these rights are:

1. Information or content
2. Communication channel
3. Format, including use of correct grammar, terms, and language
4. Level of understanding
5. Technology

It is a professional responsibility to transmit a correct, credible, properly delivered message. The appropriate communication channel must be selected, using the appropriate chain of command to convey the message. The correct format is essential for decision-making. One must decide whether to use an interdepartmental memorandum or a formal letter. The nature of the message dictates the format or type of communication. Correct grammar, terminology, and language are essential to present a professional image. Knowing the level of understanding of your intended audience is vital so that they can process the information. This means using the appropriate reading level and vocabulary. And finally, selecting the appropriate technology is important. Without the appropriate technology, recipients may not even receive your message.

Virtual Group Meetings

Groups are traditionally viewed as necessitating face-to-face meetings. This situation has changed. Technology now allows groups to meet electronically, whether in real time or asynchronously. Electronic communications have provided the means for **virtual meetings,** by which people connect with others not in the same physical environment. Virtual meetings can be used by work, educational, therapeutic, or professional groups. The group is still focused with a common goal, and members interact with some leadership present to organize and maintain the group. Ideas can be exchanged, experiences and information shared, and a common concern discussed. Many nursing groups now have Web sites and provide opportunities for students and professionals in groups to "discuss" core issues. Clients can interact with other clients and professionals via e-mail, chat rooms, and scheduled Internet meetings.

Virtual groups meet the same characteristics as face-to-face groups, in terms of group structure (formal or informal), composition (membership), roles (leader as facilitator and participants), and focus (work-related, educational, therapeutic, or professional). The virtual group experiences the same five stages of group development—initial, conflict, norming, working, and termination. The same set of evaluation criteria can be used to assess effectiveness of the virtual group. The role of the leader is more intense as a facilitator in the group process. The leader must employ a variety of the group-building roles, time and distance being major considerations.

Like those of distance learning, the advantages of virtual meetings are savings in time and travel and, perhaps, the opportunity for involvement in which the travel distance would have been prohibitive. Because these groups do not meet face-to-face, preparation time and follow-up are more intensive to allow all group members to have equivalent information and participation opportunities.

Disadvantages of virtual meetings include the need for all members to have access to similar technologies and the individual's comfort level with their application. Analyzing the functional and nonfunctional roles of the members as virtual participants can be a bit challenging without the face-to-face assessment of interactions. The functional role of a participant can be identified in the text or content communicated, for example as information giver/seeker or elaborator. The nonfunctional members—dominator, monopolizer, blocker, aggressor and recognition seeker—may appear to have a smaller impact (after all, members can delete their messages), but the leader must still address the underlying issues.

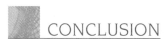 CONCLUSION

Any group—whether virtual or traditional, organizational, work, professional, educational, or therapeutic—demands the use of skills in observation, interpersonal communication, and group process that are essential characteristics of the involved professional nurse. These skills are tailored to the developmental stage of the group and the unique characteristics of its individual members. Professional nurses function as both members and leaders of such groups, and constant attention to these skills allows them to be integral components of effective groups in the profession and throughout the health-care delivery system.

Group process involves verbal and nonverbal communication between and among members of the group. One can deliberately stimulate or provoke certain responses or help individual members recognize their behaviors and move toward change and the common goals of the particular group. Learning about these group characteristics will make the nurse an effective member and leader in group situations and collaborative practice.

Key Points

- A group consists of three or more individuals with some commonality, such as shared goals or interests. Groups to consider in professional nursing practice include professional, work, educational, family, and therapeutic groups, each with specific goals and membership.
- Group process is described as the dynamic interplay of interactions within and between groups of humans.
- Groups are classified according to structure (formal or informal), composition, group roles, and focus (professional, work, educational, and therapeutic).
- The composition of a group may be homogeneous, with the group members sharing similar characteristics, or heterogeneous, with a mix of individuals.
- The issues to be addressed in establishing a group are the need and objectives for change and basic setup activities, including specifying and aligning the group purpose with the intended membership and determining the appropriate environment and group size.
- Effective groups are able to accomplish their goals in a manner that allows all members to participate, whereas ineffective groups become fragmented or dysfunctional.
- Group leaders structure the sessions to promote communication and participation by all members.
- Conflict situations within a group may be intrapersonal, interpersonal, or interorganizational, and conflict resolution is a process that requires problem-solving for effective group process.

(continued)

(continued)
- Groups go through predictable developmental stages: forming, storming, norming, working, and adjourning. These stages are similar to the stages of therapeutic relationship, which has initial, working, and termination stages. The leader modifies her or his approach according to the group's current stage.
- Traditional group leadership styles are democratic, autocratic, and laissez-faire. However, group leaders often use a combination of styles or modify their styles, depending on the group membership or topic being discussed.
- Functional group roles facilitate the group process and the ultimate effectiveness of the group. They include both functional task roles and functional group-building roles. Nonfunctional group roles are disruptive of the group-building, task accomplishment, and progress toward goal attainment.
- Organizational groups may be interorganizational or intraorganizational, depending on whether they exist between organizational systems or within an organization.
- Even though technology has provided the opportunty for virtual groups, group process skills are still applicable at a distance in a real-time or asynchronous environment.

Thought and Discussion Questions

1. Identify at least three groups of which you are a member. Consider the membership, goals, leader, composition, and focus of each group. What are the similarities and differences? Contrast the leadership styles and skills in the three groups.
2. Be prepared to discuss in class the advantages and disadvantages of heterogeneous and homogeneous groups.
3. Observe the members of the next departmental committee or nursing study group you attend.
   - Determine whether the group leader is the designated leader or a member who has assumed this role. If the leader was designated, who made the designation (external or internal designation)? Describe any effect this designation has had on the group function.
   - Describe the roles other members have assumed. Are these group roles different from these individuals' interactions in other settings?
   - Evaluate whether the members appear satisfied with the group's outcomes.
   - Evaluate whether this group or committee meets the characteristics of an effective group.
4. Review the Chapter Thought located on the first page of the chapter and discuss it in the context of the contents of this chapter.

Interactive Exercises

1. Locate three groups on the Internet and specify their structure, composition, leadership, and focus. Be prepared to participate in an online or class discussion, to be scheduled by your instructor.

2. Complete the Characteristics of Different Group Types Exercise on the Intranet site. Be prepared to participate in an online or class discussion, to be scheduled by your instructor.

3. Select a type of group you would like to lead. Complete the Group Leadership Exercise on the Intranet site. Be prepared to participate in an online or class discussion, to be scheduled by your instructor.

4. Attend a community support group. After the group meeting, describe the group process and complete the Community Support Group Exercise on the Intranet site. Be prepared to participate in an online or class discussion, to be scheduled by your instructor.

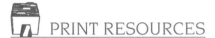 PRINT RESOURCES

References

Arnold, E. (2003). Communicating in groups. In E. Arnold & K. Boggs (Eds.), *Interpersonal relationships: Professional communication skills for nurses* (4th ed., pp. 301–331). Philadelphia: W. B. Saunders.

Berlo, D. K. (1960). *The process of communication: An introduction to theory and practice.* New York: Holt, Rinehart, & Winston.

DeWine, S., Gibson, M. K., & Smith, M. J. (2000). *Exploring human communication.* Los Angeles: Roxbury.

Lundin, W., & Lundin, K. (1995). *Working with difficult people.* New York: American Management Association.

McKay, M., Davis, M., & Fanning, P. (1995). *Messages: The communications skills book* (2nd ed.). Oakland, CA: New Harbinger.

Smith, T. E. (2001). *Meeting management.* Upper Saddle River, NJ: Prentice Hall.

Streibel, B. J. (2003). *The manager's guide to effective meetings.* New York: McGraw-Hill.

Tappen, R. M. (2001). *Nursing leadership and management: Concepts and practice* (4th ed.). Philadelphia: F.A. Davis.

Tuckman, B. (1965). Developmental sequence in small groups. *Psychological Bulletin, 63,* 384–387.

Turniansky, B., & Hare, A. P. (1998). *Individuals in groups and organizations.* London: Sage.

Wilson, M. (1985). *Group theory/process for nursing practice.* Bowie, MD: Brady Communications.

Yalom, I. (1995). *Theory and practice of group psychotherapy* (4th ed.). New York: Basic Books.

Bibliography

Arredondo, L. (2000). *Communicating effectively.* New York: McGraw-Hill.

Barnard, S. (2001). Running an effective meeting. In S. Barnard, P. J. Casella, C. Coffin, T. Hughes, J. W. Hurst, J. S. Rasey, D. Redding, R. J. Robillard, D. St James, & S. C. Ullery, *Writing, Speaking, and Communication Skills for Health Care Professionals* (pp. 293–304). New Haven: Yale University.

Berne, E. (1963). *The structure and dynamics of organizations and groups.* New York: Grove Press.

Clark, C. C. (1995). The nurse as group leader (3rd ed.). New York: Springer.

Corey, M. S., & Corey, G. (2002). *Groups: Process and practice* (6th ed.). Belmont, CA: Wadsworth.

Dana D. (2001). *Conflict resolution: Mediation tools for everyday worklife.* New York: McGraw-Hill.

Hall, R. H. (1999). *Organizations: Structures, processes, and outcomes* (7th ed.). Upper Saddle River, NJ: Prentice-Hall.

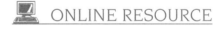 ONLINE RESOURCE

The Conflict Resolution Network (CRN). (2003). *http://www.crnhq.org.*

Genevieve M. Bartol
Rebecca S. Parrish

9
chapter

Critical Thinking

> *The whole of science is nothing more than a refinement of everyday thinking.*
> Albert Einstein, *Physics and Reality*, 1936

Chapter Objectives

On completion of this chapter, the reader will be able to:

1. Define concepts in the process of critical thinking.
2. Explain the identifying assumptions of critical thinking.
3. Discuss the judgments needed in clinical decision-making.
4. Apply the components of critical analysis to a given nursing practice situation.
5. Analyze problem-solving skills needed in nursing practice case studies.

Key Terms

Critical thinking	Hypothesis testing	Concept formation
Reflective thinking	Moral reasoning	Interpretation of data
Reactive thinking	Induction	Application of principles
Problem identification	Deduction	Interpretation of feelings,
Data collection	Assumption identification	attitudes, and values

What is *critical thinking*? What images do the words bring to mind? Do you visualize a person who finds fault with everyone and everything? Or do you visualize Rodin's famous sculpture *The Thinker*? You may see it as only the current craze of educators and the newest chapter title for nursing textbooks. Then again, you may have been taught that thinking should not be critical but inclusive, with all sides of an issue given equal weight. At this point you may want to get on with more practical matters, but we hope you are curious enough to explore the term a bit more.

Some suggest that **critical thinking** is just the latest buzzword (Cassel & Congleton, 1993). The proliferation of journal articles, monographs, essays, conference papers, and books devoted to exploring critical thinking testifies to the current interest but also suggests that a closer look at the term is warranted. The denotative meanings of *critical* include "inclined to find fault or to judge with verity, often too readily" (*Random House Unabridged Dictionary*, 1993). *Thinking* is defined as "rational reasoning; thoughtful, reflective" (*Random House Unabridged Dictionary*, 1993). One may surmise that critical thinking is a special type of thinking designed for a specific purpose.

The concept of **critical thinking** dates back at least to Socrates in ancient Greece. Dewey (1910, 1933) prompted educators to pay attention to how we think and to teach students how to think. Glaser's (1941) and Black's (1952) writings represent efforts to integrate clinical thinking into education (cited in Cassel & Congleton, 1993). Paul (1990) reviewed the efforts to teach reasoning in the 1930s and the 1960s. McPeck (1990) pointed out that before 1980, few schools were concerned with teaching critical thinking and even fewer theoretical analyses of the concept existed. McPeck (1990) writes that he had to search disparate sources to find any sustained published discussions of critical thinking (p. 1) when he researched the topic in 1979–1980.

In 1990, Facione gathered a panel of 48 educators and scholars, including leading fig-

ures in critical thinking theory, to work toward a consensus on the role of critical thinking in educational assessment and instruction. Facione and Facione (1996) reported that the expert researchers and theoreticians described *critical thinking* as the purposeful, self-regulatory judgment that results in interpretation, analysis, evaluation and inference as well as the explanation of the evidential, conceptual, methodologic, criteriologic, or contextual considerations on which that judgment was based (p. 129).

As you read this chapter, you will see that despite this consensual statement, the literature is replete with definitions and descriptions of critical thinking. Rubenfeld and Scheffer (1999) wrote an interactive textbook on critical thinking that uses Paul's description of critical thinking: the art of thinking about your thinking while you are thinking in order to make your thinking better: more clear, more accurate and more defensible (p. xi). It is in the spirit of this definition, we hope, that you will read this chapter.

CRITICAL THINKING IN NURSING

Nurses have long been taught to use the nursing process to guide their practice. The nursing process provides a structure for using knowledge and thinking to provide holistic care for individuals, families, groups, and communities. The process can be used with all theoretical frameworks and clients in all settings. Although its components may be expressed in slightly different ways, the nursing process is basically a problem-solving method that has served nurses well by helping them use empathic and intellectual processes with scientific knowledge to assess, diagnose, plan, implement, and evaluate nursing care and client outcomes. When used appropriately, the nursing process involves critical thinking.

The growing diversity and complexity of nursing practice and the exponential growth of knowledge require nurses who can think critically. Nurses must master the reasoning skills needed to process growing volumes of information. When nurses assess clients, the data they gather need to be organized into meaningful patterns. Nurses must evaluate responses to treatment and care continuously to determine whether the nursing diagnosis was appropriate and the intended outcome achieved. Even one additional piece of information related to the client may change the whole configuration and require redefinition of the problem. In nursing, situations change so rapidly that reliance on conventional methods, procedure manuals, or traditions to guide judgments about the appropriate nursing action required is insufficient.

Critical thinking requires attention to many factors. Complex legal, ethical, organizational, and professional factors are involved in seemingly simple decisions and require critical thinking skills. For example, nurses consider ethical factors (e.g., keeping client information confidential) and scheduling factors (e.g., when to admit visitors) when they decide not to admit visitors to a unit between 10 AM and 12 noon because patients are participating in a support group in the commons room during that time.

Nurses make inferences, differentiate facts from opinions, evaluate the credibility of the sources of information, and make decisions, all skills needed for critical thinking. Because each of these skills can be learned, at least to some extent, individual potential to become an effective critical thinker can be enhanced.

CRITICAL THINKING OUTLINED

What is critical thinking? Some nursing educators would argue that it is really the same as the nursing process (Jones & Brown, 1993; Kintgen-Andrews, 1991; White and colleagues, 1990; Woods, 1993). Others insist that although the nursing process requires critical thinking, critical thinking is much more. It is generally maintained, however, that critical thinking is a valuable skill or set of skills capable of being learned and

taught (Facione & Facione, 1996, 2000; Smith, 1990).

Definitions

Critical thinking is often considered a special, even rare, skill. Because the characteristics of critical thinking match those of sound clinical judgments (Case, 1994), critical thinking is viewed as a highly desirable skill. A review of the nursing literature indicates that there is no general agreement about what critical thinking is. Definitions abound in the nursing literature; Table 9–1 gives a sampling of several classic and currently accepted definitions. Experts are currently leaning toward description rather than definitions. The definitions have common elements. Critical thinking is viewed as engaging in a purposeful cognitive activity directed toward establishing a belief or map of action. Each definition speaks to the need for a person to actively process and evaluate information, to validate existing knowledge, and to create new knowledge. Each echoes Dewey (1933) in urging the use of **reflective thinking** of the kind that turns a subject over in the mind and gives it serious and consecutive consideration (p. 3). All are consistent with Dewey's definition of *reflective thinking* as active, persistent, and careful consideration of any belief or supposed form of knowledge in light of the grounds that support it and the further conclusions to which it tends (Dewey, 1933, p. 9). All suggest using a thought chain (Dewey, 1993, p. 4) that aims at conclusions.

Different elements are also evident in the definitions and descriptions offered in the nursing literature. Some seem to equate critical thinking with reactive thinking (Kataoka-Yahiro & Saylor, 1994; Kintgen-Andrews, 1991). **Reactive thinking** implies a response to what is, and not to what may yet be. Most view critical thinking as a focused, rational analysis of existing knowledge with very specific steps (Bandman & Bandman, 1995; Kataoka-Yahiro & Saylor, 1994; Kintgen-Andrews, 1991). One refers to creating new knowledge (Case, 1994), whereas another implies that only existing knowledge is uncovered (Bandman & Bandman, 1995).

TABLE 9–1
Classic Definitions and Descriptions of Critical Thinking

Definition/Description	Source, Date
"The rational examination of ideas, inferences, assumptions, principles, arguments, conclusions, issues, statements, beliefs and actions."	Bandman & Bandman, 1995, p. 5
"Reflective and reasonable thinking about nursing problems without a single solution and is focused on deciding what to believe and do."	Kataoka-Yahiro & Saylor, 1994, p. 352
"A process and cognitive skill that functions in identifying and defining problems and opportunities for improvement; generating, examining and evaluating options; reaching conclusions and decisions, and creating and using criteria to evaluate decisions."	Case, 1994, p. 101
"Reasonable and reflective thinking that is focused on deciding what to believe or do."	Kingten-Andrews, 1991, p. 152

The discussion about critical thinking continues. Jones and Brown (1993) examine alternative views on critical thinking, arguing that it is both a philosophical orientation toward thinking and a cognitive process characterized by reasoned judgment and reflective thinking (p. 72). Woods (1993) insists on the importance of recognizing the role feelings and attitudes have in critical thinking. The many definitions and descriptions suggest that nursing has not reached a consensus on the role of critical thinking.

Descriptions

The following statements gleaned from the literature and our own perspectives attempt to provide a fuller description of critical thinking:

- "Critical thinking is directed toward taking action. Although it is often associated with scientific reasoning, which includes **problem identification**, **data collection**, and **hypothesis testing**, it is not limited to that activity. Critical thinking also includes the affective processes of **moral reasoning** and development of values to guide decisions and actions" (Woods, 1993).
- Critical thinking presumes a disposition

toward thinking analytically. Uncritical acceptance of all data is antithetical to critical thinking. An attitude that welcomes intellectual skepticism and honesty is essential.
- Critical thinking embraces thinking about how we think. We need to monitor our approach to the problem and our reasoning process. An error in reasoning may be as serious a barrier to finding a solution as a miscalculation in determining a proper drug dose. We should critique the process as well as the proposed solution.
- Critical thinking assumes maturity. Psychology reminds us that our thinking styles evolve as we grow and develop. We think concretely before we think abstractly. The ability to think abstractly is requisite to critical thinking. We accept many beliefs as children simply because an adult told us they were true. Only as we grow do we question and examine those beliefs.
- Critical thinking requires knowledge. A broad educational foundation and a healthy intellectual curiosity are prerequisite. Nursing is sometimes described as a "boundary discipline" because nurses draw knowledge from many other disciplines (Bartol & Richardson, 1998). Moreover, this solid educational foundation needs to

be informed by common sense and experience as well as knowledge of one's own biases and limitations. (Alfaro-Lefevre, & Hunt, 2003).

- Critical thinking requires skills. We need to know how to gather and evaluate the quality of data. We need to distinguish facts from opinions and probe the assumptions behind a line of reasoning. We need to know how to draw inferences from facts and observations, evaluating them as tenable or not. Precision is key. Knowing a fact is insufficient; we need to know how that fact was obtained and from where it was derived. We need to identify what data is missing. Throughout the process, we need to suspend judgment until all the evidence is weighed. There are many ways to view a problem. The way we view a situation influences our proposed solutions.

- Critical thinking, however, is more than a set of skills. Syllogistic thinking, inductive and deductive reasoning, analysis, and synthesis are used, but other styles of thinking are also needed. According to Lonergan (1977), the imagination is the highest function of the intellect and precedes all other thinking activities. Certainly, critical thinking uses imagination. Using a metaphor such as a computer or a holograph to describe a function of the brain, for example, can provide additional insight into the process. Critical thinking is creative. We reach original solutions by drawing from past experiences and making creative applications to new situations.

- Critical thinking includes feelings because they are inseparable from all thinking and behavior. Feelings cannot be eliminated or viewed as an inconvenience that complicates the activity of critical thinking, but are an integral part of all we do.

- Critical thinking frequently involves finding fault. Questions, disagreements, and even arguments may be included in the process. Critical thinking always challenges the status quo.

- Critical thinking considers the complexity and ambiguity of issues. At the same time, critical thinking seeks to identify the essential elements and exclude whatever is irrelevant to the matter being considered. Valid conclusions cannot be drawn or appropriate action taken unless one knows what is to be considered.

- Critical thinking is a contextual activity. We must be aware of our own context and how it influences our thinking. Our social environment, past and present, may bias our thinking, and we must be aware of how this occurs and deal with it appropriately. We do not do our thinking in a vacuum.

- Critical thinking is inseparable from language because it is applied to language and expressed through language (Smith, 1990). Attention should be directed to the meaning of words.

- Critical thinking is not always a self-conscious activity. We may not be aware of when we are engaging in critical thinking, or even alert to its absence. Moreover, we often unconsciously work on problems and reach solutions without knowing precisely how we arrived at them until we reflect on the process.

- Critical thinking is not an esoteric activity. It is something everyone does to some degree at least some of the time. Written guidelines, decision trees, algorithms, and critical pathways formalize the critical thinking process but cannot contain it wholly.

- Critical thinking is a habit that improves with proper use and withers with disuse. In the beginning, we use structure to guide our practice. As we gain proficiency, structure diminishes, but we must continue practicing to improve or even maintain our ability to think critically.

- Thinking critically is a social, not a solitary activity. We expose our beliefs and actions, and the thinking that helped us arrive at those beliefs and actions, to the scrutiny of others. We invite this criticism in different ways, for example, by sharing with colleagues in a discussion or writing a report. We often need others to help us see our errors.

All these characteristics of critical thinking are present during the process of critical thinking. We may be more conscious of one particular characteristic at a specific point during the process, but the others remain in the background, influencing the outcome.

Measures of Critical Thinking

How do you know whether you are thinking critically? Evaluation takes into account the purpose for which the information is gathered, and then a suitable technique is chosen. Many paper-and-pencil objective tests have been designed to measure generic competency in critical thinking, but not specifically in nursing. The Watson-Glaser Critical Thinking Appraisal (W-GCTA), the California Critical Thinking Inventory, and the Cornell Critical Thinking Tests, Level X and Z, are the most widely known and used (Norris & Ennis, 1989). The central aspects of critical thinking—**induction**, **deduction**, and **assumption identification**—are included in all three, but only the California Critical Thinking Inventory (Facione, 2000) attempts to measure the disposition toward critical thinking. Probably the best way to improve your critical thinking ability is to critique how you are thinking and practice critical thinking.

Developing Critical Thinking Skills

Critical thinking skills can be developed. Nursing is a practice discipline. A body of knowledge is gained from classes and study and applied in the clinical setting. Information drawn from personal experience in the clinical setting informs this body of knowledge. Information must be cultivated, organized, and conscientiously arranged by using critical thinking.

Raingruber and Haffer (2001) suggest four strategies that nurses can use to develop critical thinking skills. First, reflect on accounts of other nurses' clinical experiences. The narratives may be in the form of oral or written accounts and may include anything from a simple story of a clinical event to a detailed case study. Such activities enable you to reach across time and space to broaden your base of knowledge before you encounter those experiences in your clinical practice.

Second, apply Brookfield's four critical thinking processes. Namely, secure contextual awareness and determine what needs to observed and considered. Explore and imagine alternatives, and question, analyze, and reflect on the rationale for decisions.

Third, use mind maps as a visual learning tool. Associations that play a major role in nearly every mental function help you identify the key elements in a situation and prompt you to generate solutions. For example, you anticipate an assignment in a clinical setting in which you have not previously worked. You are experiencing some anxiety before the assignment. You recall being in similar situation in the past and take steps to reduce your anxiety. You may call a friend for support, review appropriate material in a nursing text, imagine several scenarios that you may encounter during the assignment, and visualize successfully providing quality care to your clients. Briefly, you rehearse caring for your clients in your mind in anticipation of actually providing care.

Fourth, keep a journal of your clinical experiences, noting your concerns about how you coped with particular situations and your reflections about what you could do to improve the care your delivered. Opportunities to reflect in writing help clarify meanings and promote understanding. Examining your reasoning and actions in writing reinforces learning and enables you to draw on knowledge gleaned from this activity in future clinical situations. Even a brief record of the verbal exchange you had with a client can help you gain insight into

ONLINE CONSULT

California Critical Thinking Inventory http://rose–hulman.edu/irpa/old/
ASSESSMENT/references/tests/crit_think_main.html

your style of communication and what you can do to improve.

THE NURSING PROCESS AND CRITICAL THINKING

Nurses can develop a meaningful concept of information and material needed to practice nursing by using logical steps of the nursing process. Taba identifies four teaching phases necessary for developing critical thinking (Maleck, 1986). The first three phases—concept formation, interpretation of data, and application of principles—focus on the cognitive domain. The fourth phase speaks to the affective domain, including interpretation of feelings, attitudes, and values.

1. **Concept formation:** Conception formation is similar to the nursing process. Nurses need to identify known data, determine common characteristics, and prioritize data.
2. **Interpretation of data:** Next, nurses are encouraged to differentiate between pieces of information, determine cause-and-effect relationships among variables, and extract meaning from what they observed.

These first two logical phases or steps in thinking prepare nurses for the third phase:

3. **Application of principles:** Nurses analyze the nature of the problem or situation. It is important to note that nurses do not ask the analytic "why" questions until this application phase. The premature use of "why" questions produce deductive conclusions, rather than inductive alternatives. The question "Why does an infection cause an elevated temperature?" tends to lead to a rote response culled from classroom lectures or the textbook. Conversely, a thought-producing question, such as "What factors related to an elevated temperature suggest an infection?" encourages nurses to sift and combine cognitive knowledge to understand an important clinical concept. Only after defining the problem are nurses able to isolate the

relationships among the data. Once these relationships are established, nurses can apply factual information to predict an outcome on the basis of cognitive principles.

4. **Interpretation of feelings, attitudes and values:** The fourth phase involves principles of interpersonal problem-solving and analysis of values. This activity, although less concrete than the other three phases, is imperative for determining the nature of attitudes and perceptions developed through one's life experiences. For example, a nurse's concern about a rising temperature in a client taking haloperidol (Haldol) may be provoked by a past experience with a client who was taking the drug and demonstrated neuroleptic malignant syndrome. At this point, the nurse needs to gather additional data to confirm or rule out the possibility that the rising temperature is a sign of malignant hyperthermia in the present client, and must not leap to a premature conclusion. Additionally, the nurse must be open to other possible explanations for the elevated temperature. Appropriate action is then taken, including gathering additional data when indicated.

These phases have been described in terms of steps, but they can occur almost simultaneously. Sequencing and pacing questions are essential in critical thinking. Sequencing questions is important because the processes of thought evolve from the simple to the complex. As mentioned earlier, asking "why" questions prematurely would only bring premature closure. The principle of pacing allows nurses to match questions to their levels of readiness and cognitive ability. To accommodate pacing, nurses must pursue each question long enough to permit a variety of responses. In this way, they become active participants in the thinking process, not simply vessels for facts.

The implementation of the nursing process requires complex clinical and diagnostic knowledge and application of critical thinking skills.

A closer look at the nursing process shows that following it appropriately involves critical thinking. The five steps of the nursing process are:

1. Assessment
2. Diagnosis
3. Planning
4. Implementation
5. Evaluation

This process provides a framework for identifying and treating client problems. The nursing process is an ongoing and interactive cycle that results in flexible, individualized, and dynamic nursing care for all clients. Assessment is the foundation of the process and leads to the identification of both nursing diagnoses and collaborative problems. Nursing diagnosis provides the primary focus for developing client-specific individualization of client goals. The planning process allows for individualization of client goals and nursing care within the context of managed care guidelines. Implementation involves providing nursing actions to treat each diagnosis. Ongoing evaluation determines the degree of success in achieving the client goals and the continued relevance of each nursing diagnosis and collaborative problem.

The implementation of the nursing process requires complex clinical and diagnostic knowledge and application of critical thinking skills. Learning and applying these skills is a continuing challenge for the nurse and requires much practice. If the nurse uses the diagnostic reasoning process appropriately, the result will be effective nursing interventions leading to desirable patient outcomes.

Nurses must be critical thinkers because of the nature of the discipline and their work. Nurses are commonly confronted with problem situations; critical thinking enables them to make sound decisions. During the course of a workday, nurses are required to make decisions of many kinds. These decisions often determine the health of clients and even their very survival, so it is essential that the decisions be sound. Critical thinking skills are needed to assess information and plan decisions. Nurses need good judgment, for example, to decide what they can manage and what should be referred to another health care provider. Nurses deal with rapidly changing situations in stressful environments. Treatments and medications are modified frequently in response to a client's condition. Routine behaviors are often inadequate to deal with the complex circumstances. Familiarity with the routine for giving medications, for example, does not necessarily help you intervene appropriately with a client who is afraid of injections. When unexpected complications arise, critical thinking ability helps nurses recognize important cues, respond quickly, and adapt interventions to meet specific needs.

Nurses use knowledge from other subjects and fields. Using insight from one subject to shed light on another subject requires critical thinking skills. Because nurses deal holistically with human responses, they must draw meaningful information from other subject areas to understand the meaning of client data and plan effective interventions. Nurses need knowledge from neurophysiology, social sciences, psychology, and nutrition, for example, to assist clients who are severely depressed.

> *When unexpected complications arise, critical thinking ability helps nurses recognize important cues, respond quickly, and adapt interventions to meet specific needs*

Case Study

CASE STUDY

APPLYING CRITICAL THINKING

Case studies offer us excellent opportunities to use critical thinking. This study contains data about Mr. Jones, a patient admitted to the same-day surgery unit for repair of a right inguinal hernia. The nurse must use critical thinking to determine appropriate data collection, assessment, nursing diagnoses, and interventions for the care of the patient and his family. Clearly, critical thinking is used in every step of the nursing process as nurses collect, cluster, and analyze data and formulate nursing diagnoses. Critical thinking enables the nurse to provide high-quality care that is appropriate, individualized, creative, sensitive, and comprehensive. In determining the appropriate care for Mr. Jones, the nurse would find it helpful to organize her thoughts and actions as follows:

1. Assessment

- List the significant assessment findings: Objective and Subjective.
- Cluster the significant assessment data by functional health patterns.
- What general problem areas does Mr. Jones have?
- Develop data clusters for each of the general problems identified.

2. Nursing Diagnosis

- From the clustered data, develop at least two diagnostic hypotheses using accepted nursing diagnosis labels.
- Evaluate each of the diagnostic hypotheses by writing and comparing the definitions and applicable defining characteristics of each diagnosis.
- Write complete nursing diagnosis statements, by priority.

3. Planning

- Plan appropriate nursing interventions.

4. Implementation

- Implement appropriate nursing interventions.

5. Evaluation

- Evaluate the outcomes.

FACTS: HEALTH HISTORY AND RANGE OF SYMPTOMS

Mr. Jones is a 45-year-old married man, employed as a supervisor with Parrish Construction Company. He is brought by his wife to the same-day surgery unit for a presurgery assessment the day before his scheduled operation. His breath smells of alcohol.

Chief Concern: "I need to get this surgery over with. We have a big job to do at work, and it will be my butt if it is not completed on schedule. I plan to cut down on my drinking. I know I drink too much sometimes, but it's because of the pain from this thing." (Patient points to area of hernia.)

History of Present Illness: Mr. Jones was referred by the nurse from the construction company to the surgeon, Dr. Judge. Mr. Jones had experienced periodic pain and swelling in his right groin area for at least 5 years and several times has seen the employee health physician, who told him he had a right inguinal hernia that should be repaired. He admits to experiencing decreased appetite and insomnia for the past 10 days.

FACTS: SOCIAL AND FAMILY HISTORY

Mr. Jones's father died of cirrhosis at the age of 52 years. His mother is 80 years old and has a history of diabetes. Mr. Jones is the youngest of six children. One brother died at birth, another died at age 6 of a tumor, and a third brother was a heavy drinker. Two sisters are alive and well. Mr. Jones has been married to his second wife for 9 years; they have no children. His second wife has three boys, aged 12, 14, and 16 years, who live with her first

(continued)

(continued)

husband and have no contact with Mr. and Mrs. Jones. He has five children by his first marriage; all are alive and well, living with his first wife. He pays $50.00 a week for child support for each child. The children visit him every other weekend. There is no family history of tuberculosis, hypertension, epilepsy, or emotional illness.

FACTS: REVIEW OF SYSTEMS

General: No current change in weight and usually feels good, except when the hernia acts up.
Skin: No symptoms.
Eyes: He wears glasses for reading.
Ears: No symptoms.
Nose: No symptoms.
Mouth and Throat: Experiences recurrent episodes of hoarseness. Denies dysphagia.
Neck: No symptoms.
Respiratory System: Denies pain, dyspnea, palpitations, syncope, and edema.
Gastrointestinal System: Reports eating only three "good meals" during the past 10 ten days. Appetite is good when not drinking. Denies food intolerance, emesis, jaundice, flatulence, diarrhea, constipation, and melena.
Genitourinary System: No symptoms.
Neurologic: See "History" and "Interview with Significant Other."

FACTS: PHYSICAL EXAMINATION

Mr. Jones is a 45-year-old white man with dark complexion and a ruddy face who appears chronically ill. He is mildly intoxicated and appears anxious. Weight is 136 pounds; height is 5 ft, 11 inches; temperature is 98.8°F, pulse is 92, and regular respirations are 20 and unlabored; blood pressure is 160/90.
Skin: Well hydrated and without lesions.
Head: Normocephalic.
Eyes: PERRLA. Vision corrected with glasses. Visual acuity decreased to 3 mm print at 18 in. on the left and 4 mm print at 18 in. on the right. Extraocular movements full; no nystagmus is noted. Visual fields are intact as tested

per confrontation. Conjunctivae are slightly injected. Sclerae clear. Lenses are without opacities bilaterally. Funduscopic examination reveals the discs normally cupped, and no vascular changes bilaterally.
Ears: External ears symmetrical, without lesions. Otic canal is clear. Tympanic membrane pearly gray bilaterally. Hearing is within normal limits per watch tick at 6 inches.
Mouth and Throat: Lips, tongue, and buccal mucosa are pink and moist. Teeth are brown, crooked. Gingivae are atrophic. No inflammation of posterior nasopharynx.
Nose: Nasal septum in the midline. Nares are patent bilaterally. Sinuses not tender.
Neck: Full mobility and no significant lymphadenopathy. Thyroid not enlarged, without nodules.
Chest: Bony thorax is without deformity or tenderness. Respiratory movement is full, and diaphragmatic excursion is adequate bilaterally. Lungs are clear to percussion and auscultation.
Cardiovascular: The PMI is in the fifth intercostal space of the LMCL. NSR without murmurs or gallops.
Abdomen: Abdomen is soft and flat. Bowel sounds are heard in four quadrants. Liver is descended 5 cm below the costal margin. No splenomegaly, tenderness, or mass. Surgical scar present in right lower quadrant.
Genitourinary: Normal male genitalia. No hernia palpated.
Rectal: Internal and external hemorrhoids noted at 5 and 7 o'clock. Normal sphincter tone. Anal canal free of tenderness. Prostate is in the midline, firm without nodules, not enlarged.
Extremities and Back: Muscular development symmetrical. Normal in appearance, color, and temperature. Peripheral pulses palpable and symmetrical. Free of varicosities or edema.
Neurologic: Speech is slurred, sensorium somewhat cloudy. Cranial nerves II through XII are intact as tested per gross screen. Moderately tremulous. Biceps, triceps, brachioradialis, patella, and Achilles reflexes are

(continued)

(continued)

symmetrical but brisk. Babinski's reflexes are down bilaterally.

FACTS: SIGNIFICANT LABORATORY FINDINGS

Blood alcohol level: 0.29 U/L.
Stool guaiac: Negative.
ECG: Sinus tachycardia, otherwise WNL
Chest x-ray: No active chest disease.
Coulter-S: Hgb 16.0 g/dL (H), HCT 48.2% (H), MCV 101 m3 (H), CL 92 mEq/L (L), uric acid 8.04 mg/dL (H), SGOT 90 U/L (H).
Liver panel: TX:GGT 66 IU/L (H).
Urine: Bacteria 21, WBC 8–12.

FACTS: INTERVIEW WITH SIGNIFICANT OTHER

According to Mrs. Jones, Mr. Jones works out of town from Monday morning to Thursday evening. When he returns home, he begins to drink. He does not drink during the work-week. Mrs. Jones related the following incidents of the past 10 days, which occurred when her husband was intoxicated: ran all of the children out of the house into the rain, scuffled with brother-in-law, and brandished a shotgun after an argument. Mrs. Jones reports that she left her husband in June but returned to him about 4 weeks ago. She has never attended Al-Anon, but has reviewed information from the Alcoholism Information Center. This is the second marriage for Mrs. Jones; her first husband and her father were alcoholics.

ANALYSIS

The nurse used critical thinking skills, appropriate interpersonal communication (see Chapter 7), and competent technical ability to develop a comprehensive database for Mr. Jones. Mr. Jones is the primary source of data, and his physical condition, developmental level, and intellectual and emotional status determined the extent of information obtained from him. As the nurse talked with Mr. Jones and made observations, she drew on data derived from experiences with other clients and her knowledge base built on clinical experiences and reading. The nurse assessed Mr. Jones holistically and identified current and potential health needs and problem areas.

The nurse organized, synthesized, compared, and analyzed the data to establish the nursing diagnoses. Formulation of nursing diagnoses, as a diagnostic process, is a complex intellectual exercise that relies heavily on the nurse's critical thinking, clinical decision-making, and interpersonal skills. The nursing diagnosis or diagnoses provided the framework for the next three nursing process steps: planning, implementation, and evaluation.

Planning includes priority setting for the nursing diagnoses, identification of Mr. Jones's goal and objectives, and establishing interventions with defined outcome criteria. After the planning stage, the nurse wrote the nursing care plan and began implementing nursing care. The delivery of the nursing care depends on the complexity and technical nature of the nursing care plan, the time and environmental limitations of the nurse, and the overall ability and condition of Mr. Jones. The evaluation phase of the nursing process begins with implementation, because the nurse reviews the goal achievement and reassesses nursing actions as they are carried out.

As a result of this process, with data collected, the nurse determines that Mr. Jones needs the hernia repair and has multiple system disturbances associated with alcoholism. He has tremors due to withdrawal, poor nutrition, potential complications with anesthesia and surgery, potential abusive behavior related to loss of control, potential difficulties in parenting of adolescents related to disruption in family structure and poor role modeling, and potential alcoholism in three adolescent boys related to a family history of alcohol problems. Engaging in the critical thinking process, the nurse continues to look for an increase in tremulousness or irritability. The nurse will notify the physician that Mr. Jones is in possible withdrawal; surgery may need to be postponed.

Because Mr. Jones shows evidence of poor nutrition related to excessive alcohol intake,

(continued)

(continued)

alcohol consumption must be eliminated, with a corresponding increase in nutritious fluid and food intake. A high-protein diet will be needed to regenerate functional liver tissue and promote healing. A high-carbohydrate diet will be needed to sustain weight and spare the use of protein for cell building. Vitamin and mineral supplements will probably be needed to correct deficiencies. A low-fat diet is indicated because bile manufacturing is reduced with chronic drinking and fats are not easily digested. This case study illustrates the essential role of critical thinking in professional nursing practice.

Key Points

- Critical thinking has been defined and described by many scholars. It is multifaceted and involves a combination of logical, rhetorical, and philosophical skills and attitudes that promote the ability to determine what we should believe and do.
- Critical thinking is essential for professional nursing practice. The need for critical thinking in nursing has greatly increased with the diversity and complexity of nursing practice.
- Reflective thinking is "active, persistent, and careful consideration of any belief or supposed form of knowledge in the light of the grounds that support it and the further conclusions to which it tends." (Dewey, 1933, p.9).
- Reactive thinking implies a response to what is and not to what may yet be.
- Critical thinking is often associated with scientific reasoning, which includes problem identification, data collection, and hypothesis testing, but it is not limited to these activities.
- The central aspects of critical thinking are induction, deduction, and assumption identification.
- Concept formation is similar to the nursing process. First, the nurse needs to identify known data, determine common characteristics, and prioritize data.
- Interpretation of data occurs when nurses differentiate between pieces of information, determine-cause and-effect relationships among variables, and extract meaning from what they have observed.
- Application of principles occurs when nurses analyze the nature of the problem or situation and apply factual information to predict an outcome on the basis of cognitive principles.
- Interpretation of feelings, attitudes, and values requires interpersonal problem-solving and analysis of values.

Thought and Discussion Questions

1. Give an example from your clinical practice for each of the descriptive statements of critical thinking.
2. Select a nursing issue, such as an open visiting policy in the surgical intensive care unit or family presence during a "code," and engage in a debate with a peer.

3. Select a problem at your place of work. Explore a solution to the problem with the help of a peer with whom you work. Analyze the problem-solving process you used to address the problem.

4. Review the Chapter Thought located on the first page of the chapter and discuss it in the context of the contents of the chapter.

Interactive Exercises

1. Rewrite the case study from Mr. Jones's point of view. Repeat the exercise from a family member point of view, the physician's point of view, and your point of view. A short story such as "The Jilting of Granny Weatherall" by Katherine Ann Porter (1930) or "The Interior Castle" by Jean Stafford (1953) may be substituted for a case study.

2. Write an argument for a change in policy or to support a request for additional funds that can be presented in 10 minutes or less. Select a health need, such as free access to a primary physician or nurse with questions about health. Prepare a fact sheet that could be presented to a legislator or an insurance provider to support the action you propose.

3. Using the case studies and format provided on the Intranet site, select at least five descriptive statements of critical thinking that you would use in working with clients in each of the practice situations. Explain your rationale for each statement.

PRINT RESOURCES

References

Alfaro-LeFevre, R. & Hunt, J. (2003). *Critical thinking and clinical judgment: A practical approach* (3rd ed.). Philadelphia: Elsevier Science.

Bandman, E. L. & Bandman, B. (1995). *Critical thinking in nursing* (2nd ed.). Norwalk, CT: Appleton & Lange.

Bartol, G. M., & Richardson, L. (1998). Using literature to create cultural competence. *Image: Journal of Nursing Scholarship*, 30, 75–79.

Case, B. (1994). Walking around the elephant: A critical thinking strategy for decision making. *The Journal of Continuing Education in Nursing*, 25(3), 101–109.

Cassel, J. F., & Congleton, R. J. (1993). *Critical thinking: An annotated bibliography*. Metuchen, NJ: Scarecrow Press.

Dewey, J. (1933). *How we think*. New York: D. C. Heath & Co.

Dewey, J. (1910). *How we think*. Boston: D. C. Heath & Co.

Facione, P. (Project director). (1990). Critical thinking: A statement of expert consensus for purposes of educational assessment and instruction. *The Delphi Report: Research findings and recommendations prepared for the American Philosophical Association* (ERIC Doc. No. ED 315 423). Washington, DC: ERIC.

Facione, N. C. (2000). *Critical thinking assessment in nursing education programs: An aggregate data analysis*. Millbrae, CA: Academic Press.

Facione, N. C., & Facione, P. A. (1996). Externalizing the critical thinking in knowledge development and clinical judgment. *Nursing Outlook*, 44, 129–136.

Jones, S. A., & Brown, L. N. (1993). Alternative views on defining critical thinking through the nursing process. *Holistic Nursing Practice*, 7(3), 71–76.

Kataoka-Yahiro, M., & Saylor, C. (1994). A critical thinking model for nursing judgment. *Journal of Nursing Education*, 33(8), 351–356.

Kintgen-Andrews, J. (1991). Critical thinking and nursing education: Perplexities and insights. *Journal of Nursing Education*, 30, 152–157.

Lonergan, B. (1977). *Insight, a study of human understanding*. New York: Harper & Row.

Maleck, C. J. (1986). A model for teaching critical thinking. *Nurse Educator*, 11(6), 20–23.

McPeck, J. E. (1990). *Teaching critical thinking*. New York: Routledge.

Norris, S. P., & Ennis, R. H. (1989). *Evaluating critical thinking*. Pacific Grove, CA: Midwest Press.

Paul, R. W. (1990). Critical thinking: Fundamental for a free society. *Educational Leadership*, 41, 44.

Porter, K. A. (1930). The jilting of Granny Weatherall. In *Flowering Judas and other stories*. New York: Harcourt, Brace, 80–89.

Raingruber, B., & Haffer, A. (2001). *Using your head to land on your feet: A beginning nurse's guide to critical thinking.* Philadelphia: F.A. Davis.

Random House unabridged dictionary (2nd ed.). (1993). New York: Random House.

Rubenfeld, M. G., & Scheffer, B. K. (1999). *Critical thinking in nursing: An interactive approach.* Philadelphia: Lippincott Williams & Wilkins.

Smith, F. (1990). *To think.* New York: Teachers College Press.

Stafford, J. (1953). The interior castle. In *The children are bored on Sunday.* New York: Harcourt, Brace, 205–217.

White, N. E., Beardslee, N. Q., Peters, D., & Supples, J. M. (1990). Promoting critical thinking skills. *Nurse Educator,* 15(5), 16–19.

Woods, J. H. (1993). Affective learning: One door to critical thinking. *Holistic Nursing Practice,* 7(3), 64–70.

Bibliography

Abegglen, J., & Conger, C. O. (1997). Critical thinking in nursing: Classroom tactics that work. *Journal of Nursing Education,* 36(10), 452–458.

Adams, B. L. (1999). Nursing education for critical thinking: An integrative review. *Journal of Nursing Education.* 38(3), 111–119.

Beckie, T. M., Lowry, L. W., & Barnett, S. (2001) Assessing critical thinking in baccalaureate nursing students: A longitudinal study. *Holistic Nursing Practice,* 15 (3) 18–26.

Billings, D. M., & Halstead, J. A. (1998). *Teaching in nursing: A guide for faculty.* Philadelphia: W. B. Saunders.

Birx, E. C. (1999). Critical thinking and theory-based practice. In J. W. Kenney (Ed.), *Philosophical and Theoretical Perspectives for Advanced Nursing Practice* (2nd ed., pp. 309–314). Boston: Jones & Bartlett.

Bitner, N. P., & Tobin, E. (1998). Critical thinking: Strategies for clinical practice. *Journal for Nurses in Staff Development,* 14, 267– 272.

Brock, A., & Butts, J. B. (1998). On target: A model to teach baccalaureate nursing students to apply critical thinking. *Nursing Forum,* 33(3), 5–10.

Broughton, V. (1998). Critical thinking: Linking assessment data and knowledge. *Nursing Connections,* 11(4), 59–65.

Brown, J. M., Alverson, E. M. (2001). The influence of a baccalaureate program on tradition, RN–BSN, and accelerated students' critical thinking abilities. *Holistic Nursing Practice,* 15(3), 4–8.

Case, B. (1995). Critical thinking: Challenging assumptions and imagining alternatives. *Dimensions of Critical Care Nursing,* 14, 274–279.

Catalano, J. T. (2003). *Nursing now! Today's issues, tomorrow's trends* (3rd ed.). Philadelphia: F.A. Davis.

Cloutterbuck, J. C., & Cherry, B. S. (1998). The Cloutterbuck Minimum Data Matrix: A teaching mechanism for the new millennium. *Journal of Nursing Education,* 37, 385–393.

Collier, I. C., McCash, K. E., & Bartram, J. M. (1996). Writ-ing nursing diagnoses: A critical thinking approach. St. Louis: Mosby.

Dillon, P. M. (2002) *Nursing health assessment: A critical thinking, case studies approach.* Philadelphia: F.A. Davis.

DeYoung, S. (2003). *Teaching strategies for nurse educators.* Upper Saddle River, NJ: Prentice-Hall.

Duchscher, J. E. B. (1999). Catching the wave: Understanding the concept of critical thinking. *Journal of Advanced Nursing,* 29, 577–583.

Fowler, L. P. (1998). Improving clinical thinking in nursing practice. *Journal for Nurses in Staff Development,* 14(4), 183–187.

Green, C. J. (2000). *Critical thinking in nursing: Case studies across the curriculum.* Upper Saddle River, NJ: Prentice-Hall.

Jones, D. (1998). *Exploring the Internet using critical thinking skills.* New York: Neal–Schuman.

Jones, D. C., & Sheridan, M. E. (1999). A case study approach: Developing critical thinking skills in novice pediatric nurses. *The Journal of Continuing Education in Nursing,* 30(2), 75–78.

Kelly-Thomas, K. J. (Ed.). (1998). *Clinical and nursing staff development: Current competence, future focus.* Philadelphia: Lippincott Williams & Wilkins.

Locsin, R. C. (2001). The dilemma of decision–making: Processing thinking critical to nursing. *Holisitic Nursing Practice,* 15(3), 1–3.

Nelms, T. P., & Lane, E. B. (1999). Women's way of knowing in nursing and critical thinking. *Journal of Professional Nursing,* 15(3), 179–186.

Nugent, P. M. (2004). *Fundamentals success: A course review applying critical thinking to test taking.* Philadelphia: F.A. Davis.

Oerman, M. H., & Gaberson, K. B. (1998). *Evaluation and testing in nursing education.* New York: Springer, 109–135.

Smith-Stoner, M. (1999). *Critical thinking activities for nursing.* Philadelphia: Lippincott Williams & Wilkins.

Spelic, S. S., Parsons, M., Hercinger, M., Andrews, A., Parks, J. & Norris, J. (2001). Evaluation of critical thinking outcomes of a BSN program. *Holistic Nursing Practice,* 15(3), 27–34.

Thiroux, E. (1999). *The critical edge: Thinking and researching in a virtual society.* Upper Saddle River, NJ: Prentice-Hall.

Walsh, C. M., & Hardy, R. C. (1999). Dispositional differences in critical thinking related to gender and academic major. *Journal of Nursing Education,* 38, 149–155.

Wilkinson, J. M. (2001) *Nursing process & critical thinking* (3rd. ed.). Upper Saddle River, NJ: Prentice-Hall.

ONLINE RESOURCES

http://www.philosophy.unimelb.edu.au/reason/critical
http://www.cjss.montclair.edu/ict/homepage.html
http://nursing.umaryland.edu/students/wjkohl/scenario/opening.htm
http://www.nln.org/testprods/pas_ct.htm

Rose Kearney-Nunnery

Teaching-Learning Process

To achieve a lasting change in observed behavior, the value of that change and the intellectual capacity to understand and process the information must first be present.

Chapter Objectives

On completion of this chapter, the reader will be able to:

1. Discuss the components of teaching and learning.
2. Examine differences in the ways people learn.
3. Describe methods to assess learning readiness and motivation.
4. Propose different teaching methods for a variety of learning needs.
5. Devise a lesson plan on a topic that contains behavioral objectives, a content outline with appropriate teaching methods, and a plan for evaluating learner outcomes.

Key Terms

Behaviorist perspective
Classical conditioning
Operant conditioning
Gestalt theory
Cognitive theories
Social learning theory
Humanism

Multiple intelligences
Teaching
Learning
Affective domain
Cognitive domain
Psychomotor domain
Learning environment

Cognitive learning
  styles
Andragogy
Readiness
Motivation
Behavioral objectives
Lesson plan

Teaching and learning are integral parts of contemporary nursing practice. Client or patient teaching has long been an expected nursing behavior. As a process, teaching and learning are much more than sharing and accepting information. Intricate parts of the process must be considered for effectiveness.

NURSING PROCESS APPLIED TO TEACHING-LEARNING PROCESS

Consider the steps in the nursing process: assessment, diagnosis, outcome identification and planning, implementation, and evaluation. These steps are also applicable to the teaching and learning process.

Assessment

Think about both the learner and the teacher. They represent more than simply the provider and receiver of information. Communication—verbal, nonverbal, and written—is a vital component in the teaching and learning process. It is a mutual process in which critical thinking is essential for both teacher and learner. Both teacher and learner obtain information, use reasoning skills, make analyses based on the data, and then move to decision-making or problem-solving on the learning need. The learner learns from the teacher—good, bad, or indifferent. But the teacher also gains awareness and skill from each interaction with learners. In the assessment stage, there is essential information we need to know for an effective teaching-learning process. Some of the following questions arise:

- What are the attributes of each individual teacher and learner?
- Are there literacy, bilingual, or information processing issues to be addressed?
- What are the learning needs of the learner?
- How does he or she learn?

- What special attributes does the learner possess?
- What is the readiness for and motivation to learn?
- What changes in behavior or attitude are perceived as being needed by both the teacher and the learner?
- What individual characteristics will enhance or inhibit learning?
- What are the teacher's teaching style and skills?
- What is the cognitive style of the learner?
- What environmental factors will enhance or inhibit learning?
- What activities and resources will enhance learning?
- How can both the teacher and the learner evaluate the effectiveness of the learning process?

Assessing for a learning deficit or teaching need incorporates many factors. Notice that the concentration of the assessment is on the process of teaching and learning, not on specific content to be included in a presentation of information. Determining content is a discrete task performed later in the process, on the basis of specific attributes and needs of the people and environment. Using this assessment information can lead to a *Diagnosis* about the learner's particular teaching need.

Outcome Identification, Planning, and Implementation

Next, developing behavioral objectives gives direction for a teaching plan and evaluation of the learning. Teaching strategies, methods, and resources to meet the diagnosed learning need, with specific content, are then planned and implemented.

Evaluation

The outcomes of the teaching-learning process are evaluated. The evaluation component focuses on how the learner met the objectives and the specific outcome behaviors from the experience. Outcome objectives can be assessed by both the learner and the teacher. Evaluation is focused on the behavioral objectives specified for the learner earlier in the process. All these considerations are important in the teaching-learning process addressed in this chapter.

TEACHING AND LEARNING THEORIES

Educators have studied learning theories for many years to understand and improve on the teaching-learning process. There are several schools of learning theories. Major examples of these theories applicable to professional nursing practice are behaviorism, gestalt, social learning theory, humanism, and multiple intelligences (Box 10–1).

Classical Conditioning

In introductory psychology courses, classic stimulus-response conditioning and operant conditioning are taught, providing a **behaviorist perspective** on learning. Pavlov's pioneering research with dogs led to our understanding of **classical conditioning**, in which the reflexive responses in behavior result from some stimulus. In classical conditioning, we saw that the pairing of food (the unconditioned stimulus) with the sound of a bell as a neutral (conditioned) stimulus led to salivation in dogs as an unconditioned response—first as an unconditioned response for the sight of the food, and ultimately as a conditioned stimulus with the sound of a bell alone. Using classical conditioning with infants, John Watson provided further insight on learning with his focus on the environment and emotional responses. Watson was a true behaviorist, looking at the development of the emotions fear, love, and rage through classical conditioning and desensitization.

Use of classical conditioning in nursing practice is limited. One situation may be in teaching clients to intervene as needed to physiologic or emotional cues, auras, or trig-

> **BOX 10–1**
> **SELECTED THEORIES OF LEARNING**
>
> - Classical conditioning
> - Operant conditioning
> - Gestalt theory
> - Cognitive development
> - Social learning theory
> - Humanism
> - Multiple intelligences

gers before an allergic, metabolic, or neural response. The individual with diabetes, a severe allergy, or epilepsy can be taught to perceive and make the association with early signs or symptoms that could lead to a larger physiologic reaction. Classical conditioning is useful for early intervention to circumvent the reaction chain. Reflexes are important in this scenario to ensure that the individual is in a safe environment and has the resources for prompt treatment. Another example is the use of distraction, focusing, and breathing in certain reflexive situations—for clients in labor, in pain, or experiencing fear, for example.

Operant Conditioning

Operant conditioning provides further clues to learning, with a focus on purposive behaviors and the role of reinforcement. In Thorndike's law of effect, reinforcement of a behavior is more likely to lead to repetition of that behavior. B. F. Skinner's research with rats and reinforcers for learned behaviors provided much additional information. In **operant conditioning**, the behavior is affected by the consequences (reinforcer), but the process is not trial and error (Skinner, 2003, p. 1). This theory introduced positive and negative reinforcers and reinforcement schedules to learning. The work of Skinner led to behavior modification programs and programmed instruction with shaping, reinforcement, and generalization of behavior.

Behavior modification programs are widely used in health care and education. They have been used effectively in certain nursing situations, such as nutritional programs that require a lifelong change in behavior. In such situations, old patterns are broken, stimuli are introduced to effect positive outcomes, responses are generalized to specific dietary items, positive and negative reinforcement are applied, and behavior is shaped over time. Another use for behavioral techniques is with adult clients who have urinary incontinence. One method of treatment includes bladder retraining with the components of education, scheduled voiding, and positive reinforcement.

Behaviorism focuses on observation and measurement of actions in response to some association or conditioning. Rigorous use of the scientific process in the laboratory setting was a major factor in this perspective. Dissatisfaction with the emphasis on conditioning and reinforcement led to the evolution of other perspectives, including gestalt theory, cognitive theories, social learning theory, and humanism. In these later perspectives, we see an increased focus on the human intellect and human emotions.

Gestalt Theory

Gestalt theory focuses on meaning and thought, holding that learning occurs through perception. In the German tradition, a "gestalt" is perception of a whole form rather than its component parts. More than 100 laws on this perspective evolved with the identification of major principles concerning the way we perceive objects related to organization, proximity, similarity, direction, simplicity, background, and closure. Gestalt theorists view learning as based on perception of and completion of patterns. Patterns are perceived and reorganized by the person. In terms of learning, this perspective focuses on how the learner perceives the information and his or her environment. Kurt Lewin's field theory and work on change (see Chapter 13) provide a major influence in this perspective. Lewin's Field Theory emphasizes the importance of the environmental field. The perception of this environmental field by the person influences how that person, as a system, responds within the larger environmental system.

The classic principle in the gestalt perspective is that the whole is not merely the sum of the parts. This principle is consistent with the holistic view of the person in professional nursing practice. Consider the importance we place on understanding how the person views the information to be learned. This involves teaching materials that are used in addition to perceptual values. Further consider the learning environment and the importance we place on client teaching in an unrushed, private, and comfortable setting when teaching (or promoting change for) specific health practices, as opposed to the hectic clinic environment where the person is distracted by children playing in the waiting room.

Cognitive Theories

Cognitive theories of learning focus on the intellect and the development of knowledge. Recall the example of Piaget's theory of cognitive development from Chapter 3. Schema were seen as patterns of thought or behavior that become more complex with the addition of more information. *Assimilation* is the acquisition of this information and incorporation into the individual's existing cognitive and behavioral structures. *Accommodation* is the change in the individual's cognitive and behavioral patterns based on the new information acquired. This acquisition of information is learning with the comprehension of concepts, memory, and analysis.

There are many different cognitive theories, mostly focusing on information processing. In nursing practice, use of cognitive theory is readily apparent with our focus on the level of cognitive development and acquisition of health-care knowledge. We use principles of cognitive development to tailor a teaching plan to the client's level of development, whether the client is an elderly diabetic or a child. We are also concerned about the way learners process information, so that we can tailor our teaching strategies to suit their learning styles. In addition, the use of behavioral objectives with our clients provides a focus for developing cognitive skills, moving from recall of knowledge to understanding, application, analysis, evaluation, and creation, as we will see later in the revised taxonomy table (Anderson et. al, 2001) that stemmed from the classic work of Bloom's (1956) taxonomy.

Social Learning Theory

Cognitive learning through observation and imitation is the basis of Bandura's **Social Learning Theory**. Through the research of Bandura and his associates, aggressive and socialization behaviors of children were documented after observation of both symbolic and actual models. An important aspect of Bandura's work is the modeling of behavior with television and the effect of visualizing vicarious reinforcement and punishment for behavior. A humanistic, rather than mechanistic, orientation is apparent in this theoretical focus. Bandura (1977) explained the emphasis of vicarious, symbolic, and self-regulatory processes on how humans learn and influence their own destiny.

Nursing applications of this learning model are prevalent in the development of psychomotor skills in clients, such as self-administration of medications, procedures, and treatments. We often demonstrate skills to clients in person and expect them to return the demonstration. We provide positive reinforcement in the coaching function during the process, by making comments such as, "That's good," "That's the way," and "What a nice job." We promote healthful practices with encouragement and the hope for positive results as a reinforcement for the behavior. We show clients videos on a procedure in which they see modeling and positive and negative reinforcement through a case scenario. These nursing behaviors are based on social learning theory and focus on the individual in the environment as a thinking, feeling, and reacting being.

Humanism

Humanism is another major perspective on learning. In this perspective, the focus is totally on the person. Abraham Maslow and Carl Rogers were major influences on this learning theory. As Maslow (1971) stated:

[T]he humanistic goal ... is ultimately the "self actualization" of a person, the becoming fully human, the development of the fullest height that the human species can stand up to or that the particular individual can come to. In a less technical way, it is helping the person to become the best that he is able to become. (p. 169)

The full range of human experiences are considered, as personally experienced and interpreted. As is discussed later in this chapter, Maslow's humanistic focus included motivation as a vital concern. Humanism is the basis of Carl Rogers's person-centered counseling. As described by his daughter, Rogers "above all, valued the worth and dignity of the individual and trusted their capacity for self direction if given the proper environment" (Rogers & Freiberg, 1994, p. iii). Personal growth and autonomy are key to the humanistic perspective.

The humanistic perspective is consistent with the concepts of professional nursing. We focus on the person and assist in empowering him or her for health (whether an emerging state or to a higher level), therefore focusing on the consumers of health care and advocating for their active involvement in the health promotion process. The environment should be considered in terms of the person and his or her unique environmental setting and culture. Consider the promotion of a healthy lifestyle with cardiac rehabilitation clients. Self-direction and insight into personal beliefs, attitudes, lifestyle, and behaviors are fundamental to the learning process. Culture, literacy, and learning or information processing deficits are also vital considerations with this perspective. As viewed in the health models in Chapter 5, cultural perspectives as a way of life must be included in any useful and humanistic teaching-learning plan. In addition, as with cognitive learning styles, deficits in learning or information acquisition or processing are humanistic factors that must be discovered, along with an understanding of adaptive patterns, for effective teaching and learning to occur.

Multiple Intelligences Theory

Another theory of learning focused on the person proposes **multiple intelligences**

(Gardner, 1993a, 1993b), all of which are considered equally important and are most often found in combination in individuals to differing degrees. This theory looks beyond cognitive capacity and encourages a view of the individual's cognitive profile. The basis for the theory is Gardner's observations of and work with children and adults, prodigies, gifted, normal, autistic, brain-damaged, and idiot savant individuals. Gardner (1993b) has characterized the seven different multiple intelligences as shown in Table 10–1.

The theory of multiple intelligences allows a greater focus on the individual and his or her unique talents and combinations of abilities. As Gardner (1993b) points out, in most people, the intelligences work together to solve problems. In addition, "owing to hereditary, early training, or in all probability, a constant interaction between these factors, some individuals will develop certain intelligences far more than others; but every normal individual should develop each intelligence to some extent, given but a modest opportunity to do so" (Gardner, 1993a, p. 278). Consider for a moment that you are caring for two clients after their hip replacement operations and are planning discharge teaching. One client is an architect who designs custom homes and meets with his customers for at least an hour before he develops the house plans to ensure that he truly understands their desires and ideas. The other

is a retired English professor who is concerned about the rehabilitation schedule and the completion of a collection of essays that he must submit to the publisher in 6 weeks. Your approach to each will differ on the basis of his unique talents and abilities.

The perspective of multiple intelligences is humanistic, focusing on the unique combinations of talents and abilities possessed by an individual. These unique individual abilities are consistent with the practice of nursing dealing with the individual and environmental influences. Given the variety of learning theories, however, application may involve selecting a more eclectic approach. Specific teaching guides involve our consideration of the person and the environment, given the particular health focus in contemporary nursing practice. Certain principles provide direction in this process.

TEACHING AND LEARNING PRINCIPLES

The philosophical and theoretical structures of any discipline reflect how the teacher and learner are viewed. In nursing, we view both the teacher and the learner as thinking, reasoning, active participants involved in the teaching-learning process. We believe individuals are influenced by and influence their environment. These environmental

---

TABLE 10–1
Seven Intelligences

Intelligence	Description	Example(s)
Linguistic	Language and verbal	Poets, writers
Logical	Mathematical cognitive skills in logic, mathematics, and science	Mathematicians, scientists
Spatial	Use of mental models of spatial world	Sailors, engineers, artists
Musical	Innate musical sense and talent	Musicians, composers
Bodily kinesthetic	Use of body in problem-solving	Dancers, athletes, craftspeople
Interpersonal	Understanding of others	Politicians, salespeople, teachers, clergy
Intrapersonal	Understanding of self	Virginia Woolf

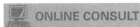

influences, including persons, events, and tangible surroundings, must be taken into account when any teaching behavior is considered. In terms of health, teaching in nursing reflects information to promote or maintain the highest level of health attainable. The teacher's and the learner's definitions of health and wellness influence physical, psychological, emotional, and spiritual health as personal determinants of behavior.

Teaching

With this in mind, several processes can be readily seen as inherent in the teaching-learning process, such as communication and critical thinking. Although the teaching-learning process is an interactive communication process, its component parts must be considered. **Teaching** is more than the transmission of information. The information must be received, understood, and evaluated by the learner. Teaching has been described as "an intentional and reasoned act" (Anderson et al., 2001). Benner (1984) has identified the teaching-coaching function of the expert nurse working with acutely ill patients. Broadening these characteristics of *the expert* could include the following:

1. Use timing to capture learning readiness and motivation
2. Assist with integration of learning into lifestyle
3. Demonstrate an understanding of client's own interpretation of the situation
4. Provide interpretations of situations and rationales for new behaviors
5. Show, through example, coaching behav-iors in culturally sensitive issues. (Benner, 1984, pp. 77–94)

These characteristics demonstrate the active roles of both teacher and learner in the process. Readiness and motivation must be present for both the teacher and the learner during the process. The best teachers are those who truly believe in the information they are sharing and can communicate this belief. They provide the excitement, or at least some reinforcement, for the learner, who wants to know more. The active role of the learner in the process is vital, because passive learning rarely results in persistent change in attitudes or behaviors. The motivation of teacher and learner are also important, as the teacher demonstrates an understanding of the learner's unique characteristics and perspective on the subject or situation. Providing information is the traditional role of the teacher, but doing so in the context of the learner's reality helps provide a rationale for behavior changes. Finally, coaching through example, with sensitivity, is the essence of expert teaching and nursing.

Teaching is an interactive process, not a unidirectional transmission of information. As Benner (1984) demonstrates in her examples of expert nurses, we also learn from those we teach.

Learning

Learning is the perception and assimilation of the information presented to us in a variety of ways. Learning contains the following characteristics:

- Perception of new information
- Initial reaction to the information
- Ability to recall or repeat the information (simple knowledge level)
- Rejection or acceptance of the information (understanding)
- Use of the information in a similar situation (application)
- Critical analysis of the information
- Incorporation of the information into the value system (evaluation)
- Use of the information in various situations and combinations (creation)

An increasing complexity emerges here as the learner moves from receiving and recalling information through:

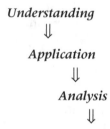

Understanding

⇓

Application

⇓

Analysis

⇓

Evaluation of the knowledge acquired and *Creation* of new applications

We see this process in the client who accepts information on breast self-examination, is able to perform the self-examination, does so on a monthly basis, teaches her daughter or mother the process, and is now investigating regular screening for colon cancer for herself and family members. This client has moved from simple knowledge to incorporation of knowledge into the value system and behaviors of herself and other family members.

Learning can be enhanced with specific strategies or approaches with learners. Babcock and Miller (1994) identify the following 16 useful principles of learning:

- Focusing intensifies learning.
- Repetition enhances learning.
- Learner control increases learning.
- Active participation is necessary for learning.
- Individual styles vary.
- Organization promotes learning.

- Association is necessary to learning.
- Imitation is a method of learning.
- Motivation strengthens learning.
- Spacing new material facilitates learning.
- Recency influences retention.
- Primacy (first items) affects retention.
- Arousal influences attention.
- Accurate, prompt feedback enhances learning.
- Application in varied contexts broadens generalization.
- Personal history shapes the perception of the experience. (pp. 45–48)

To increase the effectiveness of the presentation and the acquisition and application of knowledge, each of these principles should be evident in a lesson plan.

Because learning is the acceptance and assimilation of information, it is incorporated into the learner's domains of knowledge and behavior. Note the difference reflected here between the knowledge and the demonstration of behaviors. We may "know" something but either consciously or unconsciously decide not to demonstrate that behavior. For example, a client may have been given a low-fat diet but decide that ice cream is a part of the diet, ignoring its fat content.

Domains

A *domain* is merely a category. There are three domains of learning or knowledge: affective, cognitive, and psychomotor.

The **affective domain** includes attitudes, feelings, and values; for example, how the client feels about the importance of or the positive effect on his life of a needed dietary change will influence whether he will make the change. Often, the nursing goal is to incorporate the value of the diet into the person's belief system. However, cultural influence, cultural differences in the individual, family, or group, and the nurse's professional influences can all either positively or negatively affect whether the goal is achieved.

The **cognitive domain** involves knowledge and thought processes within the individual's intellectual ability. Using the same example of the client and the low-fat diet, the cognitive domain involves understanding the information received about nutrition, diet, health conditions, and indications. The ability to conceptualize types of foods, gram counts, and dietary needs involves comprehension, application, and synthesis at an intellectual level before the actual behaviors are performed.

The **psychomotor domain** is the processing and demonstration of behaviors; the information has been intellectually processed, and the individual is displaying motor behaviors. To continue with the example, psychomotor skills are demonstrated by how the client has performed on the changed diet, as seen in food diary reporting, preparing and ingesting appropriate foods, and even laboratory reports evaluating bodily functions.

It is important to consider these three domains in the teaching-learning process. Behavioral objectives, teaching content and methods, and evaluation of learning can be very different for the three domains and should be distinct. Remember, to achieve a lasting change in observed behavior (psychomotor domain), the value of that change (affective domain) and the intellectual capacity to understand and process the information for behavioral changes (cognitive domain) must first be present.

Consistent with the philosophical focus of nursing, the **learning environment** is important in any teaching or learning activity. Physical comfort as well as respect and acceptance of the learner are humanistic factors. The consumer of health care may also have physical, sensory, or psychological deficits that can interfere with comfort in the learning environment or in the teaching-learning process. Comfort measures should be validated with the client before and during the process. Physical comfort can include such things as the temperature of the room and the height or firmness of the chairs in addition to specific effects of acute or chronic health problems. Sensory concerns include the extraneous sensory stimuli perceived by the teacher or learner in the learning environment, such as sounds, smells, and sights. In addition, the client may have sensory deficits that may interfere with learning or may require more

resources, such as visual, hearing, or information processing problems. Psychological deficits, including fear, problems with cognition, attention span, effects from medications, and worry, can be major inhibitors to teaching and learning. Receptivity of the learner to new and different ideas is vital. Creative measures taken by the teacher to provide for an environment conducive to learning are essential.

> *To achieve a lasting change in observed behavior (psychomotor domain), the value of that change (affective domain) and the intellectual capacity to understand and process the information for behavioral changes (cognitive domain) must first be present.*

COGNITIVE LEARNING STYLES

The *cognitive learning process* is a broad area that examines how meaning is perceived, evaluated, remembered, reinforced, and demonstrated. Piaget gave us information on childhood cognition through observations of his own and other children. The different stages of cognitive development are sensorimotor, preoperational thought, concrete operations, and formal operations. Piaget provided us with the concepts of assimilation and accommodation in cognitive development. Recall that assimilation is the acquisition and incorporation of new information into the individual's existing cognitive and behavioral structures, and accommodation is the change in the individual's cognitive and behavioral patterns based on this new information.

> *Stemming from a basis in Jung's theory of the unconsciousness and personality, the Myers-Briggs Inventory was developed and has been used widely in education and business applications for learning styles. This personality inventory uses the following four scales to identify 16 personality types that can be further classified for learning preferences:*
>
> * Introversion–Extroversion
> * Sensing–Intuition
> * Thinking–Feeling
> * Judging–Perceptive

In the mid-1980s, Kolb (1981) identified specific learning styles as concrete experience, reflective observation, abstract conceptualization, and active experimentation.

Cognitive styles are further applied in cognitive mapping. Joseph Hill has used testing procedures to develop individualized cognitive maps illustrating how students and teachers acquire and transmit meaning. And the research continues as we seek to understand better how individuals acquire meaning and knowledge.

Increasingly we are concerned with the involvement of the learner in the process, for learning to truly occur. **Cognitive learning styles** or preferences are the ways learners perceive, think, organize, use, and retain knowledge. To understand this concept, merely recall colleagues in the same learning environment—those who took copious notes, those who just listened, and those who made notes or drawings on what they interpreted the message in the lecture to be. Understanding the differences in cognitive styles can help teachers and learners make more informed decisions about which learning activities will be useful or productive to them as individuals and as members of learning groups or communities.

Teaching and learning strategies have developed to match the learner with the teaching resources most effective for his or her learning style or to develop strategies to adjust to the prevalent teaching style. For example, some learners are highly visual in the way they perceive information and derive meaning. For these learners, structured lectures with few visual aids is a less desirable learning environment than one enhanced by visual aids. Others learn better through the written word, either by reading or note-taking. Learners who are highly auditory in their learning preference derive greater meaning from just listening to the information. The theory of multiple intelligences can be useful in this situation, to tailor the learning further to the individual's talents.

Assessment data on learning style may be obtained from the client in a nursing interview rather than formal testing inventories used with larger groups. In essence, good assessment of the learner is vital to ensure the

most effective teaching and efficient and enjoyable learning.

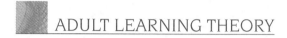

ADULT LEARNING THEORY

Most consumers of nursing care are adults: parents, couples, individual adult or aging clients, families, community groups, and even professional peers. Learning in adults requires the teacher to make some adjustments to meet the different characteristics of learners. Adult learners differ from children in that they have past experiences, good and bad, with both teaching and learning.

Malcolm S. Knowles was a major force in adult learning in the United States, providing a theoretical model, **andragogy**. The term *andragogical model* was borrowed from European education (Knowles, 1990; Knowles et al., 1985). Expanding the traditional pedagogical learning models used with children to incorporate learning characteristics and needs of adults, this developmental model proposes that the accumulated life experiences of adults give them different teaching and learning needs from younger learners. In the pedagogical model, learners are generally dependent or passive, have few prior experiences to build on, and have external pressures from parents and others to learn something (Knowles et al., 1985, pp. 8–9). Adult learners are self-directing, have experiences that have shaped their identity, experience life events or a learning need that triggers their readiness to learn, have internal motivators, and demand an available, knowledgeable resource to assist them with practical problems and identified needs (Knowles et al., 1985).

As Knowles and associates (1985) have pointed out, adult learners often initially assume the comforting and passive learner roles of pedagogy, but then an inner conflict develops with their self-directing nature. The adult's ego system is based on his or her self-concept and accumulated knowledge and experiences, whereas a child is gratified by impressing a parent, teacher, or peer. Knowles's developmental focus is demonstrated further with his identification of life problems by age group in early, middle, and later adult life groups. He specified life problems in the areas of vocation and career, home and family life, personal development, enjoyment of leisure, health, and community living (Knowles, 1990). Health promotion and maintenance are a consistent theme of adult health problems in all age groups.

Adult teaching and learning depend on both physical and psychological climates. Physical climate relates to the learning environment. The setup of the room should not replicate a stilted lecture setting and should promote comfort so that the learners can focus on learning needs and problem-solving. Knowles emphasized the need for adults to feel at ease in the learning environment, which leads to the psychological climate for the adult learner. Knowles identified seven characteristics of the psychological climate conducive to adult learning: mutual respect, collaborativeness, mutual trust, supportiveness, openness and authenticity, pleasure, and humanness (Knowles et al., 1985, pp. 15–17). Knowles views the teacher as the catalyst and facilitator. A common thread running through teaching and learning strategies for adults is mutuality in diagnosing, planning, learning, and evaluating.

One key to successful teaching and learning in adults is their active involvement throughout the process. Knowles has suggested that adult learners should be involved in the planning, needs identification, development of learning objectives and contracts, and evaluation of learning (Knowles, 1980; Knowles et al., 1985). Adults must be able to apply information to past experiences and have self-identified or mutually agreed on learning needs or some future desire or informational inquiry. On the basis of Knowles's work, Vella (1994) has identified the following 12 principles for effective adult learning:

- Participation of the learners in naming what is to be learned
- Safety in the environment and the process
- Sound relationship between teacher and learner for learning and development
- Careful attention to sequence of content and reinforcement

- Praxis: action with reflexion or learning by doing
- Respect for learners as subjects in their own learning
- Cognitive, affective, and psychomotor aspects: ideas, feelings, actions
- Immediacy of the learning
- Clear roles and role development
- Teamwork and use of small groups
- Engagement of the learners in what they are learning
- Accountability: how do they know they know? (pp. 3–4)

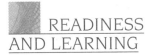

READINESS AND LEARNING

Readiness is an important concept in learning, regardless of the learner's chronologic age. Readiness relates to the developmental needs and tasks of individuals. Consider the views of two developmental theorists: Erikson (1963) described readiness as critical periods, whereas Havighurst (1972) referred to readiness as sensitive periods or the "teachable moment." For teaching to be effective and learning to take place, the readiness of the learner must be a prime consideration. A good example is the issue of compliance and noncompliance in the client group.

Compliance is an often misused and misunderstood concept. We talk about patients being noncompliant when they do not follow their discharge or health-care teaching. The reasons and background for the behavior in the client group must first be realized and understood, not assumed. Compliance is yielding to the desire of others, possibly as a result of threats or force. But as we see later in the change process, threats and force do not bode well for a permanent change in behavior. Human behavioral change is more effective when one is personally involved in the process. Specifically, how do learning and the readiness apply to receiving and accepting information for a change in lifestyle? Consider the teenager undergoing dialysis who carefully monitors his sodium intake after dialysis but fills up on fast food the day or morning before the scheduled dialysis. Is this truly noncompliance or developmental maneuvering with peer pressure and dietary restrictiveness? Now consider the adult cardiac client with a strict dietary sodium restriction. Is noncompliance by this individual due to a stubborn adherence to food preferences, culture, or custom, or perhaps failed health teaching for change because of a failure to achieve learning readiness?

The learner must be willing to change and accept the learning need. When this occurs, readiness for learning is apparent. This can be seen in terms of King's (1981) theory of goal attainment: Both the nurse and the client must be focused on and sensitive to the same goal. Readiness for the learning and teaching is then present. Ultimately, the effectiveness of the teaching methods and content is evaluated on the basis of the learning that did or did not take place. Learning readiness involves the following factors: human motivation, understanding or cognitive level, and applicability or acceptability.

Literacy and language issues are an additional consideration in readiness. For the individual with a low literacy level, years of adaptive behavior may disguise the inability to read basic information. Likewise, an individual who speaks English as a second language may perceive information differently. In each situation, the individual may be unwilling to indicate to the nurse that he or she did not fully understand or accept the information the nurse presented. The readiness to learn is inhibited by additional factors in these cases.

Motivation

Motivation in humans is a manifestation of internal and external personal and environmental factors that cause people to respond to a situation in the way that they do. Motivation has been classically viewed as needs, drives, and impulses that cause behavior. One view of motivation in humans is Maslow's Theory of Human Motivation, based on the hierarchy of basic needs. Maslow (1954) made the following 16 propositions about human desires or motivation:

1. The individual is an integrated, organized whole.
2. Hunger is a specific physiologic drive, not a classic motivation paradigm.
3. Desire for something is often a means to another end, rather than the end itself.
4. Culture affects desires.
5. Multiple motivations are often present.
6. Motivation is a constant state, but fluctuating and complex.
7. Relationships among motivators must be considered.
8. Human drives are varied and are not mutually exclusive or isolated.
9. Fundamental goals and needs are the basis for classification of motives.
10. Care must be present when animal data are used to understand human motivation.
11. Motivation is affected by the individual's environment and culture.
12. Humans may display integrated or segmented responses in reactions.
13. Not all behavior or reactions are motivated by needs.
14. Humans are motivated by the conscious possibility of attainment.
15. The influence of reality on unconscious impulses must be considered.
16. Motivation theory includes both positive and negative cases (pp. 63–79).

These propositions imply a complex interrelationship in human motivation based on internal and external factors as personally interpreted by the individual. Maslow's work indicates that the hierarchy of human needs is based on motivation. But motivation is as intricate as the person, not merely inherent impulses and drives.

The concept of motivation, then, considers the person's interpretations of the situation. Readiness, therefore, involves motivation and understanding. *Understanding* is the cognitive ability to perceive and intellectualize the content and consequences of information. Bandura (1977) defines this cognitively based motivation as how behavior is activated and maintained (p. 160). He believes that most actions are under anticipatory control, as humans use symbolic representation to envision future outcomes of behavior. The way the person views these future consequences of behavior becomes the motivation to behave or proceed in the present. This concept relates well to health teaching, in that the client can be motivated to learn with a realistic anticipation of the situation and consequences. Nurses can recognize client anticipation in the assessment phase, through interview data, diagnosis of the teaching and learning needs, and development of behavioral objectives. During this process, motivation can be assessed and stimulated by the client as well as by the professional nurse.

Cognitive Level

A person's cognitive level is a component of understanding; the content provided must be at the person's level of understanding. Piaget's theory of cognitive development describes the differences in learning levels between the sensorimotor infant developing object permanence and the older child who is able to learn abstract mathematical skills through formal operations. Information is available to the person at his or her cognitive level for processing and development of knowledge. The person may require concrete examples to envision future consequences or may be able to handle more abstract or even philosophical examples. A further consideration here is the client's state of health. Current physiologic or psychological functioning and medications may interfere with reasoning and understanding as well as the attention span. Readiness for health teaching in this instance may be at different levels, depending on physical and emotional functioning.

Applicability and Acceptability

A third component of readiness for the teaching-learning process is applicability and acceptability of the information. The person must perceive that the information is applicable to him or her, as an individual, a member of the family, or a member of a group. If the person denies that a health problem exists, he or she will not be ready for health teaching in that area. The information is not perceived as personally applicable. *Acceptability* means that the information must be within the person's worldview. Cultural influences are important, because values and belief systems influence understanding and acceptability of information. The health problem and readiness must be seen in the context of the individual's belief system. This is an important relationship, as we see in the health belief model. Cultural assessment data provide important information on the client's belief system that should be incorporated into the teaching-learning process.

 PRACTICAL TEACHING TIPS

Developing behavioral objectives sets the stage for the teaching-learning process and leads to the preparation of the lesson plan, selection of appropriate teaching strategies and methods, and evaluation of both the learning outcomes and the teaching process.

Writing Behavioral Objectives

The purpose of writing **behavioral objectives** is to provide a frame of reference for the intended outcomes of the teaching-learning activity for both the teacher and the learner. The use of behavioral objectives gives us a focus on learners and evaluation of their experiences with specific measures for behaviors. Behavioral objectives are the intended outcomes of the learners, not the teacher's goals for the activity.

Think of behavioral objectives in terms of the learner's "who, what, where, when, and how." In viewing the individual components of behavioral objectives, consider those listed at the start of this chapter. Initially, there is the stem statement, "On completion of this chapter, the reader will be able to ..." This provides the "who"—the reader of the chapter—and the "when"—after completion of the chapter. The "what" and "how" are the action-oriented outcomes that the learner will demonstrate in the listed behaviors. Behavioral objectives do not address all the content that will ultimately be included in the teaching plan—the specific "what" we wish to impart to the learner. Rather, the "what" in the behavioral objectives is the outcome we can evaluate after the teaching has occurred. Consider the chapter objectives to determine the "how" and "what" information:

1. Discuss (how) the components of teaching and learning (what).
2. Examine (how) differences in the ways people learn (what).
3. Describe (how) methods to assess learning readiness and motivation (what).
4. Propose (how) different teaching methods for a variety of learning needs (what).
5. Devise (how) a lesson plan on a topic that contains behavioral objectives, a content outline with appropriate teaching methods, and a plan for evaluating learner outcomes (what).

This example focuses on the learner at the end of the prescribed learning activity, with action verbs—discussing, examining, describing, proposing, and devising—as their outcome ability; describing "how" they should perform.

The next focus is on the complexity you as the evaluator (whether learner or teacher) wish to see demonstrated at the end of the activity. This is the degree that can be measured, or the "where." The type and complexity of the outcome behavior are determined by the level of the learning domain.

When developing behavioral objectives, be sure to consider the domains of knowledge. Further, within each domain there is a leveling process, or progress in attainment of increasingly complex skills. From the work of Bloom and other teaching and learning theorists, a revised two-dimensional taxonomy has been developed. The revised taxonomy table considers the interrelationship of two dimensions, knowledge and cognitive processes (Anderson et al., 2001). This is the knowledge or the "what" you wish the learner to acquire, and the cognitive process is the demonstration or "how" the learning is evaluated. The taxonomy table allows objectives to be developed that address both knowledge and processes. Consider that the nursing goal for the client is to be at the procedural knowledge level to apply a dressing change at home

but also at the factual knowledge level to evaluate signs of infection or monitor the response to a prescribed medication.

Knowledge Dimension

In this revised taxonomy table, the knowledge dimension represents the four rows of the table with the following knowledge categories:

- Factual, as the basic elements
- Conceptual, or the interelationships among elements
- Procedural, demonstration of a set of skills
- Metacognitive, as the highest level or awareneess of the thought processes (Anderson et al., 2001).

Consider the difference of these categories in nursing practice, as in the case of a sterile field. "Factual" is simply the knowledge of the components. "Conceptual" would be the understanding of the interrelationship, as with spillage and contamination of the field. "Procedural knowledge" would be in the performance of a dressing change and maintenance of the field. "Metacognitive knowledge" would occur during practice with an unanticipated occurence and resolution using critical thinking skills. In patient education, we strive for the procedural level, for the return demonstration of a set of skills, as in the dressing change needed at home and the protection of the surgical site.

Cognitive Processes Dimension

In the revised taxonomy table, the cognitive process dimension is represented in the six columns of the table as the following levels of increasing complexity:

- Remember, as recognizing and recalling
- Understand, as interpreting, exemplifying, classifying, summarizing, inferring, comparing, and explaining
- Apply, as executing and implementing
- Analyze, to include diffentiating, organizing, and attributing
- Evaluate, or making judgments based on certain criteria to

- Create, or developing a new process (Anderson et al., 2001).

Cognitive processes in this taxonomy build from the simple recall of facts to the extrapolation into a new process. Continuing to use our example, we want the nurse in a preceptor position for a senior student or a new graduate to use congnitive skills through evaluation for the maintenance of the sterile field in all practice applications with the novice nurse or nursing student. However, in advanced practice, the nurse would consistently use all processes in the domain for the specialty area, including the creation of new processes within the selected scope of practice. In the scenerio of patient education, the goal would be for the client to be able to remember, understand, and apply specific skills, and to analyze and evaluate when professional intervention is needed, as in the case of potential infection or a complication, on the basis of specific standards or criteria taught as part of the teaching-learning process.

In the cognitive processes dimension, we first have the knowledge received through recall or recognition. Next, we proceed to an understanding of the information. The final levels of the cognitive domain are applying the information, analyzing, evaluating the information, and finally creating for application of the knowledge in other situations. Consider the levels in the cognitive processes domain with the following action words in your behavioral objectives for teaching a client about his or her condition:

1. *Knowledge* implies simply that the learner has perceived the information and can report it back to the teacher. Action verbs such as *identifies*, *recalls*, *recognizes*, and *repeats* are useful for behavioral objectives at this knowledge level of the cognitive domains, such as the ability to recall a list of the signs of infection in a learning situation.
2. At the next level, the learner demonstrates *understanding* of the knowledge, based on the four levels of the knowledge dimension. Action verbs for behavioral objectives at this level include *explains* and *compares*, as illustrated by the client who can explain

how to look for redness indicating infection in a surgical wound.
3. The third level of the cognitive domain is *application*, demonstrating the ability to relate the learning to a situation. The following action verbs are appropriate for behavioral objectives for the learner's outcomes at this point: *applies*, *demonstrates*, *employs*, and *uses*. For example, "the client uses the dressing change skill at home after discharge."
4. Further critical thinking occurs at the next cognitive level of *analysis*. The learner steps back and analyzes the information objectively. Action verbs useful at this level of complexity include *assesses*, *appraises*, *organizes*, and *differentiates*. Now the client has determined the need to call the physician's office for evaluation of potential complications from the surgery.
5. *Evaluation* occurs at the next level of cognitive processes in which judgment is an essential component. Action verbs appropriate for this level include *evaluating*, *testing*, *monitoring*, and *critiquing*.
6. *Creation* is the highest level of the cognitive domain, in which the learner manipulates the concepts from the learning in new combinations and situations. Action verbs addressing this level of complexity in the taxonomy include *creates*, *designs*, *devises*, *constructs*, and *generates*.

Both the cognitive and psychomotor domains are readily apparent in the taxonomy table with the focus on knowledge and the cognitive process. The psychomotor domain is easily apparent in the application of the knowledge. However, it is important to include behavioral objectives at the various knowledge levels to measure client progress from simple to complex skills. For example, you have taught a newly diagnosed diabetic client to self-administer insulin. As the teacher, you must be able to see how the learner-client has accomplished this task, beyond the simple return demonstration with saline injections you observe. At the next level of manipulation of the psychomotor skill, the learner demonstrates the entire procedure of proper injection of insulin, from filling the syringe to properly disposing of the supplies. Precision of the psychomotor skill is demonstrated when the learner can perform the injection on schedule with a sense of comfort in his or her ability in the process, expressed with the phrase "Demonstrates skill in the procedure." Articulation, or full use of the skill, is demonstrated when the diabetic client is able to manage at home with insulin, including testing blood glucose for additional needs during stressful periods. This is reflected in the phrase "Uses results of blood glucose monitoring to regulate. ..."

The highest level of skill acquisition comes when the individual has a sense of competence and the skill has become a natural part of his or her routine; the individual can determine signs of hyperglycemia or hypoglycemia and self-test as naturally as he or she dresses or bathes. The individual has incorporated the process sufficiently to spend a month traveling with a sense of independence, comfort, and control in the process. Action terms reflecting this level include "Independently monitors and effectively regulates administration of insulin."

The affective domain is less apparent in the revised taxonomy table but is inferred in the higher levels of knowledge and cognitive processes. In fact, the creators of the revised taxonomy propose that "nearly every cognitive objective has an affective component" (Anderson et al., 2001). For the affective domain, complexity progresses from receiving to responding, valuing, organizing values, and finally characterizing or standing for certain values transmitted. Consider the newly diagnosed diabetic client. Acceptance of his or her condition is vital to developing long-range personal care skills. But this is a difficult domain to measure because values and attitudes are more difficult to assess than knowledge or psychomotor skills. Although action verbs for the affective domain include *receiving, responding, valuing, organizing values*, and *characterizing*, this is a difficult domain of learning to evaluate. We must rely on the individual to communicate his or her attitudes, feelings, and values honestly through verbal and nonverbal behaviors.

Behavioral objectives are the intended action-oriented outcomes of an educational process, they contain all the "who" (the learner), "when" (on completion of the learning activity), and "how" (the action verb) used to identify the "what" (the behavior) that the learner will demonstrate as the outcome, or "where" (at a specified point), of learning. These objectives are tools for teaching, learning, and evaluating. Evaluation data can provide useful feedback on whether the learner has achieved the objective or requires repetition, reinforcement, or revision.

Developing Lesson Plans

Once the assessment of learners and teachers takes place and the behavioral objectives have been developed, we must plan for the specific content and how it will be transmitted to the client group. As the **lesson plan** evolves, it defines content.

Initially, when you think of lesson plans, you may picture primary school teachers with their attendance books and plans or activities for the day. This is far from the content of the professional nurse's lesson plan for a teaching activity. The primary school teacher has some advantages over the nurse: a consistent audience of 20 to 25 7-year-old students and subject matter identified in a curriculum guide. The nurse, in contrast, has a variable audience of clients, with variable health and teaching needs. The nurse interacts not only with an individual or group of client learners but also, in many cases, with family members, community groups, and professional colleagues.

Babcock and Miller (1994) describe a client education lesson plan as consisting of the client, objectives, content, setting, strategies, materials, and the means of evaluation (p. 176). The assessment data obtained earlier in this process have been used to define and describe the client, including characteristics, attributes, learning assets and deficits, readiness, and specific needs to be addressed. This procedure was conducted with the client as an individual, family, or group to diagnose the learning needs and prepare for continuation of the process. Next, behavioral objectives were identified to guide the process and plan for the evaluation of outcomes. Now we must plan the content, teaching strategies and methods of delivery, learning resources, and specific evaluation procedures.

Traditional lesson plans are frequently prepared in a column format (FIG. 10–1). The first column contains the behavioral objectives developed for the learning activity. Subsequent columns contain learning content, teaching strategies, perhaps teaching principles, learning resources, evaluation methods, and timing, which all can be easily viewed in relation to the behavioral objectives. A sample format is posted on the Intranet site for this text. The learning content is the specific content outline designed to meet the objective. Teaching strategies relate to the objective and the specific content, including variations for the learning setting and clients. Suggested learning resources and materials are proposed to enhance the teaching strategy and meet the learner's cognitive style, especially if a group

or lecture presentation is appropriate for the general audience but may not meet the needs of individual learners.

All of the lesson plan so far is the proposal for the teaching-learning activity. Before implementing it, one must specify evaluation methods along with a proposed time-frame for the process. Implementation of the teaching-learning process can then proceed using the strategies identified in the lesson plan. Evaluation of the teaching-learning process is essential and is designed to address the behavioral objectives at the level of the taxonomy specified for acquisition of affective, cognitive, and psychomotor behaviors.

Consider the simple example of a 56-year-old white female outpatient with unstable hypertension without angina. She has come to the health clinic after being denied health insurance last week because of the prepolicy examination requirement. Blood pressure measurements ranged from 210/105 to

Behavioral Objectives	Learning Content	Teaching Strategies	Learning Resources	Evaluation Methods	Time Frame

FIG. 10–1. Sample lesson plan. Develop a lesson plan on a topic that includes behavioral objectives, a content outline with appropriate teaching methods, and a plan for evaluating learner outcomes.

185/100 on the two consecutive visits. She has had no serious illness or hospitalizations, but she is leaving town in 5 weeks to visit family abroad for a month. Today, her doctor prescribed daily antihypertensive medication (Sular) and a low-sodium diet. The client has verbalized the need to lower her blood pressure for insurance purposes. She also reported that she has used a salt substitute for the past 3 days and has continued to play tennis three times a week. Her descriptions of nutritional intake indicate high dietary fat and sodium content in meals prepared at home and selected in restaurants. She volunteers much information about cooking for her family as well as attending gourmet cooking classes at the local college, which she signed up for because she wanted to watch the teacher and ask questions rather than just read the cookbooks.

The assessment data indicate a teaching deficit, learning readiness, and the motivation to adhere to a treatment plan within a confined time frame. You and the client determine that you will schedule individualized teaching sessions with her for her next four weekly visits. Behavioral objectives for this teaching-learning process might include the following:

1. Explains food selection and food preparation techniques to maintain a low-sodium diet.
2. Monitors blood pressure regularly.
3. Uses Sular as prescribed, monitoring for side effects, adverse effects, and toxicity.
4. Uses appropriate food choices and preparations for maintenance of a low-sodium diet.
5. Organizes activities including maintenance of her exercise program.
6. Reapplies for health insurance coverage.

The learning content, in the second column, addresses the behavioral objectives by teaching food selections and revisions needed with food preparation, periodic assessment of blood pressure, administration of medication, monitoring for side effects and toxicity, and maintenance of a healthy nutritional and exercise program. Teaching strategies are then selected for the individualized cognitive style of the client, using resources such as videos

and written information to take home. Evaluation methods are proposed to address each of the behavioral objectives at the following four weekly visits, specifying the time frame for each activity.

Teaching Strategies And Methods

Teaching strategies and methods are geared toward accomplishing the behavioral objectives in light of the audience. Selection is also based on how the content can best be delivered and addresses the affective, cognitive, and psychomotor domains of learning. Teaching methods generally are lecture presentations, demonstrations, discussions, modeling, role-playing, individualized instruction, programmed instruction, computer-assisted instruction (CAI), other simulations, and group activities. As Bastable (2003) has described, the instructional strategy is the overall plan for the learning experience whereas instructional methods are the techniques or approaches to bring the learner into contact with the content to be learned (p. 356).

Selection of a teaching strategy, and some combination of teaching methods, depends on the client. For a client group of 24, a lecture format followed by breaking out into four small groups to apply the lecture content may be quite appropriate for presenting information on child development and wellness practices. For a group of three new mothers on the postpartum unit, a lecture would be impersonal and less effective than a small-group discussion on plans for returning home with their healthy neonates. In our example of the client with hypertension, individualized teaching would be most effective, because the client prefers the interaction with a teacher and has a limited time frame to accomplish the behavioral outcome objectives. The characteristics of the client group and their intended outcomes, therefore, guide the selection of appropriate teaching methods. For further information on selected instructional methods, refer to Table 10–2.

Enhancing the delivery of content and improving learning on the basis of the cognitive style of the client require careful selection of learning resources. Teaching aids change as

TABLE 10–2
Teaching Methods

Method	Advantages	Disadvantages
Lecture	Easier to organize and transfer large amount of information Predictable, quicker, more efficient, cost-effective, and useful for a large group Allows teacher control over material being presented Easy to focus material	Lacks opportunity for feedback Risk of information overload Sustaining interest may be difficult Difficult to tailor material for the group
Group discussion	Allows for continual feedback, attitude development, and modification Flexible, able to be modified according to the motivation of the audience Able to identify confusion and resolve difficulties Serves as a vehicle for networking	Increases chance of getting off the focus Risk of discussion becoming pointless Allows participants to be dominant or passive Time-consuming
Demonstration	Activates many senses Clarifies the "whys" as a principle Commands interest Correlates theory with practice Allows for problem identification Helps learner receive directed practice	Time-consuming Does not cover all aspects of cognitive learning
Modeling	Facilitates active learning Bypasses defenses Effective with children	Ineffective without rapport Learning not always visible Risk for learner ambivalence
Programmed or computer-assisted instruction	Allows learning at a self-directed pace Learner can repeat sections at will Breaks down information into manageable increments Saves teacher time	Effectiveness depends on learner motivation Does not account for unplanned feedback, which can distance the learner Variable quality of programs
Simulated environments, games, activities, and role-playing	Greatest transfer of learning Facilitates learning of what is needed to cope with problem or environment Allows for practice that is most transferrable	Facilitates unpredictable occurrences May be threatening to learner Time-consuming Achievement of outcomes is more difficult
Team teaching	Uses competencies of more than one teacher Allows for learning among the teachers Accentuates divergent points of view	Lacks continuity and internal consistency Requires more planning Group processing slower Eliminates teacher autonomy

Adapted with permission from Babcock, D. E., & Miller, M. A. (1994). *Client education: Theory and practice.* St. Louis: Mosby.

our available technology changes. In 1978, Guinee listed teaching aids as display boards (bulletin, magnetic, felt or flannel, chalk), projectors (overhead, micro), textbooks, models, equipment, specimens, exhibits, films, slides, filmstrips, audiotapes, and closed-circuit television. Some of these are still appropriate and readily available, but others have been displaced as our technology has grown to include multimedia presentations, presentation graphics, teleconferencing, computer simulations, and sychronous and asynchronous use of technology, such as courses, chatrooms, and bulletin boards.

Teaching aids and instructional technology are frequently used in client teaching situations to enhance the content and actively involve the learner in the teaching-learning process. Using assessment data, consider how the client told you she or he best learned information in the past. When preparing for larger group presentations, consider how smaller group activities or assignments will address the needs of learners who do not do their best in the large group setting. Remember, adults learn best when actively involved in the process. Think of ways to move the client from a passive to an active learning situation.

A major consideration is how to enhance the content for the learner's own cognitive style. Some learners are highly perceptive in one or several senses in learning information. They may be highly visual, auditory, tactile, or perceptive in some combination of these senses. Recall the usefulness of understanding multiple inlelligences. When you select teaching resources, consider whether the learners are highly visual and obtain and process information mainly through observation of the world around them. These learners do well with visual aids that enhance the content presented in the teaching strategy, such as with presentation graphics or with information presented through pamphlets, handouts, and online searches.

Compare a visual style to the learner whose auditory sense is the most perceptive. Effective auditory teaching aids include videotapes, audiotapes, and recordings with well-developed sound presentations. In addition, this learner may do well using a recorder to take notes and reinforce learning through review later. For the individual who prefers to touch and manipulate new information, plan for active involvement in the teaching and learning through demonstrations, models, and samples.

> *Adults learn best when actively involved in the process. Think of ways to move the client from a passive to an active learning situation.*

Another consideration is whether the learner prefers to be an individualist or to have other people in the learning environment for interaction and stimulation. Some people learn in a very individualistic way. They prefer to obtain information and then go their own way to process, analyze, and synthesize the material. Having a group discussion to evaluate and apply information directly after it is presented in a lecture is stressful, if not torture, to this individual, who needs time before he or she can share thoughts or apply the information. Alternatively, some learners enjoy interactions and learning in a stimulating group environment. A large, impersonal lecture is deadly boring to this learner, who thrives on group discussion to work on questions posed in a case study. But learners are generally not easy to classify; these characteristics can be combined over a wide range. Pure types are rare, and the challenge is to find those teaching strategies and resources that enhance the teaching content and promote learning. Resources for different cognitive styles are presented in Table 10 –3.

In our example of the client with hypertension, we decided on individualized teaching because she prefers the interaction and has a limited time frame to accomplish the outcome objectives. Teaching aids in this case include short videos shown in the office during or before the teaching session, followed by discussion using charts and models. Pamphlets and handouts to take home for reinforcement and discussion with family and friends would also be useful, along with *appropriate* online sources for her to access. Clients need infor-

TABLE 10–3
Teaching Methods and Resources to Enhance the Cognitive Style of the Learner

Cognitive Style	Teaching Methods	Teaching Resources
Highly visual	Small-group lecture and discussion, role-playing, simulations, modeling, demonstrations, programmed instruction, computer simulations	Multimedia presentations, videos, slides, charts, posters, models, photographs, white/bulletin boards, publications, handouts, reading lists, computer-assisted instruction (CAI) with effective graphics, e-mail, chatrooms
Highly auditory	Lecture and discussion, role-playing, simulations, modeling, demonstrations	Videotapes, recordings (prepared audiotapes or self-recorded tapes made during teaching), CAI with auditory reinforcers, telephone follow-up
Highly tactile	Small-group activities, individualized teaching, role-playing, simulations, modeling, demonstrations, programmed instruction, computer simulations	Models, bulletin boards, samples, books, pamphlets, prepared handouts, CAI requiring responses to cues, chatrooms, e-mail
Highly interpersonal	Small-group lecture and discussion, role-playing, simulations, modeling, demonstrations, programmed instruction, computer simulations	Videotapes, audiotapes, charts, posters, models, photographs, pamphlets, CAI, teleconferencing techniques, chatrooms, e-mail
Highly individualistic	Lecture, simulations, modeling, demonstrations, programmed instruction, computer simulations, computer searches	Multimedia presentations, videos, audiotapes, slides, charts, overhead projections, posters, models, photographs, books, handouts, paper and pencils for notetaking, CAI, e-mail

mation on valid and reliable online sources. Recall that one of the five core competencies for health professionals was the use of informatics for both information and communication. The use of e-mail for follow-up is a powerful medium now available to both the health professional and clients.

In addition to client teaching, contemporary nursing practice consists of collegial teaching and learning opportunities such as educational programs, lectures, demonstrations, group discussions, professional and clinical conferences, case studies, clinical receptorships, grand rounds, and chatrooms, just to mention a few. The same steps are involved in this process as with assessment, diagnosis of learning needs, development of behavioral objectives, preparation of a lesson plan, selection of teaching strategies and resources, and evaluation. The difference generally lies in the size of the group, which can range from a one-to-one collegial or the unit staff to a large interdisciplinary group of professionals who are interested in the latest research on a selected topic. With the larger group, it is essential to assess the prevalent characteristics of the learner population. This includes the overall learning need that will become the topic for the presentation. Behavioral outcomes should address what the learners are expected to have gained as knowledge and skills at the end of the program or teaching session, because they will be the ones providing the evaluation data. Teaching strategies may include a team approach, especially for presentations across disciplines to foster the development of knowledge and collaboration. Although active learning in small groups is highly effective with professional colleagues, this can effectively occur as a small-group breakout phase after the basic information has been presented in a large group presentation format. Highly effective learning resources in this case include multimedia presentations with presentation graphics, videotapes, posters, models, photographs, pamphlets, handouts, and reading lists. However, a word of warning with presentation graphics: Do not read the entire presentation from the screen. Present the pertinent points graphically to engage the audience rather than lose their attention (Box 10–2). After the program or presentation, the teacher or program coordinator receives completed evaluation forms from the program participants and then develops an overall analysis based on the evaluation data the participants provide.

Evaluation of Outcomes

Evaluating outcomes is a vital component of the teaching-learning process. It may be ongoing and may lead to important information for revisions needed in subsequent sessions. Although evaluation strategies focus on both the teaching and the learning that occurred, the primary focus is on the learner. Is the learner able to demonstrate the outcomes envisioned at the beginning of the process? As in the nursing process, the evaluation phase of the teaching-learning process is used to assess the effectiveness of the process and whether the client has resolved a knowledge deficit.

BOX 10–2
TIPS FOR PRESENTATIONS

- Do not read from the screen. Presentation graphics should be used to engage the audience. Use the information on the screen as talking points to keep you on track, not the audiance distracted.
- Do not use all capital letters—they imply shouting and are not visually engaging.
- Use a clear font, not a fancy script that is hard to read and distracting for the audience.
- Limit the information on a slide or screen; for example, use only four or five lines on the screen that must be legible from the back of the room.
- Keep it simple. Limit the graphics and displays to important information without distracting background colors or graphics.
- Consider the essential number of slides or displays, in terms of content, allotted time, essential information, and printing costs if you are planning on handouts.
- Carefully proofread to avoid spelling and grammatical errors without reliance on the spell-checker function (e.g., *three*, *their*, and *there* are all in the dictionary).
- If you plan on distributing copies of your presentation as handouts or electronically, make sure the copies are readable, have the same information as your presentation, and include appropriate citations, if applicable.
- Remember your highly auditory learner—speak to him or her, while assisting your visual learner, who is watching the display rather than you.
- For the active learner, consider a follow-up activity to reinforce the content you presented.

Clients are more difficult to evaluate than traditional student learners. Cognitive domain learning activities of students are easily measured with paper-and-pencil tests and computer-adaptive testing that assesses knowledge and cognitive processes. In the client teaching situation, such tests are rarely used except in research or large group situations. Client evaluation can be complex, with problems related to timing, access, continuity, measurement, and other factors. In addition, recall that adult learners should be involved in evaluating their own learning. Normally, client evaluation is done with methods such as return demonstrations, observation, diaries, rating scales, discussion, and electronic communication.

We used different action verbs to address the three domains of learning and levels, or taxonomy, within each. Capturing evaluation data requires specificity in the behavioral outcome objective. The behavioral objectives are the intended action-oriented outcomes of an educational process and contain the "who" (the learner), the "when" (on completion of the learning activity), and the "how" (the action verb) used to identify the "what" (the behavior) that the learner will demonstrate as the outcome "where" (at a specified point) of learning. The objectives should also indicate how you are measuring the outcomes of the teaching-learning process.

The affective domain consists of attitudes, feelings, and values. Evaluation data should show how the learner progressed from receiving to internalizing the values mutually agreed on for the learning. In our example of a newly diagnosed diabetic client, the teacher and the learner must be able to measure or see attitudinal or value changes through verbal and nonverbal behaviors. The action verbs in the affective domain were *receiving, responding, valuing, organizing values*, and *characterizing specific values*. We need the individual to communicate his or her attitudes, feelings, and values in verbal and nonverbal behaviors. Methods of evaluation in this area include interviews, discussions, and observations that demonstrate certain beliefs and values. Another means of evaluating affective learning is a diary in which the client can record feelings and problems that arise between teaching sessions. Analyzing the content of the diaries can provide useful information on the affective domain as well as knowledge gaps in cognitive processes. And with the availability of electronic communication, cognitive and affective domains can be evaluated via e-mail or electronic postings.

In the cognitive domain, knowledge builds from simple recall to understanding, application, analysis, evaluation, and synthesis or creation of information. Interviews and discussion with clients can be used to evaluate whether the learner can repeat or report back the information imparted by the teacher. For understanding, the client describes, explains, and compares information during the interview. Application of the information can be evaluated as the client demonstrates and uses the information, providing specific examples of how this was done. Critical thinking and analysis take this one step further, as the client explains problems and difficulties that arose and steps taken to solve problems without the presence of the teacher. Evaluation by the learner occurs when the client determines which method worked best. Creation involves manipulating the learning in new combinations and effectively applying the information to a similar problem or situation. The learner has devised a new way of handling a situation on the basis of information obtained in another area. Occasionally, post-tests are used in client teaching, but test anxiety is a major deterrent to their use for some clients. The evaluation strategies most useful for both teachers and client-learners to gauge cognitive learning are discussion, questioning, and allowing for description, whether through face-to-face or electronic means.

Evaluating client outcomes in the psychomotor domain is easiest through direct observation of skill attainment. At the simplest level of psychomotor skill attainment is the client's ability to imitate, as seen in a return demonstration. This allows one to assess understanding and the ability to perform a specific skill, such as testing one's blood glucose. But demonstration of a skill in a clinical setting can be artificial, because the client's own environment often has additional factors not present in the health-care agency, such as shared bathrooms or medication storage problems in a home with toddlers. Flow charts, diaries, and check sheets are easy for clients to use as reminders and reinforcers in the home, and they can then be discussed at the next clinic visit or teaching session interview. The level of psychomotor skills can be assessed with a checklist or flow chart in terms of following instructions to proper scheduling, precision, and problem-solving in the procedure. The client can be encouraged to note problems encountered and how they were handled, to demonstrate skills in both cognitive and psychomotor domains. Consider the use of electronic calendars or personal digital assistants (PDAs) in some client situations. This will provide evaluation data for both the client, as the learner, and the nurse, as the teacher.

In our example of the client with hypertension, we implemented an individualized teaching strategy within a limited time frame to accomplish the outcome objectives. Objectives were developed to address learning in the cognitive and psychomotor domains. One method of evaluation would be for the client to maintain a diary, including daily food intake and exercise, and list daily blood pressure measurements, medications taken, and effects on a check sheet. This evaluation method provides visual data that address the initial five behavioral objectives agreed on by both the client and the nurse. At each of the four client visits or teaching sessions, the information in the diary is reviewed and discussed. When both the learner and the teacher are satisfied that these objectives have been met, control of the hypertension problem may be present. A health certificate can then be provided by the primary care provider so that the last objective, reapplication for health insurance coverage, can be attempted with an outlook for success. At the final teaching visit, the client and the nurse discuss the strategies and resources used during the 4-week process, to evaluate the teaching that took place. Electronic communication provides an additional resource for follow-up and evaluation.

Evaluation data can provide useful feedback that objectives have been met or that repetition, reinforcement, or revision is needed. Teaching strategies, like methods and resources, should be evaluated by both the teacher and the learner. Discovering what worked and what may have worked better helps the learner view the process and reinforce the learning while sharing with the teacher ways to improve and strategies for the future. Important factors here are encouragement and openness for honest and constructive evaluation data from both teacher and learner.

ONLINE CONSULT

Communicating Health
http://odphp.osophds.dhhs.gov/projects
Health information and toll-free numbers
http://www.health.gov/nhic/
Literacy
http://www.nifl.gov

Key Points

- There are several schools of learning theories. Major examples of these theories are behaviorism, gestalt, social learning theory, humanism, and multiple intelligences.
- Teaching is more than transmitting information. The information must be received, understood, and evaluated by the learner.
- Learning is the perception and assimilation of the information presented to us in a variety of ways.   *(continued)*

(*continued*)

- Characteristics of learning include:
  - Perception of new information
  - Initial reaction to the information
  - Ability to remember or repeat the information
  - Rejection or acceptance of the information (understanding)
  - Use of the information in a similar situation (application)
  - Critical analysis of the information
  - Incorporation of the information into the value system (evaluation)
  - Use of the information in various situations or combinations (creation)
- The three learning domains are:
  - Affective: attitudes, feelings, and values
  - Cognitive: knowledge and thought processes
  - Psychomotor: demonstration of behaviors
- Cognitive learning styles look at how information is interpreted, influences from others, and reasoning methods. Teaching and learning strategies can then be developed to match the learner's needs and resources.
- Andragogy is the model used to focus on the characteristics of the adult learner: self-direction, experiential background, readiness triggers, internal motivation, and demand for knowledgeable resources.
- Teaching-learning skills depend on the physical and psychological climate for the adult learner. Physical climate is the environment. The seven characteristics of the psychological climate conducive to adult learning are mutual respect, collaborativeness, mutual trust, supportiveness, openness and authenticity, pleasure, and humanness (Knowles et al., 1985, pp. 15–17).
- Readiness occurs when the learner is willing to change and view the learning need. Learning readiness includes human motivation, understanding, and applicability or acceptability. Motivation in humans is a manifestation of internal and external personal and environmental factors that cause people to respond to a situation the way they do. In addition, to achieve learning readiness, the person must perceive the information at his or her level of cognitive functioning, and it must be applicable and acceptable to the person as an individual, a member of the family, or a member of a group.
- The purpose of writing behavioral objectives is to provide a frame of reference for the intended outcomes of the teaching-learning activity for both the teacher and the learner. The focus of the objective is on the learner and the knowledge and cognitive process demonstrated as learning outcomes.
- A lesson plan is frequently prepared in a column format containing the following components: the behavioral objectives, content outline, teaching strategies, learning resources, evaluation methods, and timing.
- Teaching strategies are geared toward accomplishing the behavioral objectives in light of the audience.
- Evaluating learning outcomes of the teaching-learning process is essential and is designed to address the behavioral objectives at the taxonomic level specified for the acquisition of affective, cognitive, and psychomotor behaviors.
- Teaching strategies as methods and resources are evaluated by both the teacher and the learner, to discover what worked and what could have worked better in a similar teaching-learning process. Evaluation of teaching strategies by the learner provides a further view of the process and reinforces the learning.

Thought and Discussion Questions

1. Explain which theory of learning and cognitive style is applicable to the way in which you learn best.
2. Remember those two clients following their hip replacement surgeries? One is an architect who designs custom homes and meets with his customers for at least an hour before he develops the house plans to ensure that he truly understands their desires and ideas. The other is a retired English professor concerned about the rehabilitation schedule and the completion of a collection of essays that must be submitted to the publisher in 6 weeks. Plan for their individualized discharge teaching using the theory of multiple intelligences.
3. Develop a staff conference as a seminar presentation on a clinical topic, with appropriate content for a unit staff of 10 registered nurses, 6 licensed practical nurses, and 15 certified assistive personnel. Propose assessment data on the learners and ways to match cognitive styles and teaching strategies for the group. Be prepared to participate in an online or class discussion, to be scheduled by your instructor.
4. Select a health promotion topic to present to a group of 30 clients. Describe the planning process, content for presentation, and evaluation methods. Complete the lesson plan provided on the Intranet. Be prepared to participate in an online or class discussion of the planning process, to be scheduled by your instructor.
5. Read the case studies in the Case Study Bank on the Intranet Site and be prepared to discuss them in class.
6. Review the Chapter Thought located on the first page of the chapter, and discuss it in the context of the contents of the chapter.

Interactive Exercises

1. Complete the lesson plan on the Intranet Site for the client with unstable hypertention described in this chapter. Be prepared to participate in an online or class discussion on the topic, to be scheduled by your instructor.
2. Select a client teaching topic and develop at least three behavioral objectives for the three learning domains (cognitive, affective, and psychomotor). Include various levels of complexity in different domain objectives. Use the taxonomy table to identify where the objectives are placed on the table for the knowledge and cognitive process domain. Propose methods for evaluation of each objective.
3. Develop a lesson plan on one of the clinical scenarios provided on the Intranet site. Include in the plan behavioral objectives, a content outline with appropriate teaching methods, and a plan for evaluating learner outcomes. Complete the lesson plan on the Intranet site.
4. Develop a 30-minute grand rounds program on a clinical topic of interest using presentation graphics for an interdisciplinary group session. Determine roles and content areas for representative presentations by nursing practice, nursing administration, medicine, and appropriate therapies in small-group breakout sessions.
5. Do an online search for the Myers-Briggs Inventory. Take the inventory to determine your four-letter type. Find the grid and discover what this means about your learning style.

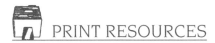

PRINT RESOURCES

References

Anderson, L. W., Krathwohl, D. R., Airasian, P. W., Cruikshank, K. A., Mayer, R. E., Pintrich, P. R.,. Raths, R. E., & Wittrock, M .C. (Eds.) (2001). *A taxonomy for learning, teaching, and assessing: A revision of Bloom's educational objectives* (abridged ed.). New York: Longman.

Babcock, D. E., & Miller, M. A. (1994). *Client education: Theory and practice.* St. Louis: Mosby.

Bandura, A. (1977). *Social learning theory.* Englewood Cliffs, NJ: Prentice-Hall.

Bastable, S. B. (2003). *Nurse as educator: Principles of teaching and learning for nursing practice.* Boston: Jones and Bartlett.

Benner, P. (1984). *From novice to expert: Excellence and power in clinical nursing practice.* Menlo Park, CA: Addison-Wesley.

Bloom, B. S. (Ed.). (1956). *Taxonomy of educational objectives.* New York: Longman.

Erikson, E. H. (1963). *Childhood and society* (2nd ed.). New York: Norton.

Gardner, H. (1993a). *Frames of mind: The theory of multiple intelligences* (2nd ed.). New York: Basic Books.

Gardner, H. (1993b). *Multiple intelligences: The theory in practice.* New York: Basic Books.

Guinee, K. K. (1978). *Teaching and learning in nursing: A behavioral objectives approach.* New York: Macmillan.

Havighurst, R. J. (1972). *Developmental tasks and education* (3rd ed.). New York: David McKay.

King, I. M. (1981). *A theory for nursing: Systems, concepts, process.* New York: John Wiley & Sons.

Knowles, M. S. (1990). *The adult learner: A neglected species* (4th ed.). Houston: Gulf.

Knowles, M. S. (1980). *The modern practice of adult education: From pedagogy to andragogy* (Rev. ed.). Chicago: Follett.

Knowles, M. S., & associates (1985). *Andragogy in action.* San Francisco: Jossey-Bass.

Kolb, D. (1981). *Learning style inventory.* Boston, MA: McBer and Company.

Maslow, A. H. (1971). *The farther reaches of the human mind.* New York: Viking Press.

Maslow, A. H. (1954). *Motivation and personality.* New York: Harper.

Rogers, C., & Freiberg, H. J. (1994). *Freedom to learn* (3rd ed.). New York: Merrill/Macmillan.

Vella, J. (1994). *Learning to listen, learning to teach.* San Francisco: Jossey-Bass.

Bibliography

Blanton, B. (1998). The application of cognitive learning theory to instructional design. *International Journal of Instructional Media, 25,* 171–175.

Boyd, M. D., Graham, B. A., Gleit, C. J., & Whitman, N. I. (1998). *Health teaching in nursing practice: A professional model* (3rd ed.). Stamford, CT: Appleton & Lange.

Briggs-Myers, I. (1980). *Gifts differing.* Palo Alto, CA: Consulting Psychologists Press.

Briggs-Myers, I., & McCaulley, M. (1992). *Manual: A guide to the development and use of the Myers-Briggs Type Indicator.* Palo Alto, CA: Consulting Psychologists Press.

Canobbio, M. M. (2000). *Mosby's handbook of patient teaching* (2nd ed.). St. Louis: Mosby.

Doak, C. C., Doak, L. G., & Root, J. H. (1995). *Teaching patients with low literacy skills* (2nd ed.). Philadelphia: Lippincott Williams & Wilkins.

Dunn, R., & Griggs, S. A. (1998). *Learning styles and the nursing profession.* Boston: Jones and Bartlett, National League for Nursing.

Fitzpatrick, J. J., Romano, C, & Chasek, R. (Eds.). (2001). *The nurses' guide to consumer health web sites.* New York: Springer.

Flynn, J. P. (1997). *The role of the preceptor: A guide for nurse educators and clinicians.* New York: Springer.

Ginsburg, H. P., & Opper, S. (1988). *Piaget's theory of intellectual development* (3rd ed.). New York: Prentice-Hall.

Glanz, K., Rimer, B. K., Lewis, F. M. (Eds.) (2002). *Health behavior and health education: Theory, research, and practice* (3rd. ed). San Francisco: Jossey-Bass.

London, F. (1999). *No time to teach? A nurse's guide to patient and family education.* Philadelphia: Lippincott Williams & Wilkins.

Redman, B. K. (2001). *The practice of patient education* (9th ed.). St. Louis: Mosby.

Reilly, D. E., & Oermann, M. H. (1990). *Behavioral outcomes: Evaluation in nursing* (3rd ed.). New York: National League for Nursing.

Skinner, B. F. (1968). *The technology of teaching.* New York: Appleton-Century-Crofts.

ONLINE REFERENCES AND RESOURCES

Ackerman, P. (1996). Child versus adult intelligence. ERIC Clearinghouse on Assessment and Evaluation, ED410228, 1–3. *http://www.ed.gov/ databases/ERIC_Digests/ ed410228.html)*

Jung. *www.cgjungpage.org*

Gardner. *http://pzweb.harvard.edu/Pls/HG.htm*

Malsow. *www.maslow.org*

Psychology. *http://tip.psychology.org*

Skinner, B.F. (2003). A brief survey of operant behavior. *http://www.bfskinner.org/operant.asp.*

Theresa M. Valiga
Sheila C. Grossman

11
chapter

Leadership

> Do not go where the path may lead. Go instead where there is no path, and leave a trail.
>
> *Anonymous*

Chapter Objectives

On completion of this chapter, the reader will be able to:

1. Differentiate between leadership and management.
2. Compare and contrast three leadership styles: democratic, authoritarian, and laissez-faire.
3. Distinguish among various theories of leadership: great man theory, traitist theory, situational theory, transformational theory, and leadership task theory.
4. Analyze the interdependence of leaders and followers.
5. Explain how each of the nine tasks of leadership as outlined by Gardner and the concept of stewardship relates to nursing practice.
6. Analyze nursing practice situations in terms of the extent to which leadership was exercised.
7. Identify your own leadership abilities or potential leadership skills.

Key Terms

Leadership Style
Authoritative Leaders
Laissez-Faire or
   Permissive Leaders
Democratic or
   Participative Leaders
Great Man Leadership
   Theory

Traitist Leadership
   Theories
Situational Leadership
   Theories
Transformational
   Leadership
   Theory

Leadership Tasks
   Theory
New Science Leadership
   Theory
Management
Stewardship

Leadership is a word that is often used, has tremendous appeal, and evokes images of greatness. When people are asked to think about individuals who have demonstrated leadership, there is likely to be agreement about individuals like Martin Luther King, Jr., Mother Teresa, Gandhi, Jesus Christ, Eleanor Roosevelt, and even Florence Nightingale. But agreement is less likely about individuals such as Adolf Hitler, Richard Nixon, Candy Lightner, and Curtis Sliwa. Agreement is even less likely when we talk about the mother who, as a member of a local PTA, led the fight to increase parents' opportunities to meet with the school board when decisions affecting their children's health and well-being are made; or about the college-age student who spearheaded the establishment of a center for multiculturalism on a relatively homogeneous campus; or about the staff nurse who mobilized her colleagues to change the governance structure on their unit. Many may see these latter people as change agents, but would they think of this mother, student, or nurse as a leader? Would the public put this mother, student, or nurse in the same category—leader—as they would put Abraham Lincoln? Perhaps not. Yet this mother, this student, and this nurse are leaders and should be thought of in that way.

Regardless of whether the name is known worldwide, in a particular region or circle of influence, or only in a local community, those who know these individuals are likely to agree that these people illustrated leadership. In other words, we know leadership when we see it. But when we try to define, describe, and explain it to someone else, it becomes more nebulous.

What is it about certain individuals that prompt others to perceive them as leaders? What is it about their character, their style, their manner of interacting with others, or the goals toward which they were striving that makes them leaders? What is it that sets them apart from ordinary citizens, politicians, and managers?

In this chapter, we explore the nature of leadership. We examine some of the hundreds of definitions of the phenomenon, explore selected leadership theories and leadership styles, analyze the concept of transformational leadership, look at leader-follower relations, analyze various components of leadership, and discuss the kind of leadership that is needed, particularly by professional nurses in the 21st century. We assert that each of us has the potential to exercise leadership in our workplaces, professional organizations, and communities.

DEFINITIONS OF LEADERSHIP

The concept of leadership has been studied extensively. As Bass (1990) notes, "There are almost as many different definitions of leadership as there are persons who have attempted to define the concept" (p. 11). Leadership has been conceptualized as a set of traits, a role that needs to be played in any group, a particular position, an art, the exercise of influence, a form of persuasion, a power relation, and a way to attain goals (Bass, 1990). After analyzing 100 years of leadership research, VanFleet and Yukl (1989) concluded, "Where once we thought of leadership as a relatively simple construct, we now recognize that it is among the more complex social phenomena" (p. 66) in our world. Bennis and Nanus (1985) spoke to the complexity of leadership and how little we truly understand about it when they wrote:

> Decades of academic analysis have given us more than 350 definitions of leadership. Literally thousands of empirical investigations of leaders have been conducted in the last seventy-five years alone, but no clear and unequivocal understanding exists as to what distinguishes leaders from nonleaders, and perhaps more important, what distinguishes effective leaders from ineffective leaders. (p. 4)

In a critique of leadership studies undertaken over the years, Rost (1991) suggested that perhaps the reason we know so little about this phenomenon, even after so much analysis, is that these studies have missed the "essential nature of what leadership is [and] the process whereby leaders and followers relate to one another to achieve a purpose" (p. 4). Indeed, many of the studies of leadership have focused more on management styles or the person of the leader and ignored or minimized the role of followers in the equation, or the interactions among the leader, the followers, and the vision or goal at hand. Because of the increasingly complex nature of our world, any exploration of leadership for the 21st century must attend to this interrelationship and interdependence.

Although it is true that leaders "cause ripples," "rock the boat," "disturb the status quo," and take risks, they are effective as leaders only when those ripples inspire others to take action, make change, and realize goals. But because leadership is more an art than a science, there is no single or simple way to go about inspiring others; instead, the leader needs to use a number of styles to mobilize a group to achieve great things.

LEADERSHIP STYLES

Style can be thought of as the way in which something is done or said or as a particular form of behavior associated with an individual. **Leadership style** can be viewed as a set of behaviors that characterize individuals as they perform their leader role. These styles differ in terms of how power is distributed among those leading and those following, how decisions are made, and whose needs are of primary concern.

Factors Influencing Style

One's style reflects forces within oneself, the group, and the situation. Forces within the leader include her or his value system (as influenced by culture, background, and family context), expectations of self and others, prior experiences in a leadership role, self-confidence, and tolerance for ambiguity and uncertainty. Forces within members of the group include their need for independence, readiness for responsibility, commitment to a common goal, expectations about sharing in decision-making, and ability to deal with the group task. These "forces" often are influenced by the culture and background of the followers, factors that must be taken into consideration when one examines leader and follower behaviors and discusses leadership styles.

Style is also determined by forces within the situation itself. These forces include the traditions and values of the organization, its size and structure, the nature of the task at hand, the time available to accomplish a goal, and the history of the relationships among members of the group.

Types of Leadership Styles

Depending on the mix of these factors, one's style can range from highly structured (or authoritative), to moderately structured (or participative), to minimally structured (or permissive). **Authoritative leaders** maintain strong control over the people in the group, give orders and expect others to obey, dominate the group, and motivate others with fear or rewards. With this style, work often proceeds smoothly, productivity is often high, and procedures are usually well defined; however, creativity, autonomy, and self-motivation are stifled, and the needs of group members go unrecognized.

Laissez-faire or permissive leaders use a nondirective style. In addition, they are generally inactive and passive. In fact, one may question whether they are leaders at all because they do not work actively to move the group forward. With this style, group members have a great deal of freedom and self-control. However, group members can become disinterested and apathetic, goals may remain unclear, group members receive little or no feedback on their contributions, and often there is confusion about the procedures that guide the work of the group. This style of leadership results in group activity that is usually unproductive, inefficient, and unsatisfying for group members.

Perhaps the most effective style is that practiced by **democratic or participative leaders**. Democratic leaders talk about "we" rather than "I," ask stimulating questions, make suggestions rather than issue commands, provide constructive criticism, and are egalitarian. The participative leader has confidence in the ability of the group members and actively stimulates and guides them to use their abilities to achieve the group's goals. In this situation, the leader and the followers are mutually responsive, communication is multidirectional, and any member of the group is expected to assume the role of leader as the situation requires (Box 11–1).

Situational details also affect the type of leadership style that is most appropriate. In times of crisis, an authoritarian style may be the most appropriate one for a leader to use. On the other hand, when there is no time pressure to complete a task and the group is a mature one, the permissive style may be most effective. Finally, when one is working to implement changes in a system, using the participative style is apt to yield the best results. Keys to effective leadership are:

- Using the style most appropriate to the group and the task or situation at hand
- Using it at the right time

- Being flexible enough to attend to the needs of the followers
- Using the talents of all group members
- Meeting the goals of the group

The participative approach to leadership reflects some of the more current theories of leadership.

THEORIES OF LEADERSHIP

Several theories of leadership have been advanced over the years. Each of these theories reflected the thinking of the time, and each has some value in helping us consider the complex nature of leadership. As we realize the limitations of each theory, we are building a new foundation to continually strive to understand the phenomenon of leadership.

Great Man Leadership Theory

One of the earliest theories of leadership was the **"great man" leadership theory**, which asserted that the individual who is born into the proper class and circumstance is the one to lead the people. This theory, which was consistent with rule by monarchs, lacks rele-

---

BOX 11–1
LEADERSHIP STYLES

These different leadership styles are illustrated beautifully in the novel *Watership Down* (Adams, 1972). This is a story of a group of rabbits that, at the urging and insistence of one member, risk leaving their familiar warren to find a safer place to live. The "leader" of the rabbits' warren of origin is authoritarian in his style; he does not listen to advice, is very efficient, is closed to new ideas, does not adapt to new situations, and is unaware of or not concerned about the needs of the followers. Along the way, the rabbits encounter a warren with a totalitarian regime and another warren that has no "chief rabbit." In the latter warren, everyone does whatever he or she wants to do, there is no common goal, and the entire warren is rather passive, with little joy evident. Finally, in the community created by the rabbits that left their warren of origin and took the journey described in this book, the unique gifts of each member are recognized and used fully, and the group works together toward common goals. In addition, the leader of this group of rabbits seeks advice from others and encourages initiative, a sense of trust exists among members of the community, and all group members feel that they own the decisions that are made because they are involved in making those decisions. There are many lessons about leadership to be learned from this classic children's story.

vance for more current, complex, democratic societies.

Traitist Leadership Theories

In an attempt to acknowledge that individuals born outside a royal lineage also provided leadership, theories were developed to outline the ideal mix of traits or characteristics that make the most effective leader—**traitist leadership theories**. Traits such as height, energy level, socioeconomic status, level of education, gender, decisiveness, and articulateness were related to effectiveness in a leader and offered some useful insights. Despite extensive research within this theoretical framework, however, no single mix of traits emerged to predict, determine, or ensure who would be the best leader in a certain situation. In essence, these theories failed to acknowledge the role of the followers, the situation, and the task at hand in determining leader effectiveness, and they also have been shown to be of little help in understanding leadership in our ever-changing, unpredictable world.

Situational Leadership Theory

Situational theories (like the one proposed by Hersey and Blanchard, 1977) clearly recognized the significance of the environment or situation as a factor in the effectiveness of a leader. They asserted that the leader was the one who was in a position to initiate change when a situation was ready for change. In addition, **situational leadership theories** acknowledged that leadership is a dynamic process that involves an interplay among (1) the personalities and maturity levels of the leader and followers, (2) the task to be accomplished, (3) the goals to be attained, and (4) the conditions within the environment.

Transformational Leadership Theory

Perhaps one of the most contemporary leadership theories is **transformational leadership theory** (Barker, 1990, 1991; Barker & Young, 1994; Marriner-Tomey, 1993). This theory asserts that leadership is longer-lasting and more far-reaching than had been thought previously. With this type of leadership, the leader engages the full person of each follower and transforms each to move beyond individual needs and interests toward higher-level concerns. The leader raises the consciousness of the followers, heightens their aspirations, and intimately involves them in determining the course of action for the group. The transformational leader operates out of a deeply held personal value system, is visionary, has strong convictions, and interacts significantly with followers to see that the vision is realized.

Leadership Tasks Theory

Among the more recent and scholarly approaches to explaining the universal, multidimensional, and complex phenomenon known as leadership is the work of John Gardner, a noted expert in the field. Gardner (1990) proposed the **leadership tasks theory**, which embodies the components of effective leadership. He asserts that individuals who consistently engage in tasks of leadership are exercising true leadership and should be recognized for their contributions to their organizations, professions, and communities. These tasks are discussed in detail later.

New Science Leadership Theory

Consistent with the interactive concepts inherent in transformational leadership theory and leadership tasks theory is what is referred to as **new science leadership theory**. This theory, proposed initially by Wheatley (1992, 1999), asserts that to understand leadership and to function as effective leaders, we must focus on relationships, connections, and holism. We also must appreciate the value of chaos and unpredictability in our world, because chaos helps us create systems that are flexible, accepting of change, attentive to the values of all members, without boundaries, constantly growing and evolving, self-renewing, and organic. Wheatley's ideas are gaining support as individuals examine ways to make organizations increasingly effective and the work of individuals in those organizations increasingly meaningful.

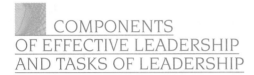

COMPONENTS OF EFFECTIVE LEADERSHIP AND TASKS OF LEADERSHIP

Because his is one of the newer theories of leadership and because it provides a framework for thinking about what leaders do, we will use Gardner's (1990) leadership tasks theory to address components of effective leadership. Each of Gardner's tasks is explained and related to the practice of professional nursing as a way to illustrate how nurses can and do provide leadership in their organizations, professional associations, and communities.

Envisioning Goals

One of the most significant tasks of leadership is envisioning new goals and possibilities. In fact, leaders are often distinguished from non-

leaders by their ability to see a different future, articulate their vision, communicate it to others in such a way that it is accepted by others, and energize others to invest the energy needed to realize the vision and create the desired future.

Does it take special training or mystical insight to envision goals? Is this a leadership task reserved for only a few elite individuals? Of course not. Each and every one of us—if we care enough about our jobs, our professions, and our communities—has some idea of how things could be done better or how "our little corner of the world" could be a better place. The leader, however, is the person who does something with or about that dream. This is the leadership task of envisioning goals. Consider the example in Box 11–2 illustrating this point.

Affirming Values

All groups and organizations are characterized by a set of values that may be clearly stated or may be inferred from the observed behaviors of members of the group. Those values may include such things as family-centered care, helping others develop to their fullest potential, and making the largest profit possible.

BOX 11–2
ENVISIONING GOALS

Several RNs are working in a community health center that provides care to a poor, underserved, multicultural population. They frequently comment to one another how discouraging it is to see women have to return to the center several times before they have all their family's health needs—such as immunizations, dental care, gynecologic examinations, vision screenings, and hypertension management—addressed. These nurses also recognize that after a while the women fail to keep appointments because it is too difficult to get back and forth to the center.

Although most of these nurses are well aware of the problem and acknowledge the serious implications of it, only one nurse begins to talk about a new approach to making appointments and scheduling visits. She envisions a "one-stop shopping" arrangement whereby the family can come to the center on one day and everyone's needs can be addressed. This nurse begins to talk about this idea to the other nurses, her supervisor, and the center's director. She develops a proposal of describing it can work; and she is willing to spearhead the effort to change the appointment scheduling process. This nurse has envisioned a goal and exercised leadership.

The individuals who run organizations assume that members of the group accept the organization's values and act in concert with them.

It is all too clear, however, that explicitly stated values, such as providing individualized, high-quality care or respecting the dignity and worth of all individuals, often conflict with the values inferred from approved policies and ongoing practices, such as a drastic reduction in the size of the professional staff. The nurse who exercises leadership serves to remind group members of the values they share, as Box 11–3 illustrates.

As Gardner (1990) notes, "Values always decay over time, however, groups that keep their values alive do so not by escaping the processes of decay but by powerful processes of regeneration" (p. 13). Leaders, such as the nurse described in Box 11–3, initiate and help sustain those processes of regeneration when they fulfill the task of leadership known as affirming values.

Motivating

Although it is critical that a leader envision new goals and help a group affirm the values underlying its existence, those tasks alone will not help organizations progress. A leader is nothing without followers, and if individuals are not motivated to choose to follow a leader, then little forward movement takes place. A leader cannot "go it alone." Thus, another important task of leadership is motivating others.

As individuals, we are motivated by internal forces, such as the desire to learn and grow and the satisfaction of knowing we did the very best we could in a situation, regardless of the outcome. We also are motivated by external forces, such as the praise we might receive from someone else, good grades, and a promotion. Both sources of motivation are valid, and both are important. It is the task of leadership to "unlock or channel" (Gardner, 1990, p. 14) the motives that drive individuals so that they can work to their fullest potential and help the group achieve its goals.

This concept is illustrated in Box 11–4. The nurse manager in this situation was most effective in getting staff to participate in activities that added new skills and new responsibilities even though they already felt overworked. Her use of incentives served to motivate the staff to learn this advanced and time-consuming skill, and they eventually became recognized as experts in the institution, serving to motivate them even further. The person who acts to inspire, encourage,

---

BOX 11–3
AFFIRMING VALUES

Nurses working in the local long-term care facility have always prided themselves on the caring environment they provide for residents and families. Elderly residents are respected, treated with dignity, and involved in their own care as much as possible. However, in recent months, one nurse has noticed that she and her colleagues seem to be spending more time complaining about their workloads, criticizing management, and "cutting corners" in their interactions with residents and families as a way to deal with the increased stresses they are feeling.

Rather than continuing to allow herself to be pulled in this direction, one nurse begins to reflect on why she has chosen to work in this kind of setting and what she finds rewarding about caring for the elderly. She then thinks about what is missing and how some of those basic values of respect and dignity seem to have eroded recently. This nurse exercises leadership when she begins to talk to her colleagues about what values they share that are related to caring for the elderly and how they can refocus their behaviors to reestablish that kind of commitment.

> **BOX 11–4**
> **MOTIVATING**
>
> In the last 3 months, the Intravenous Therapy Department at the local community hospital has been decentralized. This means that staff nurses will have to be educated and responsible for starting their own patients' peripheral lines. Many of the nurses are already feeling overworked and are, in their own words, "not excited about having to do such a time-consuming skill that they did not yet feel confident doing." The nurse manager of one renal medical unit decides to provide an incentive—a complimentary continuing education unit offering on intravenous therapy management—for every nurse who enrolls in the educational program during the first phase of training. The manager further motivates the staff with a complimentary family pack movie pass at the local movie theater after the nurse has successfully started 20 intravenous lines.
>
> This nurse manager is quite creative in motivating the staff initially with tangible awards. Interestingly, since so many of the unit's nurses sign up for the first phase of IV Insertion Training, this unit's staff becomes recognized as Resource IV Starters for the rest of the hospital. Soon the staff is so motivated to be experts on intravenous insertion and management, that they start a hospital-wide committee for protocol development and are considered the experts.

and energize others is fulfilling an important task of leadership, namely, motivating.

Managing

Management is as much a part of effective leadership as the other tasks described, because if one cannot manage a situation to "make things happen," visions will not be realized, and motivated individuals will soon become frustrated. According to Gardner (1990), the managing task of leadership involves a number of dimensions:

- Planning and setting priorities
- Creating processes and structures that will allow a vision to be realized
- Providing resources, delegating, and coordinating the group's activities
- Making decisions, even difficult ones

We often think that managing functions are the responsibility only of the person who holds some administrative position in an organization. Such persons do need good management skills, but the individual who is providing leadership within a group—and who may not occupy any hierarchical position of authority—also must be able to plan,

organize, delegate, and so on. This is the managing task of leaders, as illustrated in Box 11–5.

Achieving a Workable Unity

There is no doubt that when a number of individuals come together in the context of complex organizations to face difficult challenges, conflict is likely to arise. That conflict can come from differences in values, miscommunication or lack of communication, uncertainty, incompatible demands placed on individuals, competition for scarce resources, poorly defined responsibilities, change, and normal human drives for success, power, and recognition. Indeed, there is rarely only one source of conflict. Traditionally, conflict has been viewed as bad and something to be avoided at any cost. In the past, the emphasis had been on resolving or getting rid of conflict. Contemporary perspectives on conflict, however, acknowledge that it can be healthy. Because moderate amounts of conflict serve as an incentive to develop, excel, change, and grow, a task of the leader is to manage conflict but not necessarily resolve it. In other words, instead of trying to eliminate conflict alto-

> **BOX 11–5**
> **MANAGING**
>
> Several weeks ago, the staff on the oncology unit decided they wanted to implement self-staffing, and the nurse manager of the unit agreed that they should pursue the idea. The nurses were excited about this new opportunity, and the nurse manager was pleased with the initiative shown by the staff. However, since the time this decision was made, no progress has occurred toward implementing this new model. Staff members thought that the nurse manager would guide them in making this change, and the nurse manager assumed that, because the idea came from and is enthusiastically endorsed by the staff, the nurses themselves are working on a plan to "make it happen."
>
> As time goes by, some nurses become discouraged, and they convince themselves that the idea was not a good one after all. Other nurses become angry with the nurse manager, thinking she is "dragging her feet" in an attempt to sabotage the new model. Still others sit passively by, waiting for the nurse manager to tell the staff what to do and when and how to do it. But one nurse realizes that if the group is to do its own staffing, several steps must be taken to make that happen.
>
> This nurse asks the hospital librarian to gather a few recent articles on self-staffing projects that have been implemented elsewhere, and she reviews the notes on change from the leadership/management course she took while in school. She then thinks about the steps that needed to be taken on the unit and at higher levels of the hospital before their dream can become a reality. Finally, she reflects on her own talents and those of her colleagues in an attempt to match everyone's strengths with the tasks that need to be done. She then writes all this up as a two-page "proposal," asks the nurse manager for time on the agenda of the next staff meeting to discuss it, presents the proposal to the group as a starting point, and succeeds in getting the group to implement self-staffing within the next 2 months. As a result of fulfilling the managing task of leadership, this nurse emerges as a leader and helps her peers reach a much-desired goal.

gether, the effective leader works to ensure that the normal conflict that exists in most situations serves to stimulate ideas and new perspectives but does not escalate to a point at which members of the group become immobilized or unproductive.

One of the important tasks of leadership, therefore, is to serve as a unifying force within the group to achieve "some measure of cohesion and mutual tolerance" (Gardner, 1990, p. 16), so that the group can move forward to achieve its goals. The leader needs to try to minimize polarization and the formation of cliques by building teams and creating a sense of community among the group. The example in Box 11–6 illustrates how a nurse can fulfill the leadership task of achieving a workable unity.

Explaining

If individuals opt to follow a leader and work with that leader to achieve a goal or realize a vision, they need to understand what the goal is, what is being expected of them, and why they are being asked to do certain things. An important task of leadership, therefore, is explaining things to followers, teaching them, and being sure they are making an informed choice to follow in the first place.

The nurse described in the situation illustrated in Box 11–7 fulfills this task of leadership in an effective way. This nurse manager explained, taught, and supported his staff. He anticipated their needs and planned, in advance, to meet them or minimize their potentially negative effect. In essence, he

> **BOX 11–6**
> **ACHIEVING A WORKABLE UNITY**
>
> Two years ago, the local medical center merged with two other acute care institutions and downsized its staff. Many of the clinical nurse specialist positions were eliminated, experienced nurses were transferred out of the in-patient setting or resigned because of the poor staffing, and units were staffed heavily with unlicensed assistive personnel. During the last 6 months, the medical center has begun hiring nurses, most of whom are relatively new graduates. On one unit, there is much unrest among staff, and there seems to be little effort among staff to work collaboratively or to support and encourage one another.
>
> One seasoned nurse, who has experienced major changes many times in the past, is troubled by the lack of cooperation among her nursing peer group. She notices that nurses are unwilling to help one another, rarely comfort one another when someone had a particularly difficult patient assignment, are quick to point out one another's faults, and seem to make more of an effort to build alliances with physicians than with their fellow nurses. All of these, she concludes, are signs of the lack of unity and cohesion on the unit. She is concerned that, not only are the nurses dissatisfied with the work they are doing but also patient care might eventually suffer. Thus, she decides to try to do something to coalesce the group.
>
> This nurse makes an effort to compliment her colleagues on the work they are doing. She makes a point to ask others for advice and suggestions on different patient situations, even though she is quite able to manage those situations on her own. She invites a colleague to lunch and takes time to reflect on why she went into nursing and what keeps her excited about her job. She muses about the many times throughout her career when the autonomy and practice of nurses were threatened, how the nurses always thought that the immediate crisis was going to be the one to sound their demise, and how the resilient nurses always came through stronger than ever.
>
> This nurse also talks with the nurse manager about ways she can keep the staff better informed. She asks the nurse manager to allow time on a staff meeting agenda for discussion of concerns and to consider contacting the advanced practice psychiatric nurse to meet with the staff. Finally, she agrees to be the first to talk at the staff meeting about the very real fears and concerns experienced by the nurses, thereby taking the risk of speaking up, a risk she thinks her colleagues might not be willing to take. As a result of these small but focused actions by this nurse, the nurses on the unit start to open up to one another, work together more as a unit, and support one another—through discussion, humor, and other means. In addition, some of the more seasoned nurses begin to mentor the less experienced ones.

exercised effective leadership in relation to the specific task of explaining. As Gardner (1990) notes, "Leaders teach. ... Teaching and leading are distinguishable occupations, but every great leader is clearly teaching—and every great teacher is leading" (p. 18).

Serving as a Symbol

One of the most significant roles leaders play and one of the most important tasks they per-form is serving as a symbol for the group they lead. In other words, when those outside the group observe, listen to, and interact with the leader, they see, hear, and experience all that the group is attempting to do or be. For example, Martin Luther King, Jr., preached nonviolence, and he acted in a nonviolent way when confronted with charges and challenges from others. Jesus Christ had a vision of a world in which people loved and respected their fellow human beings regardless of who they were or how much or little they

> **BOX 11–7**
> **EXPLAINING**
>
> After extensive study and consultation, the nursing management team of the nearby rehabilitation center decides to institute computerized bedside charting throughout the institution within the next 6 months. The system has been selected, the infrastructure has been laid, the hardware has been ordered, and all nurse managers have been trained in the new system. The management team has outlined a plan for implementation, on a unit-by-unit basis, that begins in 1 month and ends 5 months later. All nurse managers have been directed to plan to bring their staff members "up to speed," and the heads of all other departments (e.g., Pharmacy, Medicine, Physical Therapy) have been directed to do the same.
>
> Knowing that his unit will be among the first ones to go online, that many of his staff members are not convinced that computerized bedside charting is "the way to go," and that many are not comfortable with computers in general, the nurse manager of one unit formulates a plan to prepare his staff appropriately.
>
> First, he arranges for some nurses from his graduate program classes, who are in institutions that have recently implemented computerized charting, to meet with his staff to talk about what the experience was like for them and how they "survived" it. The nurse manager also gathers a few articles about computers and their use in health care, and he shares these with the staff. He gains approval for his staff to go to the local university school of nursing to practice patient care documentation in its computer lab and arranges schedules so they have the time to go. In addition, he plans time during several upcoming unit staff meetings to talk about the difficulty of dealing with change, the need for the new computer system, the benefits to patients and staff of such a system, and individuals' fears and concerns about their new responsibilities. Finally, he plans for ongoing resources and opportunities for the staff to raise questions, make suggestions, express fears, and receive support throughout the implementation process and until they feel comfortable with the new system.

had; he lived his life among the poor and persecuted, shared what he had with those in need, and held no king above any peasant. Likewise, Florence Nightingale asserted that a healthy environment was critical to the recovery and well-being of the soldiers wounded in battle, and whenever she had the opportunity to speak to health officials, supervise a hospital, or write about the care of the ill, she was consistent in her message.

No less can be expected of the nurse who is providing leadership in today's world. Consider the nurse who serves as a symbol described in Box 11–8. Serving as a symbol means reflecting the group's values and collective identity in whatever one says and does. Admittedly, this is a serious responsibility for a leader to assume, but it is one that will make him or her more effective in helping a group achieve its goal.

Representing the Group

A leader often must serve as the spokesperson for the group, argue on its behalf, and represent its wishes and desires to others. When we think of "representing a group," we may conjure up an image of the corporate chief executive officer or the President of the United States giving his or her "state of the union" address to an audience. This leadership task, however, occurs at all levels and in all types of areas, as Box 11–9 illustrates. The nurse described in this account is an excellent example of the task of leadership that Gardner (1990) refers to as representing the group. She exhibited that "distinctive characteristic of the ablest leaders [namely, that she did not] shrink from external representation. [She saw] the long-term needs and goals of [her] constituency in the broad-

BOX 11–8
SERVING AS A SYMBOL

Nurse educators teach students about the value of research, the need to base their practice on research findings, the importance of participating in professional organizations, and the significance of lifelong learning, among other things. Additionally, they expect students to internalize these values as they begin or pursue new directions in their professional nursing careers. How many of these educators, however, "practice what they preach" and serve as symbols of that kind of behavior?

Often the educator who is thought of as a leader by her students and her peers is the one who lives these values and integrates them into her teaching. The teacher who tells students about what she learned from a conference, the book she read, or the research presentation she heard is conveying to students that she, too, must continue to learn. By supporting her class presentations with research findings and helping students identify gaps in nursing knowledge and areas in need of further study, the nurse educator is not merely telling students how important research is, she is living that value. Finally, the nurse educator who continually revises the teaching strategies she uses because the latest pedagogic research has shown a certain strategy to be effective in facilitating student learning demonstrates to students how one's practice needs to change continually in response to new knowledge.

BOX 11–9
REPRESENTING THE GROUP

The nurses who worked in the outpatient clinics at the medical center feel they are spending more time on paperwork and clerical duties than on patient care. They are angry, frustrated, and feeling abused.

One nurse in this group—who shares the feelings of anger and frustration—begins to keep track of specific incidents that she and others experience rather than just the vague, general complaints that are often expressed. She also makes an effort to talk with her colleagues about what they think are ways to avoid negative incidents and use their professional expertise better. When she has collected a number of such ideas, she shares them with her peers to validate whether her accounts are accurate and fair. She then asks the group if they want her to speak with the clinic director about their concerns and their suggested solutions, and she asks for their commitment to invest the time and energy needed to make changes in how the work gets done if the clinic director challenges them with that charge.

With the support of her peers, this nurse makes an appointment with the clinic director, calmly and rationally presents specific complaints, offers reasonable and well-thought-out solutions to solving these problems, and suggests that the nursing staff prepare a more comprehensive proposal of ways to deal with these issues. The clinic director is so impressed by the nurse's approach and her ability to speak confidently on behalf of the entire group that he enthusiastically supports the efforts of the staff to explore operational changes that will use their expertise better.

est context, and [she acted] accordingly" (Gardner, 1990, p. 20).

Renewing

Perhaps most significantly, "leaders must foster the process of renewal" (Gardner, 1990, p. 21). They must constantly provide members of the group with new challenges, reinforce the importance of the goal toward which all are striving, encourage and help group members to reach their fullest potential, be willing to change the course of action when it no longer serves the intended purpose, and provide opportunities for members of the group to assume the role of leader. Such actions keep the group stimulated, excited, and energized.

An illustration from the perspective of involvement in professional organizations (Box 11–10) helps illustrate the process of renewal and its positive impact on a group and an entire organization. Although the process of renewal should be a continuous one to keep a group alive and healthy, leaders often must implement strategies to revitalize a group that has been allowed to stagnate, as

---

BOX 11–10
RENEWING

A staff nurse who works for the visiting nurse service that serves an inner-city community has recently been elected president of a local professional nursing organization. From her involvement in the organization to date, she has observed that in recent years, those who held office and served on committees repeated programs from previous years, "recycled" the same people from one position to another, and structured all meetings in the same way. Additionally, she notes that there has been little, if any, reflection on the purpose of the organization or discussion of where the organization wants to be in the next 5 to 10 years.

Because this nurse believes so strongly in the purposes of this organization and in the value of organizational work itself, she launches a personal campaign to revitalize the group during her term of office. She goes back to the organization's mission statement and bylaws to note what its stated purpose and goals are. She then asks her friends, work colleagues, and members of the organization to share their ideas about what those goals might suggest in terms of programs and activities they could sponsor in the current health care climate.

This nurse approaches some of the new graduates who are working at her agency, and she speaks to the faculty member who has students at the agency for clinical experiences. In each instance, she extends an invitation to them to come to the next meeting of the organization and to consider joining the organization and serving on a committee.

She then reflects on the kinds of health-care and patient care problems she sees in practice every day and reads about in newspapers and professional journals, and she looks at all the flyers posted on the bulletin boards at work announcing conferences, programs, and community projects. This gives her a whole repertoire of possible program topics, speakers, and brochure formats.

Armed with these ideas, she approaches the executive committee of the organization and presents them with a variety of ways to revitalize themselves. She makes sure to acknowledge how the expertise of those on the executive committee matches some of the ideas suggested, recognize the valuable contributions made by members over the years, ensure the group that it does not have to take on many new things all at once, and commits her time and resources to work with others to "make it happen."

was the case here. Once that renewal starts, however, the task of leadership may become keeping the energy focused and reasonably controlled.

Stewardship

Although Gardner (1990) does not include it among his tasks of leadership, a discussion of the concept of leadership would be incomplete without considering the leader's responsibility for sound **stewardship**. Stewardship involves serving others and advancing their best interests, rather than advancing one's own interests. Block (1993) describes stewardship as a desire and willingness to be accountable for the well-being of the overall group or organization by "operating in service to, rather [than] in control of, those around us" (p. xx). It comprises the following principles (Block, 1993, p. xxi):

* Power is balanced and everyone is involved in decision-making.
* The primary commitment is to the group, organization, or larger community, not to an individual's or small group's own "agenda."
* The organizational culture and overall vision are defined by everyone, not by a select few.
* A more "balanced and equitable distribution of rewards" exists.

Thus, leaders have responsibility for keeping "the big picture," the good of the group or organization, and the ultimate goal or vision in mind. Leadership, in essence, is broadly focused and externally oriented.

NURSING LEADERSHIP IN THE 21ST CENTURY

It is obvious from this discussion of the tasks of leadership that leadership and management are not the same phenomenon. One hopes that an effective manager will also be a leader and carry out all nine of the tasks of leadership as well as be an effective steward, but this is not always the case. One should not assume that everyone in a position of authority—a nurse manager, the vice president for nursing, the dean of a school of nursing, and the president of a professional organization—is automatically a leader.

By the same token, and perhaps more significantly, leadership is not limited to those in positions of authority. Each of us has the potential to exhibit leadership at various points in our professional careers, regardless of our title, position, or academic credentials. The only barrier to our exercise of leadership is our own unwillingness to take on the challenge. There is no doubt that leadership is hard work; it takes time and sustained energy, and the rewards for those efforts often are not immediate. But if nurses and nursing are to assume the kind of position in the health-care delivery system of the 21st century that we deserve and can manage, each of us must be willing to take on the risk of being a leader.

> *Leadership is not limited to those in positions of authority. Each of us has the potential to exhibit leadership at various points in our professional careers, regardless of our title, position, or academic credentials.*

Leaders must be aware of the four kinds of futures (Valiga, 1994) that are available to each of us. The *probable future* is what is likely to happen if current situations and directions remain unchanged. For example, it is quite probable that there will continue to be concern primarily for the "bottom line," with only "lip service" given to concerns for quality care. The *possible future* refers to what might happen with only minimal changes. For example, it is possible that more and more unlicensed health-care workers will be created and used to provide direct care, and nurses will hold only oversight and coordinator positions, being minimally involved in the direct care of patients and families. The *plausible future* refers to what could occur if focused efforts are made to accomplish specific goals. For example, it is quite plausible that nurses will be expected to take the lead in interdisciplinary team efforts because of their holistic perspective on patient care. Finally, leaders must attend to—and, indeed, create—the *pre-*

ferred future, the state of affairs we want to exist. For instance, nurses should be significant participants in shaping health care policy to ensure that quality patient and family care takes priority over cost containment and that nurses hold positions of influence in designing that care.

Nursing leaders in the 21st century will have to create our preferred future. In order to do this, they will need a clear vision of what will best serve the profession and the individuals, families, and communities for whom nurses care. They must be proactive, fight for excellence, and be unwilling to accept mediocrity. They must be flexible, willing to change, and able to deal with uncertainty and ambiguity in order to prevent blind-sided reactions to change (Clampitt & DeKoch, 2001).

The nurses we will look to for leadership in the 21st century must be self-assured and self-confident but always open to new ideas and interested in growth and self-improvement. They must be collegial in their interactions with other nurses; acknowledge the strengths, capabilities, and achievements of others; men-

tor others; and help others take advantage of opportunities to facilitate their own growth. If nursing is to be a powerful force in health care in the 21st century, we will need leaders who are articulate, whose actions are consistent with their words, who are competent and credible, and who can work collaboratively within an interdisciplinary team. Leaders will be needed who are visionary, can ignite followers to join in the effort to turn visions into realities, and can sustain and continually challenge a group as it strives to implement change and face the challenges presented along the way.

Such leaders now exist among our students, staff nurses, professional association staff, nurse educators, nurse administrators, nurse scientists, and nurse entrepreneurs. Each of us must incorporate the tasks of leadership into our professional practice repertoire and perform those tasks as needed (Grossman & Valiga, 2000). This kind of behavior on the part of many nurses will ensure the profession's strong future, and nursing will be a significant player in the health-care arena of the 21st century.

Key Points

- Leadership is not the same as management, nor is it tied to a position of authority. Leadership is more an art than a science.
- The relationship between leaders and followers is interactive and mutually beneficial.
- Keys to effective leadership include the use of the appropriate style at a particular time and flexibility to attend to the needs of the followers, use the talents of the group members, and meet the goals of the group.
- Leadership style can be viewed as a set of behaviors that characterize individuals as they perform their leader role. These styles differ in terms of how power is distributed among those leading and those following, how decisions are made, and whose needs are of primary concern.
- There is no single widely accepted definition or theory of leadership.
- Leaders "cause ripples," "rock the boat," "disturb the status quo," and take risks.
- Leaders are visionary. They envision goals and possibilities.
- Leaders help members of a group reflect on their shared vision when they fulfill the leadership task known as affirming values.
- Leaders motivate others to work toward group goals. Motivation includes attending to both internal and external forces that drive individuals to achieve their fullest potential and help a group accomplish its goals.

(continued)

(continued)

- Leadership involves managing situations to achieve goals: planning carefully, using creative processes, providing resources, and making decisions.
- Leaders help a group coalesce as a unified whole so that it can move forward to achieve its goals.
- Effective leaders teach and explain so that followers can make informed choices.
- Leaders serve as symbols and spokespersons for a group by reflecting the group's values and collective identity and by representing the group.
- The effective leader exercises good stewardship, a combination of accountability and partnership that best serves the clients (patients), the group, and the profession.
- A group or organization must constantly be renewed to remain viable and strong.
- The role of the follower is critical, for without followers there can be no leaders.

Thought and Discussion Questions

1. Read the children's story *The Little Engine that Could* (Piper, 1961), or Rudyard Kipling's poem "If." How does the little engine or "being a man" relate to leadership and the challenges inherent in the role of leader?
2. Review the Chapter Thought located on the first page of the chapter, and be prepared to discuss its meaning in the context of the contents of this chapter.

Interactive Exercises

1. Think about a nurse in your workplace whom you think of as a leader. What do you think makes that person a leader? How does that individual carry out each of Gardner's tasks of leadership and function as a good steward? Use the Interactive Exercise on the Intranet site entitled Nursing Leaders to consider this leader's specific style and traits.
2. Read about or watch a documentary about someone in history who is often thought of as a leader. What did that person do to prompt us to affix the label "leader" to him or her? Fill in the Interactive Exercise on the Intranet entitled Actions of a Leader.
3. Using Gardner's nine tasks of leadership and the concept of stewardship, think about how well you "measure up." For those areas you see as strengths, what could you do to reinforce them? For those areas you think are not as well developed, what specific strategies could you employ to enhance your leadership abilities? Complete the Leadership Self-Assessment located in the Interactive Exercises section of the Intranet site.
4. Either in your work setting or as a student in the clinical setting, choose three consecutive days/shifts and write your observations of how nurses and other health care providers make decisions. Identify the decision, and classify it as client-centered or workplace-centered. Describe the outcomes of the decision and whether they were positive or negative. Offer some recommendations

regarding how the process by which the decision was made could be improved. Complete the two-part Decision-Making Journal located in the Interactive Exercises section of the Intranet site.

5. What do you see as the probable, possible, plausible, and preferred futures at your place of employment or in your student clinical experience? Be sure to include the roles of the nurse and other health-care providers, the role of the patient/client and family, and the nature of the health-care system itself. Complete the Interactive Exercise on the Intranet site entitled Probable Possible Plausible Preferred Futures.

6. Go to the Keirsey Web site (http://www.keirsey.com) and read about "The Four Temperaments" and their relationship to leading. Complete the Keirsey Temperament Sorter II test as a way to learn more about yourself. What patterns do you notice in your temperament? What kind of impact does or could this have on your role as a leader and in your performing the tasks of leadership? How might your temperament affect the way in which others respond to you, whether they would choose to follow you, and so on?

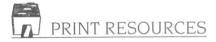
PRINT RESOURCES

References

Adams, R. (1972). *Watership down.* New York: Avon.

Barker, A. M. (1991). An emerging leadership paradigm: Transformational leadership. *Nursing & Health Care,* 12(4), 204–207.

Barker, A. M. (1990). *Transformational nursing leadership: A vision for the future.* Baltimore: Williams & Wilkins.

Barker, A. M., & Young, C. E. (1994). Transformational leadership: The feminist connection in postmodern organizations. *Holistic Nursing Practice,* 9(1), 16–17.

Bass, B. M. (1990). *Bass & Stogdill's handbook of leadership: Theory, research, and managerial applications* (3rd ed.). New York: The Free Press.

Bennis, W., & Nanus, B. (1985). *Leaders: The strategies for taking charge.* New York: Harper & Row.

Block, P. (1993). *Stewardship: Choosing service over self-interest.* San Francisco: Berrett-Koehler.

Clampitt, P. G., & DeKoch, R. J. (2001). *Embracing uncertainty: The essence of leadership.* Armonk, NY: M. E. Sharpe.

Gardner, J. W. (1990). *On leadership.* New York: The Free Press.

Grossman, S., & Valiga, T. M. (2000). *The new leadership challenge: Creating a preferred future for nursing.* Philadelphia: F.A. Davis.

Hersey, P., & Blanchard, K. (1977). *Management of organizational behavior: Utilizing human resources* (3rd ed.). Englewood Cliffs, NJ: Prentice-Hall.

Marriner-Tomey, A. (1993). *Transformational leadership in nursing.* St. Louis: Mosby.

Piper, W. (1961). *The little engine that could.* New York: Platt & Munk.

Rost, J. C. (1991). *Leadership for the twenty-first century.* Westport, CT: Praeger.

Valiga, T. M. (1994). Leadership for the future. *Holistic Nursing Practice,* 9(1), 83–90.

Van Fleet, D. D., & Yukl, G. A. (1989). A century of leadership research. In W. E. Rosenbach & R. L. Taylor (Eds.), *Contemporary issues in leadership* (2nd ed., pp. 65–94). Boulder, CO: Westview Press.

Wheatley, M. J. (1992). *Leadership and the new science: Learning about organizations from an orderly universe.* San Francisco: Berrett-Koehler.

Wheatley, M. J. (1999). *Leadership and the new science: Discovering order in a chaotic world* (2nd ed.). San Fransicso: Berrett-Koehler.

Bibliography

Bennis, W. (1989). *On becoming a leader.* Reading, MA: Addison-Wesley.

Bennis, W., Spreitzer, G. M., & Cummings, T. G. (Eds.). (2001). *The future of leadership: Today's top leadership thinkers speak to tomorrow's leaders.* San Francisco: Jossey-Bass.

Boman, L., & Deal, T. (1995). *Leading with soul: An uncommon journal of the spirit.* San Francisco: Jossey-Bass

Bruderle, E. R. (1994). The arts and humanities: A creative approach to developing nurse leaders. *Holistic Nursing Practice,* 9(1), 68–74.

Burns, J. M. (1978). *Leadership.* New York: Harper Torchbooks.

Cassidy, V. R., & Kroll, C. J. (1994). Ethical aspects of transformational leadership. *Holistic Nursing Practice,* 9(1), 41–47.

DePree, M. (1989). *Leadership is an art.* New York: Dell Publishing.

DiRienzo, S. M. (1994). A challenge to nursing: Promoting followers as well as leaders. *Holistic Nursing Practice,* 9(1), 26–30.

Greenleaf, R. K. (1977). *Servant leadership: A journey into the nature of legitimate power and greatness.* New York: Paulist Press.

Kelley, R. E. (1992). *The power of followership: How to create leaders people want to follow and followers who lead themselves.* New York: Doubleday Currency.

Koestenbaum, P. (2002). *Leadership: The inner side of greatness.* San Francisco: Jossey-Bass.

Kouzes, J. M., & Posner, B. Z. (2002). *Leadership challenge* (3rd ed.). San Francisco: Jossey-Bass.

Nanus, B. (1992). *Visionary leadership: Creating a compelling sense of direction for your organization.* San Francisco: Jossey-Bass.

Rosenbach, W. E., & Taylor, R. L. (Eds.). (1998). *Contemporary issues in leadership* (4th ed.). Boulder, CO: Westview Press.

Rost, J. C. (1994). Leadership: A new conception. *Holistic Nursing Practice,* 9(1), 1–8.

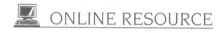 ONLINE RESOURCE

Keirsey, D. (1999, December 20). The four temperaments. http://www.keirsey.com/

Rose Kearney-Nunnery

12
chapter

Management in Organizations

> *Organizational goals and values must be translated, tranmitted, and reinforced throughout the system.*

Chapter Objectives

On completion of this chapter, the reader will be able to:

1. Apply systems theory to an organizational scenario.
2. Examine the structure, functions, goals, and culture of selected organizations.
3. Analyze factors included in motivational and humanistic management theories.
4. Examine the various managerial roles for and skills of nurses in a health-care organization.
5. Apply methods for appropriate and effective delegation in a health-care scenario.

Key Terms

Organization
Organizational
  Subsystems
Organizational Structure
Centralization
Decentralization
Flat Organizational
  Structures
Tall Organizational
  Structures

Organizational
  Functions
Management
Managerial Roles
Motivational Theories
Theory X
Theory Y
Hygiene Factors
Motivational Factors
Theory Z

Management-by-
  Objectives
Executive
Organizational
  Culture
Power
Negotiation
Delegation

253

Max Weber (1947), the renowned German sociologist, described an organization in economic and social terms as "a system of purposive activity of a specified kind" (p. 151). An **organization** is simply an arrangement of human and material resources for some purpose, as in the creation of some institution or agency to meet a stated aim. Organizations range from the single-purpose association to multipurpose, monolithic institutions. They have been studied for years in an effort to improve on outputs as the intended mission or purpose. Organizations can be viewed in terms of their structure, function, and people. Most simply, they can be envisioned as the open system described in Chapter 3, with inputs, throughput or transformations, and outputs. But understanding organizations, especially health-care organizations, becomes more complex as organizations expand, contract, and redefine themselves.

We examine how organizations are structured and how they are managed to meet their intended mission. In nursing, management in an organization must have a broad environmental, interpersonal, and dynamic vision, beyond patients and health-care providers with equipment in an isolated hospital or agency.

Principles of scientific management and management theory have undergone continued investigation and change. Many writers have defined management, but no one definition of management has been universally accepted. Grohar-Murray and DiCroce (2003) propose that management "is a process with both interpersonal and technical aspects through which the objectives of an organization (or part of it) are accomplished by efficiently and effectively using resources" (p. 150). Use of management theories and effective management skills are a critical component of professional practice. Communication, negotiation, and delegation are important factors, as are the leadership concepts described in the previous chapter. Applying these concepts of contemporary nursing practice is vital for the operation of a successful organization and an effective health-care system.

ORGANIZATIONAL THEORY: ORGANIZATIONS AS SYSTEMS

Systems theory provides a useful perspective for viewing the internal and external influences with any organization. In fact, Bertalanffy (1968), who provided the foundations of general system theory, stated that the only meaningful way to study an organization is as a system (p. 9). In nursing, Dienemann (1998) advocates the use of a systems model to understand organizations, emphasizing the structure of the work and people and the formal and informal interaction process among work and people (p. 269). She further suggests that for analysis and use in their organization, nursing administrators select from one of four models: open systems, organizational life cycle stages, organizational environments, and organizational participants. The actual selection of a particular systems model depends on the complexity and uniqueness of the organization. It requires careful assessment of the organization, examining mission and goals, present structure, and the prevailing leadership and management styles being used to guide practice and address organizational goals.

Health-care delivery systems are complex open environmental systems. The organization must be examined at the system level, with its component subsystems, as well as the macrosystem, which includes the client system as the consumer group. Agency administrative policy and operational structures internally influence and guide the system. The surrounding environmental system of the organization is the health-care arena that provides the professional, specialization, economic, and additional value structures for the organizational unit and its members. The broader social environment or macroenvironment reflects societal norms and values through the real and potential needs of health-care consumers. Direct or indirect linkages among all system parts are assumed to be essential for effectiveness and continuity. But look further at this complex system and the internal environment.

A useful perspective for viewing the intricacies of a health-care organization is to envision it as a system affected by other systems and within the larger health-care and societal systems (environmental suprasystem or macrosystem). Kast and Rosenzweig (1985) regard organizations as open, sociotechnical systems that structure and integrate human activities around various technologies (p. 113). This approach is particularly applicable to health-care organizations, with their focus on people and the dynamic influence of technology. The system in this model is further composed of five **organizational subsystems**: goals and values, technical, psychosocial, structural, and managerial (FIG. 12–1). The subsystems and their inherent internal forces can be described as follows.

Subsystems

Goals and values are implied in a statement of purpose or philosophy and are the basis of the organization's existence. The institutional mission statement and original or revised

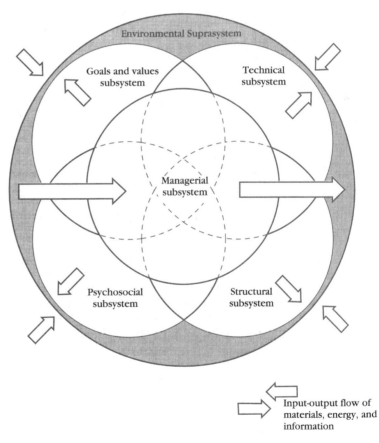

FIG. 12–1. The organizational system. (From Kast, F. E., & Rosenzweig, J. E. [1985]. *Organization and management: A systems and contingency approach* [4th ed.]. New York: McGraw-Hill, with permission.)

incorporation papers contain valuable information on how people within the organization are viewed, as customers, staff members, and administrators. Humanistic versus mechanistic values are apparent in these statements of mission, philosophy, and purpose.

The *technical subsystem* represents the knowledge and skills of the people providing service in the system as well as the physical resources. Specialized knowledge and the expertise of professional and nonprofessional labor forces are represented in this subsystem. Physical resources include operating and investment capital, equipment, information systems, services, and tangible assets.

The *psychosocial subsystem* contains the interpersonal and interdisciplinary relationships unique to the organization—role relationships, attitudes, and values of people and groups within the system. Examine the expected behaviors of each member of the organization and the interrelationships, in both formal and informal interactions. This subsystem can be further visualized as the organizational culture.

The *structural subsystem* is the institutional or agency design intended to accomplish the system's mission to provide the intended services. This structure may be complex or simple, centralized or decentralized, tall or flat. The structural subsystem also relates to the hierarchy or lines of authority, as demonstrated by the bureaucratic or organic structure. The system structure is described in formal documents and further interpreted in operation through informal sources, such as technical staff, to determine how tasks are actually accomplished in the organization.

The *managerial subsystem* is the management style pervasive in the organization. As seen later in this chapter, it may be directed from the topmost governing board or corporate officers downward, as in a bureaucratic organization operating under Theory X. Alternatively, it may be more flexible and participatory, as in Theory Z organizations.

External Environment

Once the subsystems are identifiable, move outward into the environmental layers of the open system, or the suprasystem. To understand the external environment, we must first reevaluate the organization's mission. As in any business, this provides us with market forces. Is a product being produced or a service being delivered, and to whom? Consider the differences between the environments of local organizations focused on a specific community and those of national or multinational conglomerates. To understand an organization's initial environmental layer, focus first on the immediate output of the system. Suppose we are looking at a home care agency. Such an agency provides home care within specific specialty parameters to an identified service area. In the environment, we initially have the local community with a specific geography, client population, health-care provider groups, payment streams, resources, and health-care needs. This local agency has additional environmental influences from state and federal regulatory bodies and agencies, professional disciplines, and the larger health-care system.

But consider these factors with a larger health-care agency, which offers more services to a larger clientele, such as a teaching hospital with a broader service menu and service area. We have to consider the geography, client population, health-care provider groups, payment streams, resources, and health-care needs across the state or perhaps across several states. Services may include not only acute and chronic care but also multispecialty clinics, research, and outreach programs. We have more care providers, including students, faculty, and visiting specialists from various health-care disciplines. There are more requirements and regulations from state and federal regulatory bodies and agencies and professional disciplines, just by virtue of the expanded services, funding streams, and service expectations. Coordination with the broader health-care system must also be considered, as people come from and return to their local areas.

In an open system, all boundary influences must be identified and relationships evaluated. All external layers and interrelating systems are important factors in a true understanding of the influences on any particular system. These environmental influences have repercussions on the system and its component subsystems. External forces include inputs of energy, information, materials, and the myriad technologies received from the environment, transformed and returned to the environment as outputs.

The health-care environment can easily be seen as highly complex, dynamic, and uncertain. Changes occur constantly. Change is influenced by consumers, technologic advances, government, and third-party payers. The external forces in the broader environment provide inputs into the system and affect internal operations and resultant outputs, such as client outcomes. Health-care organizations must respond to external forces in a rapid, dynamic, and innovative manner and cannot remain static. A humanistic philosophy, with its focus on the people in an organization who create, define, and fulfill organizational goals, is needed for a contemporary and innovative health-care organization. This brings us to an examination of the various structures of organizational systems.

ORGANIZATIONAL STRUCTURES

Mintzberg (1983b) has defined **organizational structure** as "the sum total of the ways in which its labor is divided into distinct tasks and then [how] coordination is achieved among these tasks" (p. 2). Generally, when we think of an organizational structure, we conceive of some type of hierarchy that tells us about positions or roles, responsibilities, status, channels of command or reporting relationships, and tasks to be accomplished. The picture that comes to mind is usually a bureaucratic structure with a multitude of "red tape" with which to contend. This is not always the case. The appropriateness of the structure depends on the organization's purposes (goals and values subsystem), the people in the organizational system (psychosocial subsystem), the skills and technology used or available (technical subsystem), how outcomes are best accomplished (managerial subsystem), and influences from the external environment(s). These system influences provide us with information on the size and complexity of the organization as the structural subsystem.

The structure demonstrates the relationships among an organization's components and presents us with its design. Looking at health-care organizations, we find two general structures: bureaucratic and organic. Mintzberg (1983b) places these two organizational designs at opposite ends of a continuum of standardization (FIG. 12–2). This range gives us a way of viewing organizational structures from the controlled, mechanistic, and standardized classic bureaucracy through a number of adaptations to the opposite extreme of a humanistic organization that contains no standardized processes, outputs, or skills across the structure. Health-care organizations generally fall somewhere between the two extremes, depending on their mission.

Bureaucratic Organizations

The most recognized and traditional organization is the bureaucratic structure. A bureaucracy is a mechanistic model focused on outcomes. Weber (1864–1920) provided the original bureaucratic model, with a high degree of efficiency and control. His work has been translated and interpreted frequently in research on organizations and organizational theory. Merton (1957) further defined a bureaucratic organization as "a formal, rationally organized social structure involving clearly defined patterns of activity in which, ideally, every series of actions is functionally related to the purposes of the organization" (p. 195). The bureaucratic organization has a

Bureaucratic Structure	Organic Structure
High standardization of processes, outputs, and skills	Absence of standardization

FIG. 12–2. Mintzberg's continuum of standardization in organizations. (Adapted from Mintzberg, H. [1983b]. *Structure in fives: Designing effective organizations.* Englewood Cliffs, NJ: Prentice-Hall.)

hierarchical structure with designated lines of authority and control. The mission of the organization is all-consuming. Actions to meet the purposes and directives are taken in lower layers, whereas policy-making, authority, and control reside primarily in the upper layers of the organization. Specific characteristics of a bureaucratic organization are as follows:

1. A clear-cut division of labor
2. Differentiated controls and sanctions
3. Roles assigned on the basis of qualifications and technical efficiency
4. Clearly stated rules and conformity to regulations
5. A premium placed on precision, speed, expert control, continuity, discretion, and optimal returns on input
6. Strict devotion to regulations
7. Depersonalized relationships (Merton, 1957, pp. 195–196)

Examples of bureaucratic health-care organizations are depicted in FIGS. 12–3 and 12–4. In these examples, management and control flow downward from the hospital board through the chief operating officer (COO) or chief executive officer (CEO), who is appointed by the board and is responsible for the organization's missions, whether for-profit or not-for-profit. To accomplish these aims, the executive layer is responsible to the COO or CEO. The executives receive mandates from the board through the COO or CEO and decide on priorities, plan implementation, and regulations. Executives, in turn, direct their administrative staffs, and on down the line. Each employee has a specific role in carrying out the organization's mission.

A bureaucratic organization is structured, standardized, controlled, and in many instances, authoritarian. Written and unwritten policies and regulations are prevalent, as are specified channels of command. Efficiency and effectiveness in achieving the organiza-

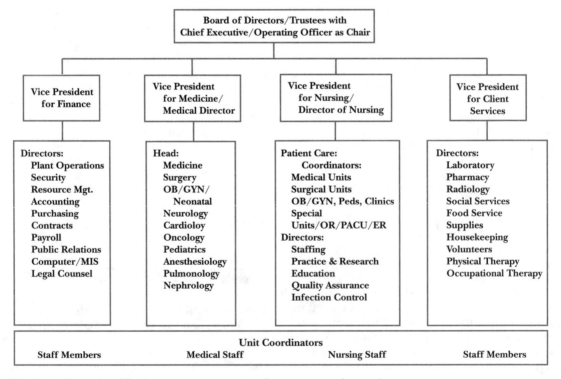

FIG. 12–3. Example of flat bureaucratic structure of a community hospital.

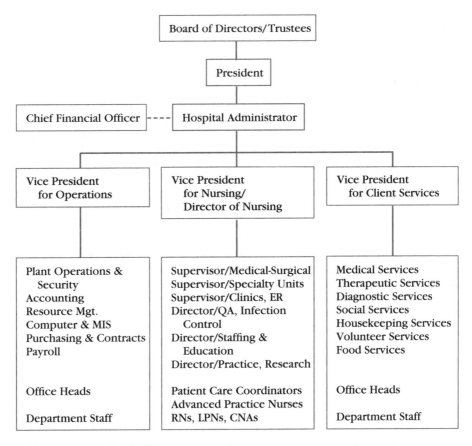

FIG. 12–4. Example of tall bureaucratic structure of a community hospital.

tional mission are organizational values. Bureaucratic organizational structures are seen in the older, traditional, and large authoritarian settings in which control and the ultimate mission of the institution are all-consuming. External influences should be predictable to obtain the most efficient functioning of the organization. Channels of command and productivity are important components of the system. But in recent years, a move toward more flexible and humanistic organizational structures, focusing on environmental influences along with employee involvement and job satisfaction for higher productivity, has led to a transformation to more innovative practices that are inconsistent with the bureaucratic design.

Organic Organizations

Organic organizational structures, or adhocracies, have evolved to meet the needs of organizations composed of humans in dynamic and sometimes complex environmental settings. The term *adhocracy* implies that the structure is a design that has been developed to meet the organizational mission and specific goals. Hall (1999) described adhocracies as dynamic organizations in which the environment is unknown and the structure can change dramatically as events demand adjustment (p. 40). These organizations represent a movement from the standardized, mechanistic bureaucracies to humanistic forms arising out of behavioral organizational research and management theories. Mintzberg (1983b) proposed that this structure is the most useful in a complex and dynamic environment in which experts, managers, and staff from different disciplines cooperate on decentralized project teams to meet a system output goal innovatively. Several organic designs are seen in health-care organizations. The most prevalent organic or adhocratic designs are functional, product, and matrix forms.

Functional Structure

A functional structure, like the bureaucracy, focuses on organizational outcomes; but unlike a bureaucracy, it has control and responsibility spread horizontally across the system to meet specific organizational functions. Daft (1998) notes that this structure is "most effective when the environment is stable and the technology is relatively routine with low interdependence across functional departments [and when] organizational goals pertain to internal efficiency and technology specialization" (p. 214). A functional form can therefore be used in an organization with a specific function, such as a rehabilitative facility. The function of the rehabilitative care across specialty lines is the organization's purpose. The people in the organization have the decision-making authority for their services in

the organization. Functional units are thus arranged in specialty areas, as illustrated in Figure 12–5.

The organization is designed to focus on the function of delivering rehabilitative care to the consumer. Two distinct functions are apparent in our example of this functional form, (1) finance and administration of the agency and (2) delivery of rehabilitative health care. An executive director or president oversees the organization with the assistance of two directors. The main organizational function of rehabilitative care delivery is structured as specialty units under the direction of the health-care director. Fragmentation and duplication of services across specialties limit this design. This limitation becomes more severe as the organization grows in size and complexity—for example, when services increase and the service area is enlarged. Daft (1998) has further described the disadvantages of the functional form as follows:

1. Has slow response time to environmental changes
2. May cause decisions to pile on top, hierarchy overload
3. Leads to poor horizontal coordination among departments
4. Results in less innovation
5. Involves a restricted view of the organizational goals (p. 215)

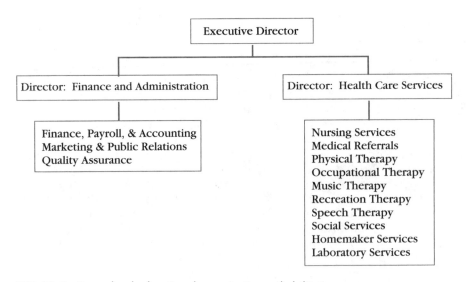

FIG. 12–5. Example of a functional organization: rehabilitative agency.

Product Structure

A product or divisional structure is similar to the functional structure except that the organization is focused on the product as the outcome, with people and processes being grouped accordingly. The goals of a product structure are external effectiveness, adaptation, and client satisfaction (Daft, 1998, p. 219). Consider the example of a large home care agency (FIG. 12–6). The product is home care services, with attention being given to the needs and desires of the home care client. The product units are organized in terms of nursing services, physical therapy, and speech therapy. Each unit has a director responsible to the president of the agency for the home care product. Vice presidents are responsible to the president for general functions of health-care referrals, contractual services, personnel, and marketing. Product units are thus arranged in specified areas (nursing, physical therapy, and speech therapy), with each being directed toward service coordination, referrals, contractual services, and marketing, to meet consumer needs.

The product structure works well with an organization whose services and marketing are directed at the consumer. This design is flexible in a dynamic or unstable environment, because consumer needs and satisfaction are of prime concern. Divisions are separated by product—nursing care, physical therapy, and speech therapy. But duplication of services is an immediate problem, especially in health-care, in which coordination of therapeutic regimens is vital for the consumer.

Matrix Structure

To address the need to coordinate consumer services, another adhocratic design combines the functional and product forms. Multidimensional decision-making and responsibility are the features of a matrix organization. In a health-care agency, this can refer to the product of state-of-the-art care and the function of provision of services to the client as the consumer. An example of the matrix design is an organization whose mission is directed at research and development and provision of care. Research managers in interdisciplinary areas, such as aging, acute infectious processes, mental health, rehabilitation, and health promotion, are located on one side of the matrix, with specialized health-care providers on the other side (FIG. 12–7). People as leaders, managers, and workers, along with tangible resources in the environment, are all represented in the matrix cells. Although this design is challenging, it is consistent with the core competency for health professionals identified in Chapter 1 for working in interdisciplinary teams.

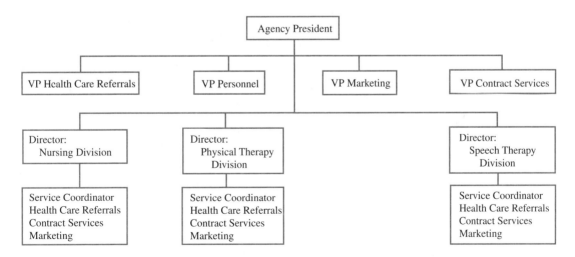

FIG. 12–6. Example of a product form organization: home care agency.

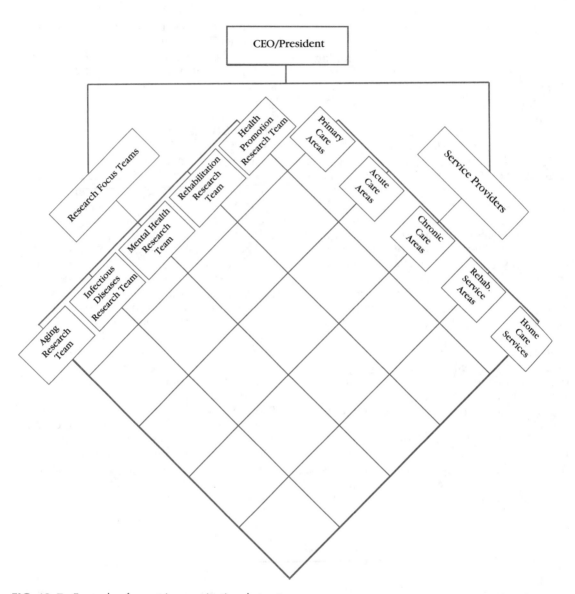

FIG. 12–7. Example of a matrix organizational structure.

Consider the example of home care for an elderly client following a hip fracture. Care for the client and the family along the continuum would move from acute care to short-term rehabilitation to home care, with interdisciplinary care providers, including home care coordinators, therapists, and specialists, all contributing to the decision-making and service provision. The complexity of this system is initially breathtaking. However, both func- tions and products must be considered in coordination of the services needed by the client. This is a collegial structure with inte- grated functions and products that require multilayered decisions. The number of people involved in the matrix for decisions varies. Larger organizations may involve only man- agers in the matrix, with traditional depart- mental structures evolving under each manager. Smaller organizations, such as the earlier example of a home care agency, could realistically involve managers and providers in the matrix according to the scope of services (product) and resources (human and material as functions).

The matrix design promotes innovative practices as a result of a consumer focus in the context of current technology, emergent practice problems, research information, and specialty practice. Research and development issues are directed at current practice, with experts from each area represented for problem-solving and decision-making. This matrix design is seen more frequently in health settings with a dual focus, such as education and service or research and service. The complexity of the design and problems with integration of all appropriate people and resources are the main disadvantages of the matrix form. Daft (1998) describes its disadvantages more fully as follows:

1. Participants experience dual authority, leading to confusion and frustration.
2. Good interpersonal skills and extensive training of participants are needed.
3. It is time-consuming, with frequent meetings and conflict resolution sessions.
4. Participants must understand and adopt collegial rather than vertical-type relationships.
5. Dual pressure from the environment is required to maintain a balance of power (p. 229)

Coordination problems are a definite disadvantage of adhocratic designs. Experts and project teams or divisions are focused on innovation and targeting of specific outcomes. This focus may represent only one piece of the mission of the organization, however. Thus, good communication and coordination are critical. But coordination problems are many times outweighed by the advantages of flexibility, innovation, and human involvement.

Structural Components for Decision-Making and Management

Organizations are also categorized by how the components are arranged, as centralized or decentralized and flat or tall. Centralized and decentralized organizational structures relate to the lines of control and decision-making within the organization. **Centralization** occurs when the span of control or management is in the classic bureaucratic style, governed from the top downward. Authority, control, and decision-making occur in upper management, with less participation from the lower levels. **Decentralization** distributes authority downward in an organization, allowing decision-making and control at local levels. Reasons suggested for decentralization are to establish a more collegial and participatory model, resulting in employee involvement, performance, and satisfaction.

Organizations can also be described as having flat or tall structures, depending on the layers of differentiation for authority, decision-making, and coordination. **Flat organizational structures** have a wide base and few layers or tiers for decision-making and authority. Decisions, controls, and governance are widely spread across the organization in a horizontal differentiation. **Tall organizational structures** have more tiers and lines of command, with less local decision-making at the lower levels. Tall organizations have more management levels, with lines of command resulting in a vertically differentiated hierarchical structure. Compare the organizational structures in Figures 12–3 and 12–4. Both are bureaucratic structures, but decisions and work functions are spread more widely across the organization in flat structures (see FIG. 12–3).

Deciding whether a centralized or decentralized, tall or flat structure is best depends on the characteristics of the specific organization. As Vecchio (1991) points out, decentralization and flat structures tend to go together, and tall organizations are more centralized. Many organizations have changed from centralized, tall structures to encourage more employee involvement. But problems can arise when communication, coordination, and monitoring of activities in the organization demand integration for effective functioning. As in his continuum of organizational standardization (see Figure 12–2), Mintzberg (1983b) suggests that centralization and decentralization be viewed as opposite ends of a continuum rather than absolutes (p. 98).

The degree of centralization or decentralization actually should depend on the organization's size, structure, technology, people, and mission. These factors are considered in four of the organization's subsystems (structural, technical, psychosocial, and goals and values) as they interact with the managerial (fifth) subsystem to determine where decisions are best made.

ORGANIZATIONAL FUNCTIONS

Tappen (2001) differentiates between two types of **organizational functions**, (1) formal and informal goals and (2) formal and informal levels of operation. These two functions represent the interaction between two organization subsystems, the goals and values subsystem and the technical subsystem.

The goals and values subsystem is described in the institutional mission and purposes statement as the basis for the organization's existence. The mission statement is the overall purpose of the organization, including whether the organization is a for-profit organization or a not-for-profit organization. Stockholders or shareholders expect to see some return on their investment in a for-profit (or proprietary) organization, and this expectation is reflected in organizational goals. Not-for-profit organizations receive funding from various sources, but there is no sense of ownership. In a not-for-profit organization, profits are generally reinvested in the organization to keep it financially competitive.

Once the mission is understood, the targets to achieve this mission become the issue. Organizational goals are specified for effective and efficient functioning. Mintzberg (1983a) has identified four types of goals that demonstrate intent and consistency of behavior in organizations: ideologic, formal, shared, and system. *Ideologic goals* relate to the values people in the organization share. This is the values component of the goals and values subsystem; an example of an ideologic goal in a health-care organization is access to and provision of high-quality health care for people of all ages. *Formal goals* are those authorized through the hierarchy from people with authority who have a power base in the organization. *Shared goals* are those set and pursued by a particular group in the organization. Involvement of family members in caregiving is an example of a shared goal that a specialty group favors and implements in the organization.

System goals are those set to maintain the system. Mintzberg (1983a) has identified system goals as survival, efficiency, control, and growth. System goals relate to continuity of the organization and contain a strong economic component. These survival system goals are driving many health-care organizations.

Organizations are now recognizing that goals that are too broad can deplete the resources and effectiveness of the intended outcomes and the system goals. We hear of companies and major industries streamlining and getting "back to basics." They seriously consider examining what they know best, and refining and focusing it, rather than diversifying. Linkages with other organizations that can better handle the diversifications may be more beneficial to both the organization and the consumer group. This development has been seen with restructuring in health-care organizations.

There are three basic reasons for the changes in health-care structures: environmental influences, changes in the provider system, and changes in consumer needs and demographics. First, external environmental influences have had a major effect on health-care organizations, as with diagnostic-related groups (DRGs) and the prospective payment system (PPS) for health-care reimbursement. Second, specialization and changes in the health-care provider system have confused consumers and legislators. Disciplinary lines between health-care providers necessarily have some overlap as we implement cross-training and focus on humanistic and holistic values for persons and groups. An example is the core competency of working in interdisciplinary teams. Coordination and collaboration are essential attributes in contemporary practice settings. Third, changes in consumer needs related to increased longevity, chronicity, personal involvement, and health promotion must drive the system to provide safe and effective health-care services.

Health-care organizations are now seeing the wisdom of a lesson learned in industry: Not every community hospital needs to have every specialty service. Community hospitals can offer services that are complementary rather than duplicated and meager. Regionalization can be accomplished by having maternal and infant or pediatric services in one agency and cardiac diagnosis, surgery, and rehabilitation in another. This arrangement prevents duplication and fosters quality. The population and the health service needs must drive the goals of the organization. A needs assessment provides the information for revision of organizational goals. Important considerations include the specific operations of the organization and the available technology.

The technical subsystem was described as representing the knowledge and skills of the people providing services in the system, along with physical resources. This subsystem provides for the formal and informal levels of operation of the organization. Specialized knowledge and expertise of professionals and nonprofessionals are represented in formal and informal functions. Formal functions are those defined by the organizational structure. Compare the different functions for a unit manager in a vertical, bureaucratic organization with decision-making in the upper levels of the hierarchy with those for the unit as a cost and decision center in a more horizontal adhocratic structure. This demonstrates a difference in formal operational functions. Informal functions facilitate goal accomplishment and include effective communication channels and how the organizational plans and tasks are actually accomplished in relation to the available resources.

Developing an appreciation of the formal and informal functions of the human and material resources in the technical subsystem is essential for understanding the operations of the organization. To do this, it is essential to be further aware of the human factor, or the individuals who coordinate the people and resources to meet the goals of the organization, the managers.

 MANAGEMENT

Management, the coordination of resources to achieve organizational outcomes, involves critical thinking, problem-solving, and decision-making. Management should not be confused with leadership. As seen in the previous chapter, a leader mobilizes a group to achieve great things, whereas a manager focuses on directing the group to meet the desired outcomes for the organization through thoughtful and careful planning, direction, monitoring, recognition, development, and representation.

An effective manager must be a good leader, and the combination of effective leadership and management skills provides the nurse with the attributes to face the multitude of challenges in the current health-care system and the various organizational structures. Understanding the foundation of effective management is essential to developing one's own management style.

Management Theories

Management has been studied extensively, with the development of several major theories that are still used to guide current practices. During the 20th century, the major themes were a focus on management science, the process, the people, and even the activities and the intended objectives. Other emerging theories and models are evolving as we attempt to understand and apply the best approaches to "getting things done" efficiently and effectively with the best possible outcomes. The concept of outcomes is an important component in the current view of management, especially in the health-care arena.

The origins of management theory are often attributed to Frederick Taylor (1911), an engineer who used time-and-motion studies to investigate and then apply efficiency principles with the bottom-line focus on productivity. In this early industrial period, training the right people for the task at hand was vital, and these people were rewarded monetarily as productivity levels rose. The focus was one of efficiency, effectiveness, and quality control. This approach was viewed as "working smarter." These principles have been used effectively with production lines, as in the early days of the automotive industry. Taylor's efficiency and productivity principles persist to this day, with the focus on organizing the proper number of trained people and activities to get a job done in the shortest time. These principles have been followed in the use and examination of nurse-patient staffing ratios and skill mix in hospitals.

In the early 20th century, Henri Fayol (1949) looked further at the process of management and the role and functions of the manager. His universalist approach highlighted the principles of authority, unity of command (one boss and a chain of command), and communication. The role of the manager in this approach encompassed five functions: planning, organizing, commanding, coordinating, and controlling. During the same period, Max Weber (1947) was addressing organizational structure and the need for consistent rules and tasks in the hierarchical structure of the bureaucratic organization.

Further managerial theories evolved, focused on individuals and the goals of organizations. **Motivational theories** are used to identify and describe the forces that motivate individuals toward a goal. Guided by these theories, an effective manager motivates individuals, thus enhancing their productivity and achieving organizational goals. Classic motivational theories have been proposed by Maslow, McGregor, and Ouchi.

As seen previously, in Chapters 3 and 10, Maslow's (1954, 1970) theory of a hierarchy of human needs was based on his 16 propositions on motivation. Motivation in humans is a manifestation of internal and external personal and environmental factors that cause people to respond to a situation in the way that they do. In these principles, the focus is on the individual in a dynamic, complex, and changing environment. Motivation is as intri-

cate as the person, and an individual's personal basic needs must be satisfied before he or she can focus on higher needs, such as self-esteem in one's position and organizational goals. Understanding individual motivation is as important as understanding the skills the individual brings to the task at hand.

McGregor (1960) critically reviewed motivation in *The Human Side of Enterprise*. He proposed his classic two "theories" about human nature. The focus during this time continued to be on the human factors of the worker and how to get the work done. In **Theory X**, individuals are viewed as lazy, needing motivation, avoiding responsibility, and needing constant direction and control by a manager to fulfill their job responsibilities and meet the organizational goals. Rewards and reinforcement are necessary for the individuals, along with a set of rules they must follow. This theory of human nature fits well with the centralized, tall, bureaucratic organizational structure. The role of the manager is one of direction and control.

Alternately, McGregor (1960) postulated **Theory Y,** in which individuals are motivated, self-directed, interested in working toward meeting organizational goals, and willing to accept responsibility without the need for constant direction and supervision. In fact, this constant "management" by the supervisor could deter their inner rewards from the job. The role of the manager in this situation should be one of coordination, guidance, and support.

Herzberg's (1966) two-factor theory organizes the individual's motivation for his or her work according to hygiene and motivational factors. **Hygiene factors** are maintenance factors in the workplace, such as salary, supervision, company policy, working conditions, status, job security, and the job's effect on personal life; these hygiene factors in the workplace can lead to satisfaction or dissatisfaction and are related to the organizational climate. **Motivational factors** are satisfiers within the job that motivate people to higher levels of performance. Motivational factors include achievement, recognition, the work itself, responsibility, and advancement. The manager helps improve job performance by ensuring that both hygiene and motivational needs of the employees are met at some level for both job satifaction and incentive to achieve the organizational goals.

In the later part of the 20th century, the Japanese style of collaborative management received much attention, with the economic successes viewed within a paticipatory approach. Ouchi (1981) described this style as **Theory Z** as an approach in which employees are trusted, empowered, and actively involved in decision-making. The components of Theory Z are collective values and decision-making, long-term or lifetime employment, slower but predictable promotions, indirect supervision, and a holistic concern for employees (Ouchi, 1981). This participatory style involves indirect supervision with the focus on the group. Ouchi (1981) believes that more creative decision-making and more effective implementation occur with the full involvement and consensus of the group (p.43). There is a "buy-in" by all team members, who are valued as individuals and as important members of the organization. Important values of this theory are trust, fairness, commitment, and loyalty to the organization, which lead to long-term employment and reduced turnover. The use of "quality circles" and "group think" emerged from this theory. However, competitiveness in some American organizations is inconsistent with this style of management.

Management-by-objectives (MBO) evolved in the business world from the work of Peter Drucker. Originally from Austria, Drucker has profoundly infuenced American businesses through his many books and observations on organizations and how they are managed. Drucker focuses on the people (both managers and work force), the organizational functions, and the results achieved in the process in line with the organizational mission. He believes that the manager's job is "to direct the resources and the efforts of the business toward opportunities for economically significant results" (Drucker, 1998, p.67). In Drucker's view, MBO focuses on the process and the team to meet the objectives of the organization. It requires the manager to be self-controlled and self-disciplined. MBO assumes that people, both management and labor, want to contribute and to be responsible (Drucker, 1974, p. 441). He proposes that management comprises a few essential principles; the first is that "its task is to make people capable of joint performance, to make their strengths effective and their weaknesses irrelevant. This is what an organization is all about, and the reason that management is the critical, determining factor" (Drucker, 1998, p. 172). More recently, Drucker (1998) has proposed replacing the term *manager* with the **executive**, "because it implies responsibility for an area, not dominion over people" (p. 188). Drucker's works on management cover a wide range of businesses, including hospitals, and look at achievement of individuals within the framework of organizational settings.

Nursing Management

The core competencies for health professionals are essential characteristics in nursing management. The focus of the nurse manager or *executive* must be on the provision of client-centered care while fostering the use of evidence-based practice and quality improvement. The complexity of the interdisciplinary team and the use of informatics will depend on the organizational system and its associated subsystems. All of these tasks involve people and managing resources for the provision of safe and effective care and positive client outcomes.

As described by Grohar-Murray and DiCroce (2003), "managers have the responsibility to help the staff become successful in their endeavors which is the work of the organization [and] this approach to management conforms with the leadership theories that empower the employee" (p. 134). But recall that Fayol (1949) identified management functions as planning, organizing, commanding, coordinating, and controlling. The question becomes one of the consistency of these functions with the humanistic view of nursing and care of clients.

Planning and organizing are indeed talents of the nurse manager. This is an outcome of the steps of assessment and planning in the provision of nursing care in any organizational context. It requires an in-depth understanding of the organization and the people, the true culture of the organization. At times, it will also involve leading the culture, as with incorporation of evidence-based practice in a particular client situation and planning for the efficient and effective use of resources.

Commanding in the context of nursing management involves ensuring that the job is done through delegation and supervision, as in the provision of care to clients. It requires knowledge of the care requirements, the clients, and external system influences. Beyond this, all levels of staffing are a vital consideration, including assistive personnel. Delegation is a skill that grows and evolves, as the nurse manager grows from novice to expert. This is an area that needs careful and ongoing professional development.

In a nursing education program, students focus on "total patient care" as they learn the interpersonal, technical, and clinical judgment skills needed in nursing practice. In the final phase of the educational program, they are engaged in obtaining leadership or management skills. This includes assignment and delegation of activities to other health-care providers, both licensed and unlicensed. Often these activities are performed with other students rather than within the interdisciplinary team in the acute care setting. However, upon graduation and initial licensure, nurses are expected to manage the health-care team effectively and to delegate activities and functions to others for the provision of efficient care to clients. Challenges in the workplace, such as economics, constantly add new twists. This leads to the need for coordination of resources, including health-care providers, for accomplishment of the organizational goals and the provision of safe and effective care for clients.

Coordination is another talent of the nurse manager, as skills in coordination of care have continued to be a component of the practice scope and setting. Controlling in nursing management is ensuring that the care to clients has been effectively and efficiently provided. Recall, however, that management is the coordination of resources to achieve organizational outcomes and involves critical thinking, problem-solving, communication, and decision-making skills. To coordinate health care and the various providers effectively, the nurse must have a thorough understanding and appreciation of the organizational culture.

ORGANIZATIONAL CULTURE

The psychosocial subsystem of the organization is termed **organizational culture**. It is perceptible as the culmination of the norms, attitudes, and values imbedded in the organizational mission and in the expected behaviors of the employees. Leininger (2002) has even classified the organizational culture of health care as a unique culture. Daft (1998) views organizational culture as having two dimensions, observable symbols (e.g., ceremonies, stories, slogans, behaviors, dress, physical settings) and the underlying values, assumptions, beliefs, attitudes, and feelings of the people (pp. 368–369).

Scrutiny of the organizational culture can provide a sense of the prevailing level of humanism present in the organization—in other words, how people are viewed as employees and consumers. New organizational values and behaviors have emerged as we redefine and recreate organizations for functioning in today's world. We moved from the belief that humans in organizations are lazy and need direction, in McGregor's (1967) Theory X, to the age of humanism with the philosophies of Theory Y and Theory Z. The humanistic perspective is a more positive one that considers the importance of the people in the organization. Still, during times of cost-cutting, a humanistic perspective can quickly disappear when the focus turns to head counts or full-time equivalents (FTEs).

Important clues on the involvement, satisfaction, and effectiveness of the people in the organization are reflected in both management styles and the behaviors and attitudes of those in the environment. In health care, the organizational culture includes both the consumers and the providers in the agency. The organizational culture is also influenced by the environment—the immediate institutional or agency environment as well as societal expectations and mandates.

As with any set of cultural expectations, the employees are expected to enculturate (adapt and adopt) and espouse the prevailing principles. Failure to enculturate results in being ostracized or terminated. These cultural expectations are the customary ways of thinking and behaving shared by members of the organization, as a form of socialization and allegiance to the norms of the organization. Incorporation of the specific expectations encompasses this organizational socialization process. An example is adopting and using a specific theory that guides the operation of the organization. At the most ideal level, if the nurse cannot view or provide care for clients in accordance with the specific model used at that agency, such as self-care, the best remedy would be to seek employment at another agency more consistent with the nurse's own worldview.

Cox (1993) applied the following six areas of behavior to cultural differences of people and groups in organizations:

- Time and space, such as territoriality in work areas and orientation to time as in rigid versus flexible schedules
- Leadership style favoring institutional procedures versus emphasis on relationships and a democratic climate
- Individualism, looking at personal goals and achievement, versus collectivism, which focuses on teamwork and attaining group goals
- Competition versus cooperativeness in social interactions and task performance
- Locus of control, as internal control over events and one's destiny versus external influences and the concept of fate affecting life events
- Communication styles related to confidence, speech anxiety, desire for discussion as sharing, and a sense of interpersonal trust (pp. 108–127)

The concepts of time and space, leadership, management, locus of control, and communication are particularly appropriate to understanding the people as individuals and groups in health-care organizations.

Time and Space

Health-care personnel generally view time as highly fixed, with set schedules. But tight schedules are often problematic because emergencies or unanticipated delays occur as a function of human events and differences. A classic example is a client's appointment for same-day surgery. We expect the client to appear on time, as scheduled, but then he or she waits in the reception area, answers repeated questions, and waits for check-ins, assessments, preparations, the actual procedure, and discharge. Time frames and perceptions vary for providers and clients and diverge further among different cultural groups and subgroups.

The concept of space is highly personal. In health-care organizations, the importance to clients of touch, space, and territoriality must be considered in light of client comfort status, both physical and emotional. The importance of touch as part of the health beliefs of selected cultural subgroups has already been illustrated. For health-care providers, work space, privacy, and territoriality are important considerations in job performance. Individual space may be at a premium in the crowded physical plant of a hospital or clinic or in an environment that favors open, shared work spaces. This may present a comforting environment for an individual or group that favors interpersonal relations and collaboration or may be unsettling for an individualist who needs "quiet time" for greater creativity and job performance.

Leadership

In Chapter 11, selected leadership styles and traits were presented. The cultural climate generally supports the predominant leadership style. But differences have been demonstrated among genders and minority groups. Cox (1993) found that women and Mexican-Americans display a marked emphasis on relationships compared with the Anglo-American male leadership tradition of institutional procedures and task accomplishment. The leadership style is nevertheless a major influence on the organizational culture or climate.

Individualism or Collectivism

Closely related to leadership style is management focus, whether on individualism and achievement or on collectivism or teamwork.

Management styles have an important influence here. Consider the differences in management with Theory X, which is focused on individual performance, versus Theory Z, which emphasizes collectivism and cooperation. The organizational focus on individualism or collectivism is apparent in promotion and evaluation structures. Administrative policies and procedures provide important clues to the organization's official position. However, subgroups or minority groups within the organization may create factions. These subgroups may set certain expectations for collectivism and cooperation in behavior or function. For example, the organization may be highly bureaucratic, with expectations and rewards valuing individual performance, competition, and task accomplishment; but if cooperation is the prevailing value in the nursing department, it will be translated into accomplishing outcomes at the upper level of management.

Locus of Control

Internal locus of control over life events is a prevailing value of Anglo-American culture and the health-care system. We promote responsible behavior and health promotion activities. But, as with health beliefs, values of different cultures may conflict with the values in the health-care system. Research has shown that external controlling factors are much stronger in Arab, Asian, African, and Latino minority and cultural groups (Cox, 1993). This finding has implications for health-care providers as well as clients in terms of motivation and confidence in life situations or work performance.

Communication

Communication of ideas and views is important in all of the cultural differences described here. Being able to communicate with clients is quite different from having your ideas heard, considered, and implemented at the organizational level. Portraying yourself as an expert and as a colleague is necessary in both client and professional interactions within the organization. Whether by ensuring that all committee or group members have the opportunity to express their opinions or by making special efforts to demonstrate recognition and give credit for another's ideas, attention to cultural differences is important. It can make the most of the talents, abilities, and skills of the human resources in the organizational system, especially in management of interdisciplinary teams.

Other Concepts in Organizational Culture

In addition to understanding the people and groups in the organizational system, other factors provide information on the organizational culture and the operational climate. On the basis of research, Vecchio (1991) identified the following six central concepts for understanding the organizational culture:

- Critical decisions of the entrepreneur or founding members
- Guiding ideals and mission
- Social structure
- Norms and values
- Remembered history and symbolism
- Institutional arrangements (pp. 553–555)

Discovering the critical decisions made in founding the organization reveals the original intent for the organization and views for the future. Closely related to the founding decisions are the current guiding ideals and mission. The guiding ideals and mission relate to the service orientation. Consider the difference between missions and the intended consumer groups in not-for-profit and for-profit organizations. This could range from elected fee-for-service care in the for-profit setting to a not-for-profit agency focusing on health care to the indigent. The philosophy of the organization provides important information about the current ideals and mission. If revisions have been made over the years, it can be quite helpful to look back at old versions to determine whether the philosophy changed in response to environmental factors.

The social structure provides information on organizational structure, leadership, and management theories and strategies used. Views of humans as clients and providers of services differ, and these differences are reflected in leadership and management styles. The norms and values of the organization are basic beliefs, attitudes, and expected behaviors. They have been translated over time and are pervasive in organizational policies and procedures that continue to interpret the organizational design and function. Remembered history and symbolism of the organization contribute additional information, for example, about an institution designed to provide hospital care for a county that has evolved into a regional referral and tertiary care center. Remembering the traditions of personalized obstetric care, a local woman's group may provide funding for a special prenatal program for indigent pregnant teenagers.

Finally, institutional arrangements and linkages, such as consortia and cooperating or referral agencies, are frequently quite complex but provide essential information on organizational relationships and interrelationships. These facts are necessary for understanding the culture and influences on the organization. But, as Hall (1999) points out, "culture is not a constant ... values and norms change as the events affect the population involved" (p. 214). The potential for change in the organizational culture requires diligent assessment and communication skills on the part of the nurse manager or executive.

COMMUNICATION UNIQUE TO ORGANIZATIONS

Communication is vital in complex, highly technologic, and dynamic organizations. As was illustrated with organizational functions, the structure of the organization plays an important role in communication channels. Formal channels are easily apparent in highly bureaucratic structures, as dictated by the organizational diagram. But informal communication channels ("grapevines") are some-

times less evident and can be highly effective in such a structure. Consider the need for supplies in some areas of an agency. Ordering can easily be handled through the computerized entry system. But what if some urgently needed item is unavailable through the system? An informal channel may be used to locate a supply from which the item may be "borrowed," to be replaced as soon as the official order is fulfilled. The departmental secretary who has an informal chain of communication may be able to use his or her knowledge of these informal systems effectively in such a procurement process.

Communication channels are important in relating subsystems to one another and to the total system. Recall the systems model with the five subsystems: goals and values, technical, psychosocial, structural, and managerial. Organizational goals and values must be translated, transmitted, and reinforced throughout the system to meet the institutional mission. The specialized knowledge, skills, and resources represented by the technical subsystem require excellent communication within the system and from external environments to be current and responsive to changes in the knowledge base and technology. Communication is the action component of the psychosocial subsystem of interpersonal and interdisciplinary roles, behaviors, and relationships in the organization system. The formal and informal communications and interactions that arise from this subsystem are the essence of the organizational culture. The structural subsystem provides the formal design, with its hierarchy or lines of authority, for the communication channels. Communications may be formally dictated in a linear manner by the bureaucratic structure, or they may be flexible and circular in adhocratic matrix designs. Informal communications must be identified to reveal the actual flow of information, decision-making, and task accomplishment. Communication of information and expectations stems from the managerial subsystem within the organization's pervasive leadership and management styles. Evaluation of the appropriate channels is vital for effective functioning in the organizational setting.

Organizations routinely use methods of communication in addition to the verbal and nonverbal interpersonal communication techniques. Consider the informatics available in organizational settings. We have computer networks, fiberoptics, satellite, and teleconferencing technology. Computers manage information storage, inventory, and rapid retrieval, data processing, data analysis, and report generation. The information we compile and the method we use to transmit it vary with the nature of the communication channel we are using. For example, a general rule in an organization is to limit memos to one page or less and disperse them to the appropriate parties; however, the sender must consider the available and appropriate technology, such as interoffice paper copies or electronic mail or messaging.

Considering the purpose of communication in an organization is indispensable. Whether we are communicating with clients or assistive personnel, the method and receiver of the information are important. Clear, concise, and timely transmission of information is necessary for an effective management process. Recall the "five rights" of organizational communications: (1) the right information or content, (2) the right communication channel, (3) the right format, including use of correct grammar, terms, and language, (4) the right level of understanding, and (5) the right technology. The appropriate communication channel must be selected, using the appropriate chain of command to convey your message.

ORGANIZATIONS, HEALTH CARE, AND NURSING MANAGEMENT

In the past two decades, health-care organizations have undergone radical change and restructuring. Pettigrew and colleagues (1992) noted changes in health-care organizations from measurement-oriented management styles in the 1980s to a focus on organizational cultures in the 1990s, with a stress on quality-based values (p. 21). We are now focused on outcomes, customer satisfaction, safety, adequacy of reimbursement for services provided, and the need to address health disparities.

Systems theory fits well with changes going on in health-care organizations. But as the system becomes more and more multilayered, the focus shifts to the openness and flexibility of the system boundaries, greater attention to environmental forces, and expanding relationships among organizations. Special attention to external influences is essential for effective planning and organizing. This includes a focus on the organization, considering its human resources, information systems, and governance structures for delegation and coordination. Ongoing feedback and evaluation become essential. Professional nurses have major roles in all steps of this process as we now focus on strategic initiatives.

Administrative nursing positions in health-care systems have been expanded at all levels. Director and supervisor roles, when still apparent in an organizational chart, have been greatly expanded. As we have seen in the chapter on leadership, nurses have major responsibility in health-care organizations. Nurses influence many different types of colleagues. Nurse managers have knowledge of people and the environmental influences on health-care needs. This is the domain of nursing. In addition, nurses are now well prepared in organizational theory, finance, and policy. We have entered the administrative arena as interdisciplinary care managers, coordinators, and leaders. Strategic planning, public relations, and cost containment have become essential skills. Nurses who have this knowledge have legitimate power in health-care organizations. But along with this power come responsibility, accountability, and the need for effective negotiation and delegation skills.

Power

Max Weber (1947) defined **power** as "the probability that one actor in a social relationship will be in a position to carry out his own will despite resistance, regardless of the basis on which this probability rests" (p. 152). More specific to organizations, Mintzberg (1983a) defines power as "the capacity to effect (or affect) organizational outcomes" (p. 4). This latter definition has much relevance for professional nursing practice, because nurses in health-care organizations are positioned to effect or affect positive health-care outcomes. These outcomes can be viewed as outputs from the health-care system, such as clients with improved health status. *Legitimate power* is the authority to effect change within one's position. The professional relationship provides the opportunity for legitimate power, and many nurses now have legitimate power by virtue of their position, role, and expertise. *Informal power* is the assertion of one's will over a situation to achieve a goal without formal or "vested" authority.

Mintzberg (1983a) identified five general bases of power (Box 12–1). These power bases are applicable to professional nursing, especially in organizational settings. First, nurses have demonstrated effective management of resources in decentralized and vertical organizations. They are being vested with responsibility especially with regard to decisions and resources needed for effective organizational functioning. Second, care of clients involves technical skills that must be performed or supervised by nurses. Third, nursing continues to develop its unique body of knowledge needed for the health of clients. The fourth base of power involves the legal prerogatives granted and implied under the practice acts, licensure, certification, and professional codes described in Chapter 1. And finally, nurses in interdisciplinary practice have access to colleagues, clients, and influential people on whom they rely for access to the other bases of power.

Negotiation for power must first be related to the goals of the organization. Nurses have the ability and responsibility to negotiate for legitimate power in organizations. Nurses certainly have access to these power sources if developed, effectively negotiated, and used.

Negotiation

As discussed in Chapter 8, conflict situations can easily arise in a group setting. And the

---

> **BOX 12–1**
> **THE FIVE GENERAL BASES OF POWER**
>
> - Control of resources
> - Control of a technical skill
> - Control of a body of knowledge
> - Exclusive rights or privileges to impose choices (legal prerogatives)
> - Access to people who have and can be relied on for the other four
>
> Data from Mintzberg, H. (1983a). *Power in and around organizations.* Englewood Cliffs, NJ: Prentice-Hall.

---

health-care organization provides the potential for many groups with different compositions, all with the potential for conflict situations to arise. This is consistent with the organizational goals and values, technical, and psychosocial subsystems. Recall that the technical subsystem consists of the knowledge and skills of the people providing service in the system, with specialized knowledge and expertise of professional and nonprofessional labor forces represented. The psychosocial subsystem contains the interpersonal and interdisciplinary relationships unique to the organization, including role relationships, attitudes, and values of people and groups within the system. The manager frequently encounters conflict among individuals or groups that necessitate artful use of interpersonal and negotiation skills. Effective conflict resolution by the manager requires **negotiation**, and ultimately, coming to some compromise. This compromise is most effective when the end result is acceptable at some level to all parties involved.

Gebelein and associates (2000) define successful negotiation as engaging people in identifying a solution satisfactory to all (p. 478). The best scenario is a "win-win" situation with confrontation and collaboration. In this situation, the solution is satisfying to both sides, who have collaborated, and each side senses some satisfaction and feeling of a "win" situation. Alternately, one side prevails ("win-loss" situation) or both sides experience a compromise that is not really satisfying to either side, thus a "loss-loss" situation.

BOX 12–2
ATTRIBUTES OF A SKILLED
NEGOTIATOR

- **C**ommunication and interpersonal skills
- **A**ssessment skills
- **V**ision and application of needed resources
- **E**ndurance
- **A**wareness
- **T**rustworthiness

An effective negotiator should consistently refine and nurture negotiation skills (Box 12–2). First, the negotiator must have excellent *communication and interpersonal skills*. The negotiator must be a skilled communicator, for understanding the concerns of both sides and promoting awareness and collaboration. Verbal and nonverbal cues are often overemphasized on both sides, although they are sometimes subtle when the negotiator is present. Focus on the facts (verbal and nonverbal) and try to diffuse emotions with effective communication. As Dana (2001) describes negotiation, a smart manager avoids power contests and rights contests, and focuses on finding ways to resolve conflicts through reconciliation of interests (p. 41).

As with any nursing care situation, *assessment skills* are needed to understand the interpersonal and situational influences from all sides. For example, consider a conflict situation that arises in the intensive care setting as the group of physicians and nurses attempt to implement a collaborative practice model. The ultimate goal is for the effective care of the client; however, the negotiator must have an understanding of all of the facts in order to uncover the common ground for all, physicians, intensivists, Advanced Practice Registered Nurses (APRNs), staff nurses, technicians, therapists, associated service providers, and the clients. The skillful negotiator must understand what is being said and what is actually occurring in the setting, and should be sensitive to all behaviors, nonverbal and expressed cues, and views. The skillful negotiator must assess not only content but also

context, culture, behaviors, and players involved.

The ability to envision what potential outcomes could be and how they would affect each side, individually and collectively, is key. The *vision* of the potential outcomes must be framed for the individuals involved, on the basis of the facts of the situation and the resources available. *Endurance* is a definite prerequisite throughout the process and during the inevitable peaks, valleys, and stalemates that can occur. There are times when the negotiation process must be halted to allow the various individuals or groups to refocus on facts and dilute emotions.

And the acute *awareness* of the negotiator must prevail throughout the entire process, from identification of conflict, alertness to all behaviors and actions throughout, to the levels of satisfaction of both parties once the resolution has been agreed upon. This awarenss of behavior and situation will have to be restated to all parties on an ongoing basis to promote focus on the facts. Another important characteristic of the negotiator is *trustworthiness*. All parties must sense the fairness of the negotiator in the process. Building trust is a necessary skill, not only to gain the cooperation of both sides during the negotiation but also to help build trust in the process and the ultimate resolution. The process is often not a smooth, linear activity when one is dealing with people, partiality, and conscious or unconsious behaviors.

Marquis and Huston (2003) identify the following destructive or manipulative negotiating tactics:

- Use of ridicule
- Inapproprite questioning
- Flattery
- Sense of helplessness
- Aggression or taking over the situation (p. 403)

These tactics are ineffective and may delay resolution or even escalate the conflict. Such tactics inhibit the building of trust and negate the collaborative process. The end result of the negotiation process must be a compromise acceptable to all at some level of satisfaction. If a compromise cannot be reached, an impasse results. In this situation, the conflict will escalate at some later point, perhaps in a different form or with different players.

Ideally, the negotiation process should take place on neutral ground, or at least in a secure environment acceptable to both parties. Specific terms are used in negotiation tactics, like "reaching a stalemate" (an impasse) and "tradeoffs" (concessions), of which the negotiator must be aware. However, once again the need for trust, well-developed communication and interpersonal skills, and a commitment to resolution acceptable to both parties are paramount throughout the process.

Marquis and Huston (2003) recommend that upon resolution of the conflict, the negotiator send a follow-up letter to both parties describing the agreed terms (p. 403). This is a follow-up as reinforcement for both recognition of individual involvement and the results of the process. The correspondence can take the form of a formal memo or an electronic communication commending the participation of both sides in the resolution and restating the agreed-upon conditions. The attributes of a successful negotiator are also essential in delegation activities.

Delegation

Delegation is defined as the "transfer of responsibility of the performance of an activity from one individual to another while retaining the accountability of the outcome" (American Nurses Association [ANA], 1997, p. 3). Classifying it as a concept, an art, a skill, and a process, the National Council of State Boards of Nursing (NCBSN) (1997c) views delegation as "a management principle used to obtain desired results through the work of others and as a legal concept to empower one to act for another" (p. 1).

Delegation activities occur when the novice nurse enters practice on the first day of professional practice. But as mentioned, educational preparation provides the concepts for the process, although seldom the opportunity to truly develop these critical skills, especially when the new nurse confronted with long-term interdisciplinary staff who may be entrenched in a certain way of providing care. The new nurse is responsible for the care of a group of clients and works with assistive personnel necessary for the provision of quality care. But delegation is a difficult activity for the novice whose skills are being developed and refined. And the accountability for the delegated act is not consistently internalized, as simple tasks are performed by others for the delivery of care. It is not a matter of simply "assigning" a list of tasks or relying on a nurse manager to make these assignments. Consider the standard practice of routine vital signs taken by assistive personnel like Certified Nursing Assistants (CNAs) or Unlicensed Assistive Personnel (UAPs). We have lost the concept of "monitoring" vital signs when the nurse assumes that the readings will be reported by the assistive personnel in a timely manner. Consider the problems with this arrangement:

- Skill of the assistive personnel
- Accuracy of readings according to a prescribed schedule
- Report on the findings
- Interpretation of readings
- Nursing judgment on readings, their accuracy, and other variables in the client's condition
- Alternate comfort measures that could have an effect on readings

And the list goes on.

Delegation is not the "hand-off" of a routine task. Application of the principles of delegation is essential to effective management as well as to client safety.

Principles of Delegation

Basic principles of degation involve awareness of the differences between assignment, delegation, responsibility, and accountability. *Assignment* is the designation of activities or tasks to be performed within the individual's licensed scope of practice (NCSBN, 1997a, p. 1), as with the division of labor of nursing care activies among the registered nurse (RN) and licensed practical nurse (LPN) staff. Also, in some states the nursing assistant is officially regulated across care settings and has a defined scope of practice based on a required level of training. *Delegation* "is the transfering to a competent individual the authority to perform a selected nursing task in a selected situation; the nurse retains accountability for the delegation" (NCSBN, 1997a, p. 2). The responsibility for completion of the task has been delegated, but not the accountability for ensuring that the task has been completed correctly by the right person and supervised appropriateley. Recall from Chapter 1 that according to the Code of Ethics for Nurses, *responsibility* is defined as accountability for performance of the duties associated with the professional role, and *accountability* is being answerable to oneself and others for one's judgments and actions in the course of nursing practice, irrespective of health-care organizations' policies or providers' directives (ANA, 2001, pp. 16–17). The nurse maintains both the responsibility and the accountability for the delegated action. However, the skillful manager must delegate some activities for necessary care of the client and to ensure patient safety.

Process of Delegation

The NCSBN envisions delegation as a pyramid, similar to the hierarcy of needs. The pyramid has four layers, beginning at the bottom with assessment, and moving up through delegation and monitoring to evaluation (NCBSN, 2002). This concept illustrates the importance of delegation as a process based on good assessment of the client, the environment, and providers who are capable and able to be delegated to provide appropriate care for the client. However, the process does not stop with the delegation. The delegation of a responsibility must be based on this assessment and must be made to the correct person, with monitoring by the nurse, who maintains the accountability for the function. The NCSBN (1998) has further described the roles of clients, licensed nurses, and assistive personnel along a continuum of care consistent with Orem's theory of Nursing (p. 1). Nursing judgment plays a role in the entire process through the evaluation phase. Nursing judgment cannot be delegated.

In addition, the NCSBN (1997b) has identified five "rights" of delegation (Box 12–3). First, the *task* must be the right one for the client. The nurse must use clinical judgment, not merely assign a CNA a group of rooms for taking vital signs. The *circumstances* must be right for the particular client and his or her care needs—again a nursing judgment. The right *person* means the right person for the care activity, nurse, technician, or assistive personel. This person who will be delegated the care of the client must clearly understand what is involved with the care to be given (*direction*). Two-way communication skills are critical. The fifth right is the provision of the correct *supervision* and evaluation of the care and the person who was delegated to provide the care. Once again, supervision and evaluation require the use of nursing judgment.

And where is the client? Consider the patient fresh from surgery who has just arrived on the floor: The nurse first makes the assessment of the client to determine status and care needs. The nurse then decides what type of monitoring of vital signs is needed for the client's well-being. The assistive person has been trained to take vital signs and has demonstrated this skill (certified to perform it). But does this nurse know that the vital signs will be taken accurately and as directed; in other words, is this the right person for the job? If this assistive person is the correct person, then the nurse gives clear, understandable directions, including the reporting cycle back to the nurse for the nurse's clinical judgment. Along with this, the appropriate supervision and evaluation of the care given must be present.

BOX 12–3
THE FIVE RIGHTS OF DELEGATION

The RIGHT
- Task
- Circumstances
- Person
- Direction/Communication
- Supervision/Evaluation

From National Council of State Boards of Nursing. (1997b). The five rights of delegation. http://www.ncsbn.org

> *Delegation involves giving responsibility, but not abdicating the accountability for the task or activity.*

The manager's knowledge of his or her staff is critical to successful delegation. The education, experience, prior performance, willingness, and expertise of the person should be considered before appropriate delegation can occur. It is the responsibility of the delegator to make an adequate assessment, which should include how long the individual will need supervision and what type of supervision. Individual Nurse Practice Acts in some states provide specific language and requirements for appropriate delegation by nurses.

Errors can easily occur in delegating. Marquis and Huston (2003) describe three common errors in delegation: underdelegation, overdelegation, and improper delegation. Whether not enough, too much, or inappropriate delegation, such errors can jeopardize the client. The correct balance is the key. Delegation is necessary to provide effective patient care. The nurse must be the one involved with the clinical judgment for the client's well-being but cannot perform all tasks involved in this process. Delegation is an essential skill of the nurse. Delegation is one of the nine provisions in the Code of Ethics for Nurses (ANA, 2001) and, specific to nurse managers and executives in the interpretative statements, it is the manager's "responsibility to provide an environment that supports and facilitates appropriate assignment and delegation" (p. 17). This environment includes appropriate orientation, mentoring, and protections for clients. Once again, we have the core competencies for the nurse as providing client-centered care that is based on evidence of efficacy and quality improvement, provided in an interdisciplinary team, and communicated with the assistance of informatics. Delegation information and tools are included on the NCSBN public Web site to assist with application in a specific organizational setting and applicable state practice act and discussion and analysis of delegation concepts and process are ongoing and occurring in professional nursing organizations.

Change for the good of clients or the health-care industry can be a result of applying principles of management in health-care organizations. As we will see in the next chapter, professional nursing practice has an integral role in this process.

 ONLINE CONSULT

Access the Delegation Resource Folder of the National Council of State Boards of Nursing at
http://www.ncsbn.org
and the American Nurses Association at
http://www.nursingworld.org

Key Points

- An organization is simply an arrangement of human and material resources for some purpose, such as creating an institution or agency to meet a stated aim. Organizations can be viewed in terms of their structure, function, and people. A useful perspective for viewing the intricacies of a health-care organization is as a system affected by other systems and within the larger health-care and societal systems (environmental suprasystem).

- Kast and Rosenzweig (1985) regard organizations as open, sociotechnical systems that structure and integrate human activities around various technologies (p. 113). The organizational system in this model is further composed of five organizational subsystems: goals and values, technical, psychosocial, structural, and managerial. *(continued)*

(*continued*)

- Organizational structure is the design of the organization, including the type of hierarchy that tells us about positions or roles, responsibilities, status, channels of command or reporting relationships, and tasks to be accomplished. The major organizational structures are bureaucratic and organic (adhocratic).

- Centralized versus decentralized organizational structures involve the lines of control and decision-making within the organization. In centralization, the span of control or management is in the classic bureaucratic style, with governance from the top downward (vertical). Decentralization distributes authority downward in an organization, with decision-making and control at local levels.

- Organizations are also described according to the layers of differentiation for authority, decision-making, and coordination. Flat organizational structures have a wide base and few layers or tiers for decision-making and authority, whereas tall organizational structures have more tiers and lines of command, with less local decision-making at the lower levels.

- Organizational functions include goals and operations to fulfill the mission of the organization. Ideologic, formal, shared, and system goals demonstrate intent and consistency of behavior in organizations (Mintzberg, 1983a). Organizational operations include formalized activities defined by the structure as well as informal functions for daily accomplishment of the organization's goals.

- Management is the coordination of resources to achieve organizational outcomes and involves critical thinking, problem-solving, and decision-making. The most successful manager is one who can motivate individuals highly, enhancing their productivity, thus addressing organizational goals.

- From a focus on the organization and increasing productivity, humanistic theories of management emerged, including the classic motivational theories proposed by Maslow, McGregor, Herzberg, and Ouchi.

- Drucker (1998) proposes that management should focus on making individuals' "strengths effective and their weaknesses irrelevant" (p. 172).

- The organizational culture involves the culmination of the norms, attitudes, and values related to the organizational mission, accompanied by the expected behaviors of people.

- Communication in organizations depends on the channels, technology, purpose, and people. The organizational communication process can also be thought of as containing five "rights": (1) information or content, (2) communication channel, (3) format, including use of correct grammar, terms, and language, (4) level of understanding, and (5) technology.

- Power is the ability to effect change in people's behavior or in the organization. Legitimate power is the authority to effect change within one's position. Power bases are built on control of resources, technical skills, and a body of knowledge as well as exclusive rights and access to other people with power.

- Effective conflict resolution requires negotiation or coming to some compromise. This compromise is most effective when the end result is acceptable at some level to all parties involved.

- Delegation is the "transfer of responsibility of the performance of an activity from one individual to another while retaining the accountability of the outcome" (American Nurses Association, 1997, p. 3).

- The five "rights" of delegation are the right task, the right circumstances, the right person, the right direction or communication, and the right supervision or evaluation (NCSBN, 1997b).

Thought and Discussion Questions

1. Characterize the organization of the institution where you work. Describe the structure, functions, lines of decision-making, communication patterns, and sources of power relative to the organizational mission. Be prepared to participate in a discussion (online or in class) to be scheduled by your instructor.
2. Considering what you have learned from this chapter and the previous one, differentiate between management and leadership. Where do the two concepts overlap?
3. Interview a member of the administrative team from a large health-care facility on the various positions held by nurses. Describe their roles, changes that have occurred, areas of legitimate power, and the skills professional nurses need in this setting. Be prepared to participate in a discussion to be scheduled by your instructor.
4. Observe the start of a shift on a nursing unit. Describe the differences between assignment and delegation. Be prepared to participate in a discussion to be scheduled by your instructor.
5. Review the Chapter Thought located on the first page of the chapter, and discuss it in the context of the contents of the chapter.

 Interactive Exercises

1. Using the format provided on the Intranet site, examine the organizational structure and discuss the components as the various subsystem structures for a health-related organization where you work or practice.
2. Obtain a copy of the organizational chart from a health-care agency. Using the format provided on the Intranet site, describe the structure, functions, lines of decision-making, communication patterns, and sources of power as illustrated on the organizational chart.
3. Complete the exercise on Use of Management Theories located on the Intranet site. Describe how these theories can be applied to a nursing unit.
4. Locate the Web sites for small, state, and national-health related organizations. Using the format provided on the Intranet site, compare their stated purposes, missions, value statements, and functions. What can you identify about the various organizational cultures, structure, and management theories that prevail in these different organizations?
5. Examine the structure, functions, and culture of a for-profit organization and a not-for-profit organization in your community. Contrast the organizations.
6. Complete the exercise on the Intranet site on Negotiation for Power in Your Organization to describe the power bases and identify areas to negotiate for additional power in interdisciplinary practice.
7. Go to ***http://www.ncsbn.org*** to locate links to the different State Boards of Nursing. Compare the Practice Act for your state and an adjacent or Compact State on specific language and requirements for delegation by nurses.

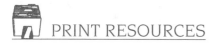
PRINT RESOURCES

References

American Nurses Association (ANA). (2001). Code of ethics for nurses with interpretive statements (Publication No. CEN21 10M 08/01). Washington, DC: American Nurses Publishing.

Bertalanffy, L. V. (1968). *General system theory: Foundations, development, applications.* New York: George Braziller.

Cox, T. (1993). Cultural diversity in organizations: Theory, research and practice. San Francisco: Berrett-Koehler.

Daft, R. L. (1998). *Organizational theory and design* (6th ed.). Cincinnati: South-Western College Publishing.

Dana, D. (2001). *Conflict resolution: Mediation tools for everyday worklife.* New York: McGraw-Hill.

Dienemann, J. A. (1998). Assessing organizations. In J. A. Dienemann (Ed.), *Nursing administration: Strategic perspectives and application* (2nd ed., pp. 267–283). Stamford, CT: Appleton & Lange.

Drucker, P. F. (1998). *Peter Drucker on the profession of management.* Boston: Harvard Business Review.

Drucker, P. F. (1974). *Management: Tasks, responsibilities, practices.* New York: Harper & Row.

Fayol, H. (1949). *General and industrial management* (C. Storrs, Trans.). London: Pittman & Sons.

Gebelein, S. H., Stevens, L. A., Skube, C. J., Lee, D. G., Davis, B. L., & Hellervik, L. W. (2000). *Successful manager's handbook: Development strategies for today's managers* (6th ed.). Minneapolis: Personnel Decisions International.

Grohar-Murray, M. E., & DiCroce, H. R. (2003). *Leadership and management in nursing* (3rd ed.). Upper Saddle River, NJ: Prentice-Hall.

Hall, R. H. (1999). *Organizations: Structures, processes, and outcomes* (7th ed.). Upper Saddle River, NJ: Prentice-Hall.

Herzberg, F. (1966). *Work and the nature of man.* Cleveland, OH: World Publishing.

Kast, F. E., & Rosenzweig, J. E. (1985). *Organization and management: A systems and contingency approach* (4th ed.). New York: McGraw-Hill.

Leininger, M. (2002). Cultures and tribes of nursing, hospitals, and the medical culture. In M. Leininger & M. R. McFarland, *Transcultural nursing: Concepts, theories, research, and practice* (3rd ed.) (pp. 181–204). New York: McGraw-Hill.

Marquis, B. L., & Huston, C. J. (2003). *Leadership roles and management functions in nursing: Theory and application* (4th ed.). Philadelphia: Lippincott Williams & Wilkins.

Maslow, A. H. (1970). *The farther reaches of the human mind.* New York: Viking Press.

Maslow, A. H. (1954). *Motivation and personality.* New York: Harper.

McGregor, D. (1967). *The professional manager.* New York: McGraw-Hill.

McGregor, D. (1960). *The human side of enterprise.* New York: McGraw-Hill.

Merton, R. K. (1957). *Social theory and social structure* (Rev. ed.). Glencoe, IL: Free Press.

Mintzberg, H. (1983a). *Power in and around organizations.* Englewood Cliffs, NJ: Prentice-Hall.

Mintzberg, H. (1983b). *Structures in fives: Designing effective organizations.* Englewood Cliffs, NJ: Prentice-Hall.

National Council of State Boards of Nursing (NCSBN). (2002). *Delegating effectively: Working through and with assistive personnel* (video). Chicago: Author.

Ouchi, W. G. (1981). *Theory Z: How American business can meet the Japanese challenge.* Reading, MA: Addison-Wesley.

Pettigrew, A., Ferlie, E., & McKee, L. (1992). *Shaping strategic change: Making change in large organizations.* London: Sage.

Tappen, R. M. (2001). *Nursing leadership and management: Concepts and practice* (4th ed.). Philadelphia: F.A. Davis.

Taylor, F. W. (1911). *The principles of scientific management.* New York: Harper & Row.

Weber, M. (1947). The fundamental concepts of sociology (A. M. Anderson & T. Parsons, Trans.). In T. Parsons (Ed.), *Max Weber: The theory of social and economic organization* (pp. 87–157). New York: Oxford University Press.

Bibliography

Drucker, P. F. (1967). *The effective executive.* New York: Harper & Row.

Locke, E. A. (1982). The ideas of Frederick W. Taylor: An evaluation. *Academy of Management Review,* 7(1), 14.

Mannering, K. (2001). *Managing difficult people: Effective management strategies for handling challenging behavior.* London: Oxford How to Books.

Marcus, L. J., Dorn, B. C., Kritek, P. B., Miller, V. G., & Wyatt, J. B. (1999). *Renegotiating health care: Resolving conflict to build collaboration.* San Francisco: Jossey-Bass.

Mintzberg, H. (1975). The manager's job: Folklore and fact. *Harvard Review,* 53, 49–61.

Spangle, M., & Isenhart, M. W. (2002). *Negotiation: Communication for diverse settings.* Thousand Oaks, CA: Sage.

Turniansky, B., & Hare, A. P. (1998). *Individuals in groups and organizations.* London: Sage.

Wywialowski, E. F. (2004). *Managing client care* (3rd ed.). St. Louis: Mosby.

Zimmermann, P. G. (2002). *Nursing management secrets: Questions and answers about nursing management.* Philadelphia: Hanley & Belfus.

Yoder-Wise, P. (2003). *Leading and managing in nursing* (3rd ed.). St. Louis: Mosby.

ONLINE RESOURCES

References

American Nurses Association. (1997a). Registered nurse education related to the utilization of unlicensed assistive personnel. *http://www.nursingworld.org/readroom/position/uap/uaprned.htm*.

American Nurses Association. (1997b). Registered nurse utilization of unlicensed assistive personnel. *http://www.nursingworld.org/readroom/position/uap/uapuse.htm*.

National Council of State Boards of Nursing. (1998). The continuum of care: a regulatory prespective. A resource paper for regulatory agencies. *http://www.ncsbn.org*

National Council of State Boards of Nursing. (1997a). Glossary—delegation terminology. *http://www.ncsbn.org*

National Council of State Boards of Nursing. (1997b). The five rights of delegation. *http://www.ncsbn.org*

National Council of State Boards of Nursing. (1997c). Role development: Critical components of delegation curriculum outline. *http://www.ncsbn.org*

Resources

Delegation Resource Folder. *http://www.ncsbn.org*

Peter F. Drucker. *http://www.peter-drucker.com*

Rose Kearney-Nunnery

13
chapter

Change

> We must always change, renew, rejuvenate ourselves; otherwise we harden.
>
> Johann von Goethe, 1749–1812

Chapter Objectives

On completion of this chapter, the reader will be able to:

1. Differentiate among the theories of change proposed by Lewin, Lippitt, Havelock, and Rogers.
2. Apply the stages of unfreezing, moving, and refreezing to a client situation for managed change.
3. Given a practice situation, describe the roles and characteristics of an effective change agent.
4. Discuss differences needed in the change process for use with individuals, families, and groups.
5. Describe the process and strategies for effective organizational change.

Key Terms

Change	Driving Forces	Internal Sources of Change
Planned Change	Unfreezing	External Sources of Change
Change Agents	Moving	
Restraining Forces	Refreezing	

Change is a part of normal daily life. We talk about changing our hair color, our attitude, someone else's mind, and so on. **Change** can be defined as a process that results in altered behavior of individuals or groups. It may be accidental or, as sometimes described, "change by drift" (Brooten et al., 1988). This type of accidental, spontaneous, or haphazard change is caused by outside forces. On the other hand, **planned change** involves conscious effort toward some goal as a deliberate and collaborative process. Change is an integral and essential component of professional nursing practice.

In today's world, change must be viewed as affecting both the individual and the group. One example of planned change would be an individual going on a diet. The result (the change) is an increase or decrease in weight. Such a change may also come about unintentionally, through outside influence. A family crisis or a normal bout of depression may lead to weight change. Or suppose the individual was eating chocolate. Gaining weight was not the intention—eating chocolate was—but weight gain was an unintended consequence. In contrast, as a planned change process, the same individual may have gone to Weight Watchers. Improved nutrition and eating practices also influence other family members through food selections and meal preparation in the home, and even may influence friends and colleagues through the individual's example.

Change is also a daily occurrence in society. Think about the number of times you have read or heard of global relations, changes in political forces, and changes in health-care organizations. And more people are beginning to embrace change since Johnson (2002) published his now classic *Who Moved My Cheese?* comparing the mice and the *Littlepeople* doing the simple things that can either work or immobilize the situation when things change. Still, making change is not an easy process for individuals or organizations.

In professional practice, we need to focus on the process of planned change, being proactive rather than reactive. Planned changes for persons or groups in the environment require structural shifts in an environmental system for improved functioning. Improved functioning involves new (changed) behaviors, attitudes, and relationships. Professional nurses are the **change agents** for people and health. Their role is to move for needed, planned change for individuals, families, community groups, and society. Such practice should occur in individual practice as well as on an organizational level.

THEORIES OF CHANGE

Understanding the theories of change applicable to individuals, families, groups, and society is the first step in moving from being reactive to unintended change to becoming proactive in creating positive, planned change.

Chinn and Benne (1976) described major groups of change strategies of three philosophies: (1) the empirical-rational nature of man, (2) normative-educative philosophy, based on human motivation and norms (attitudes, values, skills, and relationships), and (3) power-coercive philosophy, based on leadership and the application of power (p. 23). The change models of Havelock and Rogers reflect the empirical-rational philosophy, whereas the normative-educative philosophy guides the models developed by Lewin and Lippitt (Chinn & Benne, 1976). These two philosophical orientations are consistent with the metaparadigm nursing concepts of person, environment, health, and nursing, focused on the nature of the person or the group in the context of the environment.

Lewin

The classic change theorist was Kurt Lewin. Lewin (1951), who developed a model based on his Field Theory, a method of analyzing causal relationships and building the scientific constructs for change (p. 45). The mathematical model in his theory merely indicates that human behavior is based on the person (or group) and his or her environment at that point in time. Lewin (1951) focused on social change, pointing out that "group life is never without change, merely differences in amount and type of change exist" (p. 199). In groups and organizations, multiple influences from individuals and their reactions to the environment cause group behaviors and norms. This Field Theory proposes that the status quo, or a state of equilibrium, is maintained when restraining forces and driving forces balance each other. To achieve change, the restraining forces must be weakened and the driving forces strengthened. Consider the illustration of change in FIG. 13–1.

Restraining forces in society resist change; they include norms, values, relations among people, morals, fears, perceived threats, and regulations. In essence, these restraining forces are the "old guard" that maintains the status quo. **Driving forces,** on the other hand, support change and include the desire to please or the desire for more novel, effective, or efficient, or merely different activities. System imbalance becomes the impetus for change. The process involves weakening the restraining forces and strengthening the driving forces. To do this, Lewin proposes three aspects of permanent change: unfreezing, moving, and refreezing of group standards.

Unfreezing involves disequilibrium, discontent, and uneasiness. Lewin (1951) states that "to break open the shell of complacency and self-righteousness it is sometimes necessary to bring about deliberately an emotional stir-up" (p. 229). The restraining and driving forces are identified, and comparisons are drawn between the ideal and the actual situation. To bring about change, participants are prepared for change (unfreezing) to make the need for change apparent and accepted. In many situations, making individuals uneasy and discontented with the environmental system is the initial step in the process. Malcontents want change, whereas individuals who are satisfied and comfortable with the current state of affairs resist changes that will create unequilibrium. Activities are centered on unfreezing the existing equilibrium.

Moving occurs when the previous structure is rearranged and realistic goals are set. The system is moved to a new level of equilibrium. Choices must be made about accepting the change agent and the roles of the group members in the change process. At this stage, group decisions are preferable for moving toward permanent change. This represents the distribution of power among the group members to make them driving forces

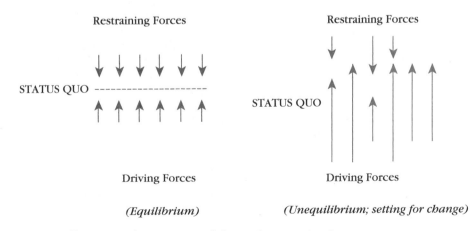

FIG. 13–1. Illustration of restraining and driving forces in the change process.

engaged in the process. The individual involved in the change process acts as a member of a group in which new social values and norms are being established.

A new status quo is established with **refreezing.** Lewin called this originally the "freezing" stage, but "refreezing" better describes the new level of equilibrium and reinforcement needed for the new patterns of behavior. The focus is on maintaining the goal achieved and highlighting the present benefits over past practices.

Consider Lewin's model with a client population. The individual with heart disease who is started on a low-salt, low-fat diet has a teaching need to bring permanent change to his diet. You discover through interviews with the client and family members that the diet at home is highly seasoned and high in animal protein and fats. *Restraining forces* in this situation are cultural values, family traditions, individual and group (family) preferences in food selection and preparation, attitudes toward diet, foods, or food preparation, fears of further illness with changes in diet, and attitudes toward restrictions on personal lifestyle.

Now consider each of these factors in relation to all members of the household and the client's work, recreation, and social environments. Think about the *driving forces:* fear of further illness without the dietary changes, respect for advice given, support network, educational presentations, role models, and so forth. *Unfreezing* involves the identification of the restraining and driving forces, motivating the client toward change, and assessing readiness for teaching. *Moving* consists of supporting a positive attitude toward change and providing nutritional information, including food selection, preparation, and presentation options.

This is a time of goal-setting with the client to bring changes that must occur after discharge, through a rehabilitation program, and lifelong. Valuable nursing theories to support nursing actions include King's Theory of Goal Attainment and Orem's Self-Care Agency. Supporting attitudinal and behavioral changes could occur through follow-up telephone or e-mail service after discharge or interviews at clinic appointments. *Refreezing* would occur with the client's stabilization,

evidenced through subjective reports (e.g., food diary), objective observations (e.g., health assessment), and laboratory findings in the rehabilitation phase. A similar application could be developed for group change using Lewin's Field Theory or the Health Belief Model.

Lippitt

As an outgrowth and expansion of Lewin's theory, Lippitt (1973) pointed out "if we want to understand, explain, or predict change in human behavior, we need to take into account the person and his environment" (p. 3). He identified several complex factors of human behavior that must be considered: motivation, multiple causation, and overrationalized habits. Looking at both individual and organizational change, he further focused on the change agent and defined seven specific phases (Figure 13–2) within an idea, similar to Lewin's change model. Thus, Lippitt described more specific activities that are still applicable to the three steps of unfreezing, moving, and refreezing.

Unfreezing

First, there is the need to collect data *and diagnose the problem* and the key people. The driving and restraining people, environmental, and organizational forces are identified, defined, and targeted. Second, the *motivation and resources* are assessed to identify the desire and capacity for change. This includes resistance and readiness of the people in the environment. In the third step, the *change agent's motivation,* commitment and resources must

7. Terminating the Relationship
6. Maintaining the Change
5. Choosing the Change Agent's Role
4. Selecting Change Objectives
3. Change Agent's Motivation and Resources
2. Assessment of Motivation and Capacity for Change
1. Diagnosis of Problem

FIG. 13–2. Lippitt's (1973) seven stages of planned change.

be assessed for the potential success of the change activity. The skills, efforts, and responsibilities are critical planning pieces in this phase of change.

Moving

Initially, *change objectives* must be selected with consideration of activities for progressive change. Lippitt uses the leverage point concept as the starting point at which receptivity for change is apparent and the objectives are initiated. Planning and evaluation are primary activities in this step. Then, following the development of an action plan with evaluation criteria, the *change agent and group roles* are selected and assigned. Acceptance and selection of an appropriate role is critical in defining the power, outcomes, and strategies of the change agent.

Refreezing

Maintaining the change occurs through ongoing training, communication, and support of the people in the environment. Communication by both driving and restraining forces advertises the success of the change using actual evaluation results. In many cases, the loudest and most visible of the restraining forces become the change agent's greatest supporters when they accept the merits of the process with evaluation. How many times have you heard someone say, "I never thought it could be done but...." or "I was behind that all along but I did not want to show it"? Finally, *terminating the helping relationship* is necessary on the part of the change agent and major players for the change to become part of the people and the environment, and not just the activity of a select individual or group. Rather, it becomes the new norm of the people or the organization.

Role of Change Agent

A major piece of Lippitt's (1973) model involves the roles for the professional change agent. He proposed four major roles for the change agent:

- Specialist
- Coordinator
- Fact finder and information link
- Consultant

Lippitt views the selection of the appropriate role for the change agent as essential in the moving phase of change. As a *specialist,* the change agent is the expert in the environment on methods and strategies for change. As a *coordinator,* the change agent functions as manager, planning, organizing, and coordinating efforts and programs for the change. The change agent as a *fact finder and information link* serves as a seeker, clarifier, synthesizer, reality-tester, and provider of information as well as a communications link among all participants in the system (Lippitt, 1973, pp. 60–61).

The consultant role is viewed as the most important role for the change agent, both inside the system and with external individuals, groups, and environments. In fact, as FIG. 13–3 illustrates, Lippitt (1973) developed a model of eight specific activity roles within this consultant role, which are viewed along a continuum from advocate through expert, trainer, alternative identifier, collaborator, process specialist, fact finder, to reflector (p. 63). The correct role for the change agent depends on the people, the environment, and how much direction is needed from the agent to implement the change. As the advocate, the change agent as consultant is highly directive in leading the group toward change. Conversely, the change agent is the least directive as a reflector, helping the group clarify and evaluate their efforts. The change agent must have knowledge, skill, and perseverance in the work-intensive process of change.

Consider, again, our example of the client who must change to a low-salt, low-fat diet. Under Lippitt's model, first, you need to collect data on meals, food preferences, and preparation at home. You identify, define, and target the environmental forces—family, friends, cultural, and collegial (work or recreational) forces. Second, you assess the motivation, resistance, readiness, and resources of the client and his family to identify the desire and capacity for change in dietary habits. In the third step, your motivation, commitment,

DIRECTIVE CONSULTATION							
Position 1	Position 2	Position 3	Position 4	Position 5	Position 6	Position 7	Position 8
Advocate	Expert	Trainer	Alternative Identifier	Collaborator	Process Specialist	Fact Finder	Reflector
Persuades client as to proper approach	Gives expert advice to client	Develops training experiences to aid client	Provides alternative to client	Joins in problem solving	Assists client in problem-solving process	Serves to help client collect data	Serves as a catalytic agent for client in solving the problem

NONDIRECTIVE CONSULTATION

FIG. 13–3. Multiple consulting approaches of a change agent. (From Lippitt, G. L. [1973]. *Visualizing change: Model building and the change process.* La Jolla, CA: University Associates; adapted from Lippitt, G. L., & Nadler, L. [August 1967]. Emerging roles of the training director. *Training and Development Journal, 9.* (pp 2–10). Permission granted by The Gordon Lippitt Foundation, Bethesda, Maryland.)

and resources must be realized as the nurse–change agent. Your skills, efforts, and responsibilities are critical in this planning phase. Lippitt's concept of leverage point occurs when the client and his family are receptive for change and the action plan is initiated with evaluation criteria. Your role as change agent is defined specific to the client and his needs. Consider the applicability of Orem's three modes of nursing, especially the supportive-educative mode, in relation to his continuum of consultant activities. Your role as change agent may alter rapidly as the client moves from the hospital setting to the home and clinic settings. Empowerment of the client and his significant others is critical for success in this type of change. And with the maintenance of the change in diet and health status that occurs through ongoing training in dietary management, communication, support, and reinforcement during the follow-up period, the client and family are moved into the termination phase, when the helping relationship is no longer necessary and the dietary changes have become part of the person and family in their environment.

Havelock

Havelock (1971) used a system and process model to depict an organization with the following major concepts: role, linkages, and communication for transfer and use of knowledge. Using the three major perspectives of problem-solving, research-development-diffusion, and social interaction, Havelock further examined the linkage process to view the broader system (Havelock & Havelock, 1973).

Building on Lewin's stages of change, Havelock added steps to the three stages, highlighting communication and interpersonal activities in these steps:

• Perception of need
• Diagnosis of the problem
• Identification of the problem
• Devising a plan of action
• Gaining acceptance of the plan
• Stabilization
• Self-renewal (Havelock & Havelock, 1973)

Unfreezing

The *perception of a need* for a change in the system is followed by *diagnosis and identification of the problem.* At this time, a reciprocal relationship develops between the user (client) system and a resource system. Linkages with needed resources are made in this initial stage before moving on the change . Havelock and Havelock (1973) stress that the problem-solver must be "meaningfully linked to outside resources" (p. 23).

Moving

Movement toward change in step 2 requires *devising a plan of action* and *gaining acceptance* of the plan in the system. This is a stage of searching for a solution and applying that solution to the identified problem, using resource linkages in the environment.

Refreezing

In the final step, refreezing, stabilization and the need for self-renewal are specified. First, *stabilization* in the system is specified to sustain change (refreezing). Havelock describes *self-renewal* as being needed to sustain the client system in the future. In essence, the values, goals, and activities of the system become the norm.

Role of Change Agent

The importance of and roles for the change agent are also a key component of Havelock's model, which lists four roles for the change agent:

- Catalyst
- Solution giver
- Process helper
- Resource linker (Havelock & Havelock, 1973, p. 60)

These roles become increasingly complex. The catalyst serves as the impetus for change to the resource linker, who brings people, environments, and resources together at the subsystem, system, and macrosystem levels (Havelock & Havelock, 1973, pp. 60–64). For effective functioning within these roles, Havelock further developed a training program for preparing effective change agents.

Havelock's model can also be used with the example of dietary change for our client with heart disease. Communication and interpersonal activities are core ingredients in the nurse–client relationship. Identifying the need for altering dietary salt and fat relates to the client's medical condition. The personal, environmental, social, cultural, and dietary habits are assessed through interview, to define the problem. A reciprocal relationship between the client system and a resource system occurs through linkages, including meeting with a nutritionist for food selection and preparation options. Informational lists on cookbooks, restaurants, and community associations advocating healthy eating with low-fat, low-salt meals are provided. Using this model, the nurse encourages linkages with outside resources such as the American Heart Association, American Association of Critical Care Nurses, and collegial relationships with nutritionists, rehabilitation specialists, and cardiologists. The plan for dietary change is devised in collaboration with the client system and includes linkages with community resources acceptable to the client and his family. Recall the concept of cultural competence and how it is necessary in this model. Linkages must be retained with the client after discharge, in the home, clinic, or rehabilitation setting. This follow-up is necessary for stabilizing the diet, given the client's physiologic and psychosocial system influences. The role of the nurse–change agent has moved from catalyst and solution giver in the initial phase of problem identification, to process helper in the planning phase, and then to resource linker. The changes in diet must become a part of the client's value system. The nurse–change agent then terminates the relationship with the client while linkages with external resources provide the client with self-renewal.

Rogers

As an outgrowth of the change model, Rogers developed the Diffusion of Innovations model. In 1971, Rogers and Shoemaker stated the following:

> Although it is true that we live more than ever before in an era of change, prevailing social structures often serve to hamper the diffusion of innovations. Our activities in education, agriculture,

medicine, industry, and the like are often without the benefit of the most current research knowledge. The gap between what is actually known and what is effectively put to use needs to be closed. (p. 1)

This is no less true today, more than 30 years later. We live in a time of even greater social change. Our information superhighways can be timelier in the transfer of information, but we must understand the innovations adopted to bridge this gap. This model was used in nursing in the 1980s to promote research-based practice and is quite appropriate today with the need for evidence-based practice.

Rogers and Shoemaker (1971) focus on communication and view *change* as the effects of a new idea or innovation being adopted and put into use or rejected. Change may occur at the level of the individual, group, organization, or society. The model was first proposed with four major steps in the process of social change: knowledge, persuasion, decision, and confirmation (Rogers & Shoemaker, 1971, p. 25). Rogers (1983) then extended the Innovation-Diffusion process to five stages:

- Knowledge
- Persuasion
- Decision
- Implementation
- Confirmation

The interest and commitment of key people and policy-makers are critical in this model.

Unfreezing

Developing a sequence of knowledge, persuasion, and decision-making is the key activity in the unfreezing stage. To *develop knowledge*, key people and policy makers are introduced to the innovation to gain understanding. Then comes *persuasion* to develop attitudes on the innovation. Rogers (1983) uses persuasion to focus on the individual whose attitudes change, either positively or negatively toward the innovation, not on the external force that changes one's mind. The *decision* to adopt or reject an innovation is the bridge between the unfreezing and moving stages in Roger's model.

Moving

Implementation applies to the stage of moving. Revisions, potential adoption, or rejection of the innovation occurs in this implementation phase.

Refreezing

Roger's fifth step, when the innovation changes from being novel to being part of the routine or norm, involves refreezing the equilibrium. He calls this step *confirmation*, in which reinforcement is sought and the key people and policy-makers decide to maintain or discontinue the innovation. Rogers (1983) admits that the research evidence shows no clear distinction between the implementation and confirmation steps. This may be related to the idea of a flexible time span between implementation and confirmation, when the process of refreezing for the innovation occurs. Rogers (1983) describes this final confirmatory stage as "routinization" of the innovation.

Throughout the entire process, five attributes determine the rate of adoption of an innovation by members of a social system:

- Relative advantage
- Compatibility
- Complexity
- Trialability
- Observability (Rogers & Shoemaker, 1971, p. 39; Rogers, 1983, pp. 238–240).

These attributes should be included in all evaluation plans and data on the change. Relative advantage is determined through comparison of the innovation with what was done in the past. The advantage may be effectiveness as well as efficiency, and the process has been described as weighing economic advantages or the cost-effectiveness. Compatibility with the values, beliefs, and needs of the group is the second factor. The complexity (difficulty in use), trialability (experimental trials), and observability (visible evidence) are all considered in the implementation stage and have a direct effect on adoption, revision, or discontinuation of an innovation.

Role of Change Agent

Rogers's model also highlights the roles of the change agent, which occur in the following sequence:

1. Develops the need for change
2. Establishes the relationship with the client system
3. Diagnoses the problems
4. Motivates the client system for change
5. Translates intent for change into the actions needed
6. Stabilizes change in system and "freezes" new behavior
7. Terminates the relationship (Rogers, 1983, pp. 315–317)

Like Lippitt, Rogers views the change agent as a professional, skilled in change for effective functioning in the role.

We take a slightly different approach with the application of Rogers' Innovation-Diffusion process model to our example of the client who needs to change his diet. You have found research studies on effective dietary compliance in cardiac rehabilitation. You now wish to bring this innovation into practice in your organization to use in client teaching programs. During the initial development of knowledge, key people and policy makers in nursing service and cardiology are introduced to the teaching program content and methods, along with the results from use with clients in other settings. Next, you need to persuade people of the effectiveness and applicability of this approach—the organization and its resources as well as the client population. The decision to adopt or reject the new teaching program is made. If it is decided to try the teaching program with a client population, the phase of implementation is entered. The teaching program may be revised, adopted, or rejected on the basis of its specificity and acceptability to the client group and the organization. If the teaching program is found to be applicable and advantageous, it is "confirmed" as the agency procedure or organizational norm. If the procedure is not adopted, the key people and policy-makers must confirm the decision to discontinue the program. These are the steps toward implementing

evidence-based practice at the organizational level.

Choosing a Model

The four models of change are summarized in Table 13–1. Selecting an appropriate model to guide practice involves how you look at the world and what is most helpful in driving your skills as an agent in the change process. Moving from the theoretical stages of change to strategies for change brings the focus to the change agent.

 CHANGE AGENTS

Our second step in becoming a major player in the change process is to develop greater understanding of the roles and attributes of a successful change agent. We have seen the importance of the change agent emerge in the models of Lippitt, Havelock, and Rogers. Table 13–2 summarizes the roles and activities of the change agent in these models. In Lewin's original model, change in humans is a function of the person and his or her environment at that point in time. Consider the roles of the change agent in the three general phases of change.

Unfreezing

Good interpersonal and assessment skills are needed to acquire data to weaken restraining forces and enhance driving forces in the present system, and both internal and external system forces must be considered. The change agent must then establish a climate that encourages and supports change. Needs assessment, diagnosis, and establishment of a professional relationship have consistently occurred during the unfreezing phase in all models. Now consider the similarity of this stage to the assessment and diagnosis activities of the nursing process.

In the nursing process, health assessment data are collected and problems are identified. Assessing the client's characteristics and current level of satisfaction with the health prob-

TABLE 13–1
Comparison of the Stages of Change Represented in Theoretical Models

Theorist	Stages						
Lewin (1951) Force Field	[1] Unfreezing	[2] Moving	[3] Refreezing				
Lippitt (1973) Planned Change	[1] Diagnosis of problem	[2] Assessment of motivation and capacity for change	[3] Change agent's motivation and resources	[4] Selecting change objectives	[5] Choosing change agent's role	[6] Maintaining the change	[7] Terminating the relation- ship
Havelock (1971) Linkages	[1] Perception of need	[2] Diagnosis of the problem	[3] Identification of the problem	[4] Devising a plan of action	[5] Gaining acceptance of plan	[6] Stabilization	[7] Self-renewal
Rogers (1983) Innovation- Diffusion	[1] Knowledge	[2] Persuasion	[3] Decision	[4] Implementation	[5] Confirmation		

TABLE 13–2.
Comparing the Roles for the Change Agent from the Different Theoretical Models

Stages of Change	Lippitt (1973)	Havelock (1973)	Rogers (1983)
Unfreezing	A specialist in the diagnosis and assessment of client system and change agent as: • Information seeker • Clarifier • Synthesizer • Reality-tester • Provider • Problem-solver	A catalyst in the identification of needs, diagnoses, and all aspects of the problem within the roles of: • Clarifier • Synthesizer • Reality-tester • Provider • Problem-solver	Range of roles from support to consultant for sharing knowledge, building persuasiveness, and leading the group toward decision making on the innovation through activities of: • Needs identification • Establishment of professional relationship with client system • Diagnosis of problems • Motivation of client system
Moving	Communication link viewed within one of eight directive toward nondirective consultative roles: • Advocate • Expert • Trainer • Alternative identifier • Collaborator • Process specialist • Fact-finder • Reflector	Solution giver and process helper as: • Clarifier • Synthesizer • Reality-tester • Provider • Problem-solver	Range of roles from support to consultant to translate intent for change into the actions needed
Refreezing	Consultation for: • Maintenance of the change • Termination of the relationship	Resource linker for stabilization and self-renewal as: • Clarifier • Synthesizer • Reality-tester • Problem-solver	Range of roles from support to consultant for: • Confirmation of change and stabilizing the adoption to prevent discontinuance and reinforce new behaviors • Termination of relationship

lem or condition is an essential component of this activity. Diagnostic statements are developed after needs identification. Asking questions and diagnosing the problem for changed client behaviors or responses, then, lead to the planning stage of the nursing process.

Moving

The change agent must help the client group set and strive for clear, realistic goals. A good deal of the change agent's time and energy is needed during this phase for strategies to deal with those who are resisting change. Again, interpersonal and motivational skills are critical. The change agent must constantly assess and evaluate resistance, conflict, and motivation in the client system and must maintain movement toward the goals and objectives of change.

As in the nursing process, the major activities of the moving stage are implementing plans, goals, and objectives and collecting evaluation data. Client data are analyzed, interpreted, and acted on. The nurse actively uses critical thinking, decision-making, interpersonal, and evaluation skills. The same skills are necessary to move toward change. This stage will probably be the most comfortable for the nurse functioning as a change agent, because skills in this area are developed through nursing practice.

Refreezing

Providing rewards and reinforcement for the change is a major part of the change agent's role in the third stage. Evaluation data for reinforcement of change must be used as supportive evidence. Activities for the change agent during this stage are supportive, initially, but involvement decreases with the need to terminate and have the client system totally involved in and responsible for the change without external intervention from the change agent.

In the nursing process, the nurse-client relationship is terminated when objectives are achieved and nursing diagnoses are resolved. The nurse has prepared the person or family

for this termination long before discharge orders are written or the person leaves the agency environment. Just as discharge planning starts with admission, this last stage must be planned for and worked toward during the entire change process, with the person, family, or group taking increasing responsibility for the new behaviors.

The interventions of a skilled change agent can make all the difference in the planned change process. Corey (1976) emphasized the concepts of enabling, understanding, and action, stating that "to be an effective change agent therefore, I should strive to enable myself and others to recognize forces in the environment, to understand the consequences of intervening among those forces, and to provide the necessary support to take planned action" (p. 273). More specifically, the skills of change agents include the following:

- Vision for the future and creativity
- Ability to look at a situation narrowly and broadly (assessment and critical thinking skills)
- Good interpersonal skills, including those of communication, motivation, assertiveness, problem-solving, and group process
- Flexibility and a willingness to consider alternative views
- Perseverance and a positive attitude
- Integrity and commitment
- Ability to manage conflict and resistance

CHANGE IN INDIVIDUALS, FAMILIES, AND GROUPS

As noted earlier, Chinn and Benne (1976) categorized change strategies into three major types: empirical-rational, normative-reeducative, and power-coercive. Power-coercive strategies are based on the application of power by legitimate authority. Nursing concerns are with the person or group and their empowerment for healthy behaviors or the creation of optimal health status. Applying power as "the authority" is inconsistent with empowering people. One can alter practices, procedures, or the environment in organizations as a coercive change, by imposing major policy, but think of the upheaval this change creates. Coercive change may be necessary in an emergency situation or when the person or family must have major assistance. The problem is that the change may not persist unless the person or group has internalized it into their value system.

The philosophical basis of nursing is consistent with the empirical-rational or the normative-reeducative strategies for change. The empirical-rational strategy assumes that people are rational and have a self-interest in change. Power for the individual or group occurs through knowledge. The normative-reeducative approach is based on social norms and the person's interaction with the environment. The normative-reeducative philosophy can be viewed as empowerment with an emphasis on interpersonal skills. Both of these philosophical orientations are consistent with nursing, but their applicability differs according to the nursing model selected for practice. For example, King's Theory of Goal Attainment, Orem's General Theory of Nursing, and Roy's Adaptation Model contain philosophical assumptions similar to the nonnative reeducative strategies, with the person viewed as a thinking, feeling, reacting being in the context of his or her environment.

Because nursing looks at both the person and interactions within the environment, several factors must be considered. These include resistance to change, empowerment or involvement of the client, and environmental, cultural, or situational factors.

A major concern of the change agent is the person's or group's resistance to change. To handle this resistance, one must evaluate what makes people resist change. People are naturally threatened by change. Change involves the loss of "near and dears" held by a person or a group. It is a threat to their value system and a loss of the comfortable status quo. They feel vulnerable and insecure. Stress is created and must be managed. The need for or the activities involved in change may also be mistrusted or misunderstood. Another innately human characteristic is the fear of failure or being unable to perform the new activities or tasks. This creates more stress.

Resistance to change can be reduced by several techniques:

- Careful planning
- Allowing sufficient time
- Support and reinforcement
- Involving the person or group

Understanding the full impact of individual or group norms and planning for a change in attitudes can lead to changes in behavior. Recall the adage, "Fools rush in." Allowing sufficient time for the change to occur and persist is essential. A gradual move toward change is more effective than a radical move. The time needed depends on the physical, psychosocial, cultural, and attitudinal characteristics of the individual or group. Patience, persistence, perseverance, and creativity are essential traits of the change agent. Another strategy for decreasing resistance to change is good communication with key and resource people throughout the entire process. In addition, a good deal of support and reinforcement will be needed. This requires excellent interpersonal skills, verbal and nonverbal, with both individuals and groups.

The involvement of the person or group is needed for lasting change. It is essential to build on their readiness, motivation, self-concept, abilities, and resources throughout the process. Involving people in planning and decision-making both reduces resistance to change and creates empowerment. Strategies for involving people include education, training, socialization and persuasion (not imposing), and facilitation. It would often be easier to make the change yourself as an external force, but the action by the client system is slower and more enduring. Note that education and training involve enlightenment and preparation rather than preaching. This creates the empowerment and sets the stage for a revision of the norm or value system.

Looking at the situation or environment is critical in the change process. First, one must understand the past or the personal history of the individual, family, or group. You include a past, personal, psychosocial, family, and environmental history in a health history. These are important basic items of information to obtain before doing the physical appraisal in any health assessment. The same thing is needed in the change process. The following questions will help in understanding the situation and people:

1. What types of change has the person or group faced in the past? Information on experience and success with change is valuable to determine whether this person is a novice with change, has embraced change throughout life, or falls somewhere between these experiential extremes.
2. How has the person or group handled change? Stress and coping factors will emerge with this information. You can then discover how to best motivate and support behaviors.
3. What resources have been available or used in previous change activities?
4. What is the person's or group's perspective on the applicability of the resources in the environment to the present situation? Human resources are included as support systems, which can be family, friends, colleagues, clergy, professionals, and even "ideal" role models. These resources may still help the person or group. If these are not available or appropriate, linking the person or group with similar resources may be effective. Remember, some people do well in support groups whereas others need more individualized support.

ORGANIZATIONAL CHANGE

To broaden the perspective from the individual, family, and community, we move to organizational change. Although organizations such as many small to medium-sized hospitals may operate as communities, both internal and external influences in contemporary health care are major considerations. Everyone within an organization has faced organizational change, from minor changes in policy to restructuring of services. Many have experienced or know a colleague who experienced a radical reorganization, with restructuring and managerial shifts, layoffs, or ownership changes. With organizational change come tension and conflict as a natural function of stress on the system, its people, and their daily activities and interactions.

Systems theory provides a useful perspective for viewing the internal and external forces of any organization. A health-care institution or agency is an open environmental system with great complexity. The organization must be considered in terms of the system with its component subsystems, as well as the macrosystem and client system. **Internal influences** come from agency administrative, policy, and operational factors guiding the system. The surrounding environmental system of the organization is the health-care arena, which provides the professional, specialization, reimbursement, and additional value structures for the organizational unit and its members. The broader social or macroenvironment reflects societal norms and values through the needs and potential needs of consumers of health care. Linkages among all system parts are assumed as necessary for effectiveness and continuity. But look further at this complex system and the internal environment.

When change is proposed for an agency or institutional system, an in-depth look at the organizational environment is needed. Recall that Kast and Rosenzweig (1979) view organizations as open, sociotechnical systems composed of five subsystems (see Chapter 12). Internal sources of change can arise from any one or some combination of these five subsystems. Consider the traditional health-care agency, the hospital. The subsystems and their associated internal forces can be described as follows:

- *Goals and values* for health care are specified for an organization as a purpose, philosophy, vision, or mission statement. Valuable information on the internal forces is apparent with this organizational view of people, health, and health care before translation into departmental or policy statements. Insight can also be obtained from the historical documents on how the institution evolved into a modem health-care organization.
- The *technical subsystem* represents the knowledge and skills of the health-care providers and physical resources in the system. Consider internal forces from the specific equipment, services, and expertise of

professional and nonprofessional labor forces in the organizational setting.

- Interpersonal and interdisciplinary relationships are a component of the *psychosocial subsystem,* with role relationships, attitudes, and values of people and groups within the system. Nurses are expected to exhibit behaviors related to the roles of health-care provider, manager, teacher, researcher, and advocate and to collaborate with members of other health-care disciplines. Direction of assistive personnel is another important aspect of this subsystem.
- The *structural subsystem* is the organizational design to provide health-care services. In addition to organizational charts, position descriptions, and policy and procedure manuals, informal sources, such as technical and clerical staff, can provide valuable information on the organization's daily operations to illustrate how tasks are accomplished in the organization.
- The *managerial subsystem* consists of the governing board and corporate officers. This organizational governance may include paid or volunteer board members, required institutional review boards, and the chief executive team or officers.

External environmental influences are the next factors to consider in terms of impact on the system and its subsystems. **External forces** include inputs of energy, information, and materials received from the environment, transformed, and returned to the environment as outputs. One input into the hospital environment is the client system. The client enters the hospital with a health-care deficit and, through the care received while hospitalized (throughput), strives for a higher level of wellness as the intended outcome (output). But environmental influences add more complexity. External forces are the broader environment providing inputs into the system. As with any open system, however, the external forces affect internal operations, and an exchange of information is returned to the environment as outputs.

External forces have a major impact on the function of the traditional hospital. Suppliers to be considered include physicians, drug and equipment companies, volunteers, and edu-cational facilities. Physicians supply patients. Drug and equipment companies compete for contracts, and organizations seek purchasing power with consortia or multiorganizational contracts. Volunteers provide valuable unsalaried transportation, recreational, and interpersonal services without which many hospitals could not survive. Educational suppliers provide additional health-care services in the present, with trainees as residents, interns, nurses, therapists, and other preparers of ancillary personnel, as well as the future workforce. In addition, new staff members bring different ideas and methods into the system.

Customers are generally thought of as the client system: in-patients, same-day surgery clients, and clinic clients. But the concept of customer can be seen more broadly to include community initiatives, educational programming, health contracts with business and industry, health maintenance organizations (HMOs), and physician practice groups. Large corporate entities, intraorganizational agreements, health insurers, and second- and third-party payers are major service and economic influences on the client system. Federal legislation, state laws, local ordinances, regulatory bodies, court precedents, insurers, and professional organizations all have a legal effect on the hospital.

On a broader, macrosystem level, consider changes predicted for the population. The increase in the elderly population, especially frail elders, has a great impact on services that will be needed. The national, state, and local economies, with their associated concerns about costs, are other societal factors that have a profound effect on hospitals and health-care organizations. All these factors, individually and combined, influence how the hospital markets and cares for its customers and personnel and meets their organizational mandates and mission.

But let us return to the change process and activities in the phases of unfreezing, moving, and refreezing. During *unfreezing,* the major change activities include assessment, diagnosis, and establishment of a professional relationship. Assessment must involve in-depth analysis and synthesis of both internal and external forces. As with individuals, families, and groups, methods for data collection include interviews and observation. But with a larger group of people, methods can include questionnaires or surveys for timely and, at times, confidential collection of data.

Like the past and personal change history obtained on a smaller scale with the person, family, or group, an organizational history provides valuable insights. The organizational history can reveal information on development and problem resolution to this point. Methods for gathering an organizational history require not only skillful interviewing of key people but also a careful review of records and documents of the organization.

Consider all environments, including the constraints, demands, and opportunities present. Resources in the environment, people and physical resources, provide major influences on any organizational change. Identifying the driving forces and individuals in the system is essential to building a base of support. Analyze external environments, especially population trends.

Diagnosis of problems becomes more complex as the volume of information and number of people increase. Whether the change agent is selected from within the organization or is an external consultant, he or she will need a high level of skill to achieve organizational change. Clear understanding of both internal and external forces will be necessary, along with a good deal of fortitude to survive the experience.

The *moving* phase in organizational change involves developing strategies to match resources with constraints, demands, opportunities, and history as part of the planning process for change to proceed. Changes in goals and values must be reflected in organizational documents. Key work groups will be needed for decision-making and policy formation. The technical subsystem will need training and educational programs to transmit knowledge of resources and to refine skills. A great deal of time and energy will be needed for the people. The psychosocial subsystem with role and status relations will require finesse and great sensitivity. Relating to the variable and altering readiness, resistance, and motivation of many individuals and groups will be quite a challenge.

People must be actively incorporated and empowered in this decision-making and implementation phase. Involvement of people in the organizational change process necessitates use of excellent leadership and skills in group dynamics, conflict management, and team building. This is especially true when the structural subsystem (how the work is accomplished) has undergone major revisions. Communication links with the managerial subsystem must be increased and reinforced as organizational members are included rather than alienated from key planners and controllers in the system. Minimizing people's stress and turmoil is a major function of the change agent in this phase.

A formalized evaluation plan must be in place and must be initiated in this moving phase. Data collection and feedback on the process communicating even small results are vital and must be ongoing. People in the system need to be continually aware of the result of their efforts. If indicated in the evaluation data, additional resources or linkages must be sought. This is the feedback loop that continues through the phase of refreezing and is essential to any successful organizational change. Evaluation data must be systematically recorded, analyzed, interpreted, and communicated. Evaluation data can be communicated through distribution of short reports, articles, or observations from various sources in newsletters and on bulletin boards, electronically, and in formal and informal discussion groups. Keeping the people on track and moving toward new organizational goals and norms requires stamina and a positive outlook despite the inevitable pitfalls and sidetracking that will occur.

> Involvement of people in the organizational change process necessitates use of excellent leadership and skills in group dynamics, conflict management, and team building.

Refreezing the change may take longer than anticipated in the multilevel organizational system. Establishing the change as the organizational norm will be related to the turmoil and differences that have arisen with the altered internal environment and the strength of external forces. Support and reinforcement are indispensable activities of the change agent, along with ongoing analysis, interpretation, and communication of the evaluation findings. The role will naturally become more consultative as termination approaches. At this point, the change should be a part of the expectations of the organization and its members. Ownership of the change is held by the people in the institutional or agency environment and not by key people or the change agent.

Consider the following example of organizational change, extending services from the traditional hospital into the community. Needs assessment, diagnosis of problems, and motivation in agency subsystems must occur in the unfreezing phase for organizational change. In addition to the traditional hospital, this change may involve outpatient departments and clinics, home care agencies, rehabilitation or nursing home settings, HMOs, physician groups, and therapy group practices.

Internal restraining and driving forces are considerations in each of the five organizational subsystems. Organizational goals and values for health care in the mission statement must change with the move from hospital to home, outpatient, or community care. The technical subsystem that represents the physical resources, knowledge, and skills of the health-care providers must now be broadened, such as intravenous and other therapies requiring periodic skilled in-home nursing care. The psychosocial subsystem will need extended interpersonal and interdisciplinary relations with a move into the community, along with coordination of services, role relationships, attitudes, and values of people. Nursing roles of health-care provider, manager, teacher, researcher, and advocate are expanded to include service facilitator and coordinator. The structural system is enlarged, with agencies providing both in-patient and community services, or it becomes more flexible and interactive with other environments providing health-care services. The managerial subsystem is similarly broadened to include overseeing corporations, resulting in buying power, larger constituencies, and overriding governing boards. This translates into augmented goals and policies, comprehensive strategic initiatives, and more controls for all members of the organization, including hospital or health-care corporations.

The external forces that drove the need for change include health-care needs of the client population, reimbursement policies, provider restrictions, and societal trends. Earlier hospital discharge and high-technology home care in the client system have driven service providers from the traditional hospital setting into the community. A good deal of this has been secondary to the reimbursement and insurance restrictions.

Organizational Change Suggestions

Organizations will continue to change and evolve in response to internal and external forces and the needs of the client system. Nurses have growing responsibility in this area. They function as members of change teams, change agents, and developers of organizational systems. This will continue and expand in interdisciplinary practice as their skills in change are recognized and sought. Remember the following steps regardless of the extent of the organizational change:

- *Always do your homework.* Be prepared with the information about and knowledge of the organization. Spend the time and acquire the information and background needed before acting or reacting. Then proceed from a solid theoretical base. Understand the change process and all the steps. Review your talents for change strategies.
- *Know your restraining and driving forces.* Take the time to understand or, at the minimum, recognize these behaviors. Share information. Make both sides aware of the situation. Take more time to understand behavioral reactions. Cultivate the driving forces and become viewed as the champion for the cause. Use all your skills in interpersonal relationships, and develop more.
- *Be sensitive to environments.* Increase your awareness of what is occurring in society and health care. Look beyond your immediate environment. Analyze internal and external forces. Imagine how your environment could be affected by these forces. Use intuition and insight as well as foresight. Be both inspired and inspiring.

- *Maintain a positive attitude and refuse to be diminished by negativity.* Negative colleagues and superiors will always be present. They are an environmental hazard. But these restraining forces should not be or become your role models. Someone will always be readily available to tell you that something never has or never can be done. If your "homework" background knowledge told you something different, become the agent of change instead of another restraining force. Have courage.
- *Be open and receptive to new ideas.* No matter how you long to keep things as they currently are, be mindful that there may be a better way of doing things. Refuse to be limited by the present, and look to the future and evidence-based practice—a core competency.
- *Be open to new people.* Venture out of your discipline. View the situation as larger than nursing care. Collaborate with other health professionals. Discuss. Debate. Interact. Try to recognize when turf issues arise, and negotiate on the basis of facts and what will be best for the client system and the organization while maintaining the integrity of your profession.
- *Involve others.* Try not to do it all yourself. Remember that the most successful and enduring changes occur when others are involved. The change has to become the norm and the expectation of the people in the environment.
- *Refine skills.* Cultivate your change agent skills. Recall the skills and roles of the change agent. Continually develop and refine these skills. Make adaptations necessary for the people and the environments. Look at yourself as objectively as you look at others. If assistance or collaboration is needed, get it. Consider this as using resources and making linkages for effectiveness of the change agent.
- *Reassess and evaluate.* Remember to evaluate activity and progress continually. Sufficient time for the change to occur and persistence are necessary components of organizational change. Recall Rogers's (1983) attributes in the diffusion of innovations, which determine the rate of adoption by members of a social system: relative advantage, compatibility, complexity, trialability, and observability. Include these attributes in your evaluation process.
- *Persevere, persevere, persevere.* Have fortitude. Use resources to cope with your stress and frustration levels. Organizational change is not easy. Look for small gains as major steps in the process. Strive for the finish line, but do not look for accolades. Terminate the relationship as the organizational norm takes hold and the organization congratulates *itself* on the accomplishment.

Remember, the philosophical basis of nursing focuses on the health of people as individuals, families, groups, and society in a complex environment. And practice must be based on the latest evidence of efficacy and acceptability. In this role, nurses can be highly effective change agents.

Key Points

- The classic change model was developed by Lewin (1951), based on his Field Theory. This model contained three phases in the change process: unfreezing, moving, and refreezing.
- Building on Lewin's work, Lippitt (1973) considered human motivation, multiple causation, and habits. He defined seven specific phases in the change process: diagnosis of the problem, assessment of motivation and capacity for change, change agent's motivation and resources, selecting change objectives, choosing the change agent role, maintaining the change, and terminating the relationship. A focus on the change agent emerged with four specific roles and skills.

(continued)

(*continued*)

- Havelock's change model contains the major concepts of role, linkages, and communication. This adds steps to the three stages of change, with heightened communication and interpersonal activities. Havelock and Havelock's (1973) seven steps in the change process are perception of the need, diagnosis of the problem, identification of the problem, devising a plan of action, gaining acceptance, stabilizing the plan, and self-renewal. Four different roles for the change agent are proposed in Havelock's model.

- Rogers's (1983) Diffusion of Innovations model has a five-stage view of change: knowledge, persuasion, decision, implementation, and confirmation. Rogers also considers five factors that influence the rate of adoption of an innovation and that may be used as evaluation criteria in the change process. Seven roles for the change agent are highlighted in this model of change.

- The roles and attributes of a skilled change agent are included in the models by Lippitt, Havelock, and Rogers. General roles for the change agent are assessor or evaluator, communicator, translator, encourager, mediator, and consultant.

- In relation to the activities in the nursing process, the phases of change are consistent with assessment, diagnosis, planning, implementation, and evaluation for resolving the problem or stabilizing the change. They can also lead to the implementation of evidence-based practice in place of traditions from the past.

- The skills of change agents include having a vision for the future and creativity, good assessment skills, good interpersonal skills, flexibility, perseverance and a positive attitude, integrity and commitment, the ability to manage conflict, and resistance.

- Strategies for reducing resistance to change include careful planning and timing, along with good communication and interpersonal skills.

- Empowerment or involvement of the client is needed for lasting change. Strategies for client involvement include education, training, socialization and persuasion, and facilitation.

- Environmental or situational factors relative to individuals, families, and groups provide additional information in the change process. Past experience, stress and coping factors, motivational clues, and resources are important data sought by the change agent.

- To view organizational change, look at internal and external forces with a multisystem approach.

- Suggestions for people involved in organizational change include (1) being knowledgeable about the organization, its restraining and driving forces, and the environments, (2) maintaining a positive attitude and being receptive to new ideas and people, (3) involving other people in the change, (4) continuing to refine skills and reevaluating the situation, and (5) persevering throughout the process.

 ## Thought and Discussion Questions

1. Recall a change that has taken place in your family. Using Lewin's theory, identify the restraining and driving forces.
2. Identify some specific sources of internal change in your organization and name the driving forces.

3. Recall a change that has taken place in your organization. Using Lippitt's theory, identify the seven stages of planned change and the roles of the change agent(s) in the process.

4. List at least six specific environmental factors that could influence change in a health-care organization. Be prepared to discuss these factors in class or online, as scheduled by your instructor.

5. Use Lewin and one additional change theorist to explain the steps of the process for permanent change to help a new 18-year-old single mother with a normal 7 lb, 9 oz full-term infant (appropriate for gestational age [AGA], Apgar score of 9) develop parenting skills and health care, including prevention and health maintenance.

6. Read *Who Moved My Cheese* by S. Johnson (2002) and determine which character you most resemble and which one you most want to be like. Be prepared to participate in a discussion on your selection of characters, either online or in class as scheduled by your instructor.

7. Review the Chapter Thought located on the first page of the chapter, and discuss it in the context of the contents of the chapter.

 Interactive Exercises

1. Two community hospitals located 6 miles apart are merging. Medical, surgical, and specialty services are being divided between the two agencies according to the resources available in each environment. Reorganization of a hospital has been mandated. As the nurse manager of a specialty unit, you must prepare your staff for expansion of their telemetry unit from 24 to 32 beds and plan for the entry of eight additional professional and ancillary staff from the other agency, whose telemetry unit is being closed. Using concepts of organizational change and systems theory, describe the system with the inputs, throughput, outputs, and feedback as outlined on the Intranet site.

2. Identify what you believe is an area for change in your organization or agency. Using concepts of organizational change and systems theory, describe the system with the inputs, throughput, outputs, and feedback as outlined on the Intranet site.

3. In a practice area of your choice, investigate current practice guidelines and research on a selected care activity. Use the Diffusion of Innovations model to describe how you, as a change agent, would approach Rogers's (1983) five phases of the process using the format provided on the Intranet site.

4. A newly appointed vice president for nursing of a 250-bed community hospital wishes a presentation of information on your care system to the medical and nursing staff members. You are hired to present your experiences. Use the sequence of roles of the change agent proposed by Rogers (1983) to describe how you, as a change agent, would approach your presentation using the format provided on the Intranet site.

5. Identify a change needed in your organization, and describe the steps you plan to take to institute the change. Using the format on the Intranet site, describe the needed change, your homework, the forces to consider, the environments, positiveness, openness, new people, involving others, refining skills, reassessment and evaluation, and perseverance.

PRINT RESOURCES

References

Brooten, D. A., Hayman, L. L., & Naylor, M. D. (1988). *Leadership for change: An action guide for nurses* (2nd ed.). Philadelphia: Lippincott.

Chinn, R., & Benne, K. D. (1976). General strategies for effecting change in human systems. In W. G. Bennis, K. D. Benne, R. Chinn, & K, E. Corey (Eds.), *The planning of change* (3rd ed.). (pp. 22–45). New York: Holt, Rinehart & Winston.

Corey, K. E. (1976). Structures in the planning of community change: A personal construct. In W. G. Bennis, K. D. Benne, R, Chinn, & K. E. Corey (Eds.), *The planning of change* (3rd ed.). (pp. 265–275). New York: Holt, Rinehart & Winston.

Havelock, R. G. (1971). *Planning for innovation through dissemination and utilization of knowledge.* Ann Arbor: Institute for Social Research, University of Michigan.

Havelock, R. G., & Havelock, M. C. (1973). *Training for change agents: A guide to the design of training programs in education and other fields.* Ann Arbor: Institute for Social Research, University of Michigan.

Johnson, S. (2002). *Who moved my cheese?* New York: G.P. Putnam's Sons.

Kast, F. E., & Rosenzweig, J. E. (1979). *Organization and management: A systems and contingency approach* (3rd ed.). New York: McGraw-Hill.

Lewin, K. (1951). *Field theory in social science.* New York: Harper & Row.

Lippitt, G. L. (1973). *Visualizing change: Model building and the change process.* La Jolla, CA: University Associates.

Lippitt, G. L., & Nadler, L. (1967, August). Emerging roles of the training director. *Training and Development Journal, 9,* 2–10.

Rogers, E. M. (1983). *Diffusion of innovations* (3rd ed.). New York: Free Press.

Rogers, E. M., & Shoemaker, F. F. (1971). *Communication of innovations: A cross-cultural approach* (2nd ed.). New York: Free Press.

Bibliography

Galvin, K., Andrews, C., Jackson, D., Chessman, S., Fudge, T., Ferris, R., & Graham, I. (1999). Investigating and implementing change within the primary health care nursing team. *Journal of Advanced Nursing, 30,* 238–247.

Gebelein, S. H., Stevens, L. A., Skube, C. J., Lee, D. G., Davis, B. L., & Hellervik, L. W. (2000). *Successful manager's handbook: Development strategies for today's managers* (6th ed.). Minneapolis: Personnel Decisions International.

Johnson, J. E., & Billingsley, M. (1998). Managing change in health care organizations. In J. A. Dienemann (Ed.), *Nursing administration: Managing patient care* (pp. 141–150). Stamford, CT: Appleton & Lange.

Tiffany, C. R., & Lutjens, L. R. J. (1998). *Planned change theories for nursing: Review, analysis, and implications.* Thousand Oaks, CA: Sage.

Joseph T. Catalano

Professional Ethics

> *The time is always right to do what is right.*
>
> Martin Luther King, Jr.

Chapter Objectives

On completion of this chapter, the reader will be able to:

1. Analyze and define the key terms used in ethics.
2. Distinguish between the two primary systems used in resolving ethical dilemmas.
3. Apply the steps of the ethical decision-making model.
4. Analyze and discuss the key ethical principles involved in (a) access to care, (b) organ transplantation, (c) euthanasia, (d) AIDS and HIV, (e) advance directives, (f) staffing and delegation, and (g) cloning.

Key Terms

Autonomy	Obligations	Utilitarianism
Justice	Legal Obligations	Deontology
Distributive Justice	Moral Obligations	Rule Deontology
Fidelity	Rights	Act Deontology
Beneficence	Welfare Rights	Code of Ethics
Nonmaleficence	Ethical Rights	Euthanasia
Veracity	Option Rights	Advance Directives
Standard of Best Interest	Normative Ethics	Cloning

As a registered nurse who has been in professional practice for some years, you are aware of the many changes occurring in the current health-care system. You have also likely encountered some of the difficult ethical dilemmas associated with these changes. By definition, ethical dilemmas present problems that defy a simple solution (Catalano, 2003).

For some reason, many nursing education programs presume that students are able to resolve ethical dilemmas from their past experiences and home moral training, and provide little training on professional ethics. As a result, nurses faced with difficult ethical dilemmas sometimes deal with them in several less than satisfactory ways (Volker, 2003). They may decide to do nothing at all, with the hope that the problem will resolve itself or someone else will solve it. If that fails, some nurses may use the "it just feels right" technique, choosing the solution that produces the least internal discomfort (Catalano, 2003).

In truth, ethical decision-making is a skill that can be learned just like inserting a catheter, starting an intravenous line, or writing a nursing diagnosis (Palviainem, 2003). And as with any learned skill, the more you practice it, the more proficient you become.

ETHICAL PRINCIPLES

No two ethical dilemmas are exactly alike, but when you begin to analyze them, you will find a few key ethical principles that seem to reoccur and serve as the underpinnings for a variety of situations. At the heart of the dilemma is often a conflict between two or more of these basic principles (Davis & Aroskar, 1997). Understanding what the principle is (Box 14–1) and how it relates to the client's situation is the beginning of resolving the dilemma.

Autonomy

Autonomy is the right of self-determination, independence, and freedom. The term refers

---

> **BOX 14–1**
> **ETHICAL PRINCIPLES**
>
> - Autonomy
> - Justice
> - Fidelity
> - Beneficence and Nonmaleficence
> - Veracity
> - Standard of Best Interest
> - Obligations
> - Rights

---

to the clients' right to make health-care decisions for themselves, even if you do not agree with those decisions (Scott, 2003). Autonomy, as with most rights, is not absolute, and under certain conditions, limitations can be imposed on it. Generally, these limitations occur when one individual's autonomy interferes with others' rights, health, or well-being. For example, a client can generally use his or her right to autonomy by refusing any or all treatments. However, in the case of contagious diseases that affect society, such as tuberculosis (TB), the individual can be forced by the health-care and legal systems to take medications to cure the disease (Aiken & Catalano, 1994). The individual can also be forced into isolation to prevent the spread of the disease.

Justice

Justice is the obligation to be fair to all people. The concept is often expanded to what is called **distributive justice**, or social justice, which refers to the individual's right to be treated equally regardless of race, sex, marital status, medical diagnosis, social standing, economic level, or religious belief (Benner, 2003). The principle of justice underlies the first statement in the American Nurses Association (ANA) *Code for Nurses*: "The nurse in all professional relationships practices with compassion and respect for the inherent dignity, worth and the uniqueness of every individual unrestricted by considerations of social or economic status, personal attributes, or the nature of health problems" (ANA, 2001). Distributive justice sometimes includes ideas such as equal access to health care for all citizens. As with other rights, limits can be placed on justice when it interferes with the rights of others.

Fidelity

Fidelity is the obligation to be faithful to commitments made to yourself and others. In health care, fidelity includes your faithfulness or loyalty to agreements and responsibilities accepted as part of the practice of the profession. Fidelity is the main support for the concept of accountability, although conflicts in fidelity might arise from obligations to different individuals or groups. For example, a nurse who is just finishing a very busy and tiring 12-hour shift may experience a conflict of fidelity when she is asked by a supervisor to work an additional shift because the unit is understaffed. The nurse would have to weigh her fidelity to herself against fidelity to the employing institution and fidelity to the profession and clients to do the best job possible, particularly if she felt that her fatigue would interfere with the performance of those obligations (Lutzen, 2003).

Beneficence and Nonmaleficence

Beneficence is a very old requirement for health-care providers that views the primary goal of health care as doing good for clients under their care (Catalano, 2003). In general, the term *good* means more than just technically competent care for clients. Good care requires a holistic approach to the client, including his or her beliefs, feelings, and wishes as well as those of the family and significant others. The main problem you will encounter in implementing the principle of beneficence is determining exactly what is good for another and who can best make the decision about this good.

Nonmaleficence requires that health-care providers do no harm to their clients, either intentionally or unintentionally. In a sense, it is the reverse side of beneficence, and it is difficult to speak of one concept without the other. In current health-care practice, the principle of nonmaleficence is often violated in the short term to produce a greater good in the long-term treatment of the client (McKenzie, 2003). For example, a client may undergo a very painful and debilitating operation to remove a cancerous growth that will prolong her or his life in the long term.

By extension, the principle of nonmaleficence also requires you to protect those from harm who cannot protect themselves. This protection from harm is particularly important in such groups as children, the mentally incompetent, the unconscious, the elderly, and others who may be too weak or debilitated to protect themselves. For example, there are strict regulations in cases of experimentation with groups such as the mentally handicapped, children, and prisoners.

Veracity

Veracity is the principle of "truthfulness." It requires you to tell the truth and not to intentionally deceive or mislead clients. As with other rights and obligations, there are limitations to this principle. The primary limitation is when telling the client the truth would seriously harm (principle of nonmaleficence) his or her ability to recover or would produce greater illness. You may often feel uncomfortable giving clients "bad news" and may avoid answering their questions truthfully. Feeling uncomfortable is not a good enough reason to avoid telling clients the truth about their diagnosis, treatments, or prognosis. Clients have a right to know this information.

Best Interest

The **standard of best interest** involves decisions made about clients' health care when they are unable to make informed decisions about their own care. The standard of best interest is based on what the health-care providers and the family decide is best for that individual (Aiken & Catalano, 1994). It is very important that you consider the individual's expressed wishes, either formally in a written declaration (such as a living will) or informally in what may have been said to family members.

The standard of best interest should be based on the principle of beneficence. Unfortunately, in situations in which clients are unable to make decisions for themselves, the dilemma may be resolved by a unilateral decision made by the health-care providers. Unilateral decisions that disregard the clients' wishes, implying that the health-care providers alone know what is best, are examples of paternalism.

Obligations

Obligations are demands made on individuals, professions, society, or government to fulfill and honor the rights of others. Obligations are often divided into two categories:

- **Legal obligations** are those that have become formal statements of law and are enforceable under the law. For example, you have a legal obligation to provide safe and adequate care for clients to whom you are assigned.
- **Moral obligations** are based on moral or ethical principles but are not enforceable under the law. For example, you are on vacation and encounter an automobile accident; in many places you may have no legal obligation, but as a nurse you have a strong moral obligation, to stop and help the victims.

Rights

Rights are generally defined as something due to an individual according to just claims, legal guarantees, or moral and ethical principles. Although the term *right* is frequently used in both the legal and ethical systems, its meaning is often blurred in everyday usage. Individuals tend to claim things as "rights" that are really privileges, concessions, or freedoms. Several classification systems for rights delineate different types of rights. The following three types of rights are included in most of these systems:

- **Welfare rights** (also called *legal rights*) are based on a legal entitlement to some good or benefit. These rights are guaranteed by laws (such as the Bill of Rights) and their violation can come under the power of the legal system. For example, citizens of the United States have a right to equal access to employment regardless of race, sex, or religion.
- **Ethical rights** (also called *moral rights*) are based on a moral or ethical principle. Ethical rights usually do not have the power of law to be enforced. Ethical rights are, in reality, often privileges allotted to certain individuals or groups of individuals. For example, in the United States and South Africa, the right to health care is really a long-standing privilege, whereas in many other industrialized countries, it is a legal right.
- **Option rights** are based on a fundamental belief in the dignity and freedom of human beings. Option rights are particularly evident in free and democratic countries, such as the United States, and much less evident in totalitarian and restrictive societies, such as North Korea. Option rights give individuals freedom of choice and the right to live their lives as they choose, but within a set of prescribed boundaries. For example, in the United States, you may wear whatever clothes you choose, as long as you do wear some type of clothing.

TWO ETHICAL SYSTEMS

Every time you interact with a client in a health-care setting, an ethical situation exists. You may not realize it, but you are continually making ethical decisions in your daily practice. This process is known as **normative ethics**. Normative ethical decisions deal with questions and dilemmas requiring a choice of actions in which the rights or obligations of the nurse and the client, the nurse and the client's family, or the nurse and the physician conflict. In resolving these ethical questions, you are probably using one of two, or perhaps a combination of two or more, ethical systems.

The two fundamental systems most used in health care–related ethical decision-making are utilitarianism and deontology (Catalano, 2003). Both systems apply to bioethics—the ethics of life (or death, in some cases). *Bioethics* and *bioethical issues* are terms that are in common use and that have become synonymous with health-care ethics, including questions not only of life and death but also of quality of life, life-sustaining and life-altering technologies, and bioscience in general (Benner, 2003). The following discussion of these two ethical systems is undertaken in the context of bioethics.

Utilitarianism

Utilitarianism (also called *teleology, consequentialism,* and *situation ethics*) is defined as the ethical system of utility. As a system of normative ethics, utilitarianism defines "good" as happiness or pleasure. It is based on two underlying principles: "the greatest good for the greatest number" and "the ends justify the means." On the basis of these two principles, utilitarianism is sometimes subdivided into rule utilitarianism and act utilitarianism. According to rule utilitarianism, you draw on your past experiences to formulate internal rules that are useful in determining the greatest good. With act utilitarianism, the particular situation that you find yourself in determines the rightness or wrongness of a particular act. In practice, the true follower of utilitarianism does not believe in the validity of any system of rules, because the rules change according to the circumstances surrounding the decision to be made (Aiken, 2003).

Situation ethics is probably the most publicized form of act utilitarianism. Joseph Fletcher, one of the best-known proponents of act utilitarianism, outlines a method of ethical thinking in which the situation determines whether the act is morally right or wrong. Fletcher views acts as good to the extent that they promote happiness and as wrong to the degree that they promote unhappiness. He defines *happiness* as the happiness of the greatest number of people, but the happiness of each person has equal weight (Fletcher, 1966). For example, abortion is considered ethical in this system in a situation in which an unwed welfare mother with four other children becomes pregnant with her fifth child. The greatest good and the greatest amount of happiness may be produced by aborting this unwanted child, for whom this mother cannot provide adequate food or care.

On the basis of the concept that moral rules should not be arbitrary but should serve a purpose, ethical decisions derived from a utilitarian framework weigh the effect of alternative actions that influence the overall welfare of present and future populations. As such, this system is oriented toward the good of the population in general, and the individual as he or she participates in that population.

Advantages

The major advantage of the utilitarian system of ethical decision-making is that many individuals find it easy to use in most situations. Utilitarianism is built around an individual's own happiness needs, of which he or she has an immediate and vested knowledge. Another advantage is that utilitarianism fits well into a society that shuns rules and regulations. The follower of utilitarianism can justify many decisions on the basis of the "happiness" principle. Its utility orientation also fits well into Western society's belief in the work ethic and the behavioristic approach to education, philosophy, and life.

For example, the follower of utilitarianism holds to a general prohibition against lying and deceiving because, ultimately, telling the truth will lead to more happiness than lying. Yet truth telling is not an absolute requirement to the follower of utilitarianism. If telling the truth would produce widespread unhappiness for a great number of people and future generations, then it would be better ethically to tell a lie. Although such behavior might appear to be unethical at first glance, the follower of strict act utilitarianism would have little difficulty in arriving at this decision as logical.

Disadvantages

Utilitarianism has some serious limitations as a system of health-care ethics or bioethics. An immediate question arises as to whether "happiness" refers to the average happiness of all or the total happiness of a few. Because individual happiness is also important, you must consider how to make decisions when the individual's happiness conflicts with the larger group's happiness. More fundamental is the question of what constitutes "happiness." Similarly, what constitutes the "greatest good for the greatest number?" Who determines what is "good" in the first place? Is it society in general? The government? Governmental policy? The individual? In health-care delivery and the formulation of health-care policy, the general guiding principle often seems to be the greatest good for the greatest number. Yet where do minority groups, such as African-Americans and Native Americans, fit into this system?

The "ends justify the means" principle has also been rejected historically as a method of justifying actions. It is generally unacceptable to allow any type of action to go forward in the hopes that the final goal or purpose is good. The Nazis used this aphorism to justify a variety of actions that were not "good."

The other difficulty with this system is in quantifying such concepts as good, harm, benefits, and greatest. This problem becomes especially acute in dealing with health-care issues that involve individuals' lives. For example, an elderly woman has been sick for a long time, and that illness has placed great financial hardship on her family. It would be ethical under utilitarianism to allow this client to die, or even to euthanize her, to relieve the financial stress created by her illness.

The use of utilitarianism as an ethical system in health-care decision-making requires the additional principle of distributive justice—such as equal access to care—as an ultimate guiding point. Nonetheless, whenever you combine an unchanging principle with this system, you negate the basic concept of pure utilitarianism. Pure utilitarianism, although easy to use as a general decision-making system, does not always work well as an ethical decision-making system in health care because of its arbitrary, self-centered nature. In the everyday delivery of health care, utilitarianism is often combined with other types of ethical decision-making to resolve ethical dilemmas.

Deontology

Deontology is a system of ethical decision-making based on moral rules and unchanging principles. This system is also called the *formalistic system*, the *principle system of ethics*, and *duty-based ethics*. A follower of a pure deontologic system of ethical decision-making believes in the ethical absoluteness of principles, regardless of the consequences of the decisions based on them. This strict adherence to an ethical theory, in which the moral rightness or wrongness of human actions is considered separately from the consequences, is based on a fundamental principle called the *categorical imperative*. It is not the results of the act that make it right or wrong, but the principles on which the act is based. These fundamental principles are ultimately unchanging and absolute and are derived from the universal values that underlie all major religions. The concern for right and wrong in the moral sense is the basic premise of the species and social cooperation. The deontologic system is also divided into rule deontology and act deontology.

Rule deontology is based on the belief that there are standards for the ethical choices and judgments made by individuals. These standards are fixed and do not change when the situation changes. The number of standards or rules is potentially unlimited, but in reality, and particularly when one is dealing with bioethical issues, many of these principles can be grouped together into a few general or "cover" principles. These principles can also be arranged into a type of hierarchy of rules, including such maxims as "Persons should always be treated as ends and never as means," "Human life has value," "One is always to tell the truth," "Above all in health care do no harm," "The human person has a right to self-determination," and "All persons are of equal value." These principles echo such fundamental documents as the Bill of

Rights and the Hospital Patient's Bill of Rights (American College of Physicians, 1998).

Act deontology places the highest value on the moral values of the individual. It requires that you make the same decision in any similar situation, regardless of time, place, individuals involved, and external circumstances. Act deontology does not depend on unchanging external rules as rule deontology does. Rather, you obtain all the data you can about the dilemma, then make the decision. The decision (act) makes it correct simply because it was made. For example, a community health nurse working in a prenatal clinic believes that birth control methods are moral and therefore gives birth control information and pills to a sexually active teenager (Lorensen, 2003). The nurse would also give the same types of information to the next sexually active teenager who came into the clinic for care, without regard to the teenager's beliefs or background.

Advantages

Rule deontology is useful in making ethical decisions in health care because it holds that an ethical judgment you make is based on principles that will be the same in a variety of similar situations, regardless of time, location, and the particular individuals involved. In addition, deontologic terminology and concepts are similar to the terms and concepts used by the legal system. The legal system also stresses rights and duties, principles, and rules. But there are significant differences between the two. Legal rights and duties are enforceable under the law, whereas ethical rights and duties usually are not. In general, ethical systems are much wider and more inclusive than the system of laws they underlie.

Disadvantages

The deontologic system of ethical decision-making is not perfect. Some of the more troubling questions are: "What do you do when the basic guiding principles conflict with each other?" "What is the source of the princi-

ples?" and "Is there ever a situation in which an exception to the rule applies?"

Although various approaches have been proposed to circumvent these limitations, it may be difficult for nurses to resolve situations in which duties and obligations conflict, particularly when the consequences of following a rule end in harm to a client. In reality, there are probably few followers of pure deontology, because most people consider the consequences of their actions in their decision-making.

Act deontology negates the underlying philosophy of the deontologic system requiring unchanging external rules, because you must obtain all the data you can about the dilemma, then make the decision. This approach is difficult to use in resolving ethical dilemmas because of its lack of rules. It requires you to judge each situation individually and arrive at the same decision in similar cases. You may not have the time or energy to analyze each situation you encounter thoroughly in providing care to clients.

APPLYING ETHICAL THEORIES

Ethical theories do not provide cookbook solutions for resolving ethical dilemmas. Instead, they give you a framework for decision-making, which you can apply to individual ethical situations. At times, you may find ethical theories too abstract or general to be of much use in specific ethical situations. Without them, however, ethical decision-making often becomes an exercise in personal emotions. Many nurses attempting to make ethical decisions use elements from both of the two theories, as presented here.

The Decision-Making Model in Ethics

Nurses, by definition, are problem solvers, and one of the important tools regularly used in problem-solving is the nursing process. The nursing process is, if nothing else, a systematic, step-by-step approach to resolving problems that deal with a client's health and well-being.

Although you routinely deal with problems related to the physical or psychological needs of clients, you may feel inadequate when dealing with their ethical problems. No matter what the health-care setting, however, you can develop the decision-making skills necessary to make sound ethical decisions if you learn and practice using an ethical decision-making model.

An ethical decision-making model provides a method for answering key questions about ethical dilemmas and organizing your thinking more logically and sequentially. Although several ethical decision-making models exist, the problem-solving method presented here is based on the nursing process. It should be a relatively easy transition for you to move from the nursing process used in resolving clients' physical problems to the ethical decision-making model to resolve ethical problems.

> Nurses, by definition, are problem solvers, and one of the important tools regularly used in problem-solving is the nursing process

The chief goal of the ethical decision-making model is to determine right from wrong in situations with no clear or readily apparent demarcations. This process presupposes that a system of ethics exists, that you know what the basic ethical principles are, and that the system applies to similar ethical decision-making problems despite multiple variables. At some point, you need to undertake the task of clarifying your own values, if you have not done it already (FIG. 14–1). You also need an understanding of the possible ethical systems that may be used in making decisions about ethical dilemmas (Catalano, 2003).

The following five-step ethical decision-making model is presented as a tool for resolving ethical dilemmas (Box 14–2).

Step 1: Collect, Analyze, and Interpret the Data

Obtain as much information as possible concerning the particular ethical dilemma you are facing. Among the issues important for you to

> **BOX 14–2**
> **STEPS OF ETHICAL DECISION-MAKING**
> 1. Collect, analyze, and interpret the data.
> 2. State the dilemma.
> 3. Consider the choices of action.
> 4. Analyze the advantages and disadvantages of each course of action.
> 5. Make the decision.

know are the client's wishes, the family's wishes, the extent of the physical or emotional problems causing the dilemma, the physician's beliefs about health care, and your own orientation to life-and-death issues.

For example, many nurses must deal with the question of whether or not to initiate resuscitation efforts when a terminally ill client is admitted to the hospital. Physicians often leave verbal instructions indicating that you really should not resuscitate the client but merely go through the motions to make the family feel better. Your dilemma becomes whether to attempt seriously to revive the client or to let him or her die quietly.

Important information that would help you make the best decision includes the mental competency of the client to make a no-resuscitation decision, the client's desires, the family's feelings, and whether the physician sought input from the client and family before leaving the orders. Many institutions have policies concerning no-resuscitation orders, and you should consider these in the data collection stage.

After collecting as much information as possible, you need to bring the pieces of information together into a form that will give the dilemma the clearest and sharpest focus.

Step 2: State the Dilemma

After you have collected and analyzed all the available information, you need to state the dilemma as clearly and succinctly as possible. Recognizing the key aspects of the dilemma helps focus your attention on the important

PART I — Rank the following from 1 to 5, with 1 being the item with the highest priority and 5 being the item with lowest priority.

A. A hospital must cut back its budget or go bankrupt. Which of the following clients should be given priority for care?
_____ A newborn with multiple birth defects who is likely to be retarded for life.
_____ A 47-year-old male scientist with an acute MI who has just discovered a new medication that might cure HIV.
_____ An 88-year-old retired female grade-school teacher who was recently diagnosed with liver cancer.
_____ A 17-year-old runaway who is addicted to cocaine and is pregnant.
_____ A 58-year-old construction worker who has severe emphysema due to his 2½ pack a day smoking habit.

B. The nurse assigned to a client who has a bleeding ulcer secondary to stress. Which aspects of his care would receive highest priority?
_____ Give him pain medications to make him comfortable.
_____ Explain the relationship between stress and ulcers.
_____ Involve him as much as possible in his self-care.
_____ Encourage him to talk about his job and family, etc.
_____ Teach him about diet and medication to control ulcers.

PART II — Rate the following statements on a scale of 1 to 5.
(1 = strongly support; 2 = support; 3 = no opinion; 4 = reject; 5 = strongly reject).
_____ 1. Abortion is always wrong, no matter what the circumstances.
_____ 2. People who receive the death penalty, deserve it.
_____ 3. Life support should be terminated for clients when they are not likely to live.
_____ 4. Street drugs should be made legal.
_____ 5. Prisoners, genetically defective, mentally retarded persons should be sterilized.
_____ 6. Premature, drug addicted newborns should be allowed to die.
_____ 7. Condoms should be given out in high schools to prevent pregnancy and HIV.
_____ 8. All hospitalized clients should be routinely screened for HIV and AIDS.
_____ 9. Scientists should be allowed to use aborted fetuses for fetal tissue research.
_____ 10. All newborn infants should be genetically screened for inherited diseases.

PART III — Complete the following sentences.

1. The one thing I have always wanted to do is _____
2. If I just inherited 5 million dollars, I would _____
3. As president of United States, I would _____
4. If I died today, I would like my obituary to say _____
5. If I could control the world and its destiny, I would _____

PART IV — Below is a partial list of things people value. Complete the list, then rank each item from 1 (highest value) to ? being the lowest value.

___ family   _____
___ career   _____
___ religion   _____
___ honor   _____
___ material possessions _____
___ health   _____
___ recreation   _____
___ professionalism _____

FIG. 14–1. Values clarification tool.

ethical principles. Most of the time, the dilemma can be reduced to a statement or two revolving around key ethical principles. These dilemmas often involve a question of conflicting rights, obligations, or basic ethical principles.

In the question of slow resuscitation versus no resuscitation, the dilemma might be stated as "The client's right to self-determination and death with dignity versus the nurse's obligation to preserve life and do no harm." In general, the principle that the competent client's wishes must be followed is unequivocal. If the client has become unresponsive before expressing his or her wishes, then the family members' input must be given serious consideration. Additional questions can arise if the family's wishes conflict with those of the client.

Step 3: Consider the Choices of Action

After you have stated the dilemma as clearly as possible, you should attempt to list, without consideration of their consequences, all the possible courses of action that you can take to resolve the dilemma. This brainstorming activity, in which you consider all possible courses of action, may require input from outside sources such as colleagues, supervisors, and even experts in the ethical field. The consequences of the different actions are considered later.

Some of the possible courses of action to consider in the resuscitation example are:

- Resuscitating the client to your fullest capabilities, despite what the physician has requested
- Not resuscitating the client at all, just going through the motions without any real attempt to revive the client
- Seeking another assignment to avoid dealing with the situation
- Reporting the problem to a supervisor
- Attempting to clarify the question with the client
- Attempting to clarify the question with the family
- Confronting the physician about the question

Step 4: Analyze the Advantages and Disadvantages of Each Course of Action

Some of the courses of actions you developed in the previous step are more realistic than others. The unrealistic actions become readily evident during this step in the decision-making process, when you consider the advantages and the disadvantages of each action in detail. Along with each option, you must consider the consequences of taking each course of action. You should evaluate the advantages and disadvantages of the consequences thoroughly.

For example, you should consider whether initiating discussion about the order would anger the physician or cause him or her to distrust you in the future. Either of these responses might make practicing at that institution difficult. The result might be the same if you successfully resuscitate the client despite orders to the contrary. Not resuscitating the client has the potential to involve you in a lawsuit if no clear order for no resuscitation exists. Presenting the situation to a supervisor may, if the supervisor supports the physician, cause you to be labeled a troublemaker and may have a negative effect on your future evaluations. The same process can be applied to the other possible courses of action.

By thoroughly considering the advantages and disadvantages of each possible action, you should be able to deduce your realistic choices of action. An important factor to include in your deliberations is the ANA's *Code for Nurses* (2001).

Step 5: Make the Decision

The most difficult part of the process is actually making the decision and living with the consequences. By their nature, ethical dilemmas produce differences of opinion, and not everyone will be pleased with your decision.

In the attempt to solve any ethical dilemma, there is always a question of the correct course of action. The client's wishes almost always supersede independent you might make. Collaborative decision-making about resuscitation that involves the client, physician, nurses, and family is the ideal solution and tends to produce fewer complications in the long-term resolution of such questions.

NURSING CODE OF ETHICS

A **code of ethics** is generally defined as the ethical principles that govern a particular profession. Codes of ethics are presented in general statements and do not give specific answers to every possible ethical dilemma that might arise. These codes do, however, offer you guidance in your ethical decisions (see Box 1–2).

Ideally, codes of ethics should undergo periodic revision to reflect changes in the profession and society as a whole. Although codes of ethics are not legally enforceable as laws, consistently violating the code of ethics is taken as an indication of an unwillingness to act in a professional manner and often results in disciplinary actions, ranging from reprimands and fines to suspension and revocation of licensure (McLeod, 2003).

The ANA Code for Nurses has been acknowledged by other health-care professions as one of the most complete ethical codes. It is sometimes used as the benchmark against which other codes of ethics are measured. Yet a careful reading of this code of ethics reveals only a set of clearly stated principles that you must apply to actual clinical situations. For example, if you are involved in the resuscitation situation described earlier, you will find no specific mention of "no resuscitation" orders. Rather, you must apply general statements, such as "The nurse provides services with respect for human dignity" and "The nurse assumes responsibility and accountability for individual nursing judgments and actions," to the particular situation.

COMMON ETHICAL DILEMMAS IN NURSING

Although the potential ethical dilemmas you might face in your career are almost unlimited, you are likely to encounter certain issues in your practice. A complete analysis of each of these issues is beyond the scope of this book, but the important ethical features are presented so that you will be able to analyze the dilemma and make an informed decision. Resolving ethical dilemmas is never an easy task, and it is likely that you will displease someone with your decision, no matter how carefully and thoughtfully you have made it.

Access to Care

Although access to health care has been a concern in the United States for many years, it is only with recent proposed changes in the health-care system that it has been pushed into the headlines as an important ethical and social issue. In today's health-care system, some individuals obtain the best care that medicine and technology can provide, whereas others can neither afford to see a physician nor purchase the medications that are prescribed. The underlying ethical principle involved in access to care is that of justice, particularly distributive justice. The basic question is whether health care is a universal right to be allotted to all citizens, or a privilege limited to those who can pay for it.

On the surface, the current health care system seems to be based on the belief that health care is a privilege. Yet the government recognizes the needs of some of those who cannot afford health care, such as the elderly, poor, and disabled, and subsidizes their health care through a variety of programs, such as Medicaid. The end result is that the United States spends more on health care than any country in the world, with most of that money coming from the pockets of taxpayers.

However, those who support universal access and health care as a basic right of every citizen are faced with the specter of health-care rationing. The reality of the situation is that if universal access becomes the law of the land, some form of restricted access to services will be likely to control the flow of money. A system of universal access to health care in the United States means that some health-care goods must be rationed.

Ideally, under the ethical principle of distributive justice, everybody should have open access to every type of health care. Because that type of access is unrealistic, a decision must be made about what health-care services will be restricted to which groups of individuals. All of the current proposals for universal coverage all would limit those health-care services that generally fall into the tertiary category—highly specialized diagnostic and treatment regimens, organ and tissue transplantation, and procedures that merely prolong life temporarily.

The group that is most often targeted for rationing of health care is the elderly, because they are a rapidly growing, easily identified group that has high health-care costs. The cost of health care for the elderly in the last year of their life has amounted to 1 percent of the total gross national product (GNP) each year since 1984 (Henderson, 2003). Also, the traditional role of the elderly in society is to care for the young and future generation, not to absorb a large portion of their heritage in the form of expensive resources.

Nevertheless, there is a strong prohibition in this country against using age alone as a criterion for restriction of services. Allocation of health-care services based on need seems to be a more equitable way to arrive at the decision. It would make more sense to restrict the use of expensive technologies by all age groups rather than all sources for the elderly only. The elderly have also contributed a great deal to this country over the years, compared with the younger members of society, and it seems only fair that they receive the care they have earned. Many nurses find it difficult to reconcile their personal and professional codes of ethics with limiting resources for just one group, such as the elderly. It is unlikely that professional groups, such as nurses, would abide by a policy that restricted care to the elderly. For example, access of the young to cardiac catherization or operations for certain malignancies is not restricted.

What is the solution to this dilemma? As with most ethical dilemmas, there is no perfect solution, yet nurses can contribute a great deal to resolving this question. Underlying any resolution to the access to care problem is the requirement for a fundamental shift in attitude and philosophy about health care. No longer can curing disease and extending life

be the primary focuses of health care. Rather, the health-care system needs to adopt caring as a central goal of health care. Nurses understand caring as a mode of treatment. Physicians and other health-care providers can learn it. Caring will refocus the goals of health care toward a more equitable and rational use of health-care resources.

Organ Transplantation

Despite the widespread public and medical acceptance of organ transplantation as a highly beneficial procedure, ethical questions remain. Whenever a human organ is transplanted, a large number of people are involved, including the donor, the donor's family, medical and nursing personnel, the recipient, and the recipient's family. Society in general could also be added to this mix, because of the high cost of organ transplantation, which is usually borne directly by tax monies or indirectly in the form of increased insurance premiums. Each one of these people or groups has rights that may conflict with the rights of the others.

Most institutions that perform transplants, or organizations that are involved in obtaining organs, have developed elaborate, detailed, and involved procedures to help deal with the ethical and legal issues involved in transplantation (McKenney, 2003). Despite these efforts, some ethical issues still arise whenever organ transplantation is considered. Consider the ethical principles involved, such as autonomy, justice, beneficence, and standard of best interest.

One particularly sensitive issue arises when a child is involved. Although parents are legally permitted to give consent for medical procedures for their children, the child must also have some input in the decision, particularly if the procedure poses a risk to her or his life, such as a kidney transplantation. By legal definition, a child younger than the age of 18 years cannot give informed consent to such a procedure. Yet it seems unethical to coerce the child into donating a kidney if she or he really did not want to do it (Casey, 2003). In the case of children, it is important to obtain both parental consent and informed assent, in which the child is aware of decisions and involved in the process.

Despite the best efforts of the medical and legal community to establish criteria for death, ethical questions about when a person is really dead remain (McKenney, 2003). Does brain death, the most widely accepted criterion for death, really indicate that a person no longer exists as a human being? Or is there some other criterion that should be examined? Such organs as heart, lungs, and liver must come from a donor whose heart is still beating. Might there be a tendency therefore to declare brain death before it actually occurs?

One of the most difficult ethical issues involved in organ transplantation is selecting recipients. The number of people who need organs far exceeds the number of available organs. Many potential ethical dilemmas arise from this fact. Should someone receive an organ because he or she is rich or famous or knows the right people? The national organ recipient list attempts to list and rank all persons who need organs in a nondiscriminatory manner. Some of the important criteria are need, length of time on the list, potential for survival, prior organ transplantation, value to the community, and tissue compatibility.

Nurses can be, and often are, involved in some aspects of the organ donation process. Many states have passed laws requiring that health-care workers ask the family members of potential organ donors whether they have ever thought about organ donation for their dead or dying loved one. Many nurses, particularly those in critical care units, provide care for clients who are potential organ donors. Nurses in operating rooms may help in the actual surgical procedures that remove organs from a cadaver and transplant them into a recipient's body. Many floor nurses provide the postoperative care for clients who have received a transplanted organ. Home health-care nurses give follow-up care to these clients at home.

Nurses working with organ transplantation must be sensitive to the potential for manipulation. Most people who are seeking organ transplantation are desperately ill or near death. They and their families can be either very easily manipulated or very manipulative. On the other side, the families of potential organ donors are usually emotionally distraught as a result of the sudden and traumatic loss of a loved one. They, too, are vulnerable to manipulation. As a general rule, neither the donor nor his or her family should play any part in selecting a recipient. Nurses must avoid making statements or giving nonverbal indications of their approval or disapproval of potential recipients. For example, a statement such as "I hope the teenager gets the kidney rather than the old lady" may prejudice the whole process.

Euthanasia

The term **euthanasia** generally means a painless or peaceful death. A distinction is often made between passive and active euthanasia. *Passive euthanasia* usually refers to the practice of allowing an individual to die without any extraordinary intervention. Such practices as do not resuscitate (DNR) orders, living wills, and withdrawal of ventilators or other life support are usually included under this umbrella definition (Anderson-Shaw, 2003). *Active euthanasia*, in contrast, describes the practice of speeding an individual's death through some act or procedure. This practice, also sometimes referred to as *mercy killing*, takes many forms, ranging from using large amounts of pain medication for terminal cancer clients to using poisons, carbon monoxide, guns, or knives to end a person's life.

Assisted suicide, brought to public attention by Dr. Kevorkian, a Michigan physician, is really a type of active euthanasia or mercy killing (Coughennower, 2003; Moody, 2003). The central issue that has been pushed to the fore by Dr. Kevorkian's public practice of assisted suicide is whether it is ever ethically permissible for health-care personnel to assist in taking a life. In all states but one the practice is illegal. The definition of *homicide*—bringing about a person's death or assisting him or her to do so—seems to fit the act of assisted suicide. Yet there is a great deal of hesitation on the part of the legal system to prosecute persons who are involved in assisted suicide for terminally ill clients.

The fundamental ethical issue is the right to autonomy or self-determination (Catalano, 2003, Patterson, 2003). In almost every other health-care situation, a client, as long as he or she is competent, can make decisions about what care is acceptable and what care he or she will refuse. Yet when it comes to the termination of life, this right no longer seems to apply. Supporters of the practice of assisted suicide hold to the belief that the right to self-determination remains intact even in the decision to end life. It is the last act of a very sick individual to control his or her own fate. Medical personnel, many believe, should be allowed to assist these clients in this procedure, just as they are allowed to assist clients in other medical and nursing procedures.

Those who oppose assisted suicide find these arguments lacking in ethical principle. Legally, ethically, and morally, suicide in American society has never been accepted. Health-care staff go to great lengths to prevent clients from injuring themselves when they are identified as suicidal. In addition, it would seem that individuals in the terminal states of a disease who are overwhelmed by pain, and depressed by the thought of prolonged suffering, might not be able to think clearly enough to give informed consent for assisted suicide. Also, the termination of life is final. It does not allow for spontaneous cures or the development of new treatments or medications.

Although nurses are unlikely to be employed in assisted suicide clinics, the reality of active euthanasia has been and will continue to be part of modern-day health care. Nurses need to remember the principle of nonmaleficence. There is a very strong obligation to do no harm to clients. Assisting in or causing the death of a client would seem to be an obvious violation of this principle.

HIV and AIDS

Few diseases have the power to raise strong opinions that human immunodeficiency virus (HIV) and acquired immunodeficiency syndrome (AIDS) do. Nurses who for years held strongly to the ethical principle that all clients, regardless of race, sex, religion, age, or disease process, should be cared for equally now question their obligation to take care of clients with AIDS.

Several ethical issues underlie the AIDS issue. One of the most important is the right to privacy. Some people believe that this issue has been carried to extremes. Many diseases that are highly contagious and sometimes fatal—TB, gonorrhea, syphilis, and hepatitis—must be reported to public health officials. Although there is a general requirement to report infection with HIV or AIDS to the Centers for Disease Control and Prevention (CDC), many states have strict laws regarding the confidentiality of the diagnosis (Botes, 2003). Revealing the diagnosis of HIV or AIDS even to other health-care personnel brings the possibility of a lawsuit against the health-care provider or institution. It is important to remember that the right to privacy is not an absolute right. If the right to privacy can be violated when the public welfare is threatened by such diseases as TB, syphilis, and gonorrhea, is it not logical to include AIDS in this group? Is it unjust to ask health-care providers to care for clients with this disease without knowing that the client has it? A parallel question involves the client's right to know when a health-care provider is infected with HIV or AIDS.

Another important ethical issue is the right to care. Can a nurse refuse to care for a client with a highly contagious and potentially lethal disease, such as HIV, hepatitis B, or medication-resistant TB? Obviously, a fundamental right of being a client is receiving care, just as a fundamental obligation of a nurse is to provide care. The first statement of the ANA *Code for Nurses* states that a nurse must provide care unrestricted by any considerations. There may be some exceptions; for example, if the nurse were pregnant, or receiving chemotherapy, or had other immunity problems, she or he might be able to refuse an assignment because of safety considerations. But in most situations, the nurse would be obligated to provide the best nursing care possible for all clients, including those with dangerous diseases.

What about the issue of justice, in light of the tremendous cost involved in treating individuals with AIDS? Studies estimate that the medical cost of treating clients with AIDS from the time of diagnosis to the time of death is in the neighborhood of $900,000 per client (Botes, 2003). In the face of this crisis, governmental agencies, who bear the brunt of the cost of AIDS treatment, will have to make some hard decisions. With more than 1 million people already infected with this disease, the cost to society is astronomical. Nurses are obligated to care for all clients, including those with AIDS, but are physicians, hospitals, and governmental agencies also held to this same precept? Is the right to health care really a privilege?

Advance Directives

Advance directives have been used in health care for a number of years. Originally developed as a means for clients to express their wishes about the type and amount of health care they desired if they became unable to make decisions at a future date (right to self-determination), advance directives are now a required part of the health care of all clients. Under the Omnibus Budget Reconciliation Act of 1990, all hospitals, nursing care facilities, home care agencies, and care providers are required by law to ask clients about advance directives and provide information about them if so desired (Aiken & Catalano, 1994).

Advance directives can take the form of living wills and medical durable power of attorney (MDPOA). A *living will* is defined as a directive from a competent individual to medical personnel and family members regarding the treatment he or she wishes to receive when he or she is no longer able to make decisions (Briggs, 2002). This directive is ideally in the form of a written document, but it may also take the form of verbal directions to a health-care provider that are documented in the client's health-care record. No standard form is accepted by all states. Some living wills are very specific as to the treatments that can and cannot be used, but other forms provide only general directions, such as "no extraordinary measures."

As a nurse, you can play an important part in identifying potential problems in a client's living will. If a client has already written a living will, you need to make sure it is signed and witnessed properly or notarized. Generally, health-care providers and the client's family members are excluded from witnessing a living will. In addition, if the living will is more than 2 years old, you should encourage the client to review it and update it if needed. Also, see how clear and detailed the statements are about which treatments are to be used or excluded. Often clients do not understand such modes of treatment as intubation, ventilation, defibrillation, medication administration, and resuscitation. Explain any new modes of treatment that may have been developed since the client first composed the living will. Finally, encourage the client to give copies of the document to his or her next of kin, primary physician, and attorney. Some states even allow the client to register a living will with certain agencies in the state, such as the secretary of state (Catalano, 2003).

Although the use of the living will seems to be a relatively simple way to resolve a complicated situation in health care, you must be aware of a number of ethical pitfalls. One of the most common ethical questions revolves around the client's level of knowledge of potential and future health-care problems he or she may encounter. Living wills are often composed while the client is in a relatively positive state of health and may be directed toward only a few "common" problems with which he or she is familiar. For example, the client may anticipate a myocardial infarction

(MI) and give specific directions for treatments to be excluded in this condition, such as "no CPR," or "no defibrillation." Suppose the client is in an automobile accident, has a crushed chest, and needs to be connected to a ventilator for proper healing of the ribs. If he is unconscious and cannot give directions to the health-care team, should they not intubate him and attach him to the ventilator because of his living will? Did he really intend to exclude this situation? In general, if there is any indication that the client did not fully understand the implications or use of possible therapies, the validity of the whole living will is in question and can probably be disregarded (Briggs, 2003).

Nurses working with clients who have a living will sometimes encounter ethical questions concerning the principles of beneficence and nonmaleficence. As defined earlier, the principle of beneficence states that your primary duty as a nurse is to do good for the client, and the principle of nonmaleficence requires you to protect the client from any harm. From the perspectives of beneficence and nonmaleficence, you may believe that following a client's living will violates these principles. Some nurses are ethically uncomfortable in situations in which implementing a client's living will involves the termination of life-sustaining treatments already in use. When you "pull the plug" on a ventilator or tube feeding, you seem to be doing definite harm to that client, namely, causing his or her death.

A third difficulty that you may encounter with a living will is actually enforcing it. The legal and ethical systems overlap a great deal in this dilemma. Strictly speaking, unless a state has enacted into law a special type of living will called a *natural death act*, the living will is not legally enforceable. Although 44 states have these acts, they vary widely in wording and requirements. Some of these laws recognize the living will only if it is in accord with the physician's plan of treatment. Other states have laws that are so specific in defining "terminal illness" that they require the client to die within a few hours of implementing the living will. Very few of these laws have any provisions to protect nurses and other health-care providers from criminal or civil actions if they do carry out the living will. You need to know not only whether your state has a natural death act but also what it says specifically about living wills.

The other form of advance directive, used less commonly than the living will, is the MDPOA, or health-care proxy. This type of advance directive allows the client to designate another person to make health-care choices if he or she becomes unconscious or otherwise unable to make decisions. Like the living will, the MDPOA has difficulties. State laws vary widely as to who can be given this power, how long it is good for, and the legal process involved in verifying the person with the power of attorney. The ethical issues surrounding MDPOA are very similar to those for living wills. In addition, some clients may designate two or more persons to have MDPOA. Making health-care decisions when these

---

ONLINE CONSULT: ADVANCED DIRECTIVES

American Academy of Family Physicians.
http://familydoctor.org/003.xml
American Bar Association.
http://www.abanet.org/aging/
American Medical Association.
http://www.ama-assn.org
Hospice Patients Alliance.
http://www.hospicepatients.org/advanced-directives.html
U.S. Living Will Registry.
http://www.uslivingwillregistry.com
OC: Also check your state's Web site for any natural death act legislation.

individuals disagree about the care they think the client wants is extremely complicated.

Staffing and Delegation

You have probably already encountered "health-care restructuring" at your workplace. No matter how it may have been presented, or how it was phrased, all restructuring has cost containment as its primary goal. Almost all health-care facilities are attempting to find ways to cut their costs while maintaining at least minimal standards of care. You may have been exposed to terms such as *managed care, resource allocation,* and *change in provider mix.* Be cautious when these terms are used, because they usually mean that the ratio between professional staff and unlicensed staff is changing, with the potential to produce ethical conflicts that challenge your role as a professional nurse. Consider the ethical principles autonomy, justice, fidelity, beneficence and nonmaleficence, veracity, standard of best interest, and obligations.

The current trend to use more unlicensed assistive personnel (UAP) poses ethical and legal concerns for you in your attempt to carry out your ethical and professional responsibilities. As a nurse, your main goal is to provide respectful, competent, and compassionate care for your clients using your expertise, knowledge, and professional skill. Professional nurses in most settings have always relied on some type of UAP help, but as the mix of professional to nonprofessional care provider changes, your ethical and legal obligations also change (Bell, 2003).

The professional nurse's primary commitment has always been, and should always be, to the health, well-being, and safety of the client. Nurses act as advocates for clients and should always be aware of, and take appropriate action regarding, situations in which incompetent, unethical, or illegal practice is performed by anyone providing care. Although it is possible for UAPs to provide safe care within their scope of practice, they may tend to carry out procedures that require skills not appropriate for their level of training. It is your ethical and legal responsibility to identify situations in which client care is adversely affected and to take action to change or eliminate the potential for harm.

Legally and ethically, professional nurses are responsible for the actions taken and judgments made by those they supervise in the provision of care. Neither physician's orders nor the employing agency's policies release nurses from the responsibility for actions taken or judgments made by subordinates (Wilkes, 2003). Nurses can protect themselves from unethical or illegal situations by constantly evaluating how staffing changes affect the safety and quality of the care being provided. By becoming involved in the formulation of institutional policies through active participation on various in-house committees, nurses can have a major influence on the staffing practices at their institution. It is also ethically permissible, and even desirable, that nurses protest and take appropriate action when they judge that UAPs are being used inappropriately or unsafely in client care situations.

Similarly, nurses are ethically and legally accountable for the appropriate delegation of nursing care activities to other health-care workers. It is important that nurses know the level of training of UAPs assigned to them and evaluate their competency when assigning client care tasks. It is ethically irresponsible to assign a nursing care function to an unlicensed assistant for which he or she is not prepared or qualified. Employer policy statements do not release the nurse from accountability for inappropriately assigning an unprepared unlicensed assistant to a task that ultimately results in harm to the client. The educator role of the professional nurse now has importance in helping to prepare and instruct UAPs in the work setting. Professional nurses will also be spending more of their time evaluating the competency of other health-care workers as they provide care in order to protect clients from harm.

In our rapidly changing health-care system, the use of UAP-type workers will only increase. Correspondingly, you will need to understand your growing professional and legal obligations regarding these workers. As with most ethical questions, there is no single right answer to the dilemma posed by UAP. You are the professional, and your judgment and accountability are not abdicated through delegation. You, as a professional nurse, must always keep in mind the ultimate goal for all clients: safe and high-quality care.

Cloning and Genetic Manipulation

With the successful birth of Dolly the sheep in Scotland in 1996, the world was awakened to the reality of cloning as a viable reproductive method. Since that time, all sorts of animals have been cloned. The concept of **cloning**, which has existed since the discovery of DNA in the 1960s by Watson and Crick, is based on the fact that every cell in an animal's body contains all the genetic information needed to reproduce every other cell in the body. In the strict scientific meaning of the word, the *cloning process* occurs when any cell in an animal's body is removed, is placed in an appropriate growth environment, and develops into an identical reproduction of the animal from which the cell came. In practice, however, scientists still do not understand what triggers some parts of a DNA strand to become active and reproduce and other parts of the DNA strand to remain dormant. Currently, if a skin cell is removed from a human being and placed in a growth medium, it will grow only new skin, not another identical person.

Although you are probably familiar with the popular term "cloning," the scientific name for the process used to produce Dolly and other animals is *somatic cell nuclear transfer technique*. First, an unfertilized ovum is removed from an animal, and then all the genetic material (DNA) is removed from the ovum. The next step requires the scientists to remove the DNA from a cell in the animal that they wish to clone and to insert it into the unfertilized, DNA-free ovum. The ovum with the new DNA is then implanted in the uterus of an appropriate animal, and it grows into an identical twin of the donor of the DNA. In the case of Dolly the sheep, the DNA donor was her mother. Therefore, Dolly is an identical twin of her mother, even though she is 6 years younger.

Another technique that may be referred to as "cloning" is really embryo splitting. After an ovum is fertilized by a sperm, either naturally or with in vitro fertilization (IVF), a single cell results, called a zygote, that contains a combination of genetic material (DNA), half from the father and half from the mother. Left alone to develop, that single cell will eventually develop into an individual who shares some of the inherited features of both parents as a result of the combination of DNA. Within 12 hours after the zygote is formed, it begins to divide into 2, then 4, then 8, and then 16 identical cells. When it reaches 16 cells, it enters the morula stage.

While the embryo is dividing up to and including the morula stage, the cells can be divided and separated. Because the cells are all identical, contain all the genetic material necessary to produce a new individual, and have fully active DNA, each cell is essentially a zygote. Once the cells are divided and separated, they can be implanted into several appropriate females and will continue to divide and develop into identical twins, or triplets, or more. Also, when the embryo is in the early four- to eight-cell stage, these cells can be separated, the genetic material removed from them, and new genetic material inserted. The cell with the new DNA will then grow into a twin of the animal from which the DNA was taken. It appears that by using the embryo-splitting procedure, scientists could produce an unlimited supply of ova for somatic cell nuclear transfer procedure.

With the IVF procedure, embryo splitting, and DNA transfer, the fertilization and early development process occur in a laboratory in a petri dish. After the cells begin to develop, they are implanted into an appropriate female for the remainder of the pregnancy. Although the cloning or embryo-splitting process is relatively simple, its success rate is at best marginal. In order to produce Dolly the sheep, more than 1000 ova were genetically treated. Of those 1000, only 29 actually began to develop, and of the 29 that developed, only one actually produced an animal (Dolly).

Ethical Issues

Shortly after the news of Dolly the sheep reached the US, a raging debate developed over whether the cloning of humans was ethical, moral, or even legal (Rapport, 2003). From the public standpoint, the three most troubling ethical issues were the loss of uniqueness of the individual, the potential misuse of the technology by diabolical scientists, and the degeneration of society as it now exists. Other, more traditional ethical concerns—such as medical risk to the mother or child (beneficence and nonmaleficence), life status of the embryos produced by the procedure, distributive justice issues of cost and availability of technology, and autonomy issues of using humans as incubators or sources of organs for donation—also remain troubling (Cassells, 2003).

The belief that genetic determinism will produce individuals who not only look but also act identically is fundamentally flawed. The fact that identical twins are exact genetic copies of each other demonstrates this result (Dinc, 2003). Although every cell in each twin's body is genetically identical to every cell in the other twin's body, experience shows us that they usually develop very individual personalities and character traits. Personality development is influenced by a wide range of environmental and experiential elements, not just genetic composition. If and when human cloning becomes a reality, cloned human babies who are born to mothers who live in different situations, although they may look the same, will likely have very different personality traits.

Similarly, the belief that there is a loss in quality each time an individual is cloned is not supported by experience. In many cases, for example, photocopies may actually be of higher quality than an original paper document. However, cloning is more than making photocopies, because the process is very different. The danger of "bad copies" from cloning that may well result in offspring of inferior quality or with congenital defects arises from the mechanical collection and transfer of the very fragile DNA strands. Scientists know that damaging even one gene sequence can produce birth defects.

As was discussed earlier, in most ethical dilemmas, motive is an important element in determining the rightness or wrongness of an act (Giarelli, 2003). There are several possible motivations to clone human beings, ranging

from egotism to helping an infertile couple have a child. The egotistical motivation conjures up images of the diabolical scientist or political leader who wants to create a "super-race" through the repeated cloning of physically and mentally superior individuals (like himself or herself, no doubt). You can imagine what Hitler might have done with this technology if it had existed at the time of the Second World War. What about cloning great inventors, brilliant leaders, or famous athletes? What owner of a football, baseball, or basketball franchise would not want a team of Terelle Davises or Mark McGuires or Michael Jordans? Could embryo factories be far behind?

A somewhat more altruistic, although still potentially objectionable, motive is the cloning of humans for the purpose of organ donation. Theoretically, the person who needs a heart transplant could donate DNA and, after a period of time, have an individual who has a heart with a perfect genetic match. However, most people have a strong abhorrence for the use of a cloned child as a means to an end, especially if harvesting the organ (as in a heart transplant) would result in the death of the child. However, some scientists in Texas have managed to clone mice without heads, whose organs were then transplanted back into the DNA donor mice. What if human clones could be created without heads? Would these headless beings truly be human, or would they just be a biological storage units for organs that could be used for donation when the need arose? Although at first glance this practice might seem abhorrent, is it really that different ethically from the sperm, egg, embryo, or organ banks that exist today?

In the past few years, several parents have decided to have children for the primary purpose of providing bone marrow for an older child who was afflicted with leukemia. In several cases, the children were an identical six-antigen match, and the bone marrow was harvested from the infant and transplanted into the sick child, who recovered completely from the disease. Is having children for this purpose so different from cloning children for use as organ transplants? What if scientists were to learn how to clone just one organ or specific tissue at a time? If a person needed a new liver, the DNA from his or her liver could be transferred to an ovum, and then a new liver grown in the laboratory. A similar procedure already exists, without ethical objections, for growing new skin used for grafting in burn patients.

Some parents might be motivated to clone a replacement child for one who has died or is going to die. These parents could "set aside" a clone through the embryo-splitting technique that could be stored in an embryo bank and could later be implanted and grown if the original child died. The underlying motivation would seem to be very selfish and self-serving—that is, to create a replacement child for relief of the parent's grief and sense of loss over the death of the first child. In reality, many couples who have lost a child to death have subsequent children to make their lives fuller and more meaningful. In addition, is the cloned child really a replacement for the child who died? Although the child would look the same, as discussed previously, his or her personality and temperament would likely be much different.

Similarly, the infertile couple who had tried all other methods and were unable to have a child might seek a cloned embryo as a last resort. This motivation may pose the fewest ethical objections. Rather than using ova, semen, or both from unknown individuals, they might opt to use their own DNA, from either the father or mother, to produce a child.

 CONCLUSION

Ethical issues and ethics are a part of your daily practice. In today's world, with rapidly advancing technology and unusual health-care situations, ethical dilemmas are increasing. You can be prepared to deal with most of these dilemmas if you keep current with the issues and are able to use a systematic process for making decisions about them. Hiding from ethical issues is not a solution. At some point, you will have to make difficult decisions. One of the most difficult parts of ethical decision-making is that someone is likely to be unhappy about your decision. But if you have made the decision after analyzing the situation on the basis of sound ethical principles, you should be able to defend it to anyone.

Key Points

- Ethical decision-making is a skill that can be learned and developed through practice.
- The steps in the ethical decision-making process are to collect and analyze the data; state the dilemma; consider the choices of action; analyze the choices and consider the consequences; and make the decision.
- Utilitarianism is a system of ethical decision-making based on the principle of the greatest good for the greatest number of people. It is situation oriented and has no established or unchanging rules. Deontology is a system of ethical decision-making based on unchanging rules and principles, without consideration of the consequences.
- The ANA *Code for Nurses* serves as the ethical guidelines for the profession of nursing. It provides the nurse with general statements about nursing ethics, which the nurse needs to interpret and apply to individual ethical situations.
- The key ethical issues involved in organ transplantation revolve around the ethical principles of distributive justice, informed consent, and determination of death.
- Ethical questions concerning end-of-life decisions often involve a conflict between the client's right to self-determination and the nurse's obligations of beneficence and nonmaleficence.

(continued)

(*continued*)

- A number of ethical principles are involved in ethical dilemmas created by the HIV and AIDS issue. These include the right to privacy, self-determination, the right to care, and distributive justice in the form of health-care workers' and society's right to protection from dangerous diseases.
- Although advance directives are now a legal part of the health-care system, a number of ethical issues still plague their use. The primary ethical concern is that of informed consent. Many clients have only a limited knowledge about the types of treatments possible for various conditions.
- A relatively new ethical concern for nurses involves current trends in health care for the increased use of unlicensed assistive personnel. Professional nurses are ethically and legally accountable for the care provided by these individuals.
- Cloning is a new technology with a promising future, but it also raises a number of disturbing ethical questions that nurses are likely to face in the future.

Thought and Discussion Questions

1. Look at the ANA *Code for Nurses*, and identify where the ethical principles come into play in its tenets.
2. Think of a recent ethical decision you have made in practice. Which ethical system do you use when making decisions? What systems do your colleagues use? How would the outcome in your earlier decision differ if you used the other system?
3. Name ten of your rights and classify them as legal, ethical, or option rights.
4. If you were to update or revise the ANA *Code of Ethics for Nurses*, what changes would you make so it is more reflective of the current health-care scenario?
5. Should people who have harmed their health by drinking, smoking, and drug use have the same right to health care as people who have taken care of themselves? What ethical issues would come into play in restricting access to care:?
6. In the specific ethical issues discussed in the chapter, what are the ethical principles that come into play in this situation? Explain the context.
7. Review the Chapter Thought located on the first page of the chapter, and discuss it in the context of the contents of the chapter.

Interactive Exercises

1. Read over the three case studies on the Intranet site, and be prepared to discuss the case study questions in a discussion to be scheduled by your instructor.
2. Participate in an on line discussion, to be scheduled by your instructor, on the topic of when the principle of veracity should or may be suspended in health care.

3. Find examples of or articles about ethical dilemmas on the Internet, and identify the ethical principles that come into play.

4. Clarify your own values using the Value Clarifications Tool shown in FIG. 14–1.

5. Look up whether or not your state has a natural death act. Does the law recognize living wills? What limits does the law place on the validity of living wills? What does your state law say about medical durable powers of attorney?

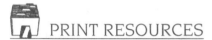 PRINT RESOURCES

References

Aiken, L. M. (2003). Critical care nurses' use of decision-making strategies. *Journal of Clinical Nursing*, 12 , 476–483.

Aiken, T. D., & Catalano, J. T. (1994). *Legal, ethical, and political issues in nursing*. Philadelphia: F. A. Davis.

American College of Physicians. (1998). Ethics manual (4th ed.). *Annual Internal Medicine*, 128, 576–594. Also available online at www.acponline.org/annuals/01apr98/ethicman.html

American Nurses Association. (2001). *Code for nurses with interpretive statements*. Washington, DC: Author.

Anderson-Shaw, L (2003). The unilateral DNR order—one hospital's experience. *Jonas Healthcare Law Ethics Regulation* 5(2), 42–46.

Bell, S. E. (2003). Ethical climate in managed care organizations. *Nursing Adminstration Quarterly* 27, 133–139.

Benner, P. (2003). Current controversies in critical care. *American Journal of Critical Care*, 12, 374–375.

Botes, A.(2003). Ethical dilemmas related to the HIV positive person in the workplace. *Nurse Ethics* 10(3), 281–294.

Briggs, L. A. (2002). End-of-life decision-making: Having those difficult discussions. *American Journal of Nurse Practitioners*, 6(8), 9–12.

Casey, J. (2003). Palliative care provisions in end-stage renal failure. EDTNA ERCA 29(1), 4–6.

Cassells, J. M. (2003). An ethical assessment framework for addressing global genetic issues in cinical practice. *Oncology Nursing Forum*, 30, 383–390.

Catalano, J. T. (2003). *Nursing now: Today's issues, tomorrow's trends*. Philadelphia: F.A. Davis.

Coughennower, M. (2003). Physician-assisted suicide. *Gastroenterology Nursing* 26(2), 55–59.

Davis, A. J., & Aroskar, M. S. (1997). Ethical dilemmas and nursing practice (4th ed.). Stamford, CT: appleton & Lange.

Dinc, L (2003). Ethical issues regarding human cloning: a nursing perspective. *Nursing Ethics*, 10, 238–254.

Fletcher, J. (1966). Situation ethics, Philadelphia: Westminster

Giarelli, E. (2003). Safeguarding being: A bioethical principle for genetic nursing care. *Nursing Ethics* 10, 255–268.

Henderson, S. (2003). Power imbalances between nurses and patients. *Journal of Clinical Nursing*, 12, 501–508.

Lorensen, M. (2003). Ethical issues after the disclosure of a terminal illness. *Nursing Ethics*, 10, 175–178.

Lutzen, K. (2003). Moral stress: Synthesis of a concept. *Nursing Ethics* 10, 312–322.

McKenney, E. (2003). Legal and ethical issues related to nonheart beating organ donation. AORN *Journal*, 77, 973–976.

McKenzie, D. R. (2002) Nursing ethics: Ethical consent in cancer treatment. VA *Nurses Today*, 11(2), 11–13.

McLeod, E. (2003). Uncovering meaning: How nursing knowledge changes policy in practice. *Nursing Science Quarterly*, 16, 115–119.

Moody, J. (2003). Euthanasia: A need for reform. *Nursing Standard*, 17(25), 40–44.

Palvianinen, P. (2003). Do nurses exercise power in basic care situations? *Nursing Ethics*, 10, 269–280.

Patterson, I. (2003). The ethics of assisted suicide. *Nursing Times*, 99(7), 30–31.

Rapport, F. (2003). Exploring the beliefs and experiences of potential egg share donors. *Journal of Advanced Nursing*, 43(1), 28–42.

Scott, P. A.(2003). Adult/elderly care nursing: Autonomy, privacy and informed consent. *British Journal of Nursing*, 12(3), 158–168.

Volker, D. L. (2003) Is there a unique nursing ethic? *Nursing Science Quarterly*, 16, 207–211.

Wilkes, L. Ethics on the floor. *Collegian*, 10(2), 34–39.

Bibliography

Catalano, J. T. (1997). Ethical decision making in the critical care patient. *Critical Care Clinics of North America*, 9(1), 45–52.

ONLINE RESOURCES

Agency for Health Care Policy and Research (AHCPR). *http://www.ahcpr.gov/ or info@ahcpr.gov/*

National Health Information Center (NHIC). *http://nhic-nt.health.org/ or NHICinfo@health.org*

AIDS Info BBS Database. *http://aidsinfobbs.org/* Contact: Ben Gardiner, *ben@aidsinfobbs.org*

American Association of Critical-Care Nurses. *http://www.aacn.org/ or info@aacn.org*

Bioethics Discussion Pages. *http://www.hsc.usc.edu/~mbernste/* Contact: Maurice Bernstein, MD, *DoktorMo@aol.com/*

Bioethics Online Service. *http://www.mcw.edu/bioethics/index.html/* Contact: Arthur R. Derse, *aderse@its.mcw.edu*

Critical Care Nurse Snapshots. *http://www.nursing.ab.umd.edu/* *students/~jkohl/scenario/opening htm/* Contact: John. Kohl, *jkohl@umabnet.ab.umd.edu*

HIV InfoWeb. *http://www.infoweb.org/*

Nurses' Station (Downsizing). *http://www.hci.net/~nursecline/* Contact: Joseph A. Cline, RN, BSN, *nursec-line@hci.net*

National Human Genome Research Institute (NHGRI). *http://www.nhgri.nih.gove/index.html*

Office of Genetics and Disease Prevention. *http://www.edc.gov/genetics*

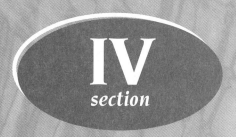

IV
section

Providing Care

Vicki L. Buchda

15
chapter

Managing and Providing Care

> Indeed, some observers believe that health-care delivery in this country will inevitably be facing a "perfect storm" over the next decade as several major environmental trends converge"
>
> McManis & Monslave Associates and AONE, 2003

Chapter Objectives

On completion of this chapter, the reader will be able to:

1. Discuss the current issues that affect planning and provision of health care for clients and groups of clients.
2. Describe the evolution and current concerns of work environments and nursing care delivery systems.
3. Contrast the various models of nursing care delivery.
4. Describe the documentation system and the taxonomy needed for selected care delivery systems.

Key Terms

Value
Cost-Effective
Outcomes of
  Care

Differentiated Nursing
  Practice
Team Nursing
Primary Nursing

Case Management
Critical Pathway
Nursing Minimum
  Data Set

Health-care management and delivery systems have evolved as health care has experienced rapid and dramatic changes in financing, reimbursement, technology, lengths of stay, and increased numbers of aging and chronically ill individuals. The Pew Health Professions Commission has observed that "over the past 50 years, nursing has changed substantially from a largely supportive role in health care to one with many independent and complex responsibilities in Health-care delivery" (O'Neil, 1998, p. 61). The changing role of the nurse is compounded by a shortage of health-care workers, including nurses, scarce resources, and concern about quality (American Hospital Association [AHA], 2002). Nurses are typically the largest segment of an acute care facility's personnel budget, so for economic reasons, nursing has become a target for redesign and restructuring. According to the AHA, many health-care workers, including nurses, are dissatisfied with their work (2002). Redesign can have positive impacts on quality, outcomes, cost-effectiveness, safety, and work satisfaction.

ORGANIZING CARE IN TODAY'S CLIMATE

It is true that economics drives health care reform and therefore has had the greatest impact on how American health care is organized and delivered (Porter-O'Grady & Wilson, 1995). Yet the demand by consumers and payers for safer care is a key component in reform as well. Articles about safety in hospitals appear almost monthly in the popular press, and consumers are being given advice about how to protect themselves. Frequently this advice involves inquiring about the registered nurse (RN)–patient ratios. New skill sets are required of nurses, including participation in continuous improvement as a routine part of clinical care (O'Neil, 1998, p. 41). Nurses are key in improving clinical care as

well as the environment in which that care is delivered.

Ultimately, care is planned, organized, and provided to meet the needs of clients, nurses, and the department or organization. The focus now in planning care has shifted. The work environment itself contributes to quality and safety. Moreover, consumers are demanding more client-focused, value-based, and outcome-oriented care.

The Role of Work Environment

The work environment is the context within which care is delivered. There are a number of reasons why work environment is vital. It contributes to the nursing shortage, quality of care issues, and patient safety concerns.

Staff nurses have identified several conditions that make a hospital a good place to work, including management style, quality of leadership, organizational structure, staffing, and personnel policies and programs (Schaffner & Ludwig-Beymer, 2003). The Institute of Medicine (IOM) convened a committee to study nurses' work environments and patient safety, and found serious threats "in all four of the basic components of all organizations—organizational management practices, workforce deployment practices, work design, and organizational culture" (IOM, 2004, p. 3). According to Aiken and colleagues (2001), nurses are very dissatisfied with their work environments, in this country, and others, and core problems in work design and workforce management threaten the provision of care (p. 43). Clearly, dissatisfaction leads to shortages.

A report published by the AHA entitled *In Our Hands* (2002) makes recommendations to address the shortages of health-care workers. Several recommendations involve the work environment and culture. The recommendations are in part:

1. Foster meaningful work by transforming hospitals into modern-day organizations, in which all aspects of the work are

designed around patients and the needs of staff to care for and support them.

2. Improve the workplace partnership by creating a culture in which hospital staff— including clinical, support, and managerial staff—are valued, have a sustained voice in shaping institutional policies, and receive appropriate rewards and recognition for their efforts.

These recommendations have themes similar to the original findings of a study conducted in 1982, which studied hospitals that seemed to be able to attract and retain nurses (McClure, et. al., 1983). These hospitals were dubbed "magnet" hospitals for their ability to attract and retain nurses, and the study noted that nurses who practiced at these hospitals experienced professional and personal satisfaction in their jobs (Box 15–1). Further, the environments supported excellence in nursing services and promoted quality patient care. The bottom line is that work environment affects the quality and safety of care provided.

> **BOX 15–1**
> **14 FORCES OF MAGNETISM**
>
> Fourteen forces of magnetism are attributed to hospitals with good work environments (McClure et al., 1983):
> - Quality of nursing leadership
> - Organizational structure
> - Management style
> - Personnel policies and programs
> - Professional models of care
> - Quality assurance
> - Consultation and resources
> - Level of autonomy
> - Community and the hospital
> - Nurses as teachers
> - Image of nursing
> - Collegial nurse-physician relationships
> - Educational development
>
> Refer to *http://nursingworld.org/ancc/magnet/process.html* for further information about the Magnet Nursing Services Recognition Program for Excellence in Nursing Services.

Client-Focused Care

As providers of care, nurses and other health-care providers recognize the need to shape a system focused on and organized around health-care consumers: clients, their families, and communities. Today an interdisciplinary plan of care is developed and implemented for each client, with goals and interventions mutually agreed on by the care providers and client. The link between client-centric care and quality and safety has been established (IOM, 2001). Consumers do not have a good way to judge the quality of their health-care and so often base their evaluation on clues such as "their care being organized around their needs rather than the doctor's schedules, the hospital's processes..." (Berry & Bendapudi, 2003, p. 102).

This shift in values also influences department organization. Historically, hospital services were organized around functions for the convenience of the staff. For example, inpatient and outpatient services were combined, requiring outpatients to navigate through inpatient facilities. In the client-focused paradigm, it is logical to organize and deliver care according to the client's needs. In the 1990s, this involved some models of restructuring and redesigning of roles so that, for example,

ONLINE CONSULT

The Institute of Medicine's second report on the quality of health care in America outlines the current concerns of health-care delivery and imperatives for the future in the United States. The report is available online at http://www.iom.edu/focuson.asp?id=8089

the admitting department admits the client at the bedside. Another trend is for facilities to form centers for outpatient care, including surgical services, for the convenience of the client.

Value

Another theme driving health-care reform is **value**. Consumers and payers are demanding value in health care, which has two essential components: cost and quality. In addition, appropriateness of care is important (IOM, 2001). Value can be expressed as "quality at a reasonable cost in a milieu of efficacy" (Pinkerton, 2001, p. 684). Understanding this concept is vital because "survival in a reformed healthcare industry will require nurses to articulate their value—i. e., nurses must demonstrate how they contribute to improving the quality of desired patient outcomes and reducing costs" (Arford & Allred, 1995, p. 64). The public expects it as well. In a national opinion survey conducted by the American Nurses Association (ANA) (1999), results indicated that when choosing a hospital, 93 percent of Americans would be more confident if they knew that the hospital had met rigorous quality standards (p. 1). Nurses are in a position to demonstrate their contribution to quality client outcomes and their ability to plan and deliver cost-effective care.

Accomplishing this involves, in part, matching needs with resources, so that the most cost-effective care provider is delivering the care. **Cost-effective** analysis examines the relationship between the cost to provide the service and the outcomes (Arford & Allred, 1995). Less expensive substitutes for professional nurses (referred to by some as "cheaper doers") therefore may not be cost-effective if outcomes are poor. However, using professional nurses to perform tasks that could be delegated is not cost-effective either (Box 15–2). As Malloch and Conovaloff (1999) have pointed out, mismatching care providers and clients has been the recurring bane of quality care (p. 50).

Outcomes

One of the most important challenges in making care more client-focused and valuable is for nurses to clearly demonstrate their contri-

**BOX 15–2
DELEGATION**

Many models of care delivery incorporate unlicensed assistive personnel (UAP). Licensed nurses must have competencies in delegation and supervision. *Delegation* is "transferring to a competent individual the authority to perform a selected nursing task in a selected situation. The nurse retains accountability for delegation" (National Council of State Boards of Nursing [NCSBN], 1995, p. 2).

The five rights of delegation (NCSBN, 1995) are:

- The right task
- The right circumstance
- The right person delegating and carrying out the right task on the right client
- The right directions or communications
- The right supervision

ONLINE CONSULT

For more information about delegation, refer to the National Council of State Boards of Nursing at
http://www.ncsbn.org.files/publications/positions/delegate.sp/

butions to **outcomes of care**. The IOM (2004) report acknowledged that "research is now beginning to document what physicians, patients, other healthcare providers, and nurses themselves have long known: how well we are cared for by nurses affects our health, and sometimes can be a matter of life and death" (p. 2). Nurses can use outcome evidence to demonstrate their value to clients and to the health-care system.

Documentation of outcomes is key because nurses can demonstrate their value only by defining the link between the quality of nursing care delivered and client outcomes. In addition, only by understanding the link between nursing care and client outcomes can we measure the effect of changing care delivery systems (ANA, 1995). Nurses need to define their contributions to the complex care delivered to ensure that their unique contributions are recognized as nursing care becomes even more highly integrated with other interdisciplinary team members.

Work to link patient outcomes with nursing care has been ongoing. A project reported by the ANA (1995) explored many of the links between nursing care and client outcomes in acute care by identifying quality indicators. This report card–type study identified 21 nursing quality indicators that have strong conceptual ties to quality nursing care. Although the study could not link all of the indicators to quality nursing care, the report emphasized the importance of such report cards and identified areas, through a review of current research and literature, where nursing is making a contribution. A review of other similar report card–type studies is included in the report. In 1997, a pilot study was conducted demonstrating the link between nurse staffing, interventions, and outcomes (ANA, 1997a). The ANA (1997, c) also funded the development of a national database for nursing-sensitive quality indicators. Data on the following 10 nursing-sensitive quality indicators are collected in this database:

- Mix of RNs, licensed practical nurses (LPNs), and unlicensed staff caring for patients in acute care settings

- Total nursing care hours provided per patient day
- Pressure ulcers
- Patient falls
- Patient satisfaction with pain management
- Patient satisfaction with educational information
- Patient satisfaction with overall care
- Patient satisfaction with nursing care
- Nosocomial infection rate
- Nurse staff satisfaction

Needleman and colleagues (2002) have demonstrated a link between a higher proportion of care provided by RNs and a greater number of hours of care by RNs per day and better patient outcomes for hospitalized patients. They studied "Outcomes Potentially Sensitive to Nursing (OPSNs)," which they selected on the basis of the literature as well as exploratory measures. They found, for example, that among medical patients, a higher portion of hours of care per day provided by RNs and a greater absolute number of hours of care per day provided by RNs were associated with a shorter length of stay (LOS) and lower rates of urinary track infections and upper gastrointestinal bleeding. The proportion of care hours provided by RNs were linked to lower rates of pneumonia, shock or cardiac arrest, and failure of rescue. There were similar findings in surgical patients (Needleman et al., 2002).

Adequate staffing levels are also key to providing quality care. Having the right numbers of the right caregivers is key to matching work with staffing. There is no one right answer to the question "How many nurses is enough?" Licensure, regulation, and legislation are regarded by some as the answer. Some states now have mandatory staffing ratios. What these ratios fail to address is the complexity of the care environment, the competence of the personnel, and the acuity and workload involved for the patient. Accreditation agencies are interested in this as well. In 2002 the Joint Commission on Accreditation of Healthcare Organizations (JCAHO) added standards addressing the assessment of the effectiveness of staffing. The purpose is to require accredited agencies to use data to assess staffing effectiveness.

ONLINE CONSULT

For more information about the Joint Commission on Accreditation of Healthcare Organizations, refer to their Web site: http://www.jcaho.org/index.htm/

The next logical step is to use outcome findings to improve practice. The responsibility to structure nursing practice on the basis of outcome data rests with nursing and poses some challenges for nurses who have followed routines for years. Taking and documenting vital signs, for example, is a firmly entrenched practice usually based on routine. Nurses are being asked to examine such practices for their contribution to the outcome. If they cannot establish a link to a positive outcome, the practice should be dropped. A move toward outcome-based practice is critical in order to offer the quality and value demanded by health-care consumers.

NURSING ROLES

It is clear that nursing contributions to client outcomes are important, but what exactly do these contributions entail? McCloskey (1995) describes two roles for the nurse: provider of care and manager of the care environment. As providers of care, nurses deliver direct and indirect care for individual clients and for groups of clients. *Direct care* is defined as those interventions "performed through interaction with the patient(s)" (Bulachek & McCloskey, 1999). *Indirect care* is performed on behalf of the client to support the direct care interventions. An example of indirect care is communication with other interdisciplinary team members.

In addition to being the provider of care, nurses play a role in managing the care environment. At the client care level, nurses' care management responsibilities include organizing, directing, and coordinating the care. The responsibility for matching needs with resources, as described earlier, is one aspect of this role. The role may also include talking with payers (including insurance companies), negotiating for client services,

and advocating within the organization on behalf of a client.

Nurses also have management responsibilities within the client care unit or department. These responsibilities include delegating and supervising other personnel and unit operations, such as staffing and scheduling. This aspect of the management role varies with the work environment, but the trend is toward flatter organizations, with direct care providers assuming more of the traditional management roles in the department (IOM, 2004).

Interdisciplinary Care Delivery

In the current system, nurses work closely with other interdisciplinary team members, such as social workers, therapists, and dietitians. The contributions of each of these highly skilled team members is coordinated and integrated into the plan of care for clients by professional nurses. As new models of work organization and structure are implemented in practice, care will be delivered to clients by groups of care providers working in highly integrated teams. Cost and quality will continue to be emphasized, and the *team* will be held accountable for the outcomes of the care.

Interdisciplinary teams, working collaboratively to deliver care, support cost-effectiveness because more often the right person with the right skills is delivering the service. This is an important step in matching needs with resources. The development of highly integrated interdisciplinary teams is not without problems, however. Some of the issues that need to be addressed are defining contributions to care, territoriality, and the shift in power. As discussed earlier, defining the contributions to care by the various providers is one of the greatest challenges facing health-care providers. It is an important step in the process, because matching the person with the knowledge, skills, and abilities to achieve the best outcome cost-effectively is the key to achieving value. The setting (e. g., intensive care unit, home health, or the whole community), the needs of the clients, and economics drive the logical providers and coordinator of care. This may lead to concerns about turf; for example, nurses may give up some responsibilities to social workers, and physicians to nurses. Some may regard this shift in accountability and power as threatening.

Differentiated Nursing Practice

The concepts of matching needs with resources and care providers with client needs may seem simplistic, but with the many levels of nursing practice, different curricula, and various education requirements, this task becomes more complex. In order to articulate contributions to care and cost-effectiveness, nursing must closely examine its own knowledge and skill sets.

Although there is agreement about the importance of the role of the registered nurse, the debate about educational preparation for professional nursing has been ongoing for almost 40 years. Currently, most nurses (62%) are employed by hospitals (U.S. Department of Health and Human Services, 2002, p. 11), and most job descriptions for registered nurses define one set of performance expectations to fulfill the role, regardless of educational preparation. With these blended job descriptions, some nurses' knowledge and skills are being underutilized and others are being asked to perform at higher levels than they were prepared for. To be seen as efficient and cost-effective in the future, nursing may benefit from differentiated nursing competencies.

The phrase "A nurse is not a nurse" is understood within nursing to acknowledge that nurses are highly skilled professionals, many of whom are subspecialized and not interchangeable with one another. Nurses themselves think of the concept in terms of whether or not they could "float to" or

practice in another area. Increasingly, however, the "recognition of the complexities of health care and the rapid expansion of knowledge is increasing the pressure to raise the level of basic education" (Nelson, 2002). It is proposed that, ultimately, "the more educated practitioner will be more cost-efficient" (Joel, 2002). Aiken and colleagues (2003) reported that surgical patients being treated in hospitals employing larger proportions of nurses with baccalaureate or higher levels had lower mortality rates and failure of rescue rates.

Levels of nursing practice were first introduced by the ANA in 1965, and **differentiated nursing practice** has been a goal of nursing professionals for a decade (American Association of Colleges of Nursing [AACN], 1995). It was recognized at that time that nurses possess a variety of skill sets, depending on educational preparation and experiential learning, and that clients and the profession would benefit from differentiating the practice. There are two types of differentiated practice: education-based practice, which is delineated according to educational credentials, and assessment-based practice, which incorporates both education and experiential learning.

One model of differentiated practice that defines roles according to educational preparation was proposed by Primm (1986). This model defines major and minor components of nursing practice, and these various components are assigned according to the nurses' educational preparation. *Technical nurses* care for clients and are responsible for meeting identified care goals in a specified work period and within structured health-care settings that provide policies and procedures as well as nursing experts for consultation and support. *Professional nurses* care for families and communities from the time of admission to after discharge, in structured and unstructured settings and in situations that may not have policies and procedures but that require independent nursing decisions (Primm, 1986).

A more sophisticated model of differentiated practice has been used at Sioux Valley Hospital, Sioux Falls, South Dakota (AACN, 1995). Roles for nurses with associate degrees, bachelor's degrees, and master's degrees are delineated within a case management model, demonstrating cost-effectiveness and quality outcomes (Koerner & Karpiuk, 1994). In addition, the hospital provides a site for nursing students from Bachelor of Science in Nursing (BSN) and Associate Degree in Nursing (ADN) programs to learn differentiated clinical practice in the real world (AACN, 1995).

More recently, in the South Carolina Colleagues in Caring project, partially funded by the Robert Wood Johnson Foundation, educational and provider group "colleagues" addressed the need to "facilitate regional workforce planning to ensure that the size and the educational mix of the nursing workforce is sufficient to meet nursing care needs across all settings" (Loquist & Bellack, 1998, i). A matrix differentiating entry level (less than 1 year) of practice by educational program type (practical nursing, associate degree, baccalaureate, and master's) was developed through the collaboration of deans and directors of educational programs. This matrix includes seven dimensions of practice by educational level:

- The average length of the program
- Curriculum purpose with expected outcome competencies related to nursing process, technical skills, communication skills, management/leadership/administrative skills, and health promotion/education skills
- Generalist (undergraduate) versus specialist (graduate) focus
- Client or recipient of care
- The time frame in which care is delivered
- The settings (structured/unstructured and traditional/nontraditional) in which care is delivered
- The type and level of complexity of

health problems (Loquist & Bellack, 1998, pp. ii–1)

Findings from this project were presented at local levels throughout South Carolina in an effort to address the workforce needs in all areas of nursing practice. In a follow-up article, Bellack and Loquist (1999) presented employer responses to differentiated nursing education. In addition, information from the matrix has been integrated in the Future Competencies Matrix of the Pew Health Profession Commission (Brady et al., 2001). The model is currently being pilot tested in selected education and practice settings in South Carolina (Brady et al., 2001). The model will be reviewed at least every 5 years, and changes will be monitored (Loquist and Brady, 2001).

> *The need for differentiated practice is compounded during times of shortage, and yet the tendency is just the opposite.*

All differentiated nursing practice models recognize the contributions of all nurses and pave the way for better delineation of outcomes with clearer job descriptions and expectations. Implementing such models increases efficiency and cost-effectiveness because it "places the highest-quality, lowest-cost provider next to the patient" (Differentiated Nursing Practice, 1995). The need for differentiated practice is compounded during times of shortage, and yet the tendency is just the opposite. During times of shortage there is a great deal of pressure to reduce educational requirements and change licensure and accreditation standards (Donley & Flaherty, 2002). In addition, the shortage of nurses makes employers shy about offending any group of nurses in the workforce (Nelson, 2002).

 ONLINE CONSULT

For further information about the South Carolina Statewide Articulation Model refer to their Web site:
http://www.sc.edu/nursing/cic/

DELIVERING CARE

Nursing care delivery systems are undergoing tremendous redesign to meet the changing needs of clients, nurses, and the organization. To be effective, the nursing care delivery system must be consistent with the mission, vision, and values of the care providers, the department, and the organization (Schaffner & Ludwig-Beymer, 2003). Schaffner and Ludwig-Beymer (2003) have identified other factors to consider by anyone redesigning a care delivery model or assessing that one is being used as follows:

- Number of RNs available in the organization and in the market area
- Fiscal resources available to fund salaries and costs such as training costs
- Nursing acceptance of the model
- Expected outcomes, such as risk reduction, fewer medication errors, fewer pressure sores, improved patient satisfaction, and improved pain management (Schaffner & Ludwig-Beymer, 2003, p. 216)

For these reasons, what may seem to be an ideal care delivery system in one organization may not work for another organization. Therefore, this section is meant to be descriptive and not prescriptive. In general, however, key factors that define success include:

- Client focus
- Cost-effectiveness
- Outcome orientation
- Safety
- Matching of needs with resources
- Documentation of care and outcomes
- Setting (work environment) that supports professional nursing practice

A comprehensive model also involves having the right caregivers available to provide care. Various acuity and/or workload systems have been developed and implemented in efforts to classify or categorize clients by needs to ensure assignment of the right caregivers. It is beyond the scope of this chapter to discuss staffing and scheduling systems, but such systems assist in the process of planning and evaluating models of care delivery.

Models of Care Delivery

Care delivery models have evolved through the years to meet the demands and challenges of the health-care arena. Many factors influence the models of care delivery existing today. This section offers a brief review of generic care delivery models. In-depth discussions of various delivery models are provided in other sources (Mayer et al., 1990; Nursing Clinics of North America, 1992; Walker, 1991; Walker et al., 1994; Hoover, 1998). Although care delivery models have undergone many changes, their underlying objectives are to "assess the patient, identify the nursing needs of the patient during hospitalization, and provide the nursing care necessary until the patient is discharged" (Lyon, 1993).

Case Method

The case method was one of the earliest models of care delivery. A nurse was assigned to provide complete care for a client or group of clients for a defined period, usually 8 hours. Sometimes referred to as *private-duty nursing*, this method was inefficient because one nurse provided all care to the client (Cohen & Cesta, 1993; Poulin, 1985). As shown by Grant and Massey (1999), this method was based on the holistic philosophy of nursing with a nurse-to-client ratio of 1:1 to 1:5, but with the disadvantage of high personnel costs (pp. 34–35).

Functional

Functional nursing evolved next, improving on the case method of assignments by using a variety of caregivers to complete the tasks (Cohen & Cesta, 1993). This model allocated tasks or functions. One nurse gave all medications, another performed all treatments, and other caregivers gave all baths. Although a variety of caregivers participated in client care delivery in this model, the functional model has been criticized because it emphasizes task completion over client needs, resulting in fragmentation of care and unmet client needs (Thomas & Bond, 1991). The lack of ongoing personal contact with the client and absence of continuity of care have been cited as distinct disadvantages of this care model (Grant & Massey, 1999, p. 35).

Team

Team nursing emerged after World War II, when there was a shortage of nurses and other personnel were recruited to deliver care (Lyon, 1993). In the team model, other health-care workers—some licensed, such as a licensed practical nurse, and some unlicensed, such as aides and orderlies—delivered care under the supervision of a registered nurse. The team was led by a team leader, who delegated the tasks and activities and provided some direct care. Team nursing provided an advantage over functional nursing by providing professional nurses to more clients, improving continuity of care, and freeing professional nurses from performing nonprofessional tasks (Cohen & Cesta, 1993). Team nursing also provided a higher level of job satisfaction for nurses over the functional method (Grant & Massey, 1999, p. 35).

Team nursing has inherent problems, however. It results in fragmented care, complex channels of communication, and shared responsibility with lack of accountability (Manthey, 1980). Care is fragmented by being divided into components delegated to appropriate caregivers, so that clients are cared for by at least three people during an 8-hour shift (RN, LPN, and nursing assistant) with a total of 9 caregivers in a day. Communication is also complex; the caregivers report to the team leader, who relays the information to the next shift team leader. In some cases, the team leader reports to a charge nurse, who relays the information to another charge nurse, who passes it on to the team leader. The information is subject to interpretation by each person in the chain.

Responsibility and accountability are major issues in team nursing. The nursing care plan, for example, is supposed to be completed and updated routinely, usually daily. The team leader bears this responsibility, as does the next shift team leader. What is not completed on one shift is completed on the next shift. According to Manthey (1980), shared responsibility equals no responsibility, and activities like completing care plans are not carried out consistently with this model.

Primary

Primary nursing evolved to meet the needs that were not addressed in the team nursing system. Manthey (1980) described primary nursing as a delivery system designed to "rehumanize" hospital care through decentralized decision-making. Responsibility for one client's care, 24 hours a day, is allocated to a primary nurse who actually provides the care whenever possible. Because one nurse has the responsibility, accountability, and authority to assess clients needs, develop a plan of care, and evaluate the clients' responses to the plan of care, a therapeutic relationship can be established between the nurse and the client (Mathews & Kamikawa, 1994; Wilkinson, 1994). The concepts of 24-hour accountability and RNs directing other RNs differentiate this model from the case method model of delivery.

The primary nursing model recognizes the contributions of various care team members but relies heavily on RNs, not only for care planning but also for delivery of care. Because of this high reliance on RNs, primary nursing was frequently perceived as a costly model of care delivery. RNs are usually very satisfied with this care delivery model (Schaffner & Ludwig-Beymer, 2003). In Great Britain, Rigby and colleagues (2001) report, primary nursing has been credited with pushing "an undervalued occupation towards greater professional recognition," but they also acknowledge that this "theoretical idea that may not be achievable in practice" (p. 530).

Patient-Focused Care

The nursing shortage of the 1980s, the cost of an all-professional staff, and obstacles to implementing primary nursing (such as 12-

hour shifts) have led some hospitals to examine alternatives to primary nursing. There are many variations of the patient-focused care model, but in general, an RN, along with an unlicensed assistant, manages a group of patients (Schaffner & Ludwig-Beymer, 2003). Some of the challenges of these types of models are role design/redesign, delegation and supervision skills of the RN, and varying levels of educational preparation of the assistive person.

Case Management

The forces in health care today have made it necessary to develop care delivery systems that go beyond the industrial model, which emphasized task completion and outputs, to integrated systems that include mechanisms to define the links between nursing care and outcomes and to demonstrate cost-effectiveness. In evaluating care delivery systems, many institutions have implemented the **case management** model because it helps organize care around the client and is in concert with interdisciplinary and intradisciplinary differentiated practice. Because this model addresses many concerns previously identified, it is discussed here is some depth. Entire texts have been written about case management, however, and you are encouraged to refer to these and other sources for further information (Powell, 2000a and 2000b).

Case management is not a new concept. Nurses and members of other disciplines have been providing case management for clients for many years. Community public health programs have had case management services since the 1900s (Lyon, 1993). Behavioral health nurses have been using many of the concepts in the community since the 1960s. Case management received more attention from other areas of health care, including acute care settings, when insurance companies began using the model. In recent years, it became one of the most frequently used care models in the country (AHA, 1990). Now the model is not only well recognized but also universally accepted (Powell, 2000a).

Case management is a care delivery model focused on the client that promotes continuity and cost-effectiveness, recognizes the contributions of the members of the interdisciplinary team, and allows for differentiation of practice within the nursing profession. There are many definitions of case management. Bower (1992) described case management as a "paradoxically simple yet complex concept" (p. 3). Simply stated, *case management* refers to "patient focused strategies to coordinate care" (Bower, 1992, p. 2). Case management has also been defined as "an approach that focuses on the coordination, integration, and direct delivery of patient services, and places internal controls on the resources used for care" (Cohen & Cesta, 1993). Gerber (2001) combines the definition of the Case Management Society of America (CMSA), and Smith's definition to provide the following descriptive definition of case management:

> Nursing case management can be defined as the application of the collaborative and interdisciplinary case management process by professional nurses to promote the delivery of high quality, holistic, cost-effective health and illness care to individuals and groups within communities and complex organizational systems through patient advocacy, communication, and effective management of available resources. (p. 693)

The purposes of case management are to ensure cost-effectiveness, quality, and continuity of care.

> *Case management is a care delivery model focused on the client that promotes continuity and cost-effectiveness, recognizes the contributions of the members of the interdisciplinary team, and allows for differentiation of practice within the nursing profession.*

Case management is often confused with other concepts, including managed care, because the terms are frequently used interchangeably, and because the historical development is similar (Cohen & Cesta, 1993). Refer to Chapter 19 for an in-depth discussion of managed care plans and financing. The entity with the most risk for expensive care and treatment of the client typically provides case management services. Managed care providers or insurance companies may provide case management services in an attempt to promote wellness and prevent hospitalization, because hospital care is usually the most costly kind of care. The hospital may also provide case management services once clients are admitted, because insurance pays only a designated amount of money, either per day or for the entire period of hospitalization, and the incentive is for hospitals to provide care as cost-effectively as possible.

Case management can be provided in a variety of settings. Lyon (1993) delineates three categories of case management in health-care settings: hospital-based case management, case management across the health-care continuum, and community case management.

Hospital-Based Case Management

Hospital-based case management began with the introduction of the prospective payment system in 1983 (Lyon, 1993). Since then, professional nurses have been responsible for clients' lengths of stay and for matching needs with resources.

The case management care delivery model can be implemented in a way that addresses some of the issues identified earlier; the care clients receive is provided by the caregivers with the right knowledge and skills, and in the right setting for the intensity, amount of care needed, and severity of illness. The role of case managers is to facilitate and integrate the contributions of the interdisciplinary team. The case manager's role also lends itself to intradisciplinary differentiation. For these reasons, this model facilitates cost-effective, quality care.

The role of case manager is carried out dif-ferently in different models. Case managers, for example, can be staff nurses who, with some additional training and education, incorporate case management activities into the planning and provision of care on a daily basis. Some organizations have designated case managers for groups of clients. Others have case managers who follow clients within the hospital, but also follow select groups of clients through the continuum of care. Some organizations assign case managers to a unit or units with clients who have common diagnoses, whereas others assign case managers to follow clients through the course of the hospital stay. Each model has advantages and disadvantages, and no one model is right for every organization. Some organizations even use case managers differently within the setting, depending on the client type and other identified needs. For example, one case manager in a hospital may be unit based and another population based, crossing units.

The case management system can be used with a variety of nursing care delivery systems—primary, team, functional, or combinations of these systems (Lyon, 1993). If it is used with one of these client care delivery systems, the case management system can be overlaid onto the existing structure, or the entire system can be reengineered. Another strength of the case management system is that it can be used with differentiated care models. For example, more experienced or baccalaureate-prepared nurses are assigned to manage a caseload of patients in addition to their other patient care responsibilities. The technical or less experienced nurse, meanwhile, might have a greater direct patient care load without the case management responsibilities.

Case managers match needs to resources

through a systematic process. The steps in the process vary with the overall model used within the organization; however, there are some common functions. The following is an example of a model in an acute care setting in which a nurse case manager is responsible for a group of clients.

There are several levels of complexity in planning and organizing care in case management models. Case managers prioritize for groups of clients, and then address the needs of individual clients. As a part of their role, nurse case managers evaluate practice patterns for appropriateness, timeliness, and medical necessity. A systematic process is used to address overutilization and underutilization of resources, inefficiencies, and delays. Care and services are coordinated and integrated.

The following steps represent an approach to a caseload model but they do not have to be carried out in this order:

1. The process used to organize a day or caseload involves reviewing payer status of the clients. Clients who are members of capitated plans, for instance, may be evaluated first, because the case manager often communicates with payers about the clients' status and anticipated length of stay. Health plans commonly need to "authorize" admissions and continued stays.
2. The case manager prioritizes review of medical records. This may be accomplished by talking with other members of the health-care team and responding to potential problems they identify, or answering referrals from other sources.
3. Clients are evaluated, usually daily, according to some criteria for appropriateness of service level, such as intensity of service and severity of illness. This evaluation is key in matching needs with resources, because some levels of care, such as intensive care, are very costly to the organization. If the client no longer meets intensity or severity criteria for the intensive care unit, the case manager facilitates transfer to an appropriate level of care. Sometimes the case manager determines that the resources a client needs are too intense for a particular unit and rec-

ommends transfer to a higher level of care. The case manager always keeps in mind the cost to quality equation.
4. The case manager also focuses on individual clients, evaluating what the client needs now, what needs are anticipated, and what resources are available. The case manager works through any obstacles to achieve the best outcome as mutually agreed upon with the client.
5. The case manager helps the team develop and implement the plan. This involves communicating with the client and family, nurses, and other members of the interdisciplinary team.
6. The case manager also has responsibility for evaluating the case management process, including productivity indicators, quality and outcome indicators, and financial information tracking.
7. The evaluation information is used to change practice, for instance, to match the care provider who has the knowledge, skills, and abilities with the care to be given. The case manager usually facilitates development of clinical pathways and ensures appropriate documentation.

Case Management Across the Continuum

Case management services can be episodic—usually initiated and completed during a hospital stay, as described in the previous section—or they can continue as the client moves back into the community. Some models that include services across the continuum report improvement in the quality of care and cost reduction (Koerner & Karpiuk, 1994; Lamb & Huggins, 1990). Sioux Valley Hospital, which uses differentiated case management, saved more than $500,000 in a six-month period through the case management of 35 complex patients (AACN, 1995). The type of service provided depends on the patient population, the goals of the program, and the provider. For example, case management for group of clients with congestive heart failure (CHF) might be performed by advanced practice nurses such as Clinical Nurse Specialists (CNSs). The CNS would follow the patient in the hospital, ensure that discharge teaching is completed, then monitor the patient with telephone calls or visits in an outpatient clinic. The goal of case management in this case is to prevent re-admission to the hospital through early detection and intervention in this chronically ill population.

Case Management in the Community

Some case management programs are community based and begin after clients are discharged from the hospital. These services are provided by nurses and other members of the interdisciplinary team. Clients are assessed, counseled, reminded of appointments for follow-up, and referred to other professionals as needed. These services are frequently provided for behavioral health clients who are reintegrating into the community. These services may be provided by the health maintenance organization (HMO) case manager, who is accountable for coordination of care overall, or by other case managers who manage "crisis and details while that patient resides in their respective level of care" (Powell, 2000a). These case managers specialize in areas such as home health, skilled nursing, and rehabilitation.

Critical Pathways

Some of the case management strategies, such as integrating and coordinating services and tracking outcomes, are not easy to implement. Tools are available, however, to facilitate the processes. One of the tools for supporting this process is a document developed to define the care for a particular client type, commonly referred to as a **critical pathway**, or CareMap^{tm}.

Critical pathways are important tools for mapping client care and expected outcomes throughout an acute episode of illness (Gibson, 1996). They define not only care but outcomes as well, and they encourage identification of variances so that new interventions can be planned. Critical pathways are different from nursing care plans, which focus on individual differences; critical pathways define the most usual care for a client type and focus on the similarities of clients. They guide health professionals to the most common ways of treating and responding to a given episode of illness. Critical pathways also allow for documentation of care provided and comparison of clients' actual status with predefined outcomes. Variances from the plan, in either the care the client is to receive or the outcomes achieved, can be tracked and analyzed.

Typical critical pathways identify the care that clients receive during a specific time frame, along with expected outcomes. Critical pathways are developed by interdisciplinary teams through a systematic process. Some maps extend across the care continuum and follow the client into the community, but most are designed for the acute care period.

Documentation

The shift in care delivery systems has also contributed to a shift in the focus of nursing documentation. In the functional model, documenting task completion was the focus. As the movement into team nursing and then primary nursing emphasized greater continuity of care, the nursing care plan gained importance as a system to document the care.

With the shift to a patient-centered care focus, the use of language in documentation also changed. Client databases, rather than nursing admission forms, are now completed at admission, and client or patient care plans, not nursing care plans, are developed. Classification systems now are increasingly focused on client outcomes.

As the environment, including reimbursement structure and risk management, continues to change, the emphasis on documentation will also continue to change. For example, under a reimbursement structure in which the provider or health-care institution is reimbursed on the basis of charges, it is extremely important to document all supplies and equipment used. Some plans will not reimburse for the use of a specialized bed, such as a low-air-loss bed, without daily documentation that the client is using the bed.

Infusion of every liter of intravenous solution must be documented, or the payer can refuse to pay for the solution, even though it was charged to the client. A payer can refuse to reimburse an entire hospital stay for failure to document administration of an antibiotic. Documentation is also important in traditional quality management monitoring and risk management.

The amount of time consumed by documentation is continually questioned. Health-care professionals are familiar with the saying "If it isn't documented, it isn't done." In a 2002 publication entitled *Principles for Documentation*, the ANA cited conscientiousness by nurses in complying with all of the documentation requirements as pulling nurses away from direct patient care. The implementation of documentation by exception, in which nurses document abnormal or significant findings, has assisted with some of the burden of documentation, but it is noted in the IOM report that 13 to 28 percent of a nurse's time in acute care is consumed in documentation, and the figure is even higher in home care because of regulatory requirements (IOM, 2004, p. 6). This time could be spent actually providing patient care and in patient monitoring. Although automated systems have improved access to information, in general, they have not reduced the time spent in documenting.

STANDARDIZED NOMENCLATURES

Standardized nomenclatures are known also as classification systems, taxonomies, and languages. According to Bulachek and McCloskey (1999), the five purposes for classification systems of nursing practice are:

- To link knowledge about diagnosis, treatments, and outcomes
- To facilitate the development of nursing and health-care information systems
- To facilitate teaching of decision-making to nursing students

- To help determine the costs of services provided by nurses
- To articulate with the classification systems of other health-care providers.

It is important for nursing to agree upon and adopt standardized nomenclature, because as discussed earlier, nurses are being asked to identify what they do and what they contribute to care. This identification requires collection of essential nursing information, including nursing diagnoses, interventions, and outcomes. Without consistent methods of documentation, national databases, or agreement of the language to be used, nurses cannot be sure that they are comparing "apples and apples." The standardized nomenclatures assist us in organizing data; ultimately that data must be "represented and managed so they can be processed using well-designed computer algorithms" (Harris et al., 2000, p. 539) to facilitate patient care and to ensure quality and cost-effectiveness.

Nursing Minimum Data Set

One goal the profession is working toward is to implement the uniform collection of essential nursing information, known as the **Nursing Minimum Data Set** (NMDS) (Moorhead et al., 1993). This database will provide large data sets allowing nursing data to be compared across populations, to complement information from other professionals. The ANA (1997c) has supported the development of the NMDS and predicts that the data set will:

- Contribute to the delivery of safe, effective nursing care
- Describe nursing practice
- Provide quality control data
- Facilitate the analysis and evaluation of health policy
- Advance nursing knowledge
- Contribute to the structure of nursing education
- Facilitate the allocation of nursing resources

ONLINE CONSULT

The ANA's position statement about a National Database to Support Nursing Practice and the use of the NMDS is available online at http://nursingworld.org/readroom/position/practice/prdatabs.htm

- Contribute toward payment reform for nursing services
- Assist in determining the cost of nursing care
- Assist in determining nursing's contributions to client care (p. 2)

Implementation of the NMDS depends on having a standardized language for four essential components: nursing diagnosis, nursing interventions, nursing outcomes, and nursing intensity (Delaney & Moorhead, 1995).

Diagnoses

Classification of client problems has been available for more than two decades through the North American Nursing Diagnosis Association (NANDA) and as a component of the Omaha System. These two systems are very different; NANDA's approach is very broad, but the Omaha System focuses on community health (Delaney & Moorhead, 1995).

Interventions

Several classifications for nursing interventions have been developed, including the Omaha System, the Home Healthcare Classification, and the Nursing Interventions Classification (NIC). A research team at the University of Iowa began work on the most comprehensive classification, NIC, in 1987. Since the initial classification was published in 1992, research has continued. Researchers constructed, validated, and coded a taxonomy. Through clinical field testing, they also identified the need for linkages between NANDA, NIC, and nursing outcomes classifi-

cations (NOC). The challenge in the clinical setting is to document both professional knowledge (for research and statistical purposes), and care delivered (for legal and reimbursement purposes).

Outcomes

A standardized language for nursing outcomes was developed by another research team at the University of Iowa. With the development of NOC, the nursing process elements of the NMDS are complete. The NOC includes outcome labels, label definitions, indicators for each outcome, and a five-point Likert-type measurement scale (Johnson et al., 2000).

> *Recently, a new data set was introduced by the American Operating Room Nurses Association (AORN), the Perioperative Nursing Data Set (PNDS). AORN (1999) has stated that the "initial goal in developing the data set was to develop a unified language so that nursing care could be systematically quantified, coded, and easily captured in a computerized format in the perioperative setting" (p. 1). This data set is based on the Perioperative Patient Focused Model that is designed to "delineate the relationships within the domains of nursing concern: nursing diagnoses, nursing interventions, and patient outcomes in continuous interaction with the Healthcare system" (AORN, 1999, p. 1).*

Intensity

The fourth component NMDS requires is standardized language for nursing intensity. *Nursing intensity* is difficult to define, and even more difficult to measure. Nursing must be able to document the resources required to provide client care and achieve defined outcomes (Delaney & Moorhead, 1995). Without this language, determining the true cost of care will be difficult, and making it cost-effective will be even more difficult.

Although it is extremely important to capture nursing's contribution to care and outcomes, it is also important to acknowledge that as we move to highly integrated interdisciplinary teams, we may not be able to use language that belongs exclusively to nursing. As integrated documentation is developed, and all professionals rely more heavily on communication in records, language that everyone can use is required.

Key Points

- Health-care planning and provision are changing dramatically as a result of shortages of care providers, economics, and changing population.
- Cost, quality, and safety are the essential components of the care that is provided.
- The economic forces and philosophical shifts experienced today are encouraging nurses to demonstrate their contributions to client outcomes.
- Roles of the interdisciplinary and intradisciplinary care providers should be differentiated by knowledge, skills, and abilities and contributions to client outcomes.
- Various care delivery models, such as team and primary nursing, are currently used to organize the delivery of care. Models must address the needs of the organization, match the organization's culture and values, and consider the content of care delivered.
- Case management is one care delivery model that addresses many of the current concerns of care delivery systems. Critical pathways are tools that assist in achieving the goals of case management.
- Documentation, an essential component of care, is changing as care delivery systems and reimbursement systems change.
- Nursing is developing taxonomies to assist in identifying what nurses do and what they contribute to care. The Nursing Minimum Data Set will assist in the uniform collection of essential nursing information.

Thought and Discussion Questions

1. Participate in a discussion on the importance of the NMDS. Why would it be helpful for the profession of nursing and health care provision in general, and what difficulties may be encountered in its use?

2. Analyze the care delivery system on a client care unit. What model is in place? Are responsibilities differentiated according to knowledge, skills, and abilities?

3. Think of some ways that your organization has made changes to focus more centrally on clients. Think about and be prepared to discuss the model of care delivery used in your organization.

4. Review the Chapter Thought located on the first page of the chapter, and discuss it in the context of the contents of the chapter (either on line or in class).

Interactive Exercises

1. Complete the exercise on the Intranet site entitled Quality Indicator Score for Acute Care Agency to identify how these indicators are addressed at your organization or an acute care facility with which you are familiar.

2. Identify a group of clients with a common diagnosis or problem. Develop a critical pathway for that client type.

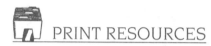

PRINT RESOURCES

References

Aiken, L. H., Clarke, S. P., Cheung, R. B., Sloane, D. M., & Silber, J. H. (2003). Educational levels of hospital nurses and surgical patient mortality. JAMA, 290(12), 1617–1623.

Aiken, L. H., Clarke, S. P., Sloane, D. M., Sochlaski, J. A., Busse, R., Clarke, H., Giovannetti, P., Hunt, J., Rafferty, A. M., & Shamian, J. (2001). Nurse's reports on hospital care in five countries. Health Affairs, 20(3), 43–53.

American Association of Colleges of Nursing. (1995). A model for differentiated nursing practice. Washington, DC: American Association of Colleges of Nursing.

American Hospital Association. (2002). In our hands: How hospital leaders can build a thriving workforce. Chicago: American Hospital Association.

American Hospital Association. (1990). Report of the hospital nursing personnel survey—1990. Chicago: American Hospital Association.

American Nurses Association. (2002). Principles for documentation. Washington, DC: ANA.

American Nurses Association. (1997a). Implementing nursing's report card: A study of RN staffing, length of stay and patient outcomes. Washington, DC: ANA.

American Nurses Association. (1995). Nursing report card for acute care. Washington, DC: American Nurses Publishing.

Arford, P. H., & Allred, C. A. (1995). Value = quality + cost. Journal of Nursing Administration, 25(9), 64–69.

Bellack, J. P., & Loquist, R. S. (1999). Employer responses to differentiated nursing education. Journal of Nursing Administration, 29(9), 4–8.

Berry, L. L, & Bendapudi, N. (2003, Feb.) Clueing in customers. Harvard Business Review, 100–106.

Bower, K. A. (1992). Case management by nurses. Washington, DC: American Nurses Publishing.

Brady, M., Leuner, J., Bellack, J. P., Loquist, R. S., Cipriano, P. F., & O'Neil. (2001). A proposed framework for differentiating the 21 Pew competencies by level of nursing education. Nursing and Health Care Perspectives, 22(1), 30–35.

Bulachek, G. M., & McCloskey, J. C. (1999). Nursing interventions: Effective nursing treatments (3rd ed.). Phildelphia: W. B. Saunders Co.

Cohen, E. L., & Cesta, T. G. (1993). Nursing case management: From concept to evolution. St. Louis: Mosby.

Delaney, C., & Moorhead, S. (1995). The nursing minimum data set, standardized language, and health care quality. Journal of Nursing Care Quality, 10(1), 16–30.

Differentiated nursing practice in all care settings. (1995). Journal of Nursing Administration, 7(8), 5–6.

Gerber, R. M. (2001). Case management: tomorrow's vision. In N. L. Chaska (Ed.), The nursing profession: Tomorrow and beyond. Thousand Oaks, CA: Sage Publications.

Gibson, S. J. (1996). Differentiated practice within and beyond the hospital walls. In E. L. Cohen (Ed.), Nurse case management in the 21st century. (pp. 222–244). St. Louis: Mosby-Year Book.

Grant, A. B., & Massey, V. H. (1999). Nursing leadership, management and research. Springhouse, PA: Springhouse Corporation.

Harris, M. R., Graves, J. R., Solbrig, H. R., Elkin, P. L., Chute, C. G. (2000). Embedded structures and representation of nursing knowledge. Journal of the American Informatics Association, 7(6), 539–549.

Hoover, K. W. (1998). Nursing work redesign in response to managed care. Journal of Nursing Administration, 28(11), 9–18.

Institute of Medicine. (2001). Crossing the quality chasm: A new health system for the 21st century. Washington, D. C. : National Academy Press.

Johnson, M., Maas, M., & Moorhead, S. (2000). Nursing Outcomes Classification (NOC) (2nd ed). St. Louis: Mosby.

Koerner, J. G., & Karpiuk, K. L. (Eds.). (1994). Implementing differentiated nursing practice: Transformation by design. Gaithersburg, MD: Aspen.

Lamb, G. S., & Huggins, D. (1990). The professional nursing network. In G. G. Mayer, M. J. Madden, & E. Lawrenz (Eds.), Patient care delivery models (pp. 169–184). Rockville, MD: Aspen.

Loquist, R. S., & Bellack, J. P. (1998). South Carolina Colleagues in Caring Project: A model for differentiated entry level nursing practice by educational program type. (Available from the South Carolina Colleagues in Caring Project, University of South Carolina College of Nursing, Columbia, SC 29208.)

Lyon, J. C. (1993). Models of nursing care delivery and case management: Clarification of terms. *Nursing Economics*, 11(3), 163–169.

Malloch, K., & Conovaloff, A. (1999). Patient classification systems, part 1: The third generation. *Journal of Nursing Administration*, 29(7/8), 49–56.

Manthey, M. (1980). *The practice of primary nursing*. Boston: Blackwell.

Mathews, B. P., & Kamikawa, C. (1994). Primary nursing. *Nursing Administration Quarterly*, 19(1), 48–50.

Mayer, G. G., Madden, M. J., & Lawrenz, E. (Eds.). (1990). *Patient care delivery models*. Rockville, MD: Aspen.

McCloskey, J. C. (1995). Recognizing the management role of all nurses. *Nursing and Health Care: Perspectives on Community*, 16(6), 307–308.

McClure, M. L., Poulin, M. A., Sovie, M. D., & Wandelt, M. A. (1983). Magnet hospitals: Attraction and retention of Professional Nurses (The Original Study). In McClure, M. L. and Hinshaw, A. S. (2002). *Magnet hospitals revisited*. Washington, DC: American Nurses Publishing.

Moorhead, S. A., McCloskey, J. C., Bulechek, G. M. (1993). Nursing interventions classification: A comparison with the Omaha System and the Home Healthcare Classification. *Journal of Nursing Administration*, 23(10), 23–29.

Needleman, J., Buerhaus, P., Mattke, S., Stewart, M., & Zelevinsky. (2002). Nurse-staffing levels and quality of care in hospitals. *New England Journal of Medicine*, 346(22), 1715–1722.

NCNA. (1992). *Nursing Clinics of North America*, 1(27).

O'Neil, E. H. (1998). *Recreating health professional practice for a new century: The fourth report of the Pew Health Professions Commission*. San Francisco, CA: Pew Health Professions Commission.

Pinkerton, S. (2001). Organizing nursing in an integrated delivery system. In Chaska, N. L. (Ed.), *The nursing profession: Tomorrow and beyond*. Thousand Oaks, CA: Sage Publications.

Porter-O'Grady, T., & Wilson, C. K. (1995). *The leadership revolution in health care: Altering systems, changing behaviors*. Gaithersburg, MD: Aspen.

Poulin, M. (1985). Configuration of nursing practice. In American Nurses Association (Ed.). *Issues in professional nursing practice* (pp. 1–14). Kansas City: American Nurses Association.

Powell, S. K. (2000a). *Case management: A practical guide to success in managed care*. Philadelphia: Lippincott-Raven.

Powell, S. K. (2000b). *Advanced case management: Outcomes and beyond*. Philadelphia: Lippincott-Raven.

Primm, P. L. (1986). Entry into practice: Competency statements for BSNs and ADNs. *Nursing Outlook*, 34(3), 135–137.

Rigby, A., Leach, C., & Greasley, P. (2001). Primary nursing: Staff perception of changes in ward atmosphere and role. *Journal of Psychiatric and Mental Health Nursing*, 8, 525–532.

Schaffner, J. W., & Ludwig-Beymer, P. (2003). *Rx for the nursing shortage*. Chicago, IL: Health Administration Press.

Thomas, L. H., & Bond, S. (1991). Outcomes of primary nursing: the case of primary nursing. *International Journal of Nursing Studies*, 28(4), 291–314.

U. S. Department of Health and Human Services. (2002). *Projected supply, demand, and shortages of registered nurses: 2000–2010*. Health Resources and Services Administration, Bureau of Health Professions, National Center for Health Workforce Analysis. Rockville, MD: HRSA.

Walker, P. H. (1991). Dollars and sense in health reform: Interdisciplinary practice and community nursing centers. *Nursing Administration Quarterly*, 19(1), 1–11.

Walker, D. D., Jones, S. L., Yamauchi, S. S., Lima, C., Archer, S., Mathews, B. P., Harris, M., Kamikawa, C., Irvine, N., Lanier, J. et al. (1994). The Queen's Medical Center Honolulu, Hawaii. *Nursing Administration Quarterly*, 19(1), 33–65.

Wilkinson, R. A. (1994). A more autonomous and independent role: Primary nursing versus patient allocation. *Professional Nurse*, 9(10), 680–684.

Bibliography

Altman G. D. (1993). Adjusting primary nursing to 12 hour shifts. *Nursing Management*, 24(2), 80–82.

American Nurses Association. (1999a). Health care and the nursing workforce issues in the United States. *Nursing Trends & Issues*, 4(1), 1–9.

AzNA awarded report card grant. (1996, May). *Arizona Nurse*, 3.

Barry-Walker, J., Bulachek, G., & McCloskey, J. C. (1994). A description of medical-surgical nursing. *MEDSURG Nursing*, 3(4), 261–268.

Daly, J. M., Mass, M., & Buckwalter, K. (1995, August). Use of standardized nursing diagnosis and interventions in long-term care. *Journal of Gerontological Nursing*, 21(8), 29–36.

Cohen, E. L. (1996). *Nurse case management in the 21st century*. St. Louis: Mosby.

Gessner, T. L. (1998). Job design and work processes in patient care. In J. A. Dienemann, (ed.), *Nursing Administration: Managing Patient Care* (pp. 359–378) (2nd ed.). Stamford, CT: Appleton and Lange.

Kerr, M. E., Hoskins, L. M., Fitzpatrick, J. J., Warren, J. J., Avant, K. C., Carpitano, L. J. Hurley, M. E., Jakob, D., Lunney, M., Mills, W. C., et al. (1992). Development of definitions for taxonomy II. *Nursing Diagnosis*, 3(2), 65–71.

Havens, D. S., & Aiken, L. H. (1999). Shaping systems to promote desired outcomes: The Magnet Hospital model. *Journal of Nursing Administration*, 29(2), 14–20.

Hyams-Franklin, E. M., Rowe-Gillespie, P., Harper, A., & Johnson, V. (1993). Primary team nursing: The 90s model. *Nursing Management*, 24(6), 50–52.

Himali, U. (1995). Managed care: Does the promise meet the potential? *American Nurse*, 27(4), 1, 14, 16.

Kayuha, A. A. (1996). Organizational systems. In C. Loveridge & S. Cummings (Eds.),. *Nursing management in the new paradigm* (pp. 24–57). Gaithersburg, MD: Aspen.

Loquist, R. S., & Bellack, J. P. (1999). *Into the future: Recreating*

South Carolina's nursing workforce for the 21st century. (Available from the South Carolina Colleagues in Caring Project, University of South Carolina College of Nursing, Columbia, SC 29208.

Malloch, K., Neeld, A. P., McMurry, C., Meeks, L., Wallach, M., Williams, S., & Conovaloff, A. (1999). Patient classification systems, part II: The third generation. *Journal of Nursing Administration, 29*(9), 33–42.

Marrelli, T. M. (1997). *The nurse manager's survival guide: Practical answers to everyday problems.* St. Louis: Mosby.

McCloskey, J. C., & Bulechek, G. M. (Eds.). (1996). *Nursing interventions classification* (NIC) (2nd ed.). St. Louis: Mosby.

McManis & Monslave Associates and American Organization of Nurse Executives. (2003, November/December). Striving for Excellence: Insights from a Key Informant Survey on Nursing Work Environment Improvement and Innovation. *Nurse Leader pp.* 13–19.

Milton, D. (1992). The evaluation of new nursing structures in single or multifacility systems. In C. Wilson (Ed.). *Building new nursing organizations: Visions and realities* (pp. 187–208). Gaithersburg, MD: Aspen.

North American Nursing Diagnosis Association. (1992). NANDA *nursing diagnosis: Definition and classification* 1992. St. Louis: North American Nursing Diagnosis Association.

Powell, S. K. (1996). *Nursing case management.* Philadelphia: Lippincott-Raven.

Rundall, T. G., Starkweather, D. B., & Norrish, B. R. (1998). *After restructuring: Empowerment strategies at work in America's hospitals.* San Francisco, CA: Jossey-Bass.

Smith, G. (1994). The paradox of collaboration. *Nursing and Health Care, 15*(7), 338–339.

Stevens, K. R., & Weiner, E. E. (2001). Informatics for nursing practice. In N. L. Chaska (Ed.), *The nursing profession: Tomorrow and beyond.* Thousand Oaks, CA: Sage Publications.

Swansburg, R. C., & Swansburg, R. J. (1999). *Introductory management and leadership for nurses* (2nd ed.). Boston: Jones and Bartlett.

Terry, D. (1999). Effective employee relations in reengineered organizations. *JONA's Health Care, Law, Ethics, and Regulation,* 1(3), 33–40.

🖳 ONLINE RESOURCES

References

American Nurses Association. (1999). Press release: Americans support rigorous standards for nursing care. *www. nursingworld.org/pressrel/1999/pr0507.htm*

American Nurses Association. (1997b). Nursing's quality indicators for acute care settings and ANA's safety and quality initiative. *Nursing Facts. www. nursingworld.org/readroom/fssafety.htm*

American Nurses Association. (1997c). Position statement: A national nursing database to support clinical nursing practice. *www.nursingworld.org/readroom/position/practice/prdatabs.htm*

AORN. (1999). Perioperative nursing data set. *www.aorn.org/research/pnds.htm*

Donley, R., & Flaherty, M. J. (2002). Revisiting the American Nurses Association's first position on education for nurses. *Online Journal of Issues in Nursing, 7*(2). *http://www.nursingworld.org/ojin/topic18_1 htm*

Institute of Medicine. (2004). Keeping patients safe: Transforming the work environment of nurses. *www. nsp.edu/openbook/0309090679/html/1.html*

Joel, L. A. (2002). Education for entry into nursing practice: Revisited for the 21st Century. *Online journal of issues in nursing, 7*(2). *http://www.nursingworld.org/ojin/topic18_4.htm*

Loquist, R. S., & Brady, M. S. (2001). South Carolina Statewide Articulation Model. *http://www.sc.edu/nursing/cic/*

National Council of State Boards of Nursing. (1995). Delegation: Understanding the concepts and decision-making process. *http://www.ncsbn.org.files/publications/positions/delegate.asp*

Nelson, M. A. (2002). Education for professional nursing practice: Looking backward into the future. *Online journal of issues in nursing, 7*(2). *http://www.nursingworld.org/ojin/topic18_3.htm*

Resources

American Nurses Association. (1997). Managed care: Challenges and opportunities for nursing. *Nursing Facts. www.nursingworld.org/readroom/fsmgdcar.htm*

American Nurses Association. (1997). Position statement: The right to accept or reject an assignment. *www. nursingworld.org/readroom/position/workplace/wkassign.htm*

American Nurses Association. (1997). Position statement: AORN official statement on RN first assistants. *www.nursingworld.org/readroom/position/joint/jtassist.htm*

Hayes, P. (1998). Managed care: Impact and relevance for regulation. *Issues,* 19 (3), 1–2. *www.ncsbn.org/files/publications/issues/vol193/mcimpact193.asp*

National Council of State Boards of Nursing. (1998). Nursing supply/demand issue brief from the policy futures panel. *Issues,* 19(3), 1–3. *www.ncsbn.org/files/publications/issues/vol193/supply193.asp*

Pila, L. (1999). How the nursing shortage jeopardizes patient care. *www.nurses.com/content/news/article asp*

Rose Kearney-Nunnery

Healthy Initiatives for At-Risk Populations

> *Wherever we look upon this earth, the opportunities take shape within the problems.*
> *Nelson Rockefeller, 1908–1979*

Chapter Objectives

On completion of this chapter, the reader will be able to:

1. Describe the national initiatives aimed at improving health and reducing health disparities.
2. Identify trends and health needs of our at-risk populations.
3. Discuss strategies for reducing health disparities for at-risk population groups.
4. Discuss the characteristics of the aging population.
5. Examine the issues to address in minority health promotion activities.
6. Contrast urban and rural community health-care needs and resources.
7. Identify the role for professional nurses in community and public health initiatives.

Key Terms

Healthy People 2000	Healthy People 2010	Disability
Priority Areas	Focus Areas	Chronicity
Health Promotion	Leading Health	Minority Health
Strategies	Indicators	Urbanized Area
Health Protection	Successful Aging	Rural Area
strategies	Usual Aging	Rural Health
Preventive Services	Pathological Aging	Community Health
Healthy Communities	Aging Adults	Nursing

Two major community health initiatives began in the last decades of the 20th century in the United States: Healthy People and Healthy Communities. The focus became one for the health of the nation as a whole through concentration on wellness and healthful initiatives for the next century. A strategic planning process began to create 10-year objectives for disease prevention and health promotion. For Healthy People 2000 (U.S. Department of Health and Human Services [USDHHS], 1992) "specificity of particular objectives for groups at higher risk had been part of the design ... [with objectives] delineated far more extensively than were the 1990 Objectives according to demographic and socioeconomic dimensions of risk" (p. vii). This focus continued as a national commitment with Healthy People 2010, which was introduced to the nation on January 25, 2000. We now see that healthy behaviors and prevention are vital for individuals, families, and society.

As a corollary to this movement, we have also seen a greater focus on consumer and public protection. In 1998, the President's Advisory Commission on Consumer Protection and Quality in the Health Care Industry presented a final report with more than 50 objectives identified to address problem areas, including avoidable errors, both underutilization and overuse of services, and variation in services. Measures proposed to strengthen the health-care industry included use of group purchasers, having informed consumers with access to services, accountability, reducing errors and increasing safety, and addressing the needs of vulnerable populations. Sources of vulnerability were identified as economic status and geographic location; health, age, and functional or developmental status; communication barriers; and unexplained vulnerability associated with race, ethnicity, and sex (The President's Advisory Commission on Consumer Protection and Quality in the Health Care Industry, 1998, pp. 130–132). At the end of the 20th century, the focus on patient safety was further highlighted with the subsequent Institute of Medicine (IOM)

reports on the current state of health care for consumers.

The nation's population profile is changing. We are older and more diverse. Although we remain a youth-oriented society, the aging of the "baby boomers" has a profound effect on the demographics and the health needs of the population. In addition, we are indeed becoming more culturally diverse and must endeavor to celebrate, respect, and embrace our differences while eliminating health disparities. Professional nursing practice has a vital role in promoting health and health initiatives and in eliminating health disparities.

 ## HEALTHY PEOPLE 2000

In **Healthy People 2000**, three general goals were stated as national health promotion and disease prevention objectives:

- Increase the span of healthy life for Americans
- Reduce health disparities among Americans
- Achieve access to preventive services for all Americans (USDHHS, 1992, p. 6)

This initiative took a major step in that it did not merely look at the health of the nation, but rather, it devised strategies for improvement. The outcome was the specification of 22 **priority areas** for health promotion and disease prevention. For each priority area, the workgroup formulated objectives with specific targets to measure success in addressing the three major goals. The priority areas were further classified as health promotion, health protection, and preventive services. Recall the discussion on levels of prevention (primary, secondary, and tertiary) in Chapter 5. The terminology from Healthy People 2000 (USDHHS, 1992) identified **health promotion strategies** as individual lifestyle, personal choices. Health promotion activities are both protective and preventive, but they require consumers to be actively involved in all levels of prevention. **Health protection strategies** consist of environmental or regulatory measures that confer protection on population groups. **Preventive services** comprise counseling, screening, immunization, and chemoprophylatic interventions. The 22 priority areas, along with a summary of the outcomes, are listed in Table 16–1. The initiative also

looked at specific age groups (infants, children, adolescents and young adults, adults, and older adults) and special populations (low-income, minorities, and people with disabilities) in order to address specific health promotion and disease prevention efforts within these divergent groups.

TABLE 16–1
Healthy People 2000: Priority Areas for Health Promotion and Disease Prevention

Category & Priority Area	Findings*
Health Promotion	
1. Physical Activity and Fitness	Decline in coronary death rates *Problems areas:* Overweight prevalence and lack of progress in physical activity
2. Nutrition	Progress toward targets in correct direction *Problem areas:* Overweight prevalence, calcium consumption, and iron deficiency
3. Tobacco	Progress demonstrated *Problem area:* Smoking cessation attempts decreased among pregnant women
4. Alcohol and Other Drugs	Alcohol-related MVA and cirrhosis deaths decreased for the total population *Problem areas:* Marijuana use in adolescents and cirrhosis deaths in selected minority groups have increased
5. Family Planning	Pregnancy, birth, and abortion rates for adolescent females declined *Problem area:* Hispanic adolescent pregnancy rates increased
6. Mental Health and Mental Disorders	Decline in suicide rate and increased use of community support services *Problem area:* Increased proportion of people who do not take steps to reduce stress
7. Violent and Abusive Behaviors	Decline in suicide, firearm death, and homicide rates *Problem areas:* Increase in child abuse and neglect
8. Educational and Community-Based Programs	Increase in average number of years of healthy life for total population and greater access for preschool children *Problem area:* Previous declines in healthy life between 1990 and 1994
Health Protection	
9. Unintentional Injuries	Reported use of seatbelts increased, and fire and drowning deaths were below baseline *Problem areas:* MVA crash and alcohol-related deaths remained stable since 1993, but below baseline data

(continued)

TABLE 16–1
Healthy People 2000: Priority Areas for Health Promotion and Disease Prevention (*continued*)

Category & Priority Area	Findings*
10. Occupational Safety & Health	Decline in work-related injuries and injury deaths and cases of hepatitis B *Problem areas:* Two leading causes of work-related injury deaths were highway crashes and homicides.
11. Environmental Health	Decline in the number of waterborne disease outbreaks *Problem areas:* Increased awareness needed of the presence and dangers of radon
12. Food and Drug Safety	Decline in outbreaks of *Salmonella enteritidis* *Problem area:* Reporting of adverse events that are serious to the Food and Drug Administration (FDA) declined
13. Oral Health	Decline in oral cancer mortality rates and increased use of the oral health care system *Problem areas:* Dental caries, gingivitis, and tooth loss in adults and screening of children prior to entry in school
Preventive	
14. Maternal and Infant Health	Decline in infant mortality and hospitalization for severe complications in pregnancy *Problem areas:* Increase in fetal alcohol syndrome, infant neural tube diseases related to low folic acid intake, and low/very-low-birthweight births
15. Heart Disease and Stroke	Decline in mortality from heart disease and stroke, yet higher among African Americans *Problem areas:* Increase in end-stage renal disease and obesity
16. Cancer	Declines in mortality from lung, female breast, and colorectal cancer *Problem areas:* Data and actions needed on limitations to sun exposure
17. Diabetes and Chronic Disabling Conditions	Declines in activity limitations due to chronic conditions, asthma, and sensory impairments *Problem areas:* Increase in rates of activity limitation due to chronic back conditions and increase in diabetes prevalence and mortality, especially in selected minority groups
18. HIV Infection	Decline in the number of AIDS cases diagnosed and the prevalence of HIV *Problem areas:* Increased AIDS incidence rates for African American, female, and Hispanic populations
19. Sexually Transmitted Diseases	Lowest rates for primary and secondary syphilis; repeat gonorrhea rate met Y2K objective; and improvement in pelvic inflammatory disease, gonorrhea, chlamydia, and hepatitis B rates *Problem area:* Clinician counseling is declining

(continued)

(continued) Category & Priority Area	Findings*
20. Immunization and Infectious Diseases	Vaccination levels in children are at the highest level recorded and incidence of vaccine-preventable diseases low *Problem areas:* Continued monitoring and measures of infectious diarrhea incidence
21. Clinical Preventive Services	Increase in the average number of years of "healthy life" and in the numbers of adults with a specific source of primary health care *Problem area:* Financial barriers to receipt of clinical preventive services
Other	
22. Surveillance and Data Systems	*Impression:* "Public health and surveillance is the systemwide collection, analysis, and use of health information" (NCHS, 1999, p. 217). *Problem area:* Consistency in measurement and collection of data nationwide

Key: AIDS, acquired immunodeficiency syndrome; FDA, U.S. Food and Drug Administration; HIV, human immunodeficiency virus; MVA, motor vehicle accident; Y2K, year 2000.

*Data from National Center for Health Statistics. (NCHS). (1999). *Healthy People 2000 review, 1998–99.* Hyattsville, MD: Public Health Service; quotation from p. 217 of same source.

Infants

Healthy People 2000 outcomes demonstrated a dramatic decline in the infant mortality rate. This decline placed the United States at a rank of 25th lowest among developed nations in infant mortality (USDHHS, 1999, p.1). Although maternal and infant health was ranked 14th in importance among the 22 priority areas, continued attention was needed in this area to maintain the decline in infant mortality and morbidity.

Children 1 to 14 Years of Age

Mortality rates in children met the Healthy People 2000 objective. In fact, the rates surpassed the year 2000 target. Childhood deaths from drowning and fire diminished, as did the incidence of nonfatal poisonings and activity limitations due to otitis media. Another good finding in the progress report was the increased use of child restraint systems in motor vehicles. A continued problem area

was the asthma hospitalization rate for children, which was still above the baseline rate and was identified as a major cause of morbidity.

Adolescents and Young Adults Ages 15 to 24 Years

Death rates in this age group declined in the 1990s, meeting the year 2000 target. Still, the leading causes of death for adolescents and young adults were motor vehicle accidents, other unintended injuries, homicide, and suicide. The proportion of students who participated in daily school physical education had not improved despite the potential for obesity implicit in a sedentary lifestyle. In addition, after a marked decline in heavy drinking reported in high school students, there was a slight increase, although the rate was still near the target. Mixed trends were noted for adolescent substance abuse. Rates of suicide, physical fighting, and weapon carrying by adolescents declined and were moving toward the targets. The prevalence of *Chlamydia trachomatis* also decreased in female adolescents and young adults.

Adults 25 to 64 Years

Although the 2000 target was not met, the mortality rate in adults declined. Mortality rates from cancer dropped below the year 2000 target, related to the declines in deaths from breast, colorectal, and lung cancers. Mixed trends were reported for the incidence of nonfatal work-related injuries. Although a decline in nonfatal work-related injuries has been reported in some professions and occupations, the rate for nursing and personal care workers moved away from the target and was higher than those for all other work areas reported.

The Aging Population

The leading causes of mortality in the aging population were heart disease, cancer, stroke, chronic obstructive pulmonary disease, diabetes, and unintentional injuries or accidents. Although limited data were available, the aging population (70 years and older) demonstrated an increase in difficulty performing two or more personal care activities, with an 16 percent increase overall and a 31 percent increase in African Americans during the 1990s (National Center for Health Statistics [NCHS], 1999, p. 17). Mortality from motor vehicle accidents and falls rose, especially in the older aging population. Although more of the aging population was involved in health promotion activities, as with influenza immunizations, mammograms, and Papanicolaou tests, a serious challenge existed in activities of daily living with advanced longevity. Visual and hearing impairments were also documented.

Selected Population Groups

Healthy People 2000 focused also on health disparities and demonstrated that a disparity exists between African Americans and the overall population with respect to average life expectancy (USDHHS, 1995). African Americans were found to have a significantly lower life expectancy (USDHHS, 2000, p. 12). Disparities included differential rates in infant mortality rate, receipt of prenatal care, maternal mortality, homicides, acquired immunodeficiency syndrome (AIDS), lung cancer, breast cancer, coronary heart disease, diabetes complications and related deaths, and immunizations. Elimination of these health disparities is a major initiative in Healthy People, 2010.

For American Indians and Alaskan natives, seven health areas were highlighted: alcoholism and substance abuse, child and family violence, diabetes, women's health, the health of the elderly, maternal and child health, and injuries. The report made particular mention of the variable infant mortality rates, with some areas below the national average and some significantly higher. Violence and injuries represented another area of particular risk, although more than half of the objectives specific to this minority group were progressing toward the year 2000 objective.

Asian Americans and Pacific Islanders were found to have a higher life expectancy than the population as a whole. However, several health problems were particularly noteworthy for these groups. Although rates of cerebrovascular diseases were rising in this group, cancer was the leading cause of death for Chinese, Korean and Vietnamese population groups. In addition, tuberculosis incidence demonstrated a slight increase, remaining well above both the year 2000 objective and its prevalence in the total population.

It was estimated that by 2010, Hispanic Americans will be the largest minority group in the United States. This group is also the largest uninsured group. Particular areas of concern included infant mortality rates, prenatal care, and receipt of preventive health screenings and care. Other areas in which population failed to meet Healthy People objectives were obesity, adolescent pregnancies, homicides, diabetes, and human immunodeficiency virus (HIV) and AIDS.

People With Disabilities

In 1994, 54 million people in the United States, or roughly 21 percent of the population, had some level of disability (USDHHS, 2000, p. 15). The two leading causes of disability (nonfatal head and spinal cord injuries) declined, whereas other conditions that lead to disability increased, including fetal alcohol syndrome, visual impairments, asthma, and complications of diabetes. The study revealed an escalating relationship between lower incomes, limitations in activity, and chronic conditions.

People With Low Income

Several areas were of particular concern in the lower-income population, including prenatal care, birth weight, food security, health care visits, immunizations, insurance coverage and health screenings, perceived health status, activity limitations, and mortality rates. Higher levels of education were associated with greater levels of prenatal care and higher birth weights of infants in this group. This group had lower levels of health insurance, perceived health status, and activity. They also had a higher mortality rate.

HEALTHY COMMUNITIES

The American Public Health Association (APHA) (1991) published *Healthy Communities 2000: Model Standards* to assist planners in adapting the Healthy People 2000 objectives to the needs and resources of individual communities. The conceptual basis of **Healthy Communities** included the following:

- Emphasis on health outcomes
- Flexibility as a planning tool
- Focus placed on the entire community
- Governmental presence at the local level
- Importance of negotiation to maintain local flexibility
- Standards (uniform objectives) and guidelines (local adaptations)

- Accessibility of services
- Emphasis on programs (APHA, 1991, pp. xvii–xix)

The Healthy People 2000 priority areas and objectives were reprinted in the document, accompanied by a model standards goal that provided flexible practical guidance for achieving the objectives. A table format was used for identification of the focus area, objectives, and indicator for an outcome measurement. Blanks were included in the objectives and guidelines to allow planners to tailor them to their local communities. The indicators promoted consistent measurement across communities.. By the final review point for Healthy People 2000, most states, the District of Columbia, and Guam had statewide objectives, some with comprehensive strategic plans and assessment projects that addressed the objectives. The strategic planning process continued in 2001 with a look to 2010, and utimately, the publication of the revised resource, *Healthy People in Healthy Communities: A Community Planning Guide Using Healthy People 2010* (USDHHS, 2001).

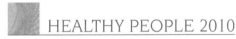 ## HEALTHY PEOPLE 2010

The prevention agenda for the nation and the associated objectives for the next decade were introduced in January 2000 as **Healthy People 2010** (USDHHS, 2000a) with two major goals:

- To increase the quality and years of healthy life
- To eliminate health disparities

Notice that these two objectives are more aggressive than the 2000 objectives. For instance, Healthy People 2000 sought to reduce health disparities, whereas Healthy People 2010 plans to eliminate them. Building upon Healthy People 2000, Healthy People 2010 specified 28 **focus areas** containing objectives and targets specified for the nation (Table 16–2) to address the specific trends of the decade, such as diversity and the aging population. Healthy People 2010 used a systematic approach to health improvement

TABLE 16–2
Healthy People 2010: Focus Areas

Focus Area	Care Components	Objectives
Access to Quality Health Services	Clinical preventive care Primary care Emergency services Long-term care & rehabilitative services	3 6 5 2
Arthritis, Osteoporosis, and Chronic Back Conditions	Arthritis Osteoporosis Chronic back conditions	8 2 1
Cancer	—	15
Chronic Kidney Disease	—	8
Diabetes:	—	17
Disability and Secondary Conditions	—	13
Educational and Community-Based Programs	School setting Worksite setting Health-care setting Community setting and select populations	4 2 3 3
Environmental Health	Outdoor air quality Water quality Toxics and waste Healthy homes and healthy communities Infrastructure & surveillance Global environmental health	4 6 5 8 5 2
Family Planning	—	13
Food Safety	—	7
Health Communication	—	6
Heart Disease and Stroke	Heart disease Stroke Blood pressure Cholesterol	6 2 4 4
HIV	—	17
Immunization and Infectious Diseases	*Diseases preventable through:* • Universal vaccination • Targeted vaccination Infectious diseases and emerging antimicrobial resistance Vaccination coverage and strategies Vaccine safety	 5 3 13 8 2

(continued) Focus Area	Care Components	Objectives
Injury and Violence Prevention	Injury prevention Unintentional injury prevention Violence and abuse prevention	12 19 8
Maternal, Infant, and Child Health	Fetal, infant, and child deaths Maternal death and illnesses Prenatal care Obstetrical care Risk factors Developmental disabilities and neural tube defects Prenatal substance exposure Breastfeeding, newborn screening and service systems	3 2 2 2 4 3 2 5
Medical Product Safety	—	6
Mental Health and Mental Disorders	Mental health status improvement Treatment expansion State activities	5 6 3
Nutrition and Overweight	Weight status and growth Food and nutrient consumption Iron deficiency and anemia Schools, worksite, and nutrition counseling Food security	4 7 3 3 1
Occupational Safety & Health	—	11
Oral Health	—	17
Physical Activity and Fitness	Physical activity in adults Muscular strength/endurance and flexibility Physical activity in children and adolescents Access	3 2 6 4
Public Health Infrastructure	Data and information systems Workforce Public health organizations Resources Prevention research	7 3 5 1 1
Respiratory Diseases	Asthma COPD Obstructive sleep apnea	8 2 2

(continued)

TABLE 16–2
Healthy People 2010: Focus Areas (continued)

Focus Area	Care Components	Objectives
Sexually Transmitted Diseases	Bacterial STD illness and disability	3
	Viral STD illness and disability	2
	STD complications (females)	3
	STD complications (fetus and newborn)	2
	Personal behaviors	2
	Community protection infrastructure	3
	Personal health services	4
Substance Abuse	Adverse consequences of substance use and abuse	8
	Substance use and abuse	7
	Risk of substance use and abuse	2
	Treatment for substance abuse	4
	State and local efforts	4
Tobacco Use	Tobacco use in population groups	4
	Cessation and treatment	4
	Exposure to secondhand smoke	5
	Social and environmental changes	8
Vision and Hearing	Vision	10
	Hearing	8

Key: COPD, chronic obstructive pulmonary disease; STD, sexually transmitted disease.

Source: U.S. Department of Health and Human Services.. (2000). *Tracking Healthy People 2010.* Washington, DC: U.S. Government Printing Office. http://www.healthypeople.gov/Document/tableofcontents.htm#acking

guided by a model with four key elements: goals, objectives, determinants of health, and health status. The objectives are to "focus on the determinants of health, which encompass the combined effects of individual and community physical and social environments and the policies and interventions used to promote health, prevent disease, and ensure access to quality health care" (USDHHS, 2000a, p. 7).

Specific objectives in each focus area are designed to address the health initiative as subgoals under the direction of a lead government agency. Objectives are both measurable (with specific set targets for which data are tracked) and developmental (for which no baseline data was available). For example, the focus area of health communications contains six objectives (Box 16–1). The first, "Increase the proportion of households with access to the Internet at home," is measurable because there was baseline information that 26 percent of homes had Internet access in 2000 (USDHHS, 2000a, pp. 11–13). The remaining five objectives are developmental in nature, because data are only collected. Availability of data and interagency collaboration are essential components of this aggressive project to address the health of the nation. This national initiative is an evidence-based approach to addressing the two major goals for a healthier nation.

ONLINE CONSULT:

Healthy People 2010.
http://www.healthypeople.gov

BOX 16–1
HEALTHY PEOPLE 2010 FOCUS AREA: HEALTH COMMUNICATIONS

Goal: Use communication strategically to improve health.
Lead Agency: Office of Disease Prevention and Health Promotion.

- Increase the proportion of households with access to the Internet at home.
- Improve the health literacy of persons with inadequate or marginal literacy skills.
- Increase the proportion of health communication activities that include research and evaluation.
- Increase the proportion of health-related World Wide Web sites that disclose information that can be used to assess the quality of the site.
- Increase the number of centers for excellence that seek to advance the research and practice of health communication.
- Increase the proportion of persons who report that their health care providers have satisfactory communication skills.

Source: U.S. Department of Health and Human Services. (2000). Healthy People 2010: Volume I (2nd ed.).
http://www.healthypeople.gov/Document/HTML/Volume1/11HealthCom.htm

Reducing health disparities involves addressing the needs of individuals or groups at risk. The needs of these at-risk populations are identifiable in the focus areas and objectives to be addressed. The demographic characteristics identified where health disparities were targeted for action were gender, age, race and ethnicity, income and educational level, disability, geographic location, and sexual orientation.

Leading Health Indicators

A new component of the Healthy People 2010 document is the identification of **leading health indicators** (Box 16–2). "The leading health indicators reflect the major public health concerns in the United States and were chosen based on their ability to motivate action, the availability of data to measure their progress, and their relevance as broad public health issues" (USDHHS, 2000a, p. 24). These 10 indicators, linked to the Healthy People 2010 objectives, have the ability to provide a "snapshot" at a point in time by which to view the health of the nation. These indicators were intended to "illuminate individual behaviors, physical and social environmental factors, and important health system

BOX 16–2
HEALTHY PEOPLE 2010: LEADING HEALTH INDICATORS

- Physical activity
- Overweight and obesity
- Tobacco use
- Substance abuse
- Responsible sexual behavior
- Mental health
- Injury and violence
- Environmental quality
- Immunization
- Access to health care

issues that greatly affect the health of individuals and communities [and] underlying each of these indicators is the significant influence of income and education" (USDHHS, 2000a, p. 24).

Physical Activity

Although the benefits of physical activity have been demonstrated, sedentary lifestyles are common in the United States. This health indicator targets perceived barriers to regular, moderate physical activity and seeks to prevent conditions associated with lack of activity. Disparities have been identified with gender, age, race, educational level, geography, and socioeconomic status. At-risk groups are females, the elderly, African Americans, Hispanics, low-income individuals, the disabled, and individuals in the southern and northeastern states (USDHHS, 2000b).

Overweight and Obesity

Increasing trends and associated conditions like heart disease, diabetes, and other chronic illnesses can be directly attributed to overweight and obesity. The interaction with physical activity is evident. The "balance between energy intake and output is influenced by metabolic and genetic factors as well as behaviors affecting dietary intake and physical activity; environmental, cultural, and socioeconomic components also play a role" (USDHHS, 2000b, 19–4). Disparities have been reported both within and among population groups, related to gender, race, ethnicity, and socioeconomic status. Obesity and overweight are becoming more and more of a concern in children and adolescents.

Tobacco Use

The use of tobacco, whether by smoking, chewing, or exposure to secondary smoke in the physical environment or in utero, has long been associated with serious complications and consequences. Objectives address use of specific products in selected groups, cessation efforts, secondhand exposure, and needed social and environmental changes for limitations or cessation in select populations. Disparities exist by age, gender, race and ethnicity, socioeconomic status, educational level, and geography.

Substance Abuse

As a leading health indicator, substance abuse is also an influence on many of the other health indicators and focus areas. Substance abuse represents more than the use of illicit drugs; it includes adverse consequences like motor vehicle and other accidents, domestic violence, intentional or unintentional overdoses, experimentation with other substances, binging, lost productivity, and associated conditions. Substance abuse crosses all ages, genders, racial and ethic groups, regions, educational levels, and socioeconomic groups. In *Healthy People 2010*, it was reported that "alcohol is the most commonly used substance, regardless of race or ethnicity" (USDHHS, 2000b, p. 26–6).

Responsible Sexual Behavior

In *Healthy People 2010*, *sexually transmitted diseases* (STDs) are described as "common, costly and preventable" (USDHHS, 2000b, p. 25–7). Although they exist in all gender, racial, ethnic, and socioeconomic groups, differences in responsible sexual behaviors have been identified within and among groups that can be used to target selected groups for intervention activities in the stated objectives. An increase in responsible sexual behaviors is the marker to reduce the incidence and complications of STDs. However, the interactions among gender, age, race, ethnicity, geography, and socioeconomic factors are further considerations as special populations are targeted, such as adolescents with the promotion of abstinence.

Mental Health

"*Mental health* is a state of successful performance of mental function, resulting in productive activities, fulfilling relationships with other people, and the ability to adapt to change and to cope with adversity" (USDHHS, 2000b, p. 18–3). Although differences have been identified within and among groups, "mental disorders occur across the lifespan, affecting persons of all racial and ethnic groups, both genders, and all educational and socioeconomic groups" (USDHHS, 2000b, p. 18–3). Co-morbidities and secondary problems are vital considerations for this indicator, as are treatment opportunities.

Injury and Violence

This leading health indicator calls for the reduction in injuries, disabilities, and deaths related to injury and violence. *Healthy People 2010* noted that "although the greatest impact in injury is human suffering and loss of life, the financial cost is staggering [including costs of] … direct medical care and rehabilitation as well as lost income and productivity" (USD-HHS, 2000b, p. 15–4). In addition, disparities in rates of injuries by age, racial and ethnic group, and economic status have been noted.

Environmental Quality

The environmental quality indicator address-es air and water quality and toxic influences in homes, at worksites, and in the comm-unity. "Potential risks include indoor air pollution; inadequate heating, cooling, and sanitation; structural problems; electrical and fire hazards; and lead-based paint hazards" (USDHHS, 2000a, p. 8–7). Individuals of cer-tain races and socioeconomic status have been identified as being at greater risk.

Immunization

Infectious diseases increased over the last decade. Strategies in this area include vacci-nation recommendations and programs, both universal and targeted, as well as concentrat-ing on selected infectious processes and antimicrobial resistence. Particular at-risk populations were identified related to age, ethnicity and race, and geography.

Access to Quality Health-Care Services

Consider the implications of this leading health indicator and its target of 100% health insurance coverage by 2010. The objectives for this indicator address clinical preventive care, primary care, emergency services, and long-term care and rehabilitative services. Disparaties have been monitored during the data collection process, with initiatives in place to address the target goals. In the June 2002 progress review, lower levels of insurance were noted in the Hispanic or Latino and American Indian or Alaska Native popula-tions. Lower levels of health insurance and ongoing sources of care were also noted in populations with lower levels of family income and education. Racial and ethnic representa-tion in the health professions is also under study with this objective, as a component of cultural competence. Little change has been demonstrated, with minority under-represen-tation persistent in the health professions.

A Work in Progress

Improving quality of life and eliminating health disparities are appropriate goals for this decade. This is a public endeavor and, as was done with Healthy People 2000, federal, state and local initiatives have been activated as part of the strategic planning process. At the local levels, Healthy Communities 2010 is involved with initiatives and data collection. At the state level, Healthy People 2010 plans specific to a state's population and geography have been initiated. For example, Alaska has implemented a "Talking Circle"; Arizona has 12 Focus Areas; Michigan is concentrating on 15 specific "Focused Indicators;" and Vermont has come up with 16 Goals of Healthy Vermonters.

At the national level, ongoing collabora-tives to address the public's health continued. For example, although not one of the leading health indicators, the focus area of diabetes was highlighted in 2003 with the start of a special initiative for people with undiagnosed diabetes. The Administration on Aging, the U.S. Food and Drug Administration (FDA), and the U.S. Department of Health and Human Services also participated in a collabo-rative effort in 2003 to highlight health dis-parities among older Hispanic Americans. Activities focused on the goals to eliminate health disparities and increase the quality and years of healthy life.

 OUR AGING POPULATION

The term *healthy life* applies not only to longevity but also to functional independence and the perception of healthy days. The three major causes of death in people 65 years and older are heart disease, cancer, and stroke. Consider the life expectancy trends reported in Table 16–3. Although life expectancies for both men and women have increased, the 10 to 13 years of functional health and independence after age 65 are less than the 15 to 19 actual remaining years of life. In addition, disparities exist by gender and race. However, trends in limitation of activities of daily living have declined, especially for those 65 years and older living in the community (NCHS, 2003).

> *The difference between healthy life and unhealthy life is the loss of independence in activities of daily life and increasing dependence on others.*

The percentage of the population aged 65 years and older has been steadily increasing. Proportional changes have been dramatic. In fact, the population 85 years and older population grew more than 500 percent from 1950 to 1990. According to the 2000 U.S. Census, there were 35 million Americans aged 65 and older, and the projections are that this number will grow to 71 million in 2030, with the number of people aged 80 and older expected to rise from 9.3 million in 2000 to 19.5 million in 2030 (CDC, 2003b, p. 1). However, this population of aging Americans is experiencing differences in health-care purchasing power and socioeconomic status, despite Medicare coverage. Consider the following information reported by the

Administration on Aging (AOA, 2002) from the 2000 Census:

> About 3.6 million elderly persons (10.4%) were below the poverty level in 2002. ... Another 2.2 million or 6.4% of the elderly were classified as "near-poor" (income between the poverty level and 125% of this level). One of every 12 (8.3%) elderly Whites was poor in 2002, compared to 23.8% of elderly African-Americans and 21.4% of elderly Hispanics. Higher than average poverty rates for older persons were found among those who lived in central cities (12.2%), outside metropolitan areas (i.e., rural areas) (11.9%), and in the South (12.7%). (p. 1)

The difference between healthy life and unhealthy life is the loss of independence in activities of daily life and increasing dependence on others for health and routine care. We now see chronic illness rather than acute illness as the major morbidity factor in aging adults. Prevention of disability and promotion of independent functioning are essential and can be aided by healthy behaviors such as smoking cessation, good nutrition, reduction of sodium intake and body weight, reduction in social isolation, regular physical activity, and availability of primary health-care services.

Approximately one third of people hospitalized are older than 65 years. Even though the average length of hospital stays has shortened, those older than 65 years need a great proportion of our health-care resources, both in and out of the acute care setting. And this proportion will increase as the population continues to age. The Centers for Disease Control and Prevention (CDC) (2003a) esti-

TABLE 16–3					
Life Expectancy (in years) At Birth and at 65 and 85 Years of Age, by Decade					
	1900	**1950**	**1970**	**1990**	**2000**
At birth	47.3	68.2	70.8	75.4	76.9
At 65 years	11.9	14.1	15.0	17.3	17.9
At 85 years	—	—	5.3	6.2	6.3

National Center for Health Statistics. (2003). Data Warehouse on Trends in Health and Aging. http://www.cdc.gov/nchs/agingact.htm.

mates that by 2030, health-care spending will increase by 25% with the increase in the older population—and this figure was calculated without adjustment for inflation or new technology costs (p. 2). However, the CDC (2003a) further recommends strategies for the health of older adults (Box 16–3) and has emphasized that "poor health is not an inevitable consequence of aging" (p. 3).

With the focus on heath promotion and quality of life for the growing aging population and the entry of "baby boomers" into this category, research has evolved in several disciplines, all proposing different theories on aging. No agreement on a specific theory has emerged. Research continues, and our knowledge of the aging process grows with biologic, sociologic, psychological, longevity, medical, and nursing theories on aging. *Biologic theories* focus on the functional capacity of cells, cell division, and organ systems, addressing genetics, immunology, connective tissues, free radicals, stresses from "wear and tear," and neuroendocrine and neurochemical factors. *Sociologic theories* focus on roles and behaviors in society, including such theories as disengagement, activity, subculture, age stratification, and person-environmental fit. *Psychological theories* of aging target human behavior and adaptation. Included in this group are theories on human needs and development. Theories on *longevity* look at the life expectancy in a cohort or age-related group for specific factors that yield longer lifespan—genetics, gender, environment, physical activity, alcohol consumption, sexual activity, nutrition, and social factors, including economics, marital status, family, religious beliefs, purpose in life, and even laughter. *Medical theories* on aging highlight disease-related influences on physiologic functioning of the person, including the single-organ theory, senescence theories, and life expectancy and functional health theory. And nursing theories propose functional consequences in which age-related changes and age-related factors are the risk factors.

Aging has also been classified as successful, usual, and pathologic (Rowe & Kahn, 1987). In **successful aging**, there is an interaction between the individual's genes and environ-

> **BOX 16–3**
> **STRATEGIES FOR HEALTH PROMOTION OF OLDER ADULTS**
>
> - Healthy lifestyles
> - Early detection of disease
> - Immunization
> - Self-management techniques for chronic diseases)
>
> From Centers for Disease Control and Prevention. (2003). Healthy aging: Preventing disease and improving quality of life among older Americans—at a glance 2003. *http://www.cdc.gov/nccdphp/aag/aag_aging. htm*

ment, both being positive. Positive genetic characteristics and positive environmental factors result in no serious detriment in functioning from the middle 20s until the early 70s. Minimal measurable changes in functioning are seen, with these individuals as the energetic and functional "survivors" in aging. They have no genetic diseases, but they represent only about 5 to 10 percent of the population. These individuals are the aging "stars" we aspire to be—those active, energetic, and involved elders we revere, admire, or respect.

Usual aging occurs in the vast majority of individuals. We observe an interaction between the person's genetic endowment and environment. A neutral or negative environment has positive or neutral genes. This raises concern for the reversible risk factors that occur with aging. The gene-environment interaction leads to obvious functional limitations, but the limitations are not serious enough to affect activities of daily living (ADLs) as long as the person makes compromises and adaptations. An example is the person whose mobility is limited but who adjusts to the limitation and is still able to live independently without assistance in daily life. With successful aging, we may also see genetic diseases, but again, adaptations are made that do not significantly interfere with independent daily functioning. This is the quality of life focus for the increasing numbers of aging adults.

At the opposite extreme is **pathologic**

aging. Here we see a negative interaction between genetic and environmental factors. Some combination of negative or neutral influences arise from both the individual's genes and the environment. We often see clinical evidence of genetic diseases in these aging individuals. This gene-environment interaction leads to serious functional limitations for the individual, such as being unable to take care of hygiene or personal needs, seriously affecting ADLs and sometimes the ability to sustain life. These functional limitations require substantial intervention, for example, in an extended-care setting. Prevention of disabilities and quality of life issues in this population are the focus of healthy initiatives.

Characterizing Aging Americans

We have acknowledged that **aging adults** represent a growing segment of our population, especially those 85 years and older and aging adults who are members of minority groups. As these population proportions increase even more, we will need to consider individual differences, needs of age groups, cultural and ethnic trends, and changing family patterns. Intergenerational issues will involve more than children, parents, grandparents, and great-grandparents. Consider the complexity of a family with two or three older adult groups, those in their middle to late 60s, 80s, and 100s, as well as the family members younger than age 60. The concern also arises as to who will be the caregiver for the frail older adult. Will the 80-year-old be caring for a frail spouse as well as a 99-year-old mother, or will the 60-year-old be caring for both the 80-year-old parents and the 99-year-old grandmother and perhaps be the head of the household also caring for grandchildren? Older women are expected to continue to outnumber men by at least three to two, according to life expectancy projections.

Residential Changes

Living arrangements are an important factor for aging adults. Most aging adults live in the community, usually with a spouse, alone, or with adult offspring. The proportion of people older than 65 who are living in nursing homes is less than 5 percent. And approximately 30 percent, or 9.7 million aging adults, live alone in the community (AOA, 2002, p.1). Decisions about living arrangements should include considerations for optimal promotion of functional independence and health. Opportunities for social interactions and access to resources and caregivers, when needed, are vital considerations.

Various housing options are considered by aging adults. In our more mobile society, being tied to a homestead may no longer be preferable, especially for urban and younger aging adults. Retirement planning may include relocating to a more temperate climate or closer to children. Instead of the large family home, smaller detached homes, condominiums, townhomes, gated retirement communities, continuing care communities, assisted-living apartments, senior homes, and group homes are options, depending on needs, affordability, and accessibility. In addition, a frail elder may relocate again to live with a child or other relative after the death of the spouse, sale of the retirement home, or growing loss of functional independence.

Physical Changes

Characteristics of aging adults continue to be as varied as the individuals themselves. Aging adults come with years of unique experiences that have molded their psychosocial profile. Physically and physiologically, aging adults also differ in development and progression of age-related changes. Aging is progressive and irreversible, but the manner in which these changes occur is variable. Appearance changes and motor activities slow down. But things do not stop without some disease process. Aging adults are more susceptible to disease and environmental factors. Maintaining homeostasis is more difficult.

Age-related changes occur in biologic systems. Skin becomes less elastic. Sweat glands, temperature receptors, pigment, and subcutaneous fat decrease. This makes the aging adults more susceptible to temperature extremes—cold and hot—and sunlight. Other senses are affected by aging as well. Visual and hearing acuity diminish. Adaptation of the lens and ocular muscles decreases, with a decrease in depth perception. Glare and driving at night become stressful, especially if the aging person looks at oncoming headlights. The home environment must be well illuminated, but with nonglare lights. For example, reducing the glare with fluorescent lights can also lower the chance of accidents, especially falls. Print may need to be larger and bolder. Eye examinations are very important. The loss of the driver's license may be devastating to an aging person, even if his or her driving is limited. Failure to pass an eye examination may even be a result of using no glasses or ones that are woefully inadequate.

Moverover, muscle mass and strength decrease, and joints may be stiff with arthritis. Muscle mass may be replaced with connective tissue. Osteoporosis occurs with calcium losses and hormonal changes, and worsens with inactivity. Low-impact, isometric, and routine exercises can prevent further immobility and loss of function. Digestion and slower motility are improved with small meals. Food may taste and smell bland. Herbs and seasoning can be used, but one must beware of hidden sodium content. Meals must be attractively displayed, well timed, and easy to digest.

Changes in level of consciousness and delirium are not normal signs of aging. Neurologic changes do occur but may indicate an underlying pathology or drug interaction. As noted in Healthy People 2010, (2000b), "In later life, the majority of people aged 65 years and older cope constructively with the changes associated with aging and maintain mental health, yet an estimated 25 percent of older people (8.6 million) experience specific mental disorders, such as depression, anxiety, substance abuse, and dementia, that are not part of normal aging" (USDHHS, 2000b, pp. 18–3—18–4). These possibilities should always be investigated further with referrals. Time rather than loss should be the first thought: It may take a little more time to remember something, but that does not mean that the memory is lost.

Sexuality and sexual intercourse continue, but adaptation may be needed as well, such as more time for arousal, excitement, and fore-play, or lubrication for vaginal dryness. Impotence should be evaluated for pathology or possible drug side effects. Counseling, erectile aids, reduction in alcohol consumption, and changes in medications all are possible treatments. Sexual activity need not stop because of advancing age, although partner availability may become an issue.

Major Health Problems of Aging Adults

Chronic illness and frailty are primary concerns of aging adults and their health-care professionals. Diseases common to aging include

- Osteoporosis
- Diabetes
- Stroke
- Depression
- Arthritis
- Alzheimer's disease
- Cancer
- Cardiovascular disease.

In 2000, 27 percent of older persons assessed their health as poor (compared with 9% in the overall population), with little difference between men and women but definite differences among minority older persons (41.6% for African Americans and 31.5% for Hispanics versus 26% for older whites) (AOA, 2002, p. 12). In addition, older individuals increasingly report limitations of daily activities as a result of at least one chronic illness—26.1 percent in individuals 65 to 74 years old and 45.1 percent for those 75 years and older (AOA, 2002, p. 12).

Consider the difference between chronicity and disability. **Disability** is the inability to do something because of a physical or mental impairment. In a national study on the health of older women, disability in old age was associated with "poor quality of life, dependence on formal and informal care providers, and often substantial medical and long-term care costs" (Fried et al, 1995, p. 2). **Chronicity** is related to duration or recurrence of a condition. The individual may have a chronic condition but, with healthy behaviors, can limit, delay, or prevent disability. Hence, health promotion behaviors and empowerment of the individual are essential for taking charge of one's own life. Unlike the irreversible normal changes of aging, risk factors can be reduced and in some cases eliminated.

Risks in aging adults include physical, environmental, psychosocial, and chemical factors. *Physical risks* affect the biologic system and related physiological function. Examples of physical risks are limitations in flexibility leading to falls and vision changes resulting in automobile accidents. *Environmental risks* can be natural or artificial. Natural environmental risks include ultraviolet radiation and weather extremes. Examples of artificial or man-made environmental risks are air quality, hazards in housing, and poor maintenance of equipment or the environment. *Psychosocial risks* are a part of everyday life, whether the aging person is isolated or active. Stress levels from illness of self, family members, or friends take an increasing toll on the individual. An inward focus on problems may make the aging person more egocentric and, as a result, more isolated. To address these risks, the special needs of aging adults should be considered.

Needs of Aging Adults

The major needs of aging adults roughly parallel the leading health indicators in Healthy People 2010. Longevity factors that have been supported by research include genetics, gender, environment, physical activity, alcohol consumption, sexual activity, nutrition, and social factors such as economics, marital status, and family, religious beliefs, purpose in life, and laughter. Positive behaviors must be directed at promoting and maintaining health and functional independence and at reducing risk factors. The aging adult also requires access to affordable health care, including transportation and acceptability of the provider to the person.

Family needs and issues are another consideration. Given the proportion of aging adults living in the community and projections for population increases, especially in the group 85 years and older, family needs are a major issue in health promotion and care activities.

Much can be found in the literature about family decisions for nursing home placement and the "sandwich generation" of caregivers. But recall that only a small proportion of older adults live in institutional settings, the great majority being cared for in the community. In addition, consider the projected increase in number of aging adults in minority groups and the importance of the extended family in some groups. Likewise, the growing older population stretches available health-care resources, placing a strain on society as a whole.

Lay Caregivers

The fact is that caring for a frail older adult takes a major toll on the caregiver and the family. The number of informal and family caregivers exceeds 23 million nationwide. Of these caregivers, 72 percent are women caring for relatives, their adult children with disabilities, or their grandchildren (AOA 2003c, p. 3). The physical and emotional toll on the caregiver can be enormous while the caregiver continues maintaining other family, social, work, and personal obligations. The physical and emotional strains on the caregiver often compromises her or his health. Financial and economic difficulties can compound the strain on the caregiver.

The concept of respite care, to give the caregiver a break, is ideal but is not perceived as always available, affordable, or even emotionally acceptable. Regardless, the caregiver will need some form of respite, and this must be determined, sought, and used regularly. The reauthorization of the Older Americans Act in 2000 supported demonstration projects on caregiving and authorized the National Family Caregiver Support Program. This program provides support and resources at the state and local levels for informal caregivers providing care for their older relatives or adults with disabilities. A user-friendly Web site is available to provide information on resources and demonstration projects and support for both caregivers and professionals. Note the 10 caregiver survival tips identified by the Support Program listed in Box 16–4.

BOX 16–4
CAREGIVER SURVIVAL TIPS

- Plan ahead.
- Learn about available resources.
- Take one day at a time.
- Develop contingency plans.
- Accept help.
- Make YOUR health a priority.
- Get enough rest and eat properly.
- Make time for leisure.
- Be good to yourself!
- Share your feelings with others.

From Administration on Aging. (2003a). National family caregivers support program. http://www.aoa.gov/prof/aoaprog/caregiver/care-fam/taking_care_of_others/survival.pdf

Societal Needs

Societal needs and issues are another consideration for aging adults. Public policy issues include the availability and allocation of health-care resources for aging adults as well as the use of these resources. Some people contend that aging adults are using the vast majority of the health-care resources with their chronic health problems. Focusing on the prevention of these health problems in the "baby boomers" is critical.

Health-care legislation and financing for aging adults occur mainly through the Social Security amendments and budget reconciliation acts, which include Medicare and Medicaid funding. With Medicaid, the role, legislation, and funding levels fall within the domain of the state of residence. But what about part-time residents who spend half the year in a state in which they do not claim primary residence? What about the issue of reverse migration of frail aging adults who, after years of retirement in a satisfactory condition in one state, lose a spouse and become increasingly frail, move to be cared for by their children? Their affluence was spent somewhere else, but when they move near the children, the new community must absorb the cost of chronic health conditions

and increasing frailty. Similar situations can have great impact on society and health-care resources.

Elder Abuse

Another area of concern at the individual, family, and societal levels is elder abuse. This includes physical neglect or violence, verbal abuse, psychological or emotional abuse, financial exploitation, and sexual abuse. It may be intended or unintended in active or passive actions of the abuser. Those aging individuals most at risk are the frail elderly who are functionally impaired and depend on others. In fact, the National Center on Elder Abuse (2003) has reported that "roughly two-thirds of all elder abuse perpetrators are family members, most often the victim's adult child or spouse [and] research has shown that the abusers in many instances are financially dependent on the elder's resources and have problems related to alcohol and drugs" (p. 1). The elders may be in dysfunctional family situations or even in nursing homes, but they often fear being alone more than the abuse or neglect they are experiencing. Assessment, reporting, education, and counseling are responsibilities of health-care providers and members of society. Elder abuse has also been related to caregiver stress. Special efforts being made to address this growing problem include the Older Americans Act and new national legislation.

MINORITY HEALTH

In pursuit of the goal to eliminate health disparities, Healthy People 2010 identified the following demographic groups within which health disparities occur: gender, race or ethnicity, education or income, disability, geographic location, and sexual orientation. In the area of race or ethnicity, Healthy People proposed that the identified disparities were "the result of the complex interaction among genetic variations, environmental factors, and specific health behaviors" (USDHHS, 2000a, p. 12). The following disparities between

ELDER ABUSE
If you suspect that an older person is being abused or neglected, you must call the adult protective services of the state where the elder is located. Proof is not required and calls made are confidential. Some states have separate reporting lines for domestic versus institutional elder abuse. Access the agency to contact in your state at *http://www.elderabusecenter.org/default.cfm?p=statehotlines.cfm*

ONLINE CONSULT

Administration on Aging.
http://www.aoa.gov
National Family Caregiver Support Program.
http://www.aoa.gov/prof/aoaprog/caregiver/caregiver.asp
National Association of State Units on Aging.
http://www.nasua.org
American Society on Aging.
http://www.asaging.org
National Center on Elder Abuse.
http://www.elderabusecenter.org/default.cfm

white and minority populations have been identified:

- Higher infant mortality rates for African Americans, Native American Indians, and Alaska Natives
- Higher incidence of cancer and heart disease for African Americans
- Higher mortality from HIV/AIDS for African Americans
- Increased diabetes-related deaths for Hispanic Americans and a higher incidence of diabetes for Native American Indians and Alaska Natives
- A higher incidence of hypertension and obesity in Hispanic Americans
- High death rates from unintentional injuries and suicide for Native American Indians and Alaska Natives
- High rates of tuberculosis in Hispanics, Asians, and Pacific Islanders
- High rates of hepatitis in Asians and Pacific Islanders (USDHHS, 2000a, p. 12).

Clearly, the reasons for the occurrence of the health disparities among ethnic groups are multifaceted and complex and the focus of many different initiatives to address the national goals. A large focus of **minority health** is on the special needs of groups characterized by race or ethnicity. The Office of Minority Health of the CDC (2004) classifies racial or ethnic minority populations as follows:

- American Indian and Alaskan Native
- Asian
- Black or African American
- Hispanic or Latino
- Native Hawaiian and other Pacific Islander

In a 2001 study conducted by the Commonwealth Fund, racial and ethnic disparities were further documented. For example:

- African Americans and Hispanics are less likely to have employee health insurance compared to Whites or Asian Americans, with the highest rate of uninsured in the Hispanic population (Collins et al., 2002, p. 2).

- African American and Hispanic adults were less likely to report excellent or very good health (Collins et al., 2002, p. 3).
- African Americans had the highest mortality rate from chronic diseases and half of the respondents reported they had been diagnosed within the past five years with at least one chronic condition (asthma, cancer, heart disease, diabetes, hypertension, obesity, or anxiety/depression) (Collins et al., 2002, p. 4).
- The incidence of chronic disease for adults aged 50 and older was 64 percent for the total population but 77% in African Americans, 68% in Hispanics, and 42% in Asian Americans (Collins et al., 2002, p. 8).
- Higher use of the emergency room or no source of regular care was documented for Hispanics (14%) and African Americans (13%) compared with the White (6%) or Asian American (8%) subjects in the study (Collins et al., 2002, p. 39).

In a study on racial and ethnic data collection processes, however, the researchers concluded, "minority data collection and reporting was inconsistent and sometimes contradictory" (Perot & Youdelman, 2001, p. 24). Stabilization was recommended. But we continue to investigate the issues and differences among population groups and the needs of the members.

Addressing the Disparities

Plans are ongoing to address current and emerging minority issues in order to achieve the goal of elimination of health-care disparities. Federal, state, and local initiatives are actively addressing the needs of the nation. In 2000, Congress passed the Minority Health and Health Disparities Research and Education Act (Public Law 106–525) establishing the National Center on Minority Health and Health Disparities under the National Institutes of Health (NIH). The NIH along with its Specialty Institutes and Centers, have integrated this initiative to eliminate health disparities into the strategic plans for the various agencies, including the National Institute of Nursing Research (Box 16–5). Initiatives continue to address not only health habits and access to care but also provider-client interactions.

In 2003, the Kaiser Family Foundation, the Robert Wood Johnson Foundation, and national heart organizations, in response to a meta-analysis research on disparities in cardiac care in different population groups,

---

BOX 16–5
RESEARCH ON STRATEGIES TO REDUCE HEALTH DISPARITIES

- Culturally sensitive interventions to modify health disparities, including studies to determine biologic and behavioral patterns and factors that prevent and influence disease outcomes.
- Development and testing of interventions at the community level and motivators of behavioral change for better health, with a focus on disparities related to gender, infants, children, the elderly, immigrants, and inner city and rural populations.
- Studies to identify stressors implicated in development of health disparities, including access to care, environmental toxins, and risks for obesity and cardiovascular disease.
- Longitudinal research on the effects of interventions and motivators of healthy behavioral change over time.
- Evaluation of the cost-effectiveness of interventions, such as nursing home visits versus clinic visits.

Source: National Institute of Nursing Research (2003).
http://www.nih.gov/ninr/research/themes.doc

led a national initiative entitled *Why the Difference,* for physician outreach about racial and ethnic disparities in medical care. This research reviewed prior rigorous studies in the literature and documented evidence of racial or ethnic differences in cardiac care, with African Americans less likely to receive certain procedures and care than their white counterparts despite similar patient character-istics (Lillie-Blanton et al., 2002). Mixed find-ings were reported for Hispanic patients.

Health-care providers and communities must address the documented disparities. However, doing so requires an understanding of the evidence and the people. Consider the documented increased infant mortality rate in the African-American population (NCHS, 2002). The CDC's Office of Minority Health has developed a fact sheet to encourage health providers and communities to promote healthy behaviors during the prenatal period in order to address the complications of preg-nancy that are more prevalent in minority populations and also to promote the reduc-tion in cases of sudden infant death syndrome (SIDS) (Box 16–6) (Office of Minority Health, 2003b). However, delivery of health-care services to specific minority populations such as the Alaskan Native and Hispanic/Latino groups is influenced by the availability, acces-sibility, and acceptability of services. Difficulty with communication, and other problems may hamper acceptance of early prenatal care

> **BOX 16–6**
> **FACT SHEET ON EFFORTS TO REDUCE INFANT MORTALITY**
>
> - Encourage health behaviors: early and regular prenatal care, good nutrition.
> - Advise clients about factors that affect birth outcomes, such as maternal smok-ing, drug and alcohol abuse, stress, chronic illness, or other medical prob-lems.
> - Parents and caregivers should place sleep-ing infants on their backs and reduce bed sharing.
>
> Adapted from Office of Minority Health, CDC. (2003). Eliminate disparities in infant mortality. (p. 1). *http://www.cdc.gov/omh/AMH/factsheets/infant.htm*

or access. Acceptability of services may be lim-ited by the clients' health-care beliefs and practices or other factors. Continuing devel-opment in cultural competence is essential for the nurse to address minority health-care dis-parities. A major resource for health-care pro-fessionals can be the faith community specific to the particular minority population.

The projection for an increase in minority populations necessitates immediate action for the health of the nation. Improved data col-lection has been designed for enhanced prac-tice based on better evidence. Initiatives for

ONLINE CONSULT

The Commonwealth Fund.
http://www.cmwf.org
The Kaiser Family Foundation.
http://www.kff.org/whythedifference/about.htm
CDC Office of Minority Health.
http://www.cdc.gov/omh
Health Resources Services Administration.
http://www.hrsa.gov
Office of Minority Health.
http://www.omhrc.gov
National Institutes of Health.
http://www.nih.gov
National Institute of Nursing Research.
http://www.nih.gov/ninr/

cultural competence in the current health-care system, improved communication, and greater diversity of health-care providers are designed to address existing disparities and perceived quality of care and health status. As the Office of Minority Health (2003a) has stated, "culturally appropriate, community-driven programs are critical for eliminating racial and ethnic disparities in health" (p.1). Collaborative efforts are growing at the national, state, and local levels. Consult the resources listed in the Online Consult to examine current initiatives and progress on the goal for the elimination of health disparities.

 ## RURAL HEALTH

Geographic location was also identified in Healthy People 2010 as a demographic characteristic for which definable health disparities exist. Until recently, there was no predominant definition of *rural*. It has been defined in several ways in the literature and at the federal level. The divergent definitions impeded research and policy-making. Most definitions have been based on population or population density of a specified area. In 2002, new criteria based on the 2000 Census were released, defining an **urbanized area** as a central city with a densely populated surrounding area of 50,000 or more. **Rural areas** are defined as areas with a population less than 2500.

Certain rural health problems have been identified as particular to people living in rural areas. In fact, Healthy People 2010 characterizes **rural health** issues as follows:

Twenty-five percent of Americans live in rural areas, that is with fewer than 2,500 residents. Injury-related death rates are 40 percent higher in rural populations than in urban populations. Heart disease, cancer, and diabetes rates exceed those for urban areas. People living in rural areas are less likely to use preventative screening services, exercise regularly, or wear seat belts. In 1996, 20 percent of the rural population was uninsured compared with 16 percent of the urban population. Timely access to emergency services and the availability of specialty care are other issues for this population group. (USDHHS, 2000a, p. 16)

Further complicating matters is the fact that rural communities may share some features but are not all the same. For example, characteristics and problems of rural residents in south Georgia may be quite different from those of rural residents in Montana or New Mexico. It is important to be aware that the large majority of rural residents are not farmers. For those who are, agriculture is a dangerous occupation with great risk of injury and illness, even for their children. Nonagricultural occupational hazards in rural areas are also an important consideration, as with water purification. More than 50 million people live in rural areas, and their health risks and access to health-care are challenged by different factors.

The National Advisory Committee on Rural Health and Human Services (2003) has characterized the differences between health-care in urban and rural areas in terms of scope and scale as follows:

The urban setting features a high volume of patients with an emphasis on technology-intensive and inpatient services. The rural setting focuses more on ambulatory care and features a much lower patient volume. Rural health care systems tend to take care of more elderly patients and patients with more advanced or chronic conditions possibly due to the delays in getting health care. Rural residents, particularly those located in more isolated and sparsely populated communities, have higher risk factors than the general population. Rural areas also face greater shortages of health care providers... [and] reimbursement for providers who practice in rural areas tends to be less than their urban counterparts. (p. 6)

The rural health literature addresses a variety of problems. However, two recurring concerns seem to predominate: chronic illness (particularly in the elderly) and inadequate prenatal care. Just consider the issue of access in rural areas, especially with challenges related to reliable transportation, limitations in activities of daily living secondary to a chronic illness, and cost factors with additional child care or loss of income from time off work. Information from the 2000 Census indicates a growth in minority population in rural areas, particularly Hispanic and Latino Americans. Not surprisingly, rural growth also was higher in the more temperate climate areas of the South and the West. Demographic factors such as age, gender, race/ethnicity, socioeconomic status, and educational level are all considerations when rural geography and health status are investigated.

Delivery of health-care services in rural communities is heavily influenced by the availability, accessibility, and acceptability of services. Rural communities have fewer health-care resources. Distance, lack of communication, and other problems may hamper access. Acceptability of services may be limited by the clients' health-care beliefs and practices or other factors. In addition, the rural community health nurse may well be the only health professional in the community, working with very limited resources. Rural residents tend to be religiously and politically conservative, self-sufficient, and wary of outsiders (especially urbanites). Thus, the community health nurse cannot expect to rush eagerly into a rural community with good intentions and gain immediate acceptance. Building rapport with residents of a rural community takes time, and showing respect for their values and beliefs is imperative. In other words, the nurse must be sensitive and must demonstrate cultural competence. A further challenge is presented when the rural residents are also members of an ethnic group that is different from that of the nurse. The rural community health nurse must beware of assuming that these clients (and their problems) are the same as those of their urban counterparts. Their ruralism may be as significant as their ethnic identity.

Under Public Law 95–210, Rural Health Clinics (RHCs) were established to provide primary care services for residents of medically underserved areas. More than 3000 of these clinics are located as permanent facilities or mobile units throughout the nation. They are certified by the Centers for Medicare and Medicaid (CMS) and have required staffing and specified reimbursement components. Federal legislation has also created the Community Health Center (CHC) program and the Migrant Health Center (MHC) program to provide primary care for medically

underserved rural populations. Agencies receiving funding under the CHC program must provide diagnostic, preventive health, transportation, and emergency medical services. The MHC program, similar to the CHC program, is limited to migrant farm workers and their families. In 2002, the President promoted expansion of centers and culturally competent services. The goal was elimination of health disparities; collaborative efforts based on the key elements of leadership, infrastructure, partnership development, and system redesign were initiated (Bureau of Primary Care, 2003).

Federal reimbursement policy is a major issue for providers of rural health care. Although some improvements have occurred, urban health-care providers are reimbursed by Medicare at a higher rate than rural providers. And an important consideration is economy of scale, in that certain key services must be available despite the low volume of service in rural health-care agencies compared with their urban counterparts. Home health care is also more costly in the rural area because of low volume and longer travel distances.

The use of telecommunications technology in health care, or *telemedicine*, has greatly increased in recent years. It is being used extensively in some areas to enhance care of rural residents. For example, a specialist at an urban medical center can consult on a patient in a remote rural area via telecommunications. And this is also occurring globally, providing consultations, preparation of imaging, or interpretation of findings. There is a tremendous potential for greater access with telemedicine, but it is not without problems. Issues such as reimbursement, liability, and credentials and licensure must be addressed.

The Rural Healthy People 2010 Project was developed as a research effort to identify disadvantages and disparities in rural communities and to address the priority health concerns of rural America with featured practice models (Gamm et al., 2003a, 2003b). As with the national Healthy People 2010 initiative, data collected through this project will provide a better understanding of

ONLINE CONSULT

National Rural Health Asssociation.
http://www.nrharural.org
Rural Healthy People 2010.
http://www.srph.tamushsc.edu/rhp2010/index.html
National Advisory Committee on Rural Health and Human Services.
http://ruralcommittee.hrsa.gov/nacpubs.htm
Migrant Health Care Program.
http://bphc.hrsa.gov/programs/MHCProgramInfo.htm
Economic Research Service, USDA.
http://ers.usda.gov/emphases/rural/

the rural population and its risk factors and will facilitate movement toward the national goals.

COMMUNITY NURSING IN THE CONTEXT OF HEALTHY PEOPLE

The nature of nursing practice in the community is different, dynamic, and responsive. **Community health nursing** crosses many traditional boundaries, is holistic, and is not limited to a particular age group, diagnostic category, or narrow set of specialized skills. Although clients include individuals and families, community health nursing may have a group or even an entire community as a client. Clients may be well or ill. Their health risks or needs may be either physical or mental in nature.

Several factors determine the roles, activities, and intervention strategies of an individual community health nurse, working in the context of Healthy People:

• Mission, philosophy, and priorities of the employing agency
• Level of prevention at which intervention is aimed
• Definition of client

The mission, philosophy, and priorities of a private agency or a faith-based organization can be quite different from those of an official government agency. The level of funding influences how well the agency is able to implement its priorities, which should be based on identified health needs in the community.

Another factor that influences the functions for the community health nurse is the agency's level of prevention focus. Community health nurses are involved in all three levels of prevention. Historically, however, these nurses have played a key role in primary prevention efforts. For more than 100 years they have been involved in health promotion and disease prevention. Over the past years, and despite initiatives like Healthy People, these traditional services have suffered under-reimbursement, with health departments compelled to provide more direct clinical services. Consequently, many public health nurses have taken on a role that is more illness-oriented. Nevertheless, Healthy People priorities clearly reflect a need for community health nurses, especially those in public health agencies, to renew and strengthen their role in primary prevention.

Community health nursing is frequently described in the literature as a synthesis of nursing and public health. Public health is unique because it broadens concerns to the "public" with a population and collaborative focus. The mission of the Public Health Nursing Section of the APHA is "to enhance the health of population groups through the application of nursing knowledge to the community" (Public Health Nursing Section, 2003, p. 1). In published standards of public health, the American Nurses Association (1999), in collaboration with several other public health nursing organizations, identified eight tenets of public health nursing and defined the practice as "promoting and protecting the health of populations using knowledge from nursing, social, and public health sciences" (p. 1). Clearly, an interdisciplinary focus is necessary to address the health of the community and the people who make up that community. One important consideration, as mentioned in Healthy People, is the environmental concerns that affect the health of the community.

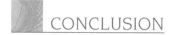

CONCLUSION

Challenges exist in many areas for professional nursing practice as we address the health needs of at-risk populations. Whether talking about the aging member of a minority population, the well elder in the community, the rural child with asthma, or the individual with diabetes, health professionals should focus on the national objectives for increasing years of healthy life and the elimination of health disparities.

Key Points

- Healthy People 2000 addressed three general goals as national health promotion and disease prevention objectives, with a focus on specific age groups and special populations in 22 priority areas.
- Healthy Communities is available to assist planners in adapting the Healthy People objectives to the needs and resources of individual communities.
- Healthy People 2010 built upon the information from the prior decade but was developed with the two major goals of increasing the quality and years of healthy life and eliminating health disparities. It uses a framework of 28 focus areas, 467 objectives, and 10 leading health indicators.
- Leading health indicators reflect the major public health concerns in the nation; they are: physical activity, overweight and obesity, tobacco use, substance abuse, responsible sexual behavior, mental health, injury and violence, environmental quality, immunization, and access to care.
- Proportional increases in the population of aging adults are predicted, with the greatest increase in those 85 years and older. Women currently account for a large proportion of this group. Predictions include an increase in minority groups represented in our aging population.
- Chronic illnesses and increasing frailty are the major causes of morbidity in aging adults. Disability is the inability to do something because of a physical or mental impairment. Chronicity is related to duration or recurrence of a condition.
- Aging has also been classified as successful, usual, or pathologic (Rowe & Kahn, 1987). In successful aging, there is an interaction between the individual's genes and environment, both being positive. Usual aging occurs in the vast majority of individuals as an interaction between the person's genetic endowment and environment. In pathologic aging, we see a negative interaction between genetic and environmental factors.
- Aging adults face physical, environmental, psychosocial, and chemical risk factors. The risks commonly affect many aging adults, creating conditions that interfere with activity. Health promotion activities are vital in this area to maintain functional ability and reduce the incidence of frailty and disability.
- Evidence that health disparities exist among ethnic groups of all ages has been documented; however, reasons for their occurrence are multifaceted and complex. Minority health is an important initiative for the health of the nation. *(continued)*

(continued)

- The CDC's Office of Minority Health (2004) classifies racial or ethnic minority populations as: American Indian and Alaskan Native, Asian, Black or African American, Hispanic or Latino, and Native Hawaiian and other Pacific Islander.
- In 2002, new criteria based on the 2000 Census were released, defining an urbanized area as a central city with a densly populated surrounding area of 50,000 or more. Rural areas are generally defined by exclusion, as other areas with a population less than 2500.
- The differences between health care in urban areas and that in rural areas have been described in terms of scope and scale of services and providers.
- Rural health clinics (RHCs) have been established to provide primary care services for residents of underserved areas. Federal legislation has also created the Community Health Center (CHC) and Migrant Health Center (MHC) programs to provide primary care for medically underserved rural populations.
- Community health nursing is frequently described in the literature as a synthesis of nursing and public health. The mission of the Public Health Nursing Section of the APHA has as its mission "to enhance the health of population groups through the application of nursing knowledge to the community" (Public Health Nursing Section, 2003, p. 1).

Thought and Discussion Questions

1. Consider goal of Healthy People 2010 "to increase the quality and years of healthy life." Be prepared to share your impressions on achievement of this national goal in a discussion to be scheduled by your instructor.
2. The second goal set for Healthy People 2010 was for the elimination of health disparities. Be prepared to participate in a discussion to be scheduled by your instructor to share your impression on achievement of this goal in the area of minority health care.
3. Review the Chapter Thought located on the first page of the chapter, and discuss it in the context of the contents of the chapter.

Interactive Exercises

1. Select one of the 10 leading health indicators in Healthy People 2010 and conduct an online search for information on the progress toward and national achievement of the objectives and targets. Use the format provided on the Intranet site to report the progress.
2. Investigate the strategies for Healthy People 2010 goals and objectives specific to your state and local community. Using the format provided on the Intranet site, compare the state objectives with the national ones. Identify the people and community groups involved in the process.
3. Interview two individuals from two different older age groups (60 to 69, 70 to 79, 80 to 89, 90 to100 years). Try to include both genders and individuals with different states of wellness. Include the questions on Core Healthy Days Measures

(CDC, 2000) in your interviews. Describe the subjects' perspectives on health and experiences with aging. Complete the needs inventory on aging adults located on the Intranet site.

4. Complete the Interactive Exercise located on the Intranet Site by suggesting interventions for specific risk factors that commonly affect aging adults and create conditions that interfere with activites of daily living.

5. Conduct an online search to identify health promotion programs and resources in your community that apply to specific at-risk population groups. Next, identify health-care services appropriate for health problems in these groups. Use the format provided on the Intranet site.

6. Conduct an online search on telemedicine. Identify at least three examples being used in a health-care agency and list the advantages, potential problems, and interpersonal and ethical issues. Be prepared to participate in an online discussion with members of your class, as scheduled by your instructor.

7. Locate a rural area with a population of 2500 people or less. Identify the health-care resources and clinics available to the population and the services they provide.

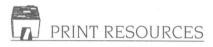

PRINT RESOURCES

References

American Nurses Association. (1999). *Scope and standards of public health nursing practice* (Publication No. 9910PH). Washington, DC: American Nurses Publishing.

American Public Health Association. (1991). *Healthy communities 2000: Model standards: Guidelines for community attainment of the year 2000 objectives.* Washington, DC: APHA. Collins, K. S., Hughes, D. L., Doty, M. M., Ives, B. L., Edwards, J. N., & Tenney, K. (2002). *Diverse communities, common concerns: Assessing health care quality for minority Americans.* New York: The Commonwealth Fund.

National Center for Health Statistics. (NCHS). (1999). *Healthy People 2000 review, 1998–99.* Hyattsville, MD: Public Health Service.

Perot, R. T., & Youdelman, M. (2001). *Racial, ethnic, and primary language data collection in the health care system: An assessment of federal policies and practices.* New York: The Commonwealth Fund.

The President's Advisory Commission on Consumer Protection and Quality in the Health Care Industry. (1998). *Quality first: Better health care for all Americans* (Final report to the President of the United States). Columbia, MD: Consumer Bill of Rights.

Rowe, J. W., & Kahn, R. L. (1987). Human aging: Usual and successful. *Science, 237,* 143–149.

U.S. Department of Health and Human Services, Office of Public Health and Science, Office of Disease Prevention and Health Promotion. (2001). *Healthy people in healthy commnities: A community planning guide using Healthy People 2010.* Washington, DC: U.S. Government Printing Office.

U.S. Department of Health and Human Services, Public Health Service. (1992). *Healthy people 2000: Summary report.* Boston: Jones & Bartlett.

Bibliography

American Cancer Society. (2003). *Cancer facts and figures for Hispanics/Latinos.* Atlanta, GA: Author.

Centers for Disease Control and Prevention. (2000). *Measuring healthy days: Population assessment of health-related quality of life.* Atlanta, GA. Author.

Coburn, A. F., & Gale, J. A. (2003). *The characteristics and roles of rural health clinics in the United States: A chartbook.* Rockville, MD: Health Resources and Services Administration.

Collins, K. S., Hall, A., & Neuhaus, C. (1999). *U.S. minority health: A chartbook.* New York: The Commonwealth Fund.

Collins. K. S., Hughes, D. L., Doty, M. M., Ives, B. L., Edwards, J. N., & Tenny, K. (2002). *Diverse communities, common concerns: Assessing health care quality for minority Americans.* New York: The Commonwealth Fund.

Health Resources and Services Administration, Office of Rural Health Policy. (2003). *The outreach sourcebook: Volume 9 rural health demonstration projects 1999 to 2002.* Rockville, MD: HRSA.

Hughes, D. L. (2002). *Quality of health care for Asian Americans.* New York: The Commonwealth Fund.

Perot, R. T., & Youdelman, M. (2001). *Racial, ethnic, and primary language data collection in the health care system: An asssessment of federal policies and practices.* New York: The Commonwealth Fund.

ONLINE RESOURCES

References

Administration on Aging. (2003a). National family care-givers support program. *http://www.aoa.gov/prof/aoaprog/caregiver/caregiver.asp.*

Administration on Aging. (2003b). Press Release: Did you know? *http://www.aoa.gov/press/did_you_know/did_you_know.asp.*

Administration on Aging (2003c). Promising pracices in the field of caregiving. *http://www.aoa.gov/prof/aoaprog/caregiver/careprof/nfcsp_projects/PromisingPractices.pdf.*

Administration on Aging (2003d). Snapshot: A statistical profile of Hispanic older Americans aged 65+. *http://www.aoa.gov/prof/Statistics/minority_aging/Facts-on-Hispanic-Elderly.pdf.*

Administration on Aging. (2002). A profile of older Americans: 2002. *http://www.aoa.gov/prof/Statistics/profile/2002profile.doc.*

Bureau of Primary Health Care. (2003). Migrant health program. *http://bphc.hrsa.gov/programs/MHCProgramInfo.htm.*

Centers for Disease Control and Prevention. (2003a). Healthy aging: Preventing disease and improving quality of life among older Americans—at a glance 2003. *http://www.cdc.gov/nccdphp/aag/aag_aging.htm.*

Centers for Disease Control and Prevention. (2003b). Public health and aging: Trends in aging—United States and worldwide. MMWR *Weekly*, 52 (06), 101–106. *http://www.cdc.gov/mmwr/preview/mmwrhtml/mm5206a2.htm*

Centers for Disease Control and Prevention. (2000). *Measuring healthy days: Population assessment of health related quality of life.* Atlanta, GA: Author. *http://www.cdc.gov/nccdphp/hrqol/pdfs/mhd.pdf.*

Economic Research Service. (2003). Rural America at a glance. *http://ers.usda.gov/briefing/rural/gallery/.*

Fried, L. P., Kasper, J. D., Guralnik, J. M., & Simonsick, E. M. (1995). The women's health and aging study: An introduction. In Guralnik, J. M., Fried, L. P., Simonsick, E.M., Kasper, J. D., & Lafferty, M. E. (eds.), *The women's health and aging study: Health and social characteristics of older women with disability* (pp. 1–6) (NIH Pub. No. 95–4009). Bethesda, MD: National Institute on Aging. *http://www.nia.nih.gov/health/pubs/whasbook/title.htm.*

Gamm, L. D., Hutchinson, L. L., Dabney, B. J., & Dorsey, A. M. (eds.). (2003a). *Rural Healthy People 2010: A companion document to Healthy People 2010.* Volume 1. College Station, TX: Texas A&M University System Health Science Research Center. *http://www.srph.tamushsc.edu/rhp2010/litrev.htm.*

Gamm, L. D., Hutchinson, L. L., Dabney, B. J., & Dorsey, A. M. (eds.). (2003b). *Rural Healthy People 2010: A companion document to Healthy People 2010.* Volume 2. College Station,

TX: Texas A&M University System Health Science Research Center. *http://www.srph.tamushsc.edu/rhp2010/litrev.htm.*

Lillie-Blanton, M., Rushing, O. E., Ruiz, S., Mayberry, R., & Boone, L. (2002). *Racial/ethnic differences in cardiac care: The weight of the evidence.* Menlo Park, CA: Kaiser Family Foundation. *http://www.kff.org/whythedifference/6040fullreport.pdf.*

Hamrick, K. (ed.). (2002). Rural America at a glance (ERS Rural Development Research Report No. RDRR94-1). *http://www.ers.usda.gov/publications/rdrr94-1/rdrr94-1.pdf*

National Advisory Committee on Rural Health and Human Services. (2003). Health care quality: The rural context. *http://ruralcommittee.hrsa.gov/QR03.htm.*

National Center for Health Statistics (NCHS 2001). Infant deaths/mortality. *http://www.cdc.gov/nchs/fastats/infmort.htm.*

National Center for Health Statistics (NCHS). (1999). Healthy People 2000: Maternal and infant progress review. *http://www.cdc.gov/nchs/about/otheract/hp2000/childhlt/childhlt.htm.*

National Center for Health Statistics (NCHS). (2003). Data Warehouse on Trends in Health and Aging. *http://www.cdc.gov/nchs/agingact.htm.*

National Center on Elder Abuse. (2003). Who are the abusers? *http://www.elderabusecenter.org/default.cfm?p=whoaretheabusers.cfm.*

Office of Disease Prevention and Health Promotion (ODPHP). (2001). Healthy People in Healthy Communities: A Community Planning Guide Using Healthy People 2010. *http://www.healthypeople.gov/Publications/HealthyCommunities2001/default.htm*

Office of Minority Health (CDC). (2004). About US: OMH vision for the 21st Century "health equality for all. *http://www.cdc.gov/omh/AboutUs/aboutUs.htm*

Office of Minority Health, CDC. (2003a). Disease burden and risk factors. *http://www.cdc.gov/omh/AMH/dbrf.htm.*

Office of Minority Health, CDC. (2003b). Eliminate disparities in infant mortality. *http://www.cdc.gov/omh/AMH/factsheets/infant.htm.*

Public Health Nursing Section, American Public Health Association (APHA). (2003). About public health nursing. *http://www.csuchico.edu/~host.*

Title 42, Chapter 35. (2000). Programs for Older Americans, Older Americans Act. Amendments of 2000. *http://www.access.gpo.gov/uscode/title42/chapter35_.html.*

U.S. Department of Health and Human Services. (2000a). Healthy People 2010: Volume I (2nd ed.). *http://www.healthypeople.gov/Document/tableofcontents.htm#volume1*

U.S. Department of Health and Human Services. (2000b). Healthy People 2010: Volume 2 (2nd ed.). *http://www.healthypeople.gov/Document/tableofcontents.htm#Volume2.*

U.S. Department of Health and Human Services. (2000c). Tracking healthy people. *http://www.healthypeople.gov/Document/tableofcontents.htm#tracking.*

U.S. Department of Health and Human Services. (1995). Healthy people 2000: Midcourse review and 1995 revisions. *http://odphp.osophs.dhhs.gov/pubs/hp2000/midcrs1.htm.*

Resources

Administration on Aging (2003). A statistical profile of Hispanic older Americans Aged 65+. *http://www.aoa.gov/prof/Statistics/minority_aging/Facts-on-Hispanic-Elderly.pdf.*

Arizona Department of Health Services, Bureau of Community and Family Health Services. (2003). Healthy Arizona 2010. *http://www.hs.state.az.us/phs/healthyaz2010.*

Doty, M. (2003). Insurance, access, and quality of care among Hispanic populations: 2003 chartpack. *http://www.cmwf.org/programs/minority/doty_hispanicchartpack_684.ppt.*

Federal Interagency Forum on Child and Family Statistics. (2003). *America's children: Key national indicators of well-being,* 2003. Washington, DC: U.S. Government Printing Office. *http://www.childstats.gov/americaschildren.*

Federal Interagency Forum on Aging-Related Statistics. (2000). *Older Americans 2000: Key national indicators of well-being.* Washington, DC: U.S. Government Printing Office. *http://agingstats.gov/chartbook2000/default.htm.*

Health Resources & Services Administration (HRSA). (2003). Promoting rural health. *http://www.hrsa.gov/.*

HRSA Workgroup on the Elimination of Health Disparities. (2000). *Eliminating health disparities in the United States.* Washington, DC: Health Resources and Services Administration. *http://www.hrsa.gov/OMH/OMH/disparities/default.htm.*

Institute of Medicine. (2003). *Unequal treatment: Understanding racial and ethnic disparities in health care.* Washington, DC: National Academy Press. *http://www.nap.edu/books/030908265X/html/*

Maine Rural Health Research Center. (2003). Rural health research in progress in the rural health research centers program (7th ed.). *http://www.rural-health.org.*

National Advisory Committee on Rural Health. (2002). A targeted look at the rural health care safety net. *ftp://ftp.hrsa.gov/ruralhealth/NACReportbb.pdf.*

National Advisory Committee on Rural Health. (2001). Key rural issues for medicare reform. *http://ruralcommittee.hrsa.gov/reform_nac.htm.*

Project HOPE Walsh Center for Rural Health Analysis. (1997). National Rural Health Policy: Recommendations from the First Eight Years of the National Advisory Committee on Rural Health. *http://www.projecthope.org/CHA/rural/nacrh.pdf.*

State of Alaska, Health and Social Services. (2003). Healthy Alaskans 2010. *http://www.hss.state.ak.us/dph/targets/ha2010/default.htm.*

State of Michigan, Department of Community Health. (2003). Critical health indicators. *http://www.michigan.gov/mdch/0,1607,7–132–2944_5327–17501—,00.html.*

U.S. Department of Health and Human Services. (2002). A demographic and health snapshot of the U.S. Hispanic/Latino population: 2002 national Hispanic health leadership summit. *http://www.cdc.gov/NCHS/data/hpdata2010/chcsummit.pdf.*

U.S. Department of Health and Human Services. (2002). Progress review: Access to quality health services. *http://www.healthypeople.gov/data/2010prog/focus01.*

U.S. Department of Health and Human Services. (2002). Progress review: Arthritis, osteoporosis, and chronic back conditions. *http://www.healthypeople.gov/data/2010prog/focus02.*

U.S. Department of Health and Human Services. (2002). Progress review: Cancer. *http://www.healthypeople.gov/data/2010prog/focus03.*

U.S. Department of Health and Human Services. (2002). Progress review: Chronic kidney disease. *http://www.healthypeople.gov/data/2010prog/focus04/.*

U.S. Department of Health and Human Services. (2002). Progress review: Diabetes. *http://www.healthypeople.gov/data/2010prog/focus05.*

U.S. Department of Health and Human Services. (2000). Healthy People 2010: Understanding and improving health. *http://www.healthypeople.gov/Document/tableofcontents.htm#uih.*

Vermont Department of Health. (2000). Healthy Vermonters 2010. *http://www.healthyvermonters.info/admin/pubs/ hv2010/hv2010.shtml*

Francoise Dunefsky

17
chapter

Quality Health Care

> Quality is everyone's responsibility.

Chapter Objectives

On completion of this chapter, the reader will be able to:

1. Discuss roles for the consumer and professional in quality appraisal in health-care settings.
2. Differentiate among terms used to assess and promote quality in health-care settings.
3. Identify quality improvement factors to be considered at the unit, organizational, and system levels.
4. Describe the steps in the processes of continuous quality improvement and total quality management.
5. Discuss the role of regulatory agencies in quality evaluation in health-care settings.
6. Select structure, process, and outcome indicators.

Key Terms

Quality Improvement	Quality Assurance	Check Sheets
Continuous Quality	Process Team	Surveys
Improvement	Flow Chart	Indicators
Benchmarking	Data Sheets	Variation

The United States is closely examining the definition of *quality* and its relationship to health-care costs. This effort has been stimulated by several factors: the necessity to compete in a global marketplace, where production costs are often significantly lower; the ongoing explosion in technologic advances; exponential expenditures for health-care services; and individual and corporate consumer pressures to improve value and safety.

Health-care institutions are attempting to understand and apply principles and techniques previously reserved for the business world. In their codes of ethics and standards of practice, professional groups, including nurses and physicians, have historically expressed the intent of ensuring that individual patients receive optimal care. The impact of structures and processes on these individual and aggregate outcomes was previously not documented nor necessarily understood.

In addition, societal forces are shifting the health-care paradigm from a paternalistic model of delivering care and services to one that responds to customer demands. Making providers accountable for evaluating the quality of care they deliver, and for communicating that quality effectively to the public, is an emerging task influenced by corporate buyers of services, who want to know what they can expect to receive for their money.

With its professional commitment to clients, responsibility for coordinating care, and roots in the psychosocial and physical sciences, nursing is poised to play an important role in the ongoing development and implementation of care delivery models that are effective and efficient, meet customer expectations, and ensure excellent clinical outcomes. The dictionary defines *quality* as "character with respect to fineness or grade of excellence." In health care, we previously defined it as being "free of mistakes" or perfect relative to process. The standard of perfection or 100 percent compliance was

focused within. The current quality movement is evolving a definition of quality that includes "meeting customer needs" and focusing on outcome.

Health-care providers have consistently looked at clinical care as the measure for quality. Traditionally, the qualifications of clinicians, state-of-the-art technology, and episodic interventions that cure illness or "do no harm" were considered indices of quality. But asking customers how they perceive "quality" enables a more complex picture to emerge. The consumer expects expert clinical care. But equally important are timely, courteous, and respectful treatment, easy access to caregivers and information, unfragmented care delivery, reasonable costs, and the ability to maneuver through the system without too many obstacles.

 ## HISTORICAL PERSPECTIVES

Human societies have always wished for excellence. Reliance on professional associations such as guilds and inspection by consumers are century-old methods of judging quality. Societal values, however, are changing the context in which quality is evaluated.

Pre–World War II health-care delivery in the United States was mostly a cottage industry. This time is referred to as the "charitable era of health care." The wealthy and fortunate rural populations relied on services delivered in the home. The poor and urban working classes were sent to hospitals in critical circumstances or died at home. A sudden growth in technology and treatment modalities and the building of hospitals stimulated by the Hill-Burton Act began the corporatization of health-care delivery. The "technologic era" lasted for more than 30 years. Extensive development of policies, procedures, standards of practice, and professional disciplines ensued. It took 20 years before the industrial model of reliance on departmental inspection and supervisory audits became part of the fabric of health care. The role of Medicare and federal and state government accelerated this growth.

The early 1970s saw the beginning of formalized measurement of clinical performance and outcomes. Organizations such as the Joint Commission on Accreditation of Healthcare Organizations (JCAHO), professional review organizations (PROs) and some state health departments played a major role in the initial movement. Retrospective audits, investigation of problems, and indicator measurements were all attempts to discover less than acceptable performance by an individual, discipline, or department. The objective was to discover the "bad apples," implement a corrective action plan, and monitor its effectiveness through ongoing measurement. It was assumed that quality was a result of the performance of individuals or groups of individuals. The tools of the corrective action plans were education, disciplinary action, and increased resources such as technology and staffing.

A gradual quality paradigm shift began in the second half of the 1980s. The "economic era" of health care was emerging. Other industries purchasing health care for their employees at rapidly rising costs challenged the health-care sector to provide "more" and "better" for "less." The Japanese were successfully invading the American marketplace as a result of quality methodologies developed by Deming, Juran, and others. Deming had persuaded the Japanese government and industry that they should focus on quality rather than price and costs. Knowing that this focus would take time and commitment, they infused their businesses with the belief that work is performed by interdependent teams, that individuals want to do a good job, that those who do the work itself know its processes better than anyone else, and that mass inspection and fear do not automatically result in quality.

Juran proposed the notion that by planning for quality, one avoids multiple trial-and-error situations and costly rework, often referred to as "the cost of poor quality." Quality could be cost-effective. Improvement required even higher goals for quality. Reliance on systems analysis and statistical methods and techniques produced better-quality products than supervision and inspection of individual human behaviors.

During the next 10 years, companies began to recognize that care is delivered by individuals who function as members of cross-functional and interdisciplinary teams, and that individuals and teams are tools for, rather than objects of, improvement. Currently a body of scientific research is emerging that tests the new theories that care is supported by environmental, managerial, support, and governance structures, and that ensuring accepted clinical outcomes is not enough to meet customer needs.

Many individuals and organizations have contributed to the quality journey over the past 30 years. The Agenda for Change at JCAHO and Donald Berwick and his group at the Institute for Healthcare Improvement are but a few that deserve recognition for being driving forces in the implementation of the new quality care models. In 1996, the Institute of Medicine (IOM), a member of The National Academies, began a multiple-phase Quality Initiative; its landmark reports include

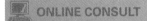

ONLINE CONSULT

For more information on accreditation initiatives visit:
The Joint Commission for Accreditation of Healthcare Organizations at
http://www.jcaho.org
The Institute for Healthcare Improvement at
http://www.ihi.org
The Institute of Medicine at
http://www4.nationalacademies.org

To Err is Human: Building a Safer Health System (2000), *Crossing the Quality Chasm: A New Health System for the 21st Century* (2001), and the study sponsored by the U.S. Department of Health and Human Services Agency for Healthcare Research and Quality, *Keeping Patients Safe: Transforming the Work Environment of Nurses* (2003). These reports focus on the quality problems and on the multiple levels of system reform needed.

Largely as a result of the IOM's activities and reports, the JCAHO has approved the 2004 National Patient Safety Goals. The requirements of these are surveyed in all health-care organizations seeking their accreditation.

The role nursing plays in all of the quality and safety work has been pushed to the forefront.

BOX 17–1
DEMING'S 14 POINTS

1. Create constancy of purpose for improvement of product and service.
2. Adopt the new philosophy.
3. Cease dependence on mass inspection.
4. End the practice of awarding business on the basis of price tag alone.
5. Improve constantly and forever the system of production and service.
6. Institute training.
7. Adopt and institute leadership.
8. Drive out fear.
9. Break down barriers between staff areas.
10. Eliminate slogans and targets in the workplace that urge increased productivity.
11. Eliminate numerical quotas for the workplace and management.
12. Remove barriers that rob people of pride in workmanship.
13. Encourage education and self-improvement for everyone.
14. Take action to accomplish the transformation.

Reprinted from *Out of the Crisis* by W. Edwards Deming by permission of the W. Edwards Deming Institute® Copyright 1986 by The W. Edwards Deming Institute®

THEORETICAL MODELS FOR QUALITY

The models used for **quality improvement** have come from industry. Some have been adapted for health care, but all share the common theme of using the scientific process.

Deming's Principles for Transformation

W. Edwards Deming was the first to challenge seriously the managerial notion that quality and increased productivity are incompatible. In doing his research and developing the 14 Points for Management, he assumed the new radical approach of listening to those who actually did the work (Box 17–1) (Deming, 1982, 1986). Deming contends that the model can be applied anywhere, including service industries. Nursing leaders at all levels of the organization can apply the principles in their quest to implement quality care. The more pervasive the quality culture in the organization, the easier the model application becomes. The stronger and more visible leadership is in its support for quality, the more rapidly a quality culture can be implemented.

The 14 Points for Management

1. *Create constancy of purpose for improvement of product and service.* Innovation is the foundation for the future. It requires a belief that there is a future and an unshakable commitment to quality and productivity. Resources must be put into education and research so we can constantly improve. The aim is to meet our mission and serve our customers, because otherwise we will not stay in business. We must address day-to-day problems without getting stuck in them. Many nurse managers fail to plan their resources, energy, and time to deal with the future. Work better, not harder, to plan new services. Meeting our customers' needs and training and

retraining personnel help deal with required change.

2. *Adopt the new philosophy.* Do not accept existing levels of mistakes or staff who are not adequately prepared to perform. Become the change agent who meets the challenge. Propose, develop, and implement improvements in systems and services.

3. *Cease dependence on mass inspection.* The inspection stage is too late to improve quality. Quality comes from improvement in production processes. Tools, such as 100 percent case review, will not improve care, are time-consuming, and require resources that could be spent better in improving design or systems. Measuring incomplete records, medication errors, or service delays, in and of themselves, will not improve the delivery of care.

4. *End the practice of awarding business on the basis of price tags alone.* The nurse manager has a responsibility to include total cost when recommending the purchase of goods or services. This includes not only the "up-front" price but also the cost of disposables and maintenance, amount of vendor support provided, ease of training in use, labor costs, and cross-functional use. It is a managerial responsibility to make well-prepared, comprehensive recommendations to the executive team. Deming believes that limiting the suppliers we deal with and establishing long-term relationships with vendors creates interdependency, which assists in the achievement of quality.

5. *Improve constantly and forever the system of production and service.* Quality must be built and incorporated during the design phase in order to avoid costly rework. Teamwork is essential in this process, especially in service industries such as health care, in which we rely on interdependent, cross-disciplinary teams to deliver the care that is our product. As our customers' needs and available resources change, we are obliged to improve existing systems. Reductions in length of stay, shifts in delivery of care along the continuum, and changing demographics all require us to seek opportunities to "do it better." It is no longer acceptable to think "we always did it this way and it worked."

6. *Institute training.* Learning must be life-long and pervasive. The principles of adult learning, and an appreciation for the fact that different people learn by different methods, apply at all layers of the organization, regardless of length of employment. All must understand the institution's mission, values, customer needs, and expectations. What the assignment is, what is acceptable work, and how we prepare people all must be defined. For the manager, this includes knowing which processes are assigned and understanding variation in these processes. We must become learning organizations.

7. *Adopt and institute leadership.* The job of management is leadership, namely, vision and communication of that vision, not supervision. The assignment is to work on quality of service, designing for quality and delivering an actual product. The leader must understand the work supervised and must remove barriers that prevent the staff members from doing their work.

8. *Drive out fear.* Fear of reprisal, fear to admit mistakes, fear of not having the needed new knowledge, and fear of not meeting the deadlines or quotas interfere with seeing opportunities for improvement. Errors, complaints, and areas that appear out of control must be studied and analyzed for opportunities to improve.

9. *Break down barriers between staff areas.* This point has proved especially difficult in health care, where the struggle to establish distinct professional domains fostered accountability, review, and disciplinary actions within professions. The emergence of matrix organizations, patient care departments, use of product or service line teams, cross-training, and decentralization of services will assist in the implementation of patient care teams focused on the patient rather than the professional. Simultaneously, this will create a new challenge to ensure that no one can hide behind or dominate the team. All professional groups must be

held accountable for their professional practice and for quality in service delivery.

10. *Eliminate slogans and targets in the workplace that urge increased productivity.* The assumption that one can improve quality and productivity by trying harder does not take into account that most problems come from systems rather than individuals. The role of management is to improve the system with results of sound statistical methods.

11. *Eliminate numerical quotas for the workforce and management.* Quotas assume that the target is correct, not too high or too low, and that all can attain them. They have a negative effect on pride in workmanship. Productivity should be studied, analyzed, and understood. Everyone should know what to do and how to do it. A sustained requirement for all to participate in setting goals and figuring out how to reach them is needed.

12. *Remove barriers that rob people of pride in workmanship.* Make clear what the job is and what the expectations are. Improving the system to make it easier for people to work well will help them invest in the organization, reducing turnover and absenteeism.

13. *Encourage education and self-improvement for everyone.* Study and development should not only focus on the immediate needs of the organization or department. Develop the organization and its members for the future as well as for the present.

14. *Take action to accomplish the transformation.* The leaders must adopt the new philosophy with pride. It must be explained often and well to a critical number of individuals. Everyone in the organization must be asked to participate. This requires substantial and sustained commitment and energy.

Deming also recognized obstacles to the transformation, which are:

- Desire to achieve instant results by hiring a consultant
- Supposition that solving problems creates transformation
- Belief that one can simply transfer systems from another organization

- Belief that the quality department takes care of quality
- Belief that your problems are different
- Poor understanding of statistical methods

More serious blocks, referred to as "deadly diseases" because of their severity and resistance to eradication, include:

- Lack of constancy of purpose
- Emphasis on short-term profits
- Evaluation of performance without long-term improvement in mind
- Mobility of management
- Management by numbers only

When considering applying Deming's principles for transformation, the nurse has to acknowledge realities in the organization. It may be necessary to maintain annual performance review, existing merit systems, strict organizational and professional hierarchies, and a focus on monthly budget fluctuations. Nevertheless, the general principles of constancy of purpose, focus on improvement, creating a learning environment, reducing fear, and removing barriers to pride in workmanship can be adopted by anyone in any setting.

Juran Trilogy

Deming offers us a framework for how to transform any organization by incorporating quality, but the Juran Trilogy focuses on the tools that organizations can use while doing the work. The two models are complementary and are often used together.

Dr. Joseph Juran (1989) defines *quality* as "fitness for use." This definition assumes both freedom from defects and presence of the multiple elements required to meet the total needs of a customer. The freedom from defect does not guarantee that this is the product the customer wants. The client assumes we can deliver care without errors. Waiting time, ease of access, and cleanliness may be crucial factors determining whether a client chooses us.

The Juran Trilogy utilizes three managerial processes, planning, control, and improvement (Box 17–2). The trilogy's proposed procedural steps and tools are unique.

> **BOX 17–2**
> **JURAN TRILOGY**
>
> A. Quality Planning
> 1. Determine who the customers are.
> 2. Determine the needs of the customer.
> 3. Develop product features that respond to the customer's needs.
> 4. Develop processes that are able to produce these product features.
> 5. Transfer the resulting plans to the operating forces.
> B. Quality Control
> 1. Evaluate actual quality performance.
> 2. Compare actual performance to quality goals.
> 3. Act on the difference.
> C. Quality Improvement
> 1. Establish an infrastructure.
> 2. Identify needs for improvement.
> 3. Establish project teams for each project.
> 4. Provide the teams with resources, motivation, and training.
>
> Adapted from Juran, J. M. (1989). Juran on leadership for quality. New York: The Free Press, with permission.

Quality Planning

Planning for programs or services requires that quality is built into them. This stage follows five distinct steps:

1. Determine who the customers of the program or service are. They can be external customers, internal customers, or both. In health care, clients, families, and payers are all external customers. Departments and providers are internal customers of one another. Nursing receives services from dietary or medical records, and those departments in turn are customers of nursing. Independent medical staff members are often considered both internal and external customers because of their ability to choose the institution and their influence and provision of services within the institution.
2. Determine the customers' needs. Surveys, focus groups, individual client interviews, complaint reviews, and market analysis can be used to determine what our customers want.
3. Develop product features that respond to the customer's needs. Consider offering services outside traditional business hours. Weekend day surgery, diagnostic procedures early and late in the day, and respite care are but a few examples.
4. Develop processes that are able to produce those product features.
5. Transfer the resulting plans to the implementation team.

For example, while teaching breast self-examination at a customer-friendly breast clinic, a nurse hears clients express concerns about the time it takes to receive mammography results. In response to complaints, the nurse, working with the department and a local women's group, initiates a formal survey of women who currently use the center and women who do not. The survey reveals that women want to receive test results within 24 hours and to be able to refer themselves for mammography. As a result, the services at the center are redesigned to incorporate these features. The clinic applies for and obtains an expanded license for self-referral. It institutes policies, procedures, and standards to ensure that the improved services are implemented and monitored.

Quality Control

The three steps of quality control involve:

1. Evaluating actual quality performance. This requires knowledge of statistical methods of measurement and analysis.
2. Comparing actual performance with quality goals.
3. Acting on the difference. This assumes understanding of common and special cause variation. Variation is part of any process. Constant reaction to it may destabilize an otherwise stable process.

Quality Improvement

Raising performance to unprecedented levels requires four steps:

1. Establishing the infrastructure needed to secure ongoing quality improvement. The infrastructure, which may comprise a quality council, departmental teams, and assigned roles, ensures that quality improvement is part of the way business is done.
2. Identifying specific needs for improvement. Data from quality control, feedback from customers, and goals of the organization help determine what needs to be improved and what needs to be prioritized.
3. Establishing a project team for each project. Responsibility must be defined clearly. This includes the objective for improvement and measures of success.
4. Providing resources, motivation, and training for the teams to diagnose causes of lesser quality, stimulate a remedy, and establish controls to hold the gains in improvements.

Juran's work has shown that most of the potential for eliminating errors and improving the system does not lie in changing workers. The 85/15, rule as it is now commonly referred to, states that 85 percent of problems can be corrected only by changing systems.

Both Deming and Juran have provided the foundation for today's quality movement in industry and in health care. The JCAHO Agenda for Change helped in the transition from quality assurance to quality improvement.

The 10-Step Model for Monitoring and Evaluation

Dr. O'Leary at the JCAHO takes the position that improvement requires effective monitoring and that effective monitoring requires good indicators.

The monitoring and evaluation process has been revised over time, but the 10 steps remain part of the foundation on which much of quality activities are based. The process requires identifying the most important aspects of care for a particular organization or division, selecting indicators that reflect these aspects, taking opportunities to improve care, taking action, and evaluating the effectiveness of that action. Elements of performance include what is done and how well it is done (JCAHO, 2003). Doing the right thing includes efficacy and appropriateness. Doing it well involves availability, timeliness, effectiveness, continuity, safety, efficiency, and providing services with respect and caring.

Step 1: Assign Responsibility

The leaders in the organization are responsible for fostering quality improvement and setting priorities for assessment and improvement. *Leaders* are defined as the leadership of the board, the executive team, including the nurse executive, the leaders of the medical staff, and department directors. This step has implications for nurse managers and other leaders in the nursing staff, because they have direct responsibility for quality.

Step 2: Delineate Scope of Care and Service

The scope of care of the organization or service must be defined in order to go on to the next step. We are not all things to all people, and we need to focus our energies on the mission and vision we have agreed on. We have to be clear about who our clients are and what we need to do for them.

Step 3: Identify Important Aspects of Care and Service

What are the key functions that warrant ongoing monitoring? Which functions need prioritization? The key function in outpatient areas are often very different from those in bedded units, as are the ones from services focusing on prevention, action, or chronic illness. Timeliness as an aspect of care may vary based on the scope of service and aspects of care of a particular service.

Step 4: Identify Indicators

Interdisciplinary teams develop and select indicators for those aspects of care that have been prioritized. As an example, turnaround time for laboratory results could be an indicator selected to reflect timeliness in an emergency department.

Step 5: Establish a Means to Trigger Evaluation

The team determines at what level and time evaluations will be triggered. Identifying thresholds that are not met after quarterly reviews is an example of how to implement evaluation. The review of every unexpected return of a patient to the surgical suite within 24 hours after surgery may be another.

Step 6: Collect and Organize Data

Defining data sources and methodology for collection, the actual data collection, and organization all are parts of this process. More often than not, too much peripheral information is collected, which actually hampers meaningful organization of data, is labor-intensive, and interferes with the next step.

Step 7: Initiate Evaluation

Once it is determined that further evaluation is needed, other feedback may be taken into consideration. Intensive evaluation should be performed by teams.

Step 8: Take Action to Improve

Actions include changes in the system, education, designation of clear authority and accountability, and development of standards.

Step 9: Assess the Effectiveness of the Actions

Whether the action improved the care or service and whether it sustained improvement are questions to be answered by evaluation of effectiveness.

Step 10: Communicate Results to Relevant Individuals and Groups

Dissemination of conclusions, actions, and results to those affected and to the leaders is necessary. This may be accomplished through team presentations, committee structures, and department or division meetings.

> *Doing the right thing includes efficacy and appropriateness. Doing it well involves availability, timeliness, effectiveness, continuity, safety, efficiency, and providing services with respect and caring.*

The 10-Step Model has been used successfully both in the traditional scope of quality assurance and in the context of quality improvement. The steps have remained the same, but the focus from within departments to processes, the level of accountability, the understanding and application of statistical methodologies, and the role of leadership have evolved significantly. Organizational leaders can no longer delegate responsibility to the quality department. Hiding behind professional or departmental boundaries is not acceptable. Leaders of boards, executive and management teams, and the medical staff are all being held accountable for delivery of quality care.

CONTINUOUS QUALITY IMPROVEMENT IN HEALTH CARE

Health-care organizations strive to embed quality in every service they provide. Their success lies in their ability to incorporate quality as a key component of their strategic mission and to implement a model by which they continually evaluate and improve quality.

Quality as Strategy

The guiding members of any organization are responsible for developing the mission, vision, and core strategies chosen to achieve the vision. Not every business will choose quality as a strategy. Competitive pricing, a customer service focus, promoting access to the product, and creating a niche market are all examples of different strategies. It is not accidental that JCAHO-accredited agencies are required to include a quality plan in their strategic plan. To survive and thrive requires a formal, well-thought-out approach with a focus on the communities we serve.

"Doing the right things right" means that we have identified what the "right things" are. They will vary according to the needs of the particular community and the mission and vision of the organization. Not every hospital can or should serve all the health-care needs of its community. Such needs may be met better by other community agencies or tertiary care centers. Once the health-care agency defines what the "right things" are, or what the scope of its services is, it must design quality into the structures and processes, monitor and analyze their performance, and identify opportunities for improvement in order to ensure that the right things are "done right" and desired outcomes result.

A successful strategic plan also requires identification of needed core competencies and methods to address existing gaps. Core competencies define the organizational capabilities as well as the subsequent employee competencies needed to achieve the vision through utilization of the strategic plan. Core competencies are not stagnant; they change with the organization's strategies. The recruitment, retention, development, and performance management of everyone working in or for the organization play a key role. Creating a "learning organization," in which skill development is dynamic, is strategic in and of itself. Understanding how to build quality into structures and processes, knowing the tools and measures to be utilized, knowing how to monitor and analyze performance, and understanding team process, group dynamics, and improvement methods require learning, which must be included in the organizational development strategies.

Quality is everyone's responsibility. It is a business strategy, or centralized philosophy, with accountability at every service level. Because quality is everyone's job, everyone must be educated and must demonstrate competence about quality—the leadership, the providers, and the customers.

Total Quality Management and Continuous Quality Improvement

The terms *total quality management* (TQM) and **continuous quality improvement** (CQI) have been used interchangeably. TQM is mostly linked with industrial models, whereas CQI has received wide acceptance in health care. Because the underpinnings of the two terms are the same, *CQI* is used through the remainder of the chapter.

The basic concepts of CQI are that quality improvement is an ongoing process that utilizes proactive and reactive strategies. The process goes beyond meeting preestablished goals or catching up to the competition; rather, it involves exceeding expectations and creating new opportunities.

Improvements can be large scale or incremental. *Quality* is defined as satisfying the needs of external and internal customers, including anticipating developing needs and introducing new services. Teamwork is the underlying framework. Improvement activities and measurement are always linked, because without measurement we cannot be sure that improvement has occurred. Additionally, measurement keeps teams focused on concrete opportunities and provides feedback regarding which core strategies helped achieve the vision and mission of the organization. **Benchmarking**, the process of comparing with the best of the industry, requires understanding of statistical methods, including the validity and reliability of the tools and measures used in both organizations, understanding systems variation, and sampling methods.

Transition From Quality Assurance To Continuous Quality Improvement

The traditional model of **quality assurance**—relying on inspection to catch problems and correcting individual performances—has already evolved in many institutions. To assume that the journey through quality assurance was wasted fails to recognize that many of the tools used in quality assurance are still used in quality improvement, and the journey helped define what constitutes quality care. However, there are many differences. CQI is widely recognized as being broader in scope, involving the leadership and many more people, and blurring boundaries. The expectation of perfection is gone, but the search for excellence is essential.

It is important to understand that the evaluation of individual performance must continue. Standards for hiring competent members of the team are more important than ever. Results of individual performance should be looked at for trends across shifts, units, and departments. Findings can be used for staff and leadership development. Individual competence remains a professional obligation. The shift in focus from individual to team does not change our standards or our accountability to those we serve.

Department- or unit-based quality programs remain valuable and should not be demolished. They are an important vehicle for teaching the concepts of CQI and provide needed mechanisms for ongoing measurement and application of standards. They also recognize that much improvement does not require large teams but can occur at the unit level.

Risk management evaluates the legal standards and their application to the delivery of care, the environment of care, and other services and functions. As with quality assurance, it relies on inspection; however, the focus is on how to protect the assets of the organization against liability. Table 17–1 highlights the differences and similarities among quality improvement, quality assurance, and risk management.

An example of how the same problem may be approached differently with the three approaches is in dealing with a medication error. In the environment of quality improvement, the investigation will search for what system weaknesses may have contributed to the error: is the dispensing system weak, are high-risk medications kept seperate, and so on. At the unit level, quality assurance may investigate the individual nurse's competencies and performance. In the risk management arena, the focus may be on documentation problems that could be discoverable in court in a malpractice claim.

Putting A Continuous Quality Improvement Structure in Place

It is now widely accepted that quality journeys are lengthy and costly. They require a well-developed structure and plan to connect the vision with the implementation. Because CQI is, first and foremost, a management philosophy, the leaders must be competent in its principles and methodologies.

The actual mechanisms of setting up the program are beyond the scope of this chapter. Creating a structure usually involves a quality council and designation of a CQI coach. The coach functions as the facilitator, educator, and expert in tools and techniques.

The function of the council is to create integration, prioritize efforts, allocate resources, develop a learning organization, and charter cross-functional teams. The journey is usually expected to take between 3 and 5 years,

TABLE 17–1 Comparing Quality Improvement, Quality Assurance, and Risk Management		
Quality Improvement	**Quality Assurance**	**Risk Management**
Broad in scope	Based at unit or departmental level	Often separate department
Organizational leadership designs and sets priorities	Often uses separate department	Looks at legally acceptable level of care or service
Purpose is improvement	Compares against standards	
Focus is on customers	Focus is on the organization	Focus is on preventing loss
Uses problems as opportunities for improvement	Continuous ongoing monitoring identifies problems (inspection)	Continuous ongoing monitoring (inspection)
Focus is on the system as a whole	Focus is on individual performance	Focus is on protecting organization's assets

depending on the resources available and the readiness for change.

Leaders and followers alike need to internalize the new beliefs and learn to use the new techniques and tools. Many organizations fail in the quest to implement the new quality organization because the efforts are all focused on the beginning of the journey. *Just-in-time learning*, the process of acquiring knowledge and skills as they are needed and used, tends to eliminate the feeling that CQI may be another managerial gimmick gone awry.

Another common mistake is the failure to prioritize efforts. Quality costs money, especially in the time and effort of human resources, and few organizations can afford to attempt to improve on all fronts at once.

TOOLS AND TECHNIQUES COMMONLY USED IN QUALITY IMPROVEMENT

An entire body of knowledge has been created in the area of valid techniques to be used for improving quality. Innovation requires team techniques such as brainstorming, boarding, decision matrices, multivoting, management of conflict, and quality communication.

Process Teams

Not all improvement projects require a **process team**. If the project or problem crosses functions and disciplines and cannot be resolved in the day-to-day operations, a process team is usually necessary.

Process teams must be chosen carefully to represent those involved in or affected by the process. If the team is very large, the project chosen may be too big and may have to be broken into steps.

How, then, does one choose an improvement project? Listen to your customers. Repeated complaints or requests for a particular service may require action. Suppose the evening charge nurse in a nonsectarian hospital receives ongoing requests for pastoral services from clients and their families. Each request requires multiple telephone calls and often results in delays. The nurse recognizes that the nursing department cannot address this problem alone. It involves not only the hospital but the community as well. The nurse develops a proposal for a process team. Other methods for selecting or recognizing processes to be improved include asking the people in the process, reviewing existing reports, and recognizing excess complexity or long delays.

Process teams require resources. Because resource allocation is a leadership function, many organizations require the development of a proposal and subsequent approval by the quality council. All teams should develop an opportunity statement (what is wrong or needs improving), define the expected output of the project, and include measures of success. Members of the team are, at a minimum, a team leader who is invested in the process, a facilitator who brings CQI skills, and a recorder or minute taker. Depending on the skills and information systems available, analytical and statistical support may be necessary.

Because process teams are groups, they will need to go through the stages of group development—forming, storming, norming, performing, adjourning. All teams must mature to perform. It is important to recognize that anxiety, testing of boundaries, competition for control, and minimal completion of work are part of the early stages. Early cohesiveness and work do not start until the norming stage. Real performance and "team" feeling belong to the performing step. Many teams also struggle with the adjourning phase— namely, meeting the final deadlines and dissolving the group.

The process team must adopt a model or method for doing its work. This model is usually organization-wide. There is value in choosing one model, because it minimizes relearning and allows different teams to communicate easily. Some common models are the Juran (1989) quality improvement project model, Deming's (1982, 1986) PDCA cycle

(Plan-Do-Check-Act), and the IMPROVE process of Ernst and Young (1990).

Quality Improvement Tools

Quality improvement (QI) tools can usually be divided into three categories, those used for:

- Process description
- Data collection
- Data analysis

Many excellent texts provide further assistance in this area. The ultimate purpose of all the QI tools is to have data that can be used and translated into information. The novice in quality improvement tools and techniques may need assistance from the CQI coach or further study of these techniques.

Process Description Tools

One tool for process description is the **flow chart,** which describes the process in detail, from beginning to end, as accurately as possible. It is a picture of the movement of information, people, or materials. The top-down flow chart (FIG. 17–1) takes the major steps in the process, writes them in a horizontal sequence, and shows the substeps to be taken under each step. Flow charts show the rework that gets done, the number of substeps or complexity in each area, the number of hand-offs between individuals and departments, and when subteams need to be formed from a particular process team. A flow chart that is too detailed makes it difficult to focus and impedes progress or action.

The cause-and-effect diagram (FIG. 17–2), also called the fishbone or Ishikawa diagram, helps identify the root causes of a problem. Typical categories are equipment, personnel,

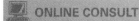

ONLINE CONSULT

For more information on the PDCA cycle, visit
http://hci.com.au/hcisite2/toolkit/pdcacycl.htm

STEP 1	→	STEP 2	→	STEP 3	→	STEP 4
Substeps		Substeps		Substeps		Substeps
....		....		....		....
....		....		....		....
....		....		....		....
....		....		....		....

FIG. 17–1. Top-down flow chart.

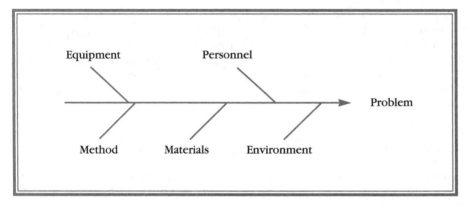

FIG. 17–2. Cause-and-effect diagram.

method, materials, and environment. The main arrow points toward the problem or desired result. It is important to remember that cause-and-effect diagrams point only toward possible causes, and more data have be collected to identify the root causes. Cause-and-effect diagrams are most effective after the process has been described, because flow charts help identify what must be included in the diagram.

Tools for Data Collection

Tools for data collection include asking the right questions, and using, among other things, data sheets, check sheets, surveys, focus groups, and interviews. Often, data are collected that turn out to be useless because the question asked was wrong, too broad, or poorly formulated. Data sheets and check sheets are both used to record data (FIG. 17–3). They differ in that **data sheets** need

further analysis. Ordinarily, a data sheet is completed for each occurrence or event in the study. The data are subsequently aggregated and then sorted according to categories of interest.

Check sheets are used to record multiple events by simply putting a mark in the appropriate box. The best check sheets are those that are easy to use, do not require much interpretation, and visually display the data. An example in which either tool could be used is the study of the delivery time of medications to a patient care unit. With data sheets, every time a medication is taken from the pharmacy, the runner uses a new data sheet. At the end of the study all the sheets are gathered and analyzed. With the check sheet, the runner could calculate the time it took to deliver the drug and check the appropriate time box on a check sheet.

There are obvious advantages and disadvantages to both tools. Data sheets tend to be more accurate because only one event is

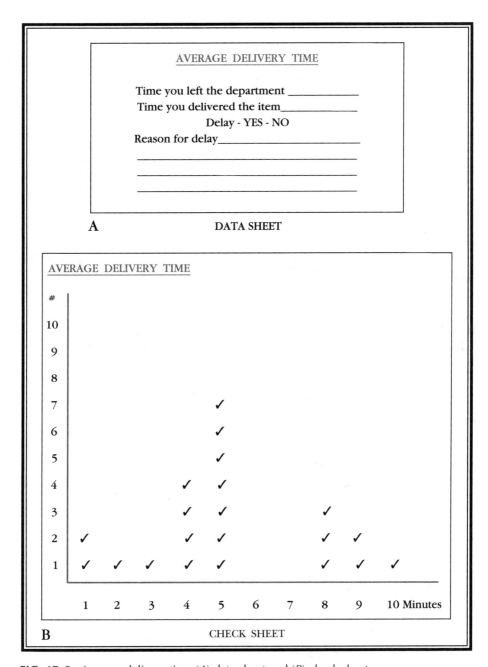

AVERAGE DELIVERY TIME

Time you left the department _____
Time you delivered the item_____
Delay - YES - NO
Reason for delay_____
_____
_____
_____

A   DATA SHEET

AVERAGE DELIVERY TIME

FIG. 17–3. Average delivery time (*A*) data sheet and (*B*) check sheet.

recorded on each. Check sheets quickly display trends as they occur without requiring a sometimes lengthy analysis. Data sheets and check sheets should be tested before project-wide work is undertaken, so that improve-ments can be made in them and only useful data are collected.

Surveys are a tool for obtaining input from large groups. The response rate and the specificity of the question affect the usefulness and quality of the information obtained. Focus groups and individual interviews are time-consuming and expensive and may require the use of experienced interviewers, but they enable one to ask open-ended questions and probe deeper, if necessary.

Data Analysis Tools

Tools for data analysis include those that compare categories. Bar and pie charts and the Pareto diagram (FIG. 17–4), for example, analyze data within a category, such as numerical and graphic summaries. The Pareto principle, sometimes called the 80/20 rule, was applied to management by Juran. It identifies the few sources of problems that contribute most to the outcome. By ranking problems on a bar graph in descending order, from left to right, Pareto diagrams focus attention on the most common problems and often build consensus about where to concentrate attention and effort.

Analysis of a particular category can include numerical summaries such as average, med-

ian, mode, and standard deviation. Graphic summaries—line graphs, histograms, scatter diagrams, and control charts—are especially valuable for working in diverse groups. They provide pictorial display of data, possible analysis and interpretation of patterns, relationships between variables, and the ability to distinguish between common and special cause variation.

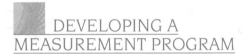

DEVELOPING A MEASUREMENT PROGRAM

As previously mentioned, improvement and measurement or evaluation are linked. Measurement of the capability of the organization, or its competence, determines the organization's ability to provide, and competence in providing, quality care. Measurement of outcome determines whether the process yielded favorable results. For example, the Breast Care Clinic use as an earlier example will not only focus its review on the ability to report examination results within 24 hours

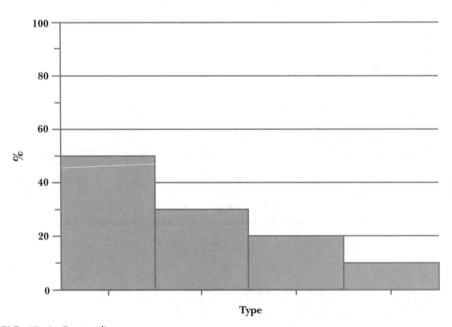

FIG. 17–4. Pareto diagram.

and on whether there is a system in place allowing women to self-refer for mammography; it will also measure whether these outcomes actually occurs.

Selecting Indicators for Measurement

Indicators are events that are measured. They are categorized by type. They can be structure, process, or outcome indicators chosen in the functions of patient care, services that support the delivery of patient care, practices, and leadership/governance. *Structure* encompasses the policies or standards regarding how service is delivered and resources made available. *Process* refers to the activities, and *outcome* is the result of activities based on policies, standards, and resources.

Practice indicators measure professional standards used in the delivery of patient care. One example of a practice indicator is measurement of documentation frequency and content and utilization of aseptic technique as required. Leadership indicators measure organizational function, namely how the system affects the delivery of care and services.

When standards are clearly written and defined, are valid, and can be measured, indicators are more easily selected and usable. Meaningful indicators are specific, relevant, reliable, valid, and measurable. They use a numerator and denominator, have a target (internal or external benchmark), relate to specific standards, and define where the data or information can be found.

Many national organizations are currently working on indicators that can be used as external benchmarks. The Maryland Indicator Project, JCAHO, the HEDIS measures from the National Council for Quality Assurance, and other professional groups continue to refine and expand the available indicators. Utilizing external performance measures exclusively is not sufficient. Internal performance indicators based on the scope of service, mission, vision, strategic plans, core competencies, organizational culture, and values ensure that overall organizational effectiveness is measured. In turn, external benchmarks compare that performance with the best in the industry.

Understanding Variation

Variation is part of any process. People, equipment, supplies, procedures, techniques, and inaccuracies in the data all contribute to variation in data from an otherwise stable process. *Common-cause variation* is the ongoing, minute variations that are part of nature. *Special-cause variation* is much larger and can be pinpointed more easily to contributors through statistical methods such as run charts and control charts. These charts can monitor processes because, even though individual data points may be unpredictable, a fluctuating pattern will emerge over time. The normal pattern is bell-shaped, meaning that most points are near the center.

The manager of a process must know when to react to particular data or situations and when it is necessary to improve the entire process. For example, suppose you have monitored medication errors on your unit for many months. When you calculate the number of errors over the number of doses administered, a percentage ranging between 0.01 and 0.02 percent emerges. This is probably the common-cause type of variation. You may want to compare that figure against those of

 ONLINE CONSULT

To learn more about indicators and benchmarks, visit the National Council for Qualiy Assurance at:
http://www.ncqa.org/Programs/HEDIS/index.htm

other institutions, of similar type or size in your region, to evaluate whether this is an acceptable error rate. If, for the first time ever, you see a rise to 0.03 percent, it would be wise to analyze the data further before taking action or deciding to wait. Are all the errors of the same type attributable to a few individuals, or have new systems been introduced? Constant tinkering with systems, without understanding what the causes of the variation are, destabilizes the process. Understanding variation is important. Common-cause variation requires an answer to the question "Is this level acceptable when looked at over time?" Special-cause variation needs careful evaluation to identify the cause and make appropriate, focused intervention.

CONTINUOUS QUALITY IMPROVEMENT IN CONTEXT

CQI in practice requires a number of cost and implementation considerations and varies significantly with the context of the health-care organization.

Relationship of Continuous Quality Improvement to Delivery Redesign

The rapid changes in health care previously discussed have also required redesign of its delivery. We have a professional obligation to ensure that the way we deliver care is evaluated along the continuum. Despite our frustration with cost containment efforts, we must prudently manage resources to enable us to provide the greatest benefit to the largest number of clients possible. We may need to develop new delivery models that optimize the role of the professional nurse, delegate tasks, and meet the needs of our customers.

Case management and work redesign are currently being used across the country for delivery redesign. The Case Management Society of America (CMSA) defines *case management* as "a collaborative process of assessment, planning, facilitation and advocacy for

options and services to meet an individual's health needs through communication and available resources to promote quality cost-effective outcomes" (CMSA, 2004, p.1). Critical pathways are tools commonly used in this process. Brainstorming, data-driven decision-making, consensus seeking, process flow charting, evaluation of costs, and satisfaction are all tools used in case management as well as in the new quality model.

Work redesign—the process of analyzing how work is done and what system changes need to be implemented to achieve effective and efficient care delivery—also requires quality to be built in up front. Professionals need to participate actively in this evolving course. Reliance on inspection and control will not ensure delivery of quality care. Simultaneously, we cannot insist on doing it the old way. The parameters set by the Robert Wood Johnson University Hospital ProACT model for work redesign include reaching comprehensive patient outcomes (including patient satisfaction) and contributing to staff satisfaction, retention, and productivity as well as to the financial integrity of the organization (Tonges, 1989). Review of studies on the implementation of redesign activities demonstrate that many focused largely on increasing efficiency and that the changes may not have been managed effectively, resulting in loss of trust in the administration and reduction of clinical nursing leadership (IOM, 2003).

> *Brainstorming, data-driven decision-making, consensus seeking, process flow charting, evaluation of costs, and satisfaction are all tools used in case management as well as in the new quality model.*

Continuous Quality Improvement in the Managed Care World

Managed care has received some favor as a methodology for controlling escalating health-care costs. Buyers of managed care, such as employers and state and federal governments, have something to say about quality, access, choice, and satisfaction with services. The more competitive the environment becomes, the more important demonstrated quality will become, to differentiate between one contract or provider and another. The managed care industry is already developing nationally accepted outcomes and indicators. Report cards on customer satisfaction with individual providers and organizations have gained popularity. Nursing must take an aggressive professional role in ensuring that the data on care delivery reflect direct nursing care delivery, coordination provided by nursing, client and family teaching, and nursing management along the continuum of care delivery.

Recommendations regarding the need to develop reliable and valid methods to measure nursing care requirements and minimum staffing levels in acute care and long-term care are considered essential (IOM, 2003).

Ongoing Role for Regulatory Agencies

Agencies such as JCAHO, the PROs, and state and federal government will continue to have a significant role in the assurance that quality, safe health care is delivered. Many of the organizations have already begun to assist in collecting benchmarking information. JCAHO, in particular, is acting as an external change agent with regard to guaranteeing that all providers accept and implement the new paradigm. The hospital associations are helping their members deal with uniform responses to the report cards required by many managed care contracts. Regulators and providers alike are struggling with the implementation of significant change in the delivery of quality health care.

Key Points

- Rapid changes in health care have prompted a new way of business.
- Purchasers require "more" and "better" for "less."
- Reliance on inspection and control against preestablished standards (the traditional quality assurance model) although of ongoing value, is no longer sufficient.
- Quality models, such as Deming's Principles for Transformation, the Juran Trilogy, and JCAHO's 10-Step Model, provide an excellent foundation for improving quality of care.
- Quality improvement is not only the result of correcting problems but also requires ongoing improvement.
- Quality journeys require a vision, a plan to turn that vision into reality, and a well-developed structure to ensure implementation.
- Most problems lie within systems, not individuals.
- To improve quality, you must improve the system.
- Specific knowledge, tools, and techniques are required to create a new quality. They include cross-functional teamwork, lifelong learning, and process improvement.
- Process teams are required for those improvement activities that cross functions and disciplines and cannot be dealt with in the day-to-day operations.
- Variation is part of all processes. It requires statistical analysis before actions that may destabilize the process are taken.
- Benchmarking is the process of comparison with the best practices in the industry.
- Tools for improvement can be divided into three categories: those used for process description, such as flow charts and cause-and-effect diagrams; those used for data collection, such as data sheets and check sheets; and those used for data analysis, such as bar and pie charts and the Pareto diagram.
- Continuous quality improvement is not a separate management tool. It is a way of doing business.

Thought and Discussion Questions

1. You are the nurse manager of an ambulatory surgery unit. Recently, you have seen a sudden rise in the number of surgical clients coming through the unit. Simultaneously, clients, physicians, and other providers have started to complain about long delays during pretesting.
   - Would you attempt to fix this problem by addressing it during a staff meeting? Why or why not?
   - Compare how to address this problem using a process team versus using the staff meeting approach.
   - Describe how you would analyze the process.
   - Explain which tools are appropriate to use for the analysis.
2. Review the Chapter Thought on the first page of the chapter, and be prepared to discuss it within the context of the chapter.

 ## Interactive Exercise

1. Complete the exercise entitled Clinical Indicators on the Interactive Exercises section of the Intranet site. Be prepared to discuss your thoughts in class.

 ## PRINT RESOURCES

References

Deming, W. E. (1982, 1986). *Out of crisis*. Cambridge, MA: Massachusetts Institute of Technology.

The Ernst and Young Quality Improvement Consulting Group. (1990). *Total quality: An executive guide for the nineties*. Homewood, IL: Business One Irwin.

IOM (Institute of Medicine). (2000). *To Err is Human: Building a Safer Health System*. Washington, DC: National Academy Press.

IOM (Institute of Medicine). (2001). *Crossing the Quality Chasm: A New Health System for the 21st Century*. Washington, DC: National Academy Press.

IOM (Institute of Medicine). (2003). *Keeping Patients Safe: Transforming the Work Environment of Nurses*. Washington, DC: National Academy Press.

Joint Commission on Accreditation of Healthcare Organizations. (2003). 2004 *comprehensive accreditation manual for hospitals*. Oakbrook Terrace, IL: Author.

Joint Commission on Accreditation of Healthcare Organizations. (1991). *An introduction to quality improvement in health care*. Oakbrook Terrace, IL: Author.

Juran, J. M. (1989). *Juran on leadership for quality: An executive handbook*. New York: Free Press.

Tonges, M. C. (1989). Redesigning hospital nursing practice: The professionally advanced care team (ProACT) model: Part 2. *Journal of Nursing Administration*, 19(8), 19–22.

Bibliography

Berwick, D. M., Godfrey, A. B., & Roessner, J. (1990). *Curing health care: New strategies for quality improvement*. San Francisco: Jossey-Bass.

Bossidy, L., & Charan, R.(2002). *Execution: The discipline of getting things done*. New York: Crown Business.

Flarey, D. L. (1995). *Redesigning nursing care delivery: Transforming our future*. Philadelphia: J. B. Lippincott.

Gale, F. (Ed.). (1994). *Tales of pursuit of quality in health care*. Tampa, FL: American College of Physician Executives.

Goodstein L., Nolan, T., & Pfeifer W. (1993). *Applied strategic planning: How to develop a plan that really works*. New York: McGraw-Hill.

Hamel, G., & Heene A. (Eds.). (1994). *Competence-based competition*. New York: John Wiley & Sons.

Juran, J. M. (1988). *Juran on planning for quality*. New York: Free Press.

Katz, J. M., & Green, E. (1997). *Managing quality: A guide to system-wide performance management* (2nd ed.). St. Louis: Mosby-Year Book.

Provance, L., Alvis, D., & Silfen, E. (1994). Quality improvement and public health—tetanus immunization in the emergency department. *American Journal of Medical Quality*, 9(4), 165–71.

Satinsky, M. A. (1995). *An executive guide to case management strategies.* Chicago: American Hospital Publishing.

Schroeder, P. (1994). *Improving quality and performance: Concepts, programs, and techniques.* St. Louis: Mosby-Year Book.

Senge, P. M. (1990). *The fifth discipline.* New York: Doubleday.

Spears, L. (Ed.). (1995). *Reflections on leadership.* New York: Wiley & Sons.

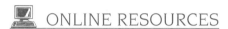
ONLINE RESOURCES

Case Management Society of America. (2004). CSMA definition and philosphy and definition. *http://www.csma.org/AboutUs/CMDefinition.aspx.*

The Institute for Healthcare Improvement (IHI). (2004). About us. *http://www.ihi.org/ihi/about.*

The Institute of Medicine at *http://www4.nationalacademies.org*

The Joint Commission for Accreditation of Healthcare Organizations at *http:// www.jcaho.org*

The Institute for Healthcare Improvement (IHI) *http:// www.ihi.org/ihi/about.*

HCi. (2004). PDCA Cycle. *http://hci.com.au/hcisite2/toolkit/pdcacycl.htm*

National Council for Qualiy Assurance. (2004). *The Health Plan Employer Data and Information Set* HEDIS®). *http://www.ncqa.org/Programs/HEDIS/index.htm* All accessed on August 14, 2004.

Julia W. Aucoin

18
chapter

Informatics and Computer Use

> *"I do not fear computers. I fear lack of them."*
>
> Issac Asimov 1920–1992

Chapter Objectives

On completion of this chapter, the reader will be able to:

1. Describe computer and informatics applications used in nursing practice, education, and research.
2. Define the basic terminology used in nursing informatics.
3. Describe the relationship between health-care provision and health management information systems.
4. Define the specialty practice of nursing informatics and the integration of that role into the nursing services of a health-care institution.
5. Identify opportunities for interdisciplinary collaboration from an informatics perspective.
6. Describe nursing career opportunities in informatics.

Key Terms

Nursing Informatics
Health Management
  Information Systems
Computerized Patient
  Record

Office Applications
Personal Digital
  Assistants
. Handheld PCs

Evidence-Based
  Practice
Minimum Data Set
  (MDS)

"**Nursing informatics** is a specialty that integrates nursing science, computer science, and information science to manage and communicate data, information, and knowledge in nursing practice" (American Nurses Association [ANA], 2001, p.vii). This specialty was first described by Graves and Corcoran in 1989, was quickly supported by several nursing graduate programs of study, was recognized as a specialty for registered nurses by the American Nurses Association in 1992, and earned credibility through the offering of a certification examination by the American Nurses Credentialing Center. Nursing informatics (NI) as a specialty grows and changes as quickly as the computer industry itself. This chapter also addresses computer applications (software uses) that support nursing activities.

OVERVIEW OF NURSING INFORMATICS

The primary interest of nursing informatics is to expand how data, information, and knowledge are used within nursing practice. Those conducting research on informatics issues are seeking to identify and explain relationships between health-care data and nursing care. Experts in nursing informatics focus their efforts on the science of information and knowledge acquisition and on the design and evaluation of the systems that process and provide data and information (Graves & Corcoran, 1989). The actual work of informatics specialists varies with settings, according to organizational needs, individual practice interests, and specific research questions. The common element in all functions within the informatics practice is the transfor-

> *The common element in all functions within the informatics practice is the transformation of data to information and, ultimately, to knowledge that supports and advances nursing practice.*

mation of data to information and, ultimately, to knowledge that supports and advances nursing practice.

Within care delivery institutions such as hospitals, long-term care facilities, and home health agencies, the NI specialist could be involved with both the tasks of nursing and improvement of the quality of care. Task-related NI activities include staffing and scheduling systems, standardization and automation of care plans, documentation systems, real-time retrieval of diagnostic results, and response to physician order entry. Clinical indicators of quality as required by Joint Commission on Accreditation of Healthcare Organizations (JCAHO, 2003) and the Centers for Medicare and Medicaid Services (CMS) require the input and retrieval of data demonstrating use of evidence-based practice guidelines. The NI specialist is instrumental in creating communication standards and pathways to provide ease in accessing necessary information for reporting to these organizations.

Nursing informatics applications in academic settings have grown to include both the use of technology in the teaching process and the teaching of an informatics-focused curriculum. Many schools of nursing use a learning platform, such as BlackBoard or WebCT, to provide Web-enhanced or totally Web-based courses, including discussion boards, chats, interactive exercises, and online testing as part of the teaching modalities (Billings, 2002). The National League for Nursing (NLN) Human Simulator Project, funded in 2003, provided eight simulators to schools of nursing to be used under research focused leadership (NLN, 2003). These simulators can be programmed to present a variety of case scenarios and respond to the students' interventions in planned ways. Information can be downloaded from the simulators to provide feedback on time management, decision-making, and nursing competence.

In addition to technology projects conducted within schools of nursing, electronic

BOX 18–1
THE VIRTUAL HOSPITAL

The Virtual Hospital is known as a digital library for health information. Established by the University of Iowa, this medical multimedia textbook takes full advantage of hypertext links to provide navigation between documents and figures embedded in the text. The seamlessly constructed links to off-site databases bring to the screen digitized audio and visual material. It is an impressive demonstration that allows professionals and consumers to quickly seek peer-reviewed information on a variety of adult and pediatric topics. This type of reference, accessible from anywhere in the world at any time of day, offers resources to support geographically isolated practitioners and teaching materials available to anyone. (Virtual Hospital, 2003.)
See *http://www.vh.org*

journals have made articles available online. These publications have gone through the peer-review process of their print counterparts but are more accessible for readers. The *Online Journal of Nursing Informatics* and the *Online Journal of Issues in Nursing* were the first for nursing professionals. Because they are exclusively online, these journals differ from the electronically accessible versions of printed journals that may be accessed through major publishers, association Web sites, and subscribers to health science libraries. Online journals can give nurses an electronic format to share findings, experience, perceptions, knowledge, and wisdom with nursing colleagues involved in all facets of their specialties. The intent is to exploit the power of cyberspace in order to create an electronic nursing community that provides both virtually accessible and timely information about nursing globally. Online journals also purport to enhance the speed of cybercommunications through an expedited editorial process that provides rapid turnaround and publication times. Downloading one copy of these electronically accessible articles is permitted for scholarly work.

Digital libraries (Box 18–1) and E-books, electronic versions of printed books, are also available. Although they are convenient ways to access reference material, their intent is not to enable you to read an entire book electronically. Libraries generally limit the window for the checkout period to hours or days. "Living books" are a newer entity similar to online journals; chapters of such books are added to the Web site as they are completed. Many textbooks come with electronic support in the form of a Web site (for access to appendices or bonus chapters) or a CD-ROM to supplement the materials. Because CD-ROMs are less expensive to duplicate, they are more efficient for distribution.

Given these advances in informatics, one might think that nursing is well evolved in the specialty. However, the Institute of Medicine (IOM) has formally identified utilizing informatics as a competency for all health professions education. This is one of the five competencies listed (Greiner & Kneibel, 2003); the other four are apply quality improvement, provide patient-centered care, work in interdisciplinary teams, and employ evidence-based practice. "Utilize informatics" encompasses the responsibility to communicate, manage knowledge, mitigate error, and support decision-making through the use of information technology. It is the only one of the five competencies to which all the Rules for Health Care in the 21st Century apply (Box 18–2) The applications of informatics discussed in this chapter are derived from the specific informatics competencies further described in the IOM report. The least developed of the five health professions education competencies is informatics, as it is not yet completely understood as a discipline. A weakness in nursing is that a number of students have been educated in colleges with underfunded computer technology. One recommendation is to have informatics courses developed by discipline, by specialty, and by stage of career progression.

Informatics tools are changing how nurses teach, deliver, and communicate nursing care. Students and practitioners are able to learn more from home, creating new opportunities for nurse educators in all settings. Updating professional skills for those residing in isolated areas and accessing expert consultation for clinicians in distant geographic areas are two more reasons to embrace technology in nursing and health care.

TRANSFORMATION OF DATA TO INFORMATION AND KNOWLEDGE

The transformation of data into information and knowledge is an important informatics concept. A *datum* is a value placed on a variable. It exists without meaning or explanation. An example is the weight of a child. The value of the weight, such as 62 pounds, is the datum for the weight. This value has little meaning until it is put into some context along with other data. For instance, if the child were 3 years old, the weight might have one interpretation, but for a 10-year-old child, 62 pounds would mean something very different. Age and weight may not be enough data to offer much information. You may also want to know the child's height, which would allow you to understand the weight's significance better. Data viewed in association with one another provide meaning. Knowledge arises from using information, often from combined sources, to determine new meanings, make new discoveries, or expand understandings. For example, patient diagnoses arise through the transformation of combined laboratory data, radiology data, symptomatology, and other information into a whole, the outcome of which is knowledge.

> *An informatics nurse is someone who has a specialty practice in nursing, not simply a computer expert who happens to be working on a nursing-related problem.*

Informatics nurses seek to create new knowledge by working first with data and then with information. Informatics specialists work as an integral part of an interdisciplinary team to support, promote, and advance the delivery of nursing care. Indeed, an informatics nurse is someone who has a specialty practice in nursing, not simply a computer expert who happens to be working on a nursing-related problem.

Some elements of nursing informatics are important for all nurses to understand. The data that are used arise from the processes involved in care delivery. To use a clinical analogy: It is important for all nurses who provide direct care to have some understanding of diabetes, yet we still use nurse specialists in diabetes to support and promote the care of diabetic patients. Nursing does not function in the exclusion of the other clinical, administrative, and managerial health professionals. Nor does nursing informatics exist independent of the larger health information management systems that hospitals, clinics, home health agencies, nursing homes, and health maintenance organizations depend on to manage their various functions (FIG. 18–1). Although these systems need to be integrated, they sometimes work as separate, noncommunicating units, creating some frustrations in the workplace. In time, these systems will operate seamlessly as we move toward full implementation of a totally computerized patient record. It is becoming more important that nurses recognize that they

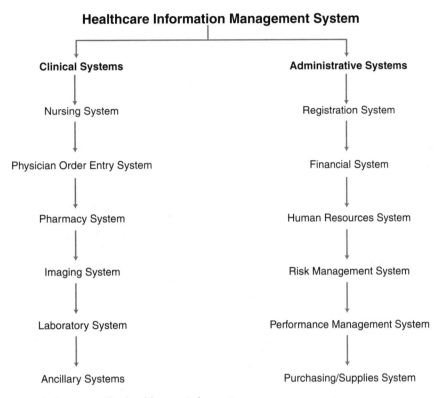

Healthcare Information Management System

Clinical Systems	Administrative Systems
Nursing System	Registration System
Physician Order Entry System	Financial System
Pharmacy System	Human Resources System
Imaging System	Risk Management System
Laboratory System	Performance Management System
Ancillary Systems	Purchasing/Supplies System

FIG. 18–1. The health-care information management system.

are contibuting data every time they carry out a nursing function. These data have the potential of providing powerful information when they are well understood within the environment of health-care delivery (Hebda et al., 2001).

HEALTH MANAGEMENT INFORMATION SYSTEMS

Because few systems can address every component of health care, there is generally an overriding information system with both clinical and administrative components. Clinical systems include those functions that directly support client care—documentation, order entry, and diagnostic reporting. Administrative systems address the financial, personnel, and managerial functions of the facility.

Together, these **health management information systems** provide all the hardware and software needed to process data into information for multiple uses.

The planning for a comprehensive information system requires an organizational strategy based on goals for efficiency, growth, utilization of resources, and technologic leadership. The system design should create workflow so that fewer people can accomplish more work. The system must be able to expand to serve new clinical facilities. Financial and human resources must be considered, as should the amount of technology the organization can support or tolerate. It is important to maintain alignment with the organization's mission and goals in all strategic planning for the information system.

The specific management information needs of health-care institutions differ according to their mode of health-care delivery, third-party payer requirements, accrediting or licensing organizations, and internal reporting protocols. An acute care facility that manages an inpatient facility, an emergency room, operating suites, extensive clinical laboratories, and a large pharmacy will have different data and information needs from those of a visiting nurse agency. Currently, no one health management information system fits all organizations. This is a significant barrier to the development of a uniform patient record, merging of patient information across institutions, and function in a managed care environment.

The nursing information system should accomplish two goals. First, it should support the way that nurses operate, giving them flexibility and permitting appropriate documentation. Second, the system should support and improve nursing practice through access to information and tools (Hebda et al., 2001). It is common now for workstations to include Internet access for searches on the World Wide Web or through a literature database such as the Cumulative Index of Nursing and Allied Health Literature (CINAHL) or the National Institute of Health's MedLine. Additionally, Intranet service often includes access to drug guides, policy and procedures, and patient teaching information. Box 18–3 describes how the integration of systems can help reduce medication errors.

Computerized Patient Record

A major national effort to develop a **computerized patient record** (CPR) has been under way for a number of years, and select institutions have had particular success in this area. The CPR is an electronic version of the patient record. The purpose of creating CPRs is to improve the ability to share client-specific information, create permanent life-long health records, and have ready access to additional information that will improve client care. Advances in the development of large data repositories held within hospitals and other health-care institutions allow linkages between an electronic patient record and administrative, bibliographic, clinical expertise, and research databases.

The IOM produced an extensive report on the importance of developing a CPR built on a set of standards shared by all involved parties in both the private and public sectors (Dick & Steen, 1991). More than a decade later, the industry still faces an interesting challenge in the development and implementation of health management information systems and

---

BOX 18–3
SYSTEM INTEGRATION TO REDUCE MEDICATION ERRORS

1. The provider enters a medication order into the order entry system, eliminating confusion from handwriting.
2. This information is transmitted to the pharmacy.
3. The pharmacy system checks for dosage, allergies, and potential interactions. Alerts are generated.
4. The medication order is filled by the pharmacy, using a barcode or robotic system.
5. The nurse checks the order against the electronic medication administration record and is alerted to administration times as well as any special considerations.
6. The nurse documents that the medication has been administered and notes the patient's response.
7. Reminders for reorders and 24-hour chart checks are generated automatically.

Cohen, M. R. (2000). *Medication errors: Causes, prevention, and risk management.* Boston: Jones & Bartlett.

the greater need for client-related information to be communicated and shared by organizations. When clients are referred for home care after hospital discharge, the referral forms are often faxed to the home care agency. When a client is transferred from a hospital to another facility, the medical record is photocopied or summarized for the receiving institution. The influx of managed care organizations has contributed greatly to the demand for the electronic transmission of health-care data. The quality of information that could be used to provide care to clients in those organizations would be enhanced by access to the entire previous record or even to all of the health records maintained over time for each client.

Creating a CPR is far more difficult than may at first be apparent. Standardized language, data collection, record format, access, confidentiality, and other ethical issues are but a few of the barriers still impeding the widespread development and use of the CPR. To build a CPR that can be shared among institutions, data must be collected and coded in a similar fashion. One issue regarding the CPR that has been and will continue to be addressed is client confidentiality. Fortunately, the Health Insurance Portability and Accountability Act (HIPAA) was implemented in 2003 in an effort to eliminate unnecessary, unwarranted, and inappropriate sharing of individual and personal information. There are now clear guidelines for when information can and cannot be shared and how to handle electronic communication (CMS, 2003). Password protection for facility and personal computers is recommended if any client identifiers—name, age, gender, social security number—will be stored in the computer.

The Center for Nursing Classification and Clinical Effectiveness (CNC), housed at the University of Iowa, has taken on the challenge of developing standardized nursing language and has published nursing interventions and outcomes with definitions to be used in documentation systems. The Center also has collaborated with the North American Nursing Diagnosis Association (NANDA) to integrate these interventions and outcomes with nursing diagnosis language. The International Council of Nurses is also working on a language and taxonomy to improve communication of nursing activities across the globe (CNC, 2003).

Computer Applications

Common **office applications**—word processing, spreadsheet, database, and graphics presentations—are also useful in nursing practice, education, and research. Specialized applications have been created to improve management and dissemination of nursing information. In practice, nurses most commonly use computers to document care and access client data. Documentation often involves selection of interventions and outcomes from a prepared list of appropriate terms, with little need for lengthy narrative comments.

Personal Digital Assistants

Increasingly, reference materials accessible through the computer have become a necessary adjunct to effective care. Handheld computer devices in the form of **personal digital**

 ONLINE CONSULT

See more about the International Council of Nurses International Classification for Nursing Practice, a standardized language, at
http://www.icn.ch/icnp.htm
For information on submitting a nursing diagnosis to the North American Nursing Diagnosis Association (NANDA), go to
http://www.nanda.org/html/diagnoses.html

assistants (PDA) and **handheld PCs** (personal computers) are becoming quite popular with direct care providers because textbook publishers now provide many common nursing references in this electronic format. Although looking up a medication in the drug guide is useful at the nurses' station, it is quite convenient to be able to scroll through an electronic guide on a PDA or handheld PC in the client's presence and answer his or her questions with confidence and competence. Hunt (2002) suggests that the PDA applications—calculator, drug reference, laboratory reference, blood gas interpretation, note taking, task lists, calendar, phone lists, e-mail, and quick search—are appropriate for today's busy nurse. Password protection helps the nurse maintain confidentiality and compliance with HIPAA regulations.

Independent Learning Activities

Computers became a quite popular way for nursing programs to provide independent learning activities; computer-assisted instruction (CAI) replaced the video, which replaced the audio-film strip. CAI consists of text, graphics, vignettes, and self-assessment quizzes. These can be loaded onto computers or played from a CD-ROM. Although distance learning has been available since the first continuing education was provided by radio in the 1920s, it has become a convenient way to complete continuing education requirements and for degree-seeking nurses (Armstrong et al., 2000). With the advent of the Internet, classes can be delivered from a server on a campus or from a business. Courses can be completed at the student's convenience, with access to numerous resources linked to the course and real-time results through online assessments. A paperless system is created for the submission of journals and assignments, and group discussion can be conducted in a synchronous (live) or asynchronous (everyone at a different time) format. Searching for information on new medications and treatments, current information on obscure conditions, and national standards and guidelines using the search engines is available.

A project known as the Simulated E-hEalth Delivery System (SEEDS) represents a successful collaboration between education and practice. Nursing students simulate the management of client cases using the live clinical system that practicing nurses are using to care for clients. The University of Missouri–Kansas City and Cerner Corporation have partnered to permit faculty to prepare clients using the nursing information system; students then respond to changes in client-status, plan client care, and document additional findings in a controlled setting (Connors, Weaver, Warren & Miller, 2002). This creative educational application of a clinical technology has already improved client care for graduates and new employees. Students tend to be satisfied with technology-enhanced learning when faculty demonstrate expertise and creativity (Bloom & Hough, 2003).

Evidence-Based Practice

Evidence-based practice implies that nursing care is delivered on the basis of knowledge generated from research. Practicing nurses have access to this knowledge—and can enhance their practice using this knowledge—by simply searching for it. The National Guideline Clearinghouse is a product of the U.S. Department of Health and Human Services; nurses can search directly at its Web site or through their professional association Web sites to find the latest guidelines on topics such as pain management, continence care, and teaching protocols for congestive heart failure. The newly launched Nursing Knowledge International serves as a repository for clinical, research, career, and continuing education resources. This is a huge managed database with links to published, proprietary, and government resources. Using the speed and power of computer search engines, this database places accurate and current information in the hands of practitioners.

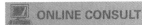

ONLINE CONSULT

Visit the National Guideline Clearing house at
www.guideline.gov.
The Nursing Knowledge International repository is located at
http://www.nursingknowledge.org/

Database Management

In addition to e-commerce, online auctions, live chats, listservs, and other computer-based services, database management and access is a growing application for computers. An agreement between major retailers and the Centers for Disease Control and Prevention (CDC) allows for the organization and reporting of information about geographic purchasing patterns related to disease management and health promotion. When the purchase of flu-related products, for instance, increases in one region, the CDC can respond with investigations and warnings for this area. Often, consumers begin purchasing over-the-counter remedies before seeking medical attention; monitoring of this activity provides information about communicable diseases before formal reporting occurs.

NURSING INFORMATICS: THE SPECIALTY

The goal of nursing informatics is to improve the health of populations, communities, families, and individuals by optimizing information management and communication (ANA, 2001). Although computers have become ubiquitous in homes and businesses, it is not unusual to see implementation of new applications in the health-care setting nearly every day. Without the aid of NI specialists, these applications might offer little improvement in client care and create inefficiencies and errors. NI specialists can guide the collection, documentation, analysis, and aggregation of data with the intent of improving client care, eliminating errors, and developing a body of

> **BOX 18–4**
> **ATTRIBUTES OF A SPECIALTY IN NURSING**
>
> - A differentiated practice
> - A defined research program
> - Organizational representation
> - Educational programs
> - A credentialing mechanism
>
> From Panniers, T. L. & Gassert, C. A. (1996). Standards of practice and preparation for certification. In M. E. Mills, C. A. Romano, and B. R. Heller (Eds.), *Information management in nursing and health care*. Philadelphia: Springhouse.

knowledge based on evidence. Educators skilled in teaching informatics or NI specialists skilled in teaching are the best people to teach nurses how to use computer applications. NI specialists possess the characteristics of a specialty (Box 18–4). The activities of the NI specialist include:

- Employment of the information systems life cycle and other tools and processes to analyze data, information, and information system requirements
- Design, development, selection, and evaluation of information technology, data structures, and decision-support mechanisms into an integrated information system
- Facilitation of the creation of nursing knowledge

Nursing informatics is interested in the nursing phenomena of client, health, environment, and nurse yet focuses on the structure of the data, information, and knowledge used by nurses in their practice and ensures that nursing's data are represented and included in the electronic processing of health information (Lange, 1997). Nurses in clinical specialties tend to focus on the content of data and information. Currently, NI specialists are working to refine nursing's language, implement efficient telehealth systems, propagate NI educational programs, and expand the use of NI in research. The National Center for Nursing Research (2003) has identified the following priorities for nursing research:

- Investigation of effective use of biotechnologies and bioinformatics to enhance adjustment to these new advances and to improve self-management, healthy behaviors, and caregivers' activities
- Managing the incorporation of telehealth into nursing interventions, such as enabling long-distance links between clients and clinicians for information exchange and measuring benefits, costs, and client/clinician satisfaction
- Developing and testing creative ways to use the Internet and determining the effectiveness of this method in providing client education and linkages with other clients and health-care providers to maintain and improve health
- Including skills training for interventions that use devices to maintain physiologic function, to ensure that clients and caregivers use these technologies to the best effect

The NI specialty is represented by several professional associations, such as the American Nursing Informatics Assocation, a working group of the American Medical Informatics Association (AMIA), a group of the International Medical Informatics Association, and other international, regional, and local organizations. Although baccalaureate programs may have a requirement for competency in computers, many offer an elective in computers in nursing. Specialization, however, is at the graduate level, with a master's degree in NI being offered first at the Universities of Maryland and Utah, and now by others, such as the University of Nebraska, University of Pittsburgh, Duke University, and Excelsior University. A 2004 Internet search yielded a limited number master's degree and certificate programs in the specialty of NI; however, more will become available as employers declare a need.

The American Nurses Credentialing Center (ANCC) offers two certifications as generalists in NI, one for a baccalaureate in nursing and the other for a baccalaureate in another field. Because the examination is offered at the generalist level, the baccalaureate degree is required. When more candidates have been prepared at the specialty level of master's, an advanced practice test can be developed. Experience and education are required for this examination, which covers systems, ergonomics, technologies, information management and generation, roles, and theories. The examination is based on, and the specialty operates from, the following overarching standards:

- Incorporate theories, principles, and concepts from appropriate sciences into informatics practice
- Integrate ergonomics and human-computer interaction (HCI) principles into

---

ONLINE CONSULT

Read the themes for nursing research at
www.nih.gov/ninr.
Learn more about the nursing informatics specialty at
www.ania.org
or
www.amia-niwg.org.
Explore nursing informatics further by reading the *Online Journal of Nursing Informatics* at
www.eaa-knowledge.com/ojni.

informatics solution design, development, selection, implementation, and evaluation
• Systematically determine the social, legal, and ethical impact of an informatics solution within nursing and health care (ANA, 2001)

CAREERS IN NURSING INFORMATICS

The diversity of informatics projects and programs has led to tremendous professional career opportunities. Managers in the rapidly changing health-care environment demand more and more information, clients receive care in many settings, and organizations have redesigned their services and care models. These changes mean continued growth for nursing and general health information systems and the creation of new positions in nursing informatics.

Many of the future informatics jobs are yet to be defined. As the technology changes, so too will the work necessary to maintain and further the acquisition of information and knowledge. Currently, informatics nurses are working in health-care organizations, for software and hardware vendors, in educational settings, and for insurance companies, to name only a few. In any position, the informatics specialist works closely with professionals from all other health-care disciplines.

Positions In Health-Care Organizations

A variety of roles exist for the specialist in nursing informatics within hospitals, home health agencies, long-term care facilities, and other health-care facilities. As organizations implement information systems, informatics nurses serve an important function in assessing the institution's information needs, evaluating available products and vendors, and assisting with product installations. As communicator and interpreter, the NI specialist serves as a liaison between the nursing staff and the information systems people. When

a system is ready for use (to "go live"), the NI specialist remains on site; later, the specialist is on call to provide expert assistance to staff. Once the system has been installed, modifications are made on the basis of user feedback, and the NI specialist is on to the next project. Informatics is a specialty that changes rapidly.

Long-term care facilities are required to make electronic reports to CMS of the **Minimum Data Set (MDS),** an assessment tool for residents of long-term care facilities. Therefore, nurses must both assess residents on an ongoing basis and report this information using the electronic tools and standardized language. The more than 16,000 long-term care facilities are required to comply with this reporting create many job opportunities for registered nurses. Performance improvement functions need NI competencies to navigate through the myriad of systems, reports, and guidelines that direct improvement activities. Compliance offices require access to all the systems in a facility. The 2004 National Patient Safety Goals (NPSG) (JCAHO, 2003) have created new requirements for training staff to better patient safety by improving, in part, data retrieval, management, and reporting. Performance improvement is concerned with NPSG, clinical indicators of quality, and evidence-based practice guidelines. From safety reporting to reimbursement opportunities, informatics skills are necessary.

Positions with Systems and Software Vendors

Many of the producers of software and information systems seek to hire NI specialists. Nurses work to develop new products, market products and services, and install systems. Experience with documentation and standardized nursing language is helpful. Clinicians with enough patient-care experience to predict barriers to implementation are most useful. NI experts serve as liaisons between the vendor and the health-care organization, because they are able to comprehend and articulate the issues for both parties.

Positions in Educational Settings

With the expectation that beginning and experienced nurses possess informatics competencies (Box 18–5), the responsibilities of educators has grown. Whether it is expertise in instructional design to create a new Web-based course or CD-ROM, or the vision required to implement the SEEDS project, this area presents many opportunities. Success in grasping these opportunities is recognized and rewarded—for instance, when Sigma Theta Tau International presents biennial awards for creativity in the use of technology in both nursing and public education. Nurse-owned companies such as Health Soft and Professional Development Software, both educational design firms, and NursingCEU.com, a continuing education company, demonstrate the opportunities for entrepreneurship in informatics. Affiliation with a professional association such as the National League for Nursing or a commercial venture such as Assessment Technologies Institute (ATI) will provide opportunities in test development and delivery.

Positions in Managed Care Organizations and Insurance Companies

As forms of managed care continue to develop, the demand for data and information will grow, as will the opportunities for informatics specialists. Informatics nurses are now working directly with care delivery institutions in developing data and information

---

BOX 18–5
INFORMATICS COMPETENCIES FOR NURSES

Beginning nurses:
- Computer literacy skills
- Information literacy skills
- Identifying, collecting, and recording data relevant to the nursing care of patients
- Analyzing and interpreting patient and nursing information as part of the planning for the provision of nursing services
- Using informatics applications designed for the practice of nursing
- Implementing public and institutional policies related to privacy, confidentiality, and security of information

Experienced nurses:
- Use system applications to manage data, information, and knowledge within their specialty
- Participate as content experts to evaluate information and assist others in developing information structures and systems to support their specialty
- Promote the integrity of and access to information, including confidentiality, legal, ethical, and security issues
- Be actively involved in efforts to improve information management and communication
- Act as advocates or leaders for incorporating innovations and informatics concepts into their specialty

Informatics nurse specialists:
- All the competencies of beginning and experienced nurses
- Operates within Standards of Practice and Professional Performance of Informatics Nurse Specialist

Adapted from American Nurses Association. (2001). *Scope and standards of nursing informatics practice.* (Publication No. NIP21 3M 05/02). Washington, DC: Author.

systems as well as with the mechanisms involved in the internal reporting processes. New roles are emerging continuously, many of which have been designed and articulated by NI specialists as this burgeoning new specialty evolves.

For more information, search the various informatics association Web sites and read the *Online Journal of Nursing Informatics*. As with many nursing specialties, nurses should look for opportunities and then create the position that will best serve the organization.

 ONLINE CONSULT

Educational design firms:
www.healthsoftonline.com
or
www.pds.com
Achievement test companies:
www.nln.org/testprods/index.htm
or
www.atitesting.com

Key Points

- Nursing informatics is a specialty that integrates nursing science, computer science, and information science to manage and communicate data, information, and knowledge in nursing practice (ANA, 2001, p.vii).
- Nursing informatics as a specialty grows and changes as quickly as the computer industry itself.
- The goal of nursing informatics is to improve the health of populations, communities, families, and individuals by optimizing the management and communication of information (ANA, 2001).
- The NI specialty is represented by several professional associations, is supported by advanced education, and is credentialed through certification.
- The primary interest of nursing informatics is to expand how data, information, and knowledge are used within nursing practice.
- Few systems can address every component of health care, so there is generally an overriding information system with both clinical and administrative components.
- In practice, nurses most commonly use computers to document care and to access client data. Yet, there are many applications for education and research.
- The diversity of informatics projects and programs has led to tremendous professional career and interdisciplinary opportunities.

 Thought and Discussion Questions

1. Since the implementation of HIPAA, what challenges have you observed regarding access to patient information?
2. What would happen in your agency if the computer system "went down"? How would the failure affect patient care?

3. What is the relationship between nursing service and health-care informatics in your facility?

4. How can handheld technology improve patient care?

5. Review the Chapter Thought on the first page of the chapter, and be prepared to discuss it online or in class.

Interactive Exercises

1. Interview someone in the information management department and someone from nursing services by asking the following questions:
   - What kinds of data are collected?
   - What types of reports are routinely generated?
   - What is the future for information systems in the facility?
   - Compare and contrast your findings. What recommendations would you make for their information system on the basis of what you have learned?

2. Evaluate your readiness for online learning. Use a search engine and look for sites that survey online learning readiness, such as **http://www. sdccdonline.net/assess.htm,** and complete the survey to see what factors are considered essential for success in online learning environments.

3. Interview a hospital risk manager, a risk manager in a physician's office, an attorney, a medical records (or clinical information) specialist, a staff nurse, an advanced practice nurse, a nursing professor, and a patient by asking the following questions:
   - What do you think are the most important issues related to the development and use of a CPR?
   - What ethical issues do you consider important in developing and using a CPR?
   - From the results of your interviews, write a brief argument for and against the further development and use of a computerized patient record.

4. Complete HIPAA training through your employer or through CMS at **http://www.cms.gov/hipaa/**

5. Go to **http://www.smartdr.com/drvisit.htm** to view a sample electronic record. Follow the links to see how the record will grow. What problems do you envision? How would you propose to fix them?

6. Review the Informatics case study located on the Intranet site, and be prepared to discuss in online or in class.

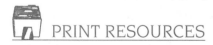
PRINT RESOURCES

References

American Nurses Association. (2001). *Scope and Standards of Nursing Informatics Practice.* (Publication No. NIP21 3M 05/02). Washington, DC: Author.

Armstrong, M., Gessner, B., & Cooper, S. S. (2000) POTS, PANS, and PEARLs: The nursing profession's rich history with distance education for a new century of nursing. *The Journal of Continuing Education in Nursing,* 31(2), 63–70, 94–95.

Billings, D. (2002). *Conversations in E-Learning.* Pensacola, FL: Pohl Publishing.

Bloom, K., & Hough, M.C. (2003). Student satisfaction with technology-enhanced learning. CIN: *Computers, Informatics, Nursing,* 21(5), 241–246.

Connors, HR, Weaver C, Warren J, Miller KL. An academic-business partnership for advancing clinical informatics. Nurs Educ Perspect. 2002 Sep-Oct;23(5):228-33.

Dick, R. S., & Steen, E. B. (1991). *The computer-based patient record: An essential technology for health care.* Washington, DC: National Academy Press.

Graves, J. R., & Corcoran, S (1989). The study of nursing informatics. *Image*, 21(4), 227–231.

Hebda, T., Czar, P., & Mascara, C. (2001). *Handbook of informatics for nurses and health care professionals.* Upper Saddle River, NJ: Prentice-Hall.

Hunt, E.C. (2002). The value of a PDA to a nurse. *Tar Heel Nurse*, 64(3), 18–19.

Lange, L. L. (1997). Informatics nurse specialist: Roles in health care organizations. *Nursing Administration Quarterly*, 21(3), 1–10.

National League for Nursing (2003). Grants. *Nursing Education Perspectives*, 24(6) , 326.

Bibliography

Armstrong, M., & Frueh, S. (2002). *Telecommunications for nurses: Providing successful distance education and telehealth.* New York: Springer.

Cohen, M. R. (2000). *Medication errors: Causes, prevention, and risk management.* Boston: Jones & Bartlett.

Mascara, C., Czar, P., & Hebda, T. (1999). *Internet resource guide for nurses & health care professionals.* Menlo Park, CA: Addison-Wesley.

Nicoll, L. (2000). *Computers in nursing's nurses' guide to the Internet.* Philadelphia: Lippincott.

Nicoll, L. (2003). Education and networking in nursing informatics. CIN: *Computers, Informatics, and Nursing*, 21(5), 275–286.

Montgomery, K., & Fitzpatrick, J. (2002). *Essentials of internet use in nursing.* New York: Springer.

Panniers, T. L. & Gassert, C. A. (1996). Standards of practice and preparation for certification. In M. E. Mills, C. A. Romano, and B. R. Heller (Eds.), *Information management in nursing and health care.* Philadelphia: Springhouse.

Thede, L. (2003). *Informatics and nursing.* Philadelphia: Lippincott.

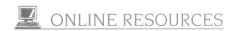 ONLINE RESOURCES

References

Centers for Medicare and Medicaid Services (2003). The Health Insurance Portability and Accountability Act of 1996. *http://www.cms.gov/hipaa/*

Center for Nursing Classification (2003). Center for Nursing Classification and Clinical Effectiveness. *http://www.nursing.uiowa.edu/cnc/index.htm*

Joint Commission on Accreditation of Healthcare Organizations (2003). *Disease-specific care certification. http://www.jcaho.org/dscc/index.htm*

National Center for Nursing Research. *Future themes of nursing research. http://www.nih.gov.ninr*

Resources

American Medical Informatics Association. *http://www.amia-niwg.org*

American Nursing Informatics Association. *http://www.ania.org*

British Computer Society—Nursing Specialty Group. *http://www.bcsnsg.org/uk*

Canadian Nursing Informatics Assocation. *http://www.cnia.org*

Health Informatics Europe. *http://hi-europe.co.uk*

Informatics Nurse Certification. *http://www.nursingworld.org/ancc*

International Medical Informatics Association. *http://www.imia.org/ni*

NLN Living Books. *http://www.nln.org/profdev/onlinecourses/livingbooks.htm*

Online Journal of Nursing Information. *http://www.eaa-knowledge.com/ojni*

Online Journal of Issues in Nursing. *http://nursingworld.org/ojin/*

PDA Software. *http://www.rnpalm.com*

Virtual Hospital. *http://www.vh.org*

Cyril F. Chang
Susan K. Pfoutz
Sylvia A. Price

19
chapter

Health-Care Economics

> *Health care is different and the free market system needs to be modified appropriately to fit the special characteristics of health care.*

Chapter Objectives

On completion of this chapter, the reader will be able to:

1. Apply the basic economic concepts of supply, demand, and market to health care.
2. Describe the structure of the American system of health-care financing and delivery.
3. Describe the roles played by the major participants of the health-care system.
4. Explore health-care issues from the perspective of economics.
5. Examine the varied health-care payment systems.
6. Explain the concept of managed care and the different forms of managed care organizations.
7. Analyze major health-care reforms.

Key Terms

Economics
Health-Care
  Economics
Demand
Supply
Provider-Driven
  System
Market-Driven
  System
Third-Party Payers

Fee-For-Service Payment
  System
Prospective Payment
  System
Diagnosis-Related
  Groups
Managed Care
Capitation
Health Maintenance
  Organization

Independent Practice
  Association
Preferred Provider
  Organization
Point-of-Service
  Plan
Health Report Card
Effectiveness
Cost-Effectiveness

Traditionally, economic and management issues have not been pivotal to nursing practice. In today's health-care market, however, a variety of economic factors are affecting nursing practice and the outcomes of nursing care. This chapter presents a broad survey of current health-care issues from an economic perspective. It prepares nurses to examine relevant economic concepts and integrate them, along with clinical, environmental, and behavioral knowledge, into their practice.

Significant changes in the health-care system, specifically, the transformation from a provider-driven system to a market-driven system, require that nurses learn the language and concepts of economics to function effectively. Nurses, as the single largest group of health-care providers and stewards of health-care resources, are increasingly challenged to defend the value of nursing care. In order to do so, nurses in a variety of practice settings are examining and analyzing such operational factors as cost, efficiency, and productivity. These economic activities, designed to link clinical outcomes to desirable financial goals, enable nurses to demonstrate the effectiveness and cost-effectiveness of nursing care.

Economics focuses on how consumers, business firms, government entities, and other organizations make choices in an environment of scarce resources. **Health-care economics**, a specialty area of economics, analyzes how the different parts of a health-care system work together to deliver service that meets the needs of patients. Nurses are critical participants in this delivery process. They must learn to conceptualize the economic and financial realities in order to achieve appropriate resource utilization, cost containment, and high-quality nursing care that the general public can afford.

Obtaining economic knowledge and applying it to nursing practice can be both personally and professionally rewarding. In personal terms, nurses who approach health care from a broader, economic perspective can compete effectively in today's health-care marketplace. In professional terms, having this additional knowledge and skills enables nurses to participate more fully in the design and delivery of health-care services and to achieve the best possible outcomes at the lowest possible cost. A good beginning point for this learning process is to review the American system of health-care delivery and explore the roles played by the system's major participants

THE AMERICAN SYSTEM OF HEALTH-CARE DELIVERY: AN OVERVIEW

The health-care system in the United States is composed of three major groups of participants (Box 19–1). The first group are clients, who are the consumers of health-care services. Only a small percentage of consumers pay for their health care out of pocket. For example, the total amount paid out of pocket by consumers accounted for approximately 15 percent of total national health-care expenditures in the year 2000 (Center for Medicare and Medicaid Service [CMS]). Most consumers are insured by private insurance companies through their employers or by a government-sponsored insurance program.

The second group of participants consists of health-care providers, such as hospitals, nurses, physicians, and other health-care workers, who participate directly and indirectly in the production and delivery of health care. The third group, called third-party payers, includes insurance companies and government health-care agencies that provide health insurance coverage to specific groups of individuals, such as employees of businesses, union members, the elderly, and low-income individuals.

In this vast and largely decentralized market for health-care services, consumers demand services to meet their health needs. Meanwhile, providers deliver the demanded services and bill the third-party payers for payment. The third-party payers collect insurance premiums or taxes to pool financial resources from a large number of individuals

ECONOMIC TERMS DEFINED

- **Capitation:** A prospective payment system that pays health plans or providers a fixed amount per enrollee per month for a defined set of services.
- **Cost-effectiveness:** An economic evaluation technique that assesses competing programs that are designed to achieve the same or similar objective.
- **Demand:** The amount of a service or a product that consumers are willing and able to buy at specific prices.
- **Diagnosis-related groups (DRGs):** The prospective payment system used by Medicare to determine payment rates for hospital services under 495 diagnosis related groups (DRGs). Each DRG represents a particular case type for which Medicare provides a flat dollar amount of reimbursement.
- **Economics:** The science that studies how consumers, businesses, government entities, and other organizations make choices to overcome the problems of scarcity.
- **Effectiveness:** The extent to which a treatment achieves its intended purpose
- **Fee-for-service (FFS) payment system:** A reimbursement system under which insurance companies reimburse hospitals and physicians after the needed services are delivered.
- **Health maintenance organization (HMO):** A managed care plan that either administers or arranges for health care to be provided to its members for a capitated monthly fee.
- **Health report card:** An on-line interactive tool designed to help users to find useful health quality information on health plans, hospitals, and other providers or the health status of a community or a region.
- **Health-care economics:** A specialty area of economics that analyzes how the different components of a health-care system work together to deliver service that meets the needs of patients.
- **Independent practice association (IPA):** An HMO model that enters into a contractual relationship with solo or group practitioners to provide physician and nurse practitioner services to enrollees.
- **Managed care:** A health-care system that combines the financing and delivery of health services into a single entity.
- **Market-driven system:** A health-care system in which most decisions are made by the impersonal forces of supply and demand and not by any particular group of individuals such as consumers, providers or third-party payers.
- **Point-of-service (POS) plan:** A managed care model that combines HMO characteristics such as capitation and coordination of service delivery with the PPO characteristics of enrollee choice of providers.
- **Preferred provider organization (PPO):** A managed care model that comprises networks of hospitals, private practice physicians, and other health-care practitioners that provide comprehensive health services to employers and their employees for a negotiated fee.
- **Prospective payment system (PPS):** A hospital payment system that sets payment rates before treatment begins.
- **Provider-driven system:** A health-care system in which most decisions are made by health-care providers.
- **Supply:** The amount of a service or a product that providers are willing to sell at particular prices.
- **Third-party payers:** Financial intermediaries such as insurance companies, health plans, and government entities that pay providers for services delivered and collect premiums from employers and their employees or taxes from taxpayers.

and businesses to raise the necessary funds to pay for the anticipated expenses. The roles played by each of the three major parties of the health-care system, along with the critical economic and health-care delivery issues, are examined later in this chapter.

Demand for Health Care

The **demand** for health care refers to the varying amount of health care that a consumer is willing and able to purchase at each of the possible prices. A number of key factors, called the *determinants of demand*, affect the amount of health care demanded:

• Consumer needs and expectations for illness cure, supportive care, preventive care, and health promotion services
• Individual values derived from the conceptualization of health, culture, ethnicity, religious beliefs, education, and gender
• Access to health care and a set of economic variables, including price of care, income, wealth, and adequacy of insurance coverage, that affect access

Consumer Need

The total demand for health care by all consumers in a country is fundamentally related to the size and health status of the general population. As the population grows large and older, the demand for health care naturally rises. The demand for health care is also influenced by the incidence of illnesses and injuries. A flu epidemic or a large natural disaster undoubtedly places greater demands on health care. Still another factor that affects the demand for health services is consumers' expectations from the utilization of various health-care services. The consumers who expect a full recovery from a particular treatment demand a greater amount of the service than those otherwise identical consumers who expect less from the same treatment.

Consumer Conceptualization

The demand for health care is also influenced by consumers' conceptualization of health care. Although good health is universally desired, it is not the only goal in one's life. Individuals routinely make tradeoffs between health and other non-health goals (rent, food, personal desires) when they conflict with one another. However, there is no universally held conceptualization of what *health* means to consumers (Fuchs, 1993). Conceptualizations of health vary widely with such individual characteristics as life expectancy, capacity for work, need for health care, and ability to perform a variety of personal and social functions. The wide variation in conceptualizations of health impedes the potential for the establishment of a public policy that can be consistently implemented and financed. In fact, the wide variations are reflected in the continuing inability of health-care reform efforts to develop and finance a national health plan.

BOX 19–1
THE THREE GROUPS OF HEALTH-CARE PARTICIPANTS

Consumers are the millions of individuals who use health care and pay for the services either out of pocket or through an insurance policy bought individually, received through employment, or offered by a government agency.

Providers are doctors, nurses, pharmacists, and other health-care professionals who work in hospitals, nursing homes, and a wide range of other health-care establishments to provide services for consumers and who receive payments from consumers directly or through a third-party payer.

Third-party payers are insurance companies, health plans, and government agencies that arrange for the services to be delivered and the necessary payments for these services.

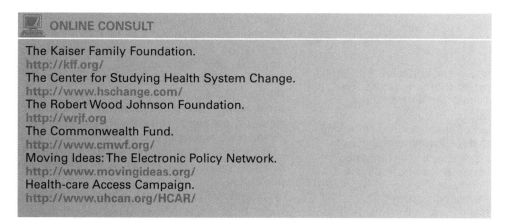

Consumer Access

The demand for health care is also influenced by consumer access to health-care services. Consumer access to health-care services—the ability of the individual physically to get to and to use health-care facilities—is influenced by geographic proximity of health-care services, eligibility for insurance benefits, income level, and individual values and preferences. Urban medical centers tend to concentrate technology and providers within a small geographic area, whereas rural areas often have a scarcity of health-care providers and limited technologic support. Some individuals cannot afford private insurance; yet their income exceeds the level that would qualify them for state-funded coverage. Access to health care has been a central value in the discussion of national health-care reform.

Delivery System Characteristics

In addition to the demand-determining factors just discussed, the amount and quality of health care actually delivered to consumers are also influenced by the characteristics of the delivery system. In a provider-driven health-care system, for example, providers dominate health-care demand. In such a system, providers not only prescribe services that they consider necessary and appropriate but also furnish them for a fee. Providers have the control over which and how many health-care services consumers use. This approach is intended to meet the needs of consumers as determined by providers on the basis of their best professional judgment. Such a system does not address the preferences and perceived demand of consumers, as is the case with most other consumer goods and services that are bought and sold every day.

In contrast, a market-driven system responds directly to the demand of the purchaser. The purchaser in this system is not the consumer or person who ultimately uses the service or product. In most cases, the purchaser is the health plan or an employer that provides insurance coverage. A market-driven system supports the emergence of competitive delivery plans that seek to attract purchasers by offering more of what consumers want—amenities as well as services and competitive prices. A good example is the attention given to quality improvement by hospitals and physician groups in response to the demand of purchaser alliances that have grown popular across the country.

It is important to note that these days, both employers who purchase health insurance and individual consumers are educated and informed. They freely voice their preferences concerning health-care issues and seek a more active part in the management of their care. It is useful to examine how different factors affect the health-care services demanded by consumers.(Box 19–2).

1. Consumer needs and expectations for illness cure, supportive care, preventive care, and health promotion services
2. Individual values derived from the conceptualization of health, culture, ethnicity, religious beliefs, education, and gender
3. Access to health care and a set of economic variables—price of care, income and wealth, and adequacy of insurance coverage—that affects access:
   - **Price** of health care is broadly defined as a wide range of sacrifices consumers must make in order to obtain the desired health-care service. It includes both the amounts of deductible, co-payments, and other out-of-pocket costs and non-cash costs such as travel time and other inconveniences involved in accessing the needed care.
   - **Income** and wealth significantly influence whether an individual can afford health insurance, which in turn affects the amount of services demanded.
   - **Insurance coverage** significantly influences the quality of health care demanded by consumers. An insured consumer demands a much greater amount of service than an otherwise identical consumer who has no insurance.

Supply of Health Care

Heath-care supply is equally as complex as health-care demand. The **supply** of health-care services refers to the ability of providers to deliver health care. The supply of health care is affected by the prevailing values of health, geographic location of both providers and consumers, availability of health-care facilities and technology, consumer and provider cultural values, and, again, the characteristics of the delivery system.

In a **provider-driven system**, the dominant providers, such as physicians and hospitals, control the location of services, types of providers, and technology available. Provider education support, provider location, and types of services offered are identified primarily by the dominant providers and secondarily by market factors. One secondary market factor, for example, is state licensing laws and available reimbursement. Each type of provider category (e.g., physician, advanced practice nurse, physician assistant, registered nurse, unlicensed assistant) must comply with such laws in order to practice.

By contrast, in a **market-driven system**, the number of providers at each level of education and the locations and types of services provided are determined by the needs and locations of consumers, rather than by the needs and location of providers. Technology is funded and provided on the basis of consumer need rather than the availability of a skilled provider. For instance, approximately 34 percent of consumers are using nontraditional health-care therapies to meet their health-care needs in addition to treatment for the same condition from a medical doctor (Eisenberg et al., 1993). As a result, nurses are supplying a growing variety of alternative services that are reimbursed by third-party payers.

A Hybrid System of Supply and Demand

The current health-care delivery system in the United States is a hybrid of the provider-dominant and market-driven systems. In general, the market forces of supply and demand are allowed to function in health care to provide the efficiency and cost savings that are customarily associated with a market-driven system. In other words, competition on the supply side is generally perceived to be healthy and appropriate for health care. However, the free-for-all type of rampant competition that often characterizes the highly competitive and sometimes volatile private sector of the U.S. economy is uniformly considered to be excessive and wasteful for health care. Hence the market-driven American health-care system is heavily tempered by rules and regulations driven by dominant providers and sanctioned by the government. The government recognizes that health care is different and that the free market system needs to be modified appropriately to fit the special characteristics of health care.

Financing Our Health-Care System

Health care is expensive and must be paid for. How we pay for health care is important because it affects both the quantity and quality of services accessible to consumers and is a critical factor in determining the cost of health care.

Role of Third-Party Payers

Very few people can afford to pay large medical bills out of their own pockets. Health care in the United States is financed primarily by employers in the private sector or by the government in the public sector. Some large employers choose to be self-insured; that is, they have elected to pay for the medical costs of their employees themselves without buying health insurance from an insurance company. But most employers, especially medium-sized and small ones, buy health coverage from insurance companies and share the costs of premiums with their employees. In health insurance terms, insurance companies and government agencies that provide insurance coverage are called **third-party payers**. This is because the consumers and providers of health care are, respectively, the first and second parties to a health-care transaction.

The major function of third-party payers is to serve as a financial intermediary. In this role, third-party payers define the services to be provided, estimate the costs of insuring a given population, and collect premiums to cover the anticipated costs of services and administration. Third-party payers play another important role—that of a health plan administrator. This role is a complex process of determining the range of services to be cov-

ered and the amounts of copayments and deductibles that enrollees must pay for each service delivered. It also involves processing the claims submitted by providers and paying providers for the services delivered. Finally, health plan administrators also monitor outcomes of services, including consumer satisfaction, clinical outcomes, quality and appropriateness of the services provided, and the cost of services.

Unlike Canada or the United Kingdom, where a single payer provides insurance coverage for the entire country (Box 19–3), a large number of health plans are evident in the American health insurance landscape. Private employers are free to choose among many private for-profit and nonprofit insurance companies, with each offering a variety of health plans to suit the needs and preferences of purchasers. In the United States, government is also involved in the provision of insurance coverage. At the federal level, for example, Medicare provides insurance coverage for elderly and disabled individuals and families. Medicaid is a government insurance program for low-income individuals that is financed jointly by the federal and state governments and is administered by the states.

The main advantages of a multiple-payer system are that it offers greater competition, choice of health plans and services, and incentives to increase efficiency and reduce health-care costs. The disadvantages, however, include multiple layers of administration and higher administrative costs, such as those imposed on providers who must deal with multiple payers and their unique administrative structures.

Payment Systems

There are two broad categories of payment for services in the American system of health-care delivery: the fee-for-service system and the prospective payment system. The fee-for-service system dominated health care for many years, but the prospective payment system has had a strong presence since the early 1980s.

> **BOX 19-3**
> **THE HEALTH-CARE SYSTEMS IN THE UK AND CANADA**
>
> The British National Health Service (NHS) is the largest national health-care system in Europe. It was set up in 1948 to provide health care for all British citizens on the basis of need, not the ability to pay. The NHS is funded by the taxpayer. This means it is accountable to Parliament. It is managed by Department of Health, which is directly responsible to the secretary of state for health. The department sets overall health policy in England, is the headquarters for the NHS, and is responsible for putting policy into practice. It also sets targets for the NHS and monitors performance through its four directors of health and social care. About 1 million people work for the NHS in England, and it cost more than £50 billion a year to run in 2002.
>
> Canada's "single-payer" health-care system has long been a source of national pride. Unlike the UK's NHS, the Canadian system is characterized by local control, doctor autonomy, and consumer choice. It is a taxpayer-supported national health-care system that covers everyone living in Canada. It is called a single-payer system because government is the only source of payment for services provided. The service is free at the point of delivery, and the ten provinces have the authority and responsibility for planning, financing, and evaluating the services for residents in each province.

Fee-for-Service Payment

The **fee-for-service (FFS) payment system**, also known as the retrospective system, gives providers maximum control of services provided to the consumer. Pre-approval by third party payers for services is usually not required in this model. Few limits are placed on the length of hospital stay, the location of the services, or the amount and type of diagnostic procedures, pharmaceuticals, or treatment procedures. Services are typically considered separately or unbundled; that is, the different services that are required for a procedure or an episode of care are billed separately, with a fee generated by each service or procedure provided. Payments to hospitals and other providers are based on providers' costs in providing the services plus an acceptable markup. Under the FFS system, all costs related to care delivery, including the costs of products, services, salaries, construction, uncompensated care, and capital equipment, are passed on to consumers and their third-party payers.

Prospective Payment System

The **prospective payment system** (PPS) has emerged in response to concerns about access to care, and spiraling health-care costs. It is a pricing model that sets payment rates for hospital services before treatment begins. The Medicare program is an example of a prospective pricing model. In 1982, Medicare transitioned to a PPS based on a diagnostic classification system called **diagnosis-related groups** (DRGs). Under the DRG system, inpatient services are grouped together, or bundled, by DRG into a package of care with a predetermined price allowed for each DRG. If the hospital can provide the service package for less than the DRG price, it can keep the difference. Conversely, if the care costs the hospital more than the allowable price, the hospital has to absorb the loss. More than 450 DRGs have been identified on the basis of the principal diagnosis, use of the operating room, age of patient, co-morbidity, and complications (Table 19-1)

The DRG system used by Medicare in the public sector of health care is the most widespread example of prospective pricing. Originally, DRGs applied only to hospital inpatient activities. Inpatient physician services and all outpatient services were excluded. In the early 2000s, different versions of DRGs were introduced in hospital outpatient care, skilled nursing home care, and home care. Private sector PPSs are gaining popularity, and a variety of models have been implemented. These

TABLE 19–1
Leading Diagnosis-Related Groups (DRGs) in 1999

DRG Code	Description	Average Days of Care	Average Cost per Discharge
005	Extracranial vascular procedures	6.1	$15,373
012	Degenerative nervous system disorders	6.2	$15,200
014	Specific cerebro-vascular disorders	3.3	$14,752
015	Transient ischemic attack and precerebral occlusions	8.1	$11,063
024	Seizure and headache, age >17 yr with Complications and Comorbidities	6.1	$12,678

From The 2001 Medicare and Medicaid Statistical Supplement to Health Care Financing Review.
http://www.cms.hhs.gov/review/supp/

include capitated managed care programs, health maintenance organizations, preferred provider organizations, independent physician associations, and physician hospital organizations.

 MANAGED CARE

More Americans are enrolled in managed care health plans than ever before. According to the Henry J. Kaiser Family Foundation (2002), approximately 80.1 million Americans, or 28.6 percent of the population, were enrolled in health maintenance organizations (HMOs) in 2000, an increase of 26.5 percent from 1999. Among the nation's 40 million Medicare enrollees, 5 million or 12.5 percent were enrolled in the "Medicare Plus Choice" managed care plan in 2002. Managed care enrollment grew even faster among Medicaid enrollees, rising from 9 percent in 1990 to 57 percent in 2001 (Henry J. Kaiser Family Foundation, 2002).

No single definition can adequately describe managed care because it encompasses a complex range of organizational forms that are still evolving. Defined broadly, however, **managed care** is a health-care system willing to be held accountable for both the clinical

and financial outcomes of an enrolled population. Payment for services is based on a capitated (fixed) payment per month per person that is determined by the covered services and enrollment size (Folland et al., 2001).

Compared with the traditional FFS health plans, managed care has two distinctive characteristics. First, it integrates the financing and delivery functions of health care into a single organized system. Second, it emphasizes the delivery of a coordinated continuum of services, from wellness care to acute care, with an emphasis on incentives to achieve cost efficiency.

> [M]anaged care is a health-care system willing to be held accountable for both the clinical and financial outcomes of an enrolled population.

Under FFS systems, insurance companies reimburse hospitals and physicians after the needed services are delivered. Providers earn more if they provide more. By contrast, under managed care, keeping patients healthy means more profit for the managed care organization. Managers of managed care plans are therefore motivated, at least theoretically, to emphasize communication and coordination of care among physicians, nurses, and other health-care providers across different delivery settings. The essence of this delivery concept is that specific patient outcomes are achieved by economizing use of resources within a fixed budget. Managed care can be defined most practically by reviewing the major participants, the concept of capitation, and the managed care models.

Major Participants of Managed Care

There are four main participants in any managed care system: managed care organizations, purchasers, enrollees, and providers. Each participant will be covered in turn.

Managed Care Organizations

Managed care organizations (MCOs) are the health-care entities that arrange for the provision of services for a group of individuals who are enrolled in the health plan. Purchasers of health plans pay MCOs a fixed monthly payment called a *capitation rate*. This rate is based on the covered services and the size of enrollment. MCOs then arrange for the delivery of services through a variety of organizations: an HMO, a preferred provider organization (PPO), a point-of-service (POS) plan, or a combination of these plans.

Purchasers

Purchasers are employers, groups of employers, trade unions, professional associations, governmental agencies, and other legal entities that buy health insurance coverage for their participating members or employees. The purchasers arrange for the necessary legal agreements to contract with MCOs for health services. They also collect the premiums, pay the MCOs, and ensure that the MCOs fulfill their financial and clinical obligations.

Enrollees

The members or enrollees of an MCO are the employees or association members

A growing number of large purchasers have in recent years chosen to insure themselves (National Center for Health Statistics, 1997; Park, 2000); they no longer buy insurance products from an insurance company. Instead, they have become their own insurers. Because the health-care costs of a large group of people can be predicted, self-insured entities save money by not paying for the expenses and profits of an outside insurance company. Many of these self-insured purchasers still contract with an insurance company or managed care organization (MCO) to manage the different health plans offered to their employees. However, the MCO in this instance is no longer an insurer; it merely provides management services like claims processing and case management for a fee.

who are insured. They receive the health services and, together with their employers or associations, pay for the covered services. They are the final consumers of health services but are not necessarily the purchasers or buyers of health care. The self-insured employers and insurance companies are the buyers of health services. In recent years, enrollees have become more sensitive to their preferences and more vocal when they are denied care or are dissatisfied with service quality. In response, Congress and many state legislatures have debated a variety of patients' rights bills designed to safeguard patients' rights to health care and to provide avenues of recourse for when services are denied or unfavorable outcomes result.

Providers

The last group of participants within a managed care system are the institutional and individual providers, such as hospitals, physicians, nurses, and other health-care professionals. They are usually organized into provider networks that deliver services to members of an MCO for specified payments. The mechanisms for payment are determined by the managed care mode. In many cities, providers are organized and represented by management services organizations (MSOs).

MSOs are paid to provide contracting and administrative services for provider organizations. They specialize in the management of all business aspects of medical practices for the providers.

Capitation

The health-care delivery system in the United States frequently uses a **capitation** system. Under this payment system, MCOs are prospectively paid a per-member-per-month (PMPM) amount for a specified range of health services for enrolled individuals. These services are delivered either directly by the MCO or through a subcontract between the MCO and independent providers, such as hospitals, clinics, doctors, and other health-care practitioners. Capitation shifts the financial risk of providing services from insurance companies to MCOs and providers, forcing them either to use health-care resources efficiently and effectively or to suffer the financial consequences.

The following discussion explains how different payment systems affect financial risk.

Fee-for-Service System

In an FFS system, the health-care provider bills the insurance company for each procedure or service delivered. As long as that service is covered, the health-care provider can expect to be paid an amount that has been agreed on. The provider always knows the potential income. The health-care provider bears no risk for the total amount of cost for services. The health-care provider increases income by increasing the number of services delivered. The incentive is for the health-care provider to provide more services. For a patient with coronary artery disease, for example, the provider would encourage diagnostic tests, invasive procedures, and prolonged rehabilitation services.

Prospective Payment System

In a prospective payment system, the health-care provider is paid one fee for an *episode of care*—a term used to measure the various health-care services and encounters rendered in connection with identified injury or period of illness. With this payment arrangement, the provider shares some financial risk, because the payment remains the same regardless of how many diagnostic tests, equipment, supplies, and institutional facilities are required. Although the amount for each episode is limited, providers could increase income by increasing the volume of episodes of care or decreasing the number of expensive services provided. With this system, treatment of a patient with coronary artery disease now would consist of only needed testing, discharge from the hospital as soon as possible, and limited rehabilitation services.

Capitated System

In a capitated system, providers bear much more financial risk. The provider is paid a specified amount per patient per month regardless of what services the patients use. The incentive here is to keep persons in good health by encouraging healthy lifestyles and aggressively treating early signs of cardiovascular risk. Critics of this system are concerned that MCOs and providers may deny some needed services in order to maintain the income of the health-care providers.

Models of Managed Care

MCOs can be for-profit or nonprofit. They may be owned by a variety of entities, including for-profit insurance companies, nonprofit companies such as Blue Cross and Blue Shield associations, physician groups, hospitals, and health management firms. MCOs can be organized in a variety of ways and are customarily classified into three major types: (1) health maintenance organization (HMO), (2) preferred providers organization (PPO), and (3) point-of-service (POS) plan.

Health Maintenance Organization

A **health maintenance organization** is a managed health plan that either administers or arranges for health care to be provided to its members for a capitated monthly fee (Fox, 2001). The philosophy of an HMO is to emphasize preventive health services, such as routine physical examinations, prenatal care, and proactive management of chronic conditions, in order to avert costly treatments that would be needed later, after disease has developed. In the United States, the number of people enrolled in HMOs jumped from 38.8 million in 1992 to 80.1 million in 2000 (Henry J. Kaiser Family Foundation, 2002).

The relationship that an HMO maintains with its providers is paramount to its success. This is because the health services provided to patients must be procured from hospitals, physicians, nurse practitioners, nurses, and other health-care providers who participate in the plan. Without providers' cooperation, HMO enrollees will not receive cost-effective health services. It is therefore critical to develop a thorough understanding of the different ways that HMOs maintain relationships with their providers. (Box 19–4).

Depending on the financial arrangement and organizational relationships with providers, HMOs can be organized in a number of ways. The major HMO models are the staff model, the group model, the independent practice association model, and the network model.

BOX 19–4
EXAMPLES OF HMO RELATIONSHIPS WITH PROVIDERS

- **Selecting, recruiting, and credentialing providers**: A successful HMO must develop an effective provider network by recruiting and selecting providers of different specialties who have the appropriate credentials and are willing to work in a managed care environment.

- **Primary care physician**: Sometimes referred to as a "gatekeeper," the primary care physician (PCP) in an HMO promotes the health of specified members. The PCP is responsible for organizing the medical care process, either by referring a patient on for specialized diagnosis and treatment or by caring for that patient then and there. Primary care physicians often participate in teams made up of specialists and other health professionals to study and improve how care is provided, particularly for patients at highest medical risk.

- **Practice guidelines**: Practice guidelines are systematically developed statements on medical practices that help a practitioner make decisions about appropriate health care for specific medical conditions. Managed care organizations commonly use these guidelines to evaluate appropriateness and medical necessity of care. Practice guidelines are developed with the "long view" of health in mind. This approach is fundamental to managed care organizations that want to keep the customers they have. Physicians in managed care environments, therefore, have the incentive to provide high-quality medicine.

Staff Model

The staff model of HMO uses its own salaried physicians, advanced practice nurses, and ambulatory care nurses. These providers deliver health services only to plan members and usually practice at clinics owned and operated by the HMO. A major advantage of this model is that it exercises tight control over the providers' practice, thereby making it easier for the HMO to monitor utilization and costs. However, a major drawback is that the physicians in a staff model, who earn a fixed income and work for a fixed number of hours to satisfy mandated encounter times, may give patients less attention than physicians working elsewhere.

Group Model

Unlike the staff model, which hires its own physicians and nurse practitioners, the group model contracts exclusively with a group of physicians and, separately, with hospitals to provide services to its enrollees. The HMO usually pays the group practice a PMPM capitation fee for the provision of health-care services. The major difference between a staff model and a group model is that the staff model HMO pays physicians directly, whereas in a group model, physicians are paid by the physician group. Physicians in a group model can maintain greater autonomy and may experience less direct pressure from the HMO to cut costs than in a staff model, because the practice group, not the HMO, pays them. However, the practice group bears the financial consequences of practice patterns that may be outside the HMO norms. For example, the cost of specialty referral services may come out of the PMPM fees, reducing the practice group's income.

Independent Practice Association Model

In the **independent practice association** (IPA), the fastest-growing HMO model, the HMO enters into a contractual relationship with solo or group practitioners to provide physician and nurse practitioner services (Chang et al., 2001, p. 307). Unlike the group model in which the HMO enters into an exclusive contract with a physician group for physician services, the IPA involves contracting with individual solo practitioners, solo practitioners in practice groups, or both, for services.

In general, the IPA receives a PMPM capitation fee through a primary capitation arrangement with the health plan purchaser and reimburses IPA physicians through a subcapitation or a discounted FFS subcontract. A *subcapitation* is a secondary capitation arrangement between the IPA and a group of physicians. This payment arrangement shifts the financial responsibilities of providing services for all or part of the enrollees of an HMO to the contracted physicians or physician group. A discounted FFS system is a payment arrangement whereby the physicians are still paid according to the services delivered— hence the term fee-for-service—but the fees are negotiated at a discount to ensure a steady flow of patients from an HMO. The arrangement for payment of specialty services is legally identified in the contract between the IPA and its providers.

Network Model

Like the IPA model, the network model HMO contracts with more than one physician group practice to provide services. Some HMOs contract with many small primary care practices (e.g., family practice, internal medicine, and pediatrics) under a subcapitation agreement that pays the physicians a fix monthly fee for each patient under the physician's care. These physician groups can make referrals to specialists but are themselves financially responsible for reimbursing these referrals. Some network model HMOs contract with broad-based multispecialty groups that can provide a wide range of services from primary care to highly specialized services. The network model allows referrals to a wider range of physicians than either the staff model or group model.

Preferred Provider Organization

A **PPO** comprises networks of hospitals, private practice physicians, and other health-care practitioners that provide comprehensive health services to an enrolled population for a negotiated fee. There are more than 1000 PPOs in the United States that serve more than 20 percent of the insured population and account for half the total enrollment in managed care plans (Fox, 2001).

A variety of entities, including insurance companies, professional organizations, hospitals, and physician groups, may sponsor PPOs. It is also common for a PPO to be jointly sponsored by a hospital and physicians. Unlike HMOs, PPOs do not assume the financial risk of arranging and providing health services; the sponsoring organizations do. In other words, it is the responsibility of the insurance companies or the professional organizations that sponsor the PPOs to bear the financial risk for the enrolled population. PPOs also do not perform many of the functions customarily assumed by HMOs, such as utilization review, quality assurance, and insurance underwriting. Put simply, PPOs are merely networks of physicians that agree to accept discounted FFS for a steady flow of patients.

For example, participating providers such as physicians and advanced practice nurses in a PPO usually are reimbursed approximately 15 to 20 percent less than the local prevailing reimbursement rates. In return for lower fees, enrollees of a PPO agree to use health-care providers and facilities with whom the PPO has established a contractual relationship.

Point-of-Service Plan

A **point-of-service plan** combines the classic HMO characteristics, such as capitation and coordination of service delivery, with characteristics of a PPO, such as enrollee choice of providers. Patients in a POS plan are required to select a primary care provider, who then manages and coordinates the health-care needs of patients under his or her care. Patients may choose a nonparticipating, out-of-plan provider at the point of receiving service. But they must receive a referral from the primary care provider, who, in addition to providing primary care, serves as a "gate-keeper." They must also pay a higher deductible or copayment for this privilege, because the out-of-plan providers are usually paid at an FFS rate. The POS plan appeals to enrollees who prefer the option of choosing providers outside the plan and are willing to pay extra for it.

The options within managed care are continually evolving to include new forms designed to appeal to purchasers and enrollees. The main goal remains the same—to reduce costs by integrating the delivery and payment of services. The managed care formats that develop to achieve this goal are responsive to health-care markets.

THE COST-QUALITY TRADEOFF

Cost issues have dominated recent public debates on health care. Managed care organizations, health-care providers including nurses, and consumers of health care often disagree about the proper role of cost containment, choice, and quality in the delivery of health-care services. In the midst of these emotion-laden debates, it is easy to lose sight of the fact that quality of care is the key to success for individual and institutional providers. Health care is different from ordinary consumer goods, in that consumers not only demand but also are willing to pay for high-quality services as long as the benefits outweigh the costs. It is critical that individual providers recognize that the winning strategy in an increasingly competitive environment is to compete in terms of quality while keeping costs at a reasonable level. The concepts of efficiency, clinical effectiveness, and cost-effectiveness play an important role in managing the relationship between quality and cost.

Recent health-care reform efforts have heightened the need for objective measures of health-care quality (Box 19–5). To this end,

> **BOX 19–5**
> **PUBLIC AND PRIVATE ENTITIES THAT MONITOR AND REPORT ON QUALITY OF HEALTH CARE**
>
> **National Center for Quality Assurance (NCQA)** is an independent, 501(c)(3) nonprofit organization whose mission is to improve health-care quality. NCQA evaluates health care in three different ways: through accreditation (a rigorous on-site review of key clinical and administrative processes); through the Health Plan Employer Data and Information Set (HEDIS, a tool used to measure performance in key areas, such as immunization and mammography screening rates); and through a comprehensive member satisfaction survey. Although participation in the accreditation and certification programs is voluntary, more than half the nation's HMOs currently participate. And almost 90 percent of all health plans measure their performance using HEDIS. *(http://www.ncqa.org/)*
>
> **The Joint Commission on Accreditation of Healthcare Organizations (JCAHO)** evaluates and accredits more than 16,000 health-care organizations and programs in the United States. An independent, not-for-profit organization, JCAHO is the nation's predominant standards-setting and accrediting body in health care. Since 1951, JCAHO has developed state-of-the-art, professionally based standards and has evaluated the compliance of health-care organizations against these benchmarks. *(http://www.jcaho.org/)*
>
> **HealthGrades.Com** is a private, for-profit, health-care quality ratings and services company. Founded in 1999, the firm is headquartered in Lakewood, Colorado, and has more than 50 employees. Its mission is to improve the quality of health care nationwide. With its proprietary, objective provider ratings and expert advisory services, HealthGrades gives clients targeted solutions that enable them to measure, assess, enhance, and market health care. *(http://www.healthgrades.com)*
>
> **Health Resources and Service Administration (HRSA) Center for Quality (CQ)** was established in the HRSA with the mission to strengthen and improve the quality of health care, especially as it relates to HRSA programs and service populations. The CQ operates jointly with the Office of the Chief Medical Officer (CMO). *(http://www.ask.hrsa.gov/Quality.cfm)*
>
> The **Institute of Medicine (IOM)** was chartered in 1970 as a component of the National Academy of Sciences. The Institute provides a vital service by working outside the framework of government to ensure scientifically informed analysis and independent guidance. The IOM's mission is to serve as adviser to the nation to improve health. The Institute provides unbiased, evidence-based, and authoritative information and advice concerning health and science policy to policymakers, professionals, leaders in every sector of society, and the public at large. *(http://www.iom.edu/)*

the federal government has made progress in increasing public disclosure of morbidity and mortality rates as well as data from facility inspections and physician malpractice and licensure actions (Blancett & Flarey, 1995). Although individual institutions monitor quality for internal review, most measures or indicators are not compiled by a centralized source of standards applicable to all institutions (Alsever et al., 1995; American Nurses Association [ANA], 1995a).

Health Report Card

Current efforts to develop comparative quality indicators that can be shared across institutions and with consumers have resulted in the "report card" phenomenon. A **health report card** is a summary of information about doctor and hospital performance and consumer satisfaction designed for consumers/patients and health-care buyers. Health plan providers, employer groups, and care providers have initiated several collaborative efforts to formulate report cards that identify and measure the quality of patient care. Examples of report cards are the ANA Nursing Report Card for Acute Care (ANA, 1995b), the Health Plan Employer Data and Information Set (HEDIS), the Leapfrog Group's Hospital Survey, and the *U.S. News and World Report*'s "America's Best Hospitals" exclusive rankings. These reports include cost benchmarks as well as selected quality indicators, but the results have been hampered by serious gaps in information and lack of standard indicators and uniform means for data collection and analysis.

The ANA has been active in the identification of nursing-sensitive outcomes—those that respond to nursing interventions. Currently, nursing-sensitive outcomes are nosocomial infections, medication errors, skin integrity, falls, patient and family complaints,

---

In addition to documenting quality, historical measures of treatment outcomes and costs must be translated into new indicators for capitated delivery models. Ongoing programs to assess patient satisfaction need to identify appropriate indicators of satisfaction and how they relate to continuing use of facility services. Traditional patient care issues, such as functional status, physiologic status, symptom management, and safety, continue to be applicable, but they should now be specifically related to patient outcomes. New quality indicators for providers and health plan managers also must be developed. These efforts assist in the development of meaningful and reportable measures of not only the effectiveness but also the cost-effectiveness of the services delivered.

---

and mortality (Aiken et al., 1994; ANA, 1995b; Blegen et al., 1998). Use of indicators from such a report card and incorporation of a nursing minimum data set (NMDS) in retrievable format can facilitate the identification of the contribution of nursing care within the larger health-care episode.

Effectiveness, Cost-Effectiveness, and Financial Performance

Effectiveness measures how well a prescribed treatment has accomplished the anticipated outcome. **Cost-effectiveness** measures whether the prescribed treatment has accomplished the desired outcome at the lowest possible cost. The delivery of effective and cost-effective services enables providers to maintain quality while keeping cost at an affordable level. Many medical services are beneficial to patients, but not all of them are cost-effective. The delivery of a non–cost-effective service may benefit a few patients but will drain scarce resources away from other patients whose needs have not been met. An emphasis on cost-effectiveness helps providers deliver the greatest possible health outcome while remaining mindful of today's financial constraints and limited resources. The attention paid to cost-effectiveness will pay dividends to providers, health plans, and, most importantly, patients.

Traditionally, financial performance in health care was evaluated on the basis of a variety of financial ratios measuring profitability, liquidity, capital structure, asset efficiency, and other aspects of the financial health of a business entity. These ratios, both individually and taken as a whole, could provide a comprehensive picture of the financial position of a hospital. The *Almanac of Hospital Financial and Operating Indicators*, published annually, includes more than 150 indicators related to these categories collected from audited financial statements, strategic operating indicator data submitted by hospitals, and Medicare cost reports (Cleverley, 1995; Medicode, 2003). New measures of financial performance for prospective capitated payments must be developed. The growing trend toward allocating resources on the basis of the number of enrolled members per month and the number of days per 1000 member-days requires new systems and processes to identify, allocate, and measure costs.

HEALTH-CARE REFORM

The preceding discussions of performance measures and quality improvement are useful for individual and institutional providers in their quest for quality improvement and cost control. But the United States as a country faces a host of health system problems, such as persistent cost inflation and racial and ethnic disparities in access to quality of health care, that can be resolved only through an effective national health reform.

With breakthrough advances in medical science such as the mapping of the human genome and better understanding of the basic disease processes, health care in the 21st century offers an array of promising technologic solutions to diseases and medical conditions. Health-care providers in the United States continue to have success in applying advanced medical technologies to previously untreatable diseases and illnesses. However, the American system of health-care delivery has persistently experienced an array of difficulties, including problems with access to care, high costs of care, and disparities in the quality and distribution of care. The United States ranks behind developed countries, such as England, Canada, and many Scandinavian countries—which spend a smaller percentage of their GDPs (gross domestic products, or total value of all goods and services produced within their borders) on health care—in basic system performance standards such as infant mortality and life expectancy (Anderson, 2003).

Numerous reform measures have been attempted in the last 30 years to improve the functioning of the American system of health-care delivery. Historically, the demand for health-care reform has come from three different sources:

- Businesses, whose employee health-care costs rise every year
- The middle class, who represent a majority of the workforce and the voting public
- Advocacy groups that lobby for the poor and the economically disadvantaged

On the supply side of the reform movement, the key players have been health policy experts, politicians at the federal, state, and local levels, and public officials who work in key health-care agencies that are charged with the responsibilities of administering public policies. In recent years, many reform measures have been pushed and implemented in three major areas of public concerns: access, cost, and quality.

Policies to Improve Access

The United States spends about 14 percent of its GDP on health care, and yet 42 million of its citizens or about 14 percent of the total population remain uninsured in any given year (Levit et al., 2004). Even among the insured populations, many people have inadequate insurance coverage or limited coverage that leaves many medical expenses uncovered. Concurrent reform efforts by federal, state, and local government have been under way to plug the holes in the insurance system and to bring health insurance to the near-universal level. These efforts include the following programs.

The Federal SCHIP Program

The State Children's Health Insurance Plan (SCHIP) was created under the Balanced Budget Act of 1997 as a new children's health insurance program under Title XXI of the Social Security Act. The purpose of the program was to encourage states to initiate and expand health insurance coverage for uninsured children. In 1999, Congress allocated $24 million over 5 years to help the states expand their insurance coverage for uninsured children. The funds cover the costs of insurance as well as outreach services to enroll children and reasonable costs for administration. Funds must be used to cover previously uninsured children and not to replace existing public or private coverage.

The statute set the broad outlines of the program's structure and established a partnership between federal and state governments. States were given great flexibility in tailoring the programs to meet their own circumstances. States could create or expand their own separate insurance programs, expand Medicaid, or combine the two approaches. States can choose among several benchmark benefit packages, develop a benefit package that is actuarially equivalent to or better than one of the benchmark plans, or use the Medicaid benefit. States also have the opportunity to set eligibility criteria regarding age, income, resources, residency, and duration of coverage within broad federal guidelines. The federal role is to provide technical assistance to the states and to ensure that programs meet statutory requirements that are designed to ensure meaningful coverage under the program.

To date, all 50 states plus the U.S. Virgin Islands have accepted the federal offers and established their SCHIP programs. The rapid expansion of this federally assisted health insurance program has recently been credited by the U.S. Bureau of Census for reducing the number of uninsured children in this country (U.S. Bureau of Census, 2003).

Individual State Initiatives

Rather than waiting for Congress and the federal government to solve their problems, many states have engaged in a variety of reforms to expand insurance coverage for their residents. These programs have been developed along two major paths, health insurance mandates and expansion of Medicaid coverage.

Insurance mandates are government laws and regulations that require the provision of certain benefits to ensure consumer access to services deemed to be desirable and necessary. State governments have issued hundreds of mandates on a wide range of health issues, including patient safety, coverage of preventive services, staffing requirements in hospitals and nursing homes, and parities of mental health care with regular health care. These state initiatives reflect the states' impatience with federal health reform, the widespread dissatisfaction with a range of health-care issues at the grass-root level, and a genuine desire for improvement in access to and quality of health care.

In addition to benefit mandates, many states have chosen to expand insurance coverage through a variety of mechanisms. One of these has been the application of the federal Section 1115 waivers to expand insurance coverage to the previously uninsured and underinsured populations. Tennessee, for example, initiated an experimental managed care program called TennCare in 1994 to add half a million previously uninsured and uninsurable individuals to its Medicaid population. The program now covers about 1.4 million individuals, or one in every four residents of

Tennessee. Since its inception, TennCare has been plagued by an assortment of administrative and cost-control problems. However, it has played a major role in reducing the percentage of individuals with no insurance in Tennessee to 11 percent, or 4.2 percentage points below the national average of 15.2 percent (U.S. Bureau of Census, 2003).

Oregon chose a different approach to Medicaid expansion, opting for an innovative rationing program called the Oregon Health Plan. The goal of the Plan was to provide insurance coverage to all residents in the state through a combination of public and private insurance programs. Central to the Oregon Health Plan is the establishment of a "prioritized list of health services," a list created by the Oregon Health Services Commission to rank more than 700 individual medical services from most to least important. Each year, the state legislature sets the funding level to cover a certain number of services on the list, but it cannot rearrange the list. Thus, in Oregon, the legislative branch of the state government determines the spending level and the predetermined priority list ensures that the most critical services are provided.

Medicare Reform and Prescription Drug Benefits

The federal Medicare program has been the nation's major health insurance program for the elderly and disabled since 1965. Despite rapid and continued increases in budget allocation for this federally funded insurance program, many critical services—such as prescription drugs, home care, and long-term care—remain uncovered or insufficiently covered. In recent years, the proposal to offer prescription drug benefits under Medicare received strong bipartisan support in Congress. During the 2000 presidential election, candidates from both political parties championed the passage of prescription drug benefits for seniors. Since capturing the White House, President George W. Bush has made the provision of prescription drug benefits a legislative priority. Throughout 2003, various versions of the prescription drug plans were proposed in both the Senate and the House of Representatives. The two houses passed sepa-

TABLE 19–2
What Do You Gain Under the Medicare Prescription Benefit?*

If Annual Medications Costs Are ($):	You Pay ($)[†]	You Save ($)	Change in Out-of-Pocket Spending
500	32.50	0	47% more[‡]
1000	857.50	142.50	14% less
1500	982.50	517.50	35% less
2000	1107.50	892.50	45% less
2500	1420.00	1080.00	43% less
3000	1920.00	1080.00	36% less
5000	3920.00	1080.00	22% less
10,000	4265.00	5735.00	57% less

*How the voluntary drug benefit, to start in January 2006, will affect individual enrollees with no other drug insurance or low-income subsidies.
[†]Includes $250 annual deductible, estimated $35 monthly premium and different levels of co-payments.
[‡]Individual enrollees with drug costs of under $810 a year would pay more out of pocket than they would get back in subsidies.
Adapted from AARP Public Policy Institute.

rate versions of prescription drug plans in the fall of 2003, and the final legislation was passed by both the House and the Senate in late November 2003 (Table 19–2).

Policies to Contain Cost

During the last three decades, federal and state governments have tried a variety of cost-containment policies to restrain the cost of health care. Some of them were designed to regulate specific targets, such as the amount of capital investment in the hospital industry and the numbers of medical and nursing school graduates. Still others regulated the prices of specific services, such as physician fees and hospital reimbursement rates. A summary of these programs follows.

Certificate-of-Need (CON) Regulation

The Certificate-of-Need (CON) program was initiated in the early 1970s to control hospital costs. It aims at regulating hospital expenditures for new beds, equipment purchases, and facility constructions. CON requires that individuals or health-care facilities seeking to initiate or expand capacity or services submit applications to a state agency. Approval must be obtained before initiation of projects that require capital expenditures above certain dollar thresholds, introduction of new services, or expansion of bed numbers or services. The rationale is that excessive hospital growth—and the resulting need to maintain underutilized facilities—is the root cause of hospital cost inflation. Further, excess supply of hospital beds presents temptations for hospital administrators and physicians to increase hospital admissions so as to raise occupancy rates for hospitals and income for physicians. The CON approach to hospital cost control has had a modest effect on hospital costs, according to many health economists who studied the program (Salkever & Bice, 1979; Conover & Sloan, 1998). It is a very conservative approach to cost control, focusing on the hospitals and large medical practices only, and it provides no new incentives to change patient or physician behavior.

The Medicare PPS Program with DRGs

As mentioned earlier, the federal government changed its method of paying hospitals for treating Medicare patients in 1983, creating an incentive for hospitals to economize. PPS pays hospitals a fixed, predetermined sum of money for a particular admission. If a hospital can provide the service at a cost below the fixed amount, it pockets the difference. If more resources and money are used than the predetermined amount, the hospital incurs a loss. Under this payment system, whereby reimbursements are determined before treatment begins, hospitals are encouraged to shorten hospital stays and reduce use of unnecessary resources in order to keep costs below the predetermined reimbursement amounts.

Diagnostic-Related Groups

The reimbursement rates under PPS are determined by DRGs. Medicare patients who need hospitalization are admitted according to their initial diagnosis, one of 495 DRGs. Each DRG defines a medical condition and the related processes of care. Each DRG is assigned a flat payment rate based on the national average costs for that DRG.

The DRG rates vary according to several factors. For example, they are modified somewhat for different regions of the country to reflect differences in local wage rates. Rates are also higher for teaching hospitals, in recognition that their teaching and training functions necessitate higher costs. Finally, the DRG rates are adjusted annually by Medicare, subject to approval by Congress, to reflect changes in the health-care environment and the resulting increases in national norms of hospital costs.

Managed Care

As already discussed, managed care helps control cost by combining the financing and delivery of health services into one entity. Managed care was credited for playing a key role in slowing down the health inflation rates in the middle and late 1990s (Staines, 1993; Levit et al., 2000). Studies published since 2000 have revealed, however, that the cost-constraining effect of managed care was mostly "one time" in nature and did not last

as long as expected (Gabel et al., 2001; Levit et al., 2003 and 2004.)

Policies to Improve Quality

Quality has always been an important issue in health care. Historically, government involvement in quality improvement focused on the regulation of the professions in terms of licensing, educational requirements, and other issues related to the quality of providers. The quality of care was mostly left to the purview of private professional groups. For example, many hospitals historically have been monitored by the Joint Commission of Accreditation of Healthcare Organizations (JCAHO), with impressive results.

A major event in government involvement in outcome regulation occurred in 1972 with the creation of professional standards review organizations (PSROs). Part of the 1972 Medicare amendment to monitor the quality of federally funded care for Medicare beneficiaries, PSROs were to ensure that beneficiaries receive the most efficient and most appropriate services. In 1983, PSROs were replaced by peer review organizations (PROs). These were private, nonprofit organizations under contract with the Health Care Financing Administration (HCFA; now CMS) for utilization review and quality of care assessments of hospitals, HMOs, and some office practices.

After the backlash in the early 1990s against managed care and media reports of managed care mistreatment of patients and other related quality issues, President Bill Clinton signed an executive order in September 1996, creating the Presidential Advisory Commission on Consumer Protection and Quality in the Healthcare Industry. The President appointed a 32-person Commission to make recommendations on how to improve quality of health service delivery and reduce medical errors. In 1999, the reputable and influential Institute of Medicine (IOM) issued a controversial report, *To Err is Human: Building a Safer Health System* (IOM, 1999), which revealed, for the first time to the

American public, that between 44,000 and 98,000 people a year die unnecessarily as a result of medical errors in hospitals. In spring 2001, the IOM released another damning report, *Crossing the Quality Chasm: A new health system for the 21st Century* (IOM, 2001), which made recommendations for achieving threshold quality improvement in health-care delivery.

> *Nurses, as the largest number of health-care professionals, can participate in the evolution of the nation's health-care system to ensure long-term effectiveness.*

Encouraged by the release of a series of government reports and taking advantage of the advancement in the World Wide Web, many private health information providers have begun to offer on-line quality data on hospitals, nursing homes, and individual physicians. Today, anyone with access to a computer and the Internet can instantly obtain information on health-care quality. An example is the HealthGrade.com Web site *(http://www.healthgrades.com)*, which offers on-line quality information on hospitals, nursing homes, and physicians.

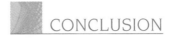

CONCLUSION

As nurses practice in the 21st century, they need to be acutely aware of the economic dimensions of providing health-care services. Nurses, as the largest number of health-care professionals, can participate in the evolution of the nation's health-care system to ensure long-term effectiveness.

Nurses are increasingly involved in the management of health-care delivery. As managers within organizations, nurses make managerial and financial decisions that affect not only the physical health of their patients but also the financial health of their organizations or agencies. To function effectively in the wider arena of health-care delivery, nurses must understand basic economic concepts such as supply, demand, market, and cost efficiency, the necessary tools to enable them to participate as well-prepared members of the health-care team. The combination of clinical expertise, knowledge of health-care delivery systems, and understanding of the economics of health care enables nurses to contribute to the design and evaluation of health care for groups of consumers.

ONLINE CONSULT

Summaries of the Institute of Medicine books can be accessed on-line as follows:

To Err is Human: Building a safer Health System
http://www.iom.edu/report.asp?id=5575

Crossing the Quality Chasm: a New Health System for the 21st Century
http://www.iom.edu/report.asp?id=5432

Keeping Patients Safe
http://www.iom.edu/report.asp?id=16173

Key Points

- Economics focuses on how consumers, business firms, government entities, and other organizations make choices in an environment of scarce resources.
- Health-care economics, a specialty area of economics, analyzes how the different parts of a health-care system work together to deliver service that meets the needs of patients.
- Demand in health care refers to the varying amount of health care that a consumer is willing and able to purchase at each of the possible prices.
- The supply of health-care service refers to the ability of providers to deliver health care.
- In a provider-driven system, the location of services, types of providers, and technology available are controlled by the dominant providers, such as physicians and hospitals.
- In a market-driven system, the providers' level of education and the locations and types of services provided are determined by the needs and location of consumers rather than the needs and location of providers.
- Third-party payers are insurance companies and government agencies that provide insurance coverage.
- The fee-for-service payment system gives providers maximum control over services provided to the consumer. Preapproval for services is usually not required in this system.
- The prospective payment system has emerged in response to concerns about access to health care and spiraling health-care costs. The federal Medicare program is an example of this system.
- A diagnosis-related group is a prospective pricing system based on a diagnostic classification system.
- Managed care, broadly defined, is a health-care system willing to be held accountable for both clinical and financial outcomes of an enrolled population.
- Managed care organizations are the entities that arrange for the provision of services for a group of individuals who are enrolled in the health plan.
- Capitation is a system in which MCOs are prospectively paid a per-member-per-month amount for a specified range of health services for enrolled individuals. These services are delivered either directly by the MCO or through a subcontract between the MCO and independent providers such as hospitals, clinics, doctors, and other health-care providers.
- A health maintenance organization (HMO) is a managed health plan that either administers or arranges for health care to be provided to its members for a capitated monthly fee.
- An independent practice association (IPA) is a type of HMO that enters into a contractual relationship with solo or group practitioners to provide physician and nurse practitioner services. IPAs are the fastest-growing type of HMO.
- A preferred provider organization (PPO) consists of networks of hospitals, private practice physicians, and other health-care practitioners that provide comprehensive health services to employers and their employees for a negotiated fee.
- A point-of-service plan combines HMO features such as capitation and coordination of service delivery with the PPO feature allowing enrollee choice of providers.
- A health report card is a summary of information of doctor and hospital performance and consumer satisfaction designed for consumers/patients and health-care buyers.
- Effectiveness measures how well a prescribed treatment has accomplished the anticipated outcomes.   (*continued*)

(*continued*)
- Cost-effectiveness measures whether the prescribed treatment has accomplished the desired outcome at the lowest possible cost.
- The American health-care system is far from ideal, and it suffers from a number of health system problems, including access, health cost, and quality disparities.
- Both the government and the private sector have experimented with a wide range of reform measures to improve access, contain cost, and improve health-care quality.

Thought and Discussion Questions

1. Discuss the values and demands for health care from the perspectives of:
   - An employer who is trying to choose a health plan.
   - An employee who will be using the services of the health plan.
2. Describe how you would evaluate the clinical effectiveness and cost-effectiveness of strategies designed to limit costs. Provide examples of nursing-sensitive patient outcomes.
3. Discuss how the movement to share with health-care providers the financial risk of providing care is changing patterns of practice in your community for:
   - Ambulatory services.
   - Hospital care.
   - Preventive services.
   - Rehabilitation.
4. Review the Chapter Thought at the beginning of the chapter, and be prepared to discuss its meaning in the context of the chapter.

Interactive Exercises

1. List the advantages and disadvantages of each of the following systems of supplying health care:
   - Provider-driven system
   - Market-driven system
   - Hybrid system
2. Form small groups or a panel for a debate or online chat. Have each member of the panel discuss the advantages and disadvantages of managed care as an organizational structure. Each group should have 5 to 6 members. Potential panel members:
   - MCO administrator
   - Executive of a large corporation that is purchasing health-care services
   - Older physician who has maintained a solo practice
   - Younger physician who is just completing residency
   - Older nurse considering retirement
   - Young hospital nurse

- Community health nurse
- Nurse assistant
- Labor union leader
- Older couple on Medicare
- Auto worker with a history of traditional fee-for-service insurance

3. Complete the Interactive Exercise Health Economics and Services Demanded By Consumers on the Intranet site. Be prepared to discuss your findings.

4. Complete the Interactive Exercise Market-Driven Forces in Your Health-care Facility located on the Intranet site. Be prepared to discuss your findings.

5. Look up the Patients' Bill of Rights. What kinds of tenets does it have? Do you believe such a bill of rights would help to resolve the problems posed by managed care?

PRINT REFERENCES

Aiken, L. H., Smith, H. L., & Lake, E. T. (1994). Lower Medicare mortality among a set of hospitals known for good nursing care. *Medical Care*, 32(8), 771–787.

Alsever, J. D., Ritchey, T., & Lima, N. P. (1995). Developing a hospital report card to demonstrate value in health care. *Journal of Health Care Quality*, 17(1), 19–25.

American Nurses Association. (1995a). *Report and recommendations on Joint Congress Task Force on Quality Indicators*. Congress of Nursing Practice and Congress on Nursing Economics, June 1995.

American Nurses Association. (1995b). *Nursing report card for acute care*. Washington, DC: American Nurses Publishing.

Anderson, F. G., Reinhardt, U. E., Hussey, P. S., Petrosyan, V. (2003) It's the prices, stupid: Why the United States is so different from other countries. *Health Affairs*, 22(3), 89–105.

Blancett, S. S., & Flarey, D. L. (1995). *Reengineering nursing and health care: The handbook for organizational transformation*. Gaithersburg, MD: Aspen.

Blegen, M. A., Goode, C. J., & Reed, L. (1998). Nurse staffing and patient outcomes. *Nursing Research*, 47(1), 43–50.

Chang, C. F., Price, S. A., & Pfoutz, S. K. (2001). *Economics and nursing: Critical professional issues*. Philadelphia: FA Davis.

Cleverley, W. O. (1995). *The 1995 almanac of hospital financial and operating indicators*. Columbus, OH: Center for Health Care Industry Performance Studies.

Conover, C. J., and Sloan, F. (1998). Does removing certificate of need regulations lead to a surge in health care spending? *Journal of Health Politics, Policy and Law*, 23, 455–481.

Eisenberg, D. M., Kessler, R. C., Foster, C., Norlock, F. E., Calkins, D. R., & Delbanco, T. L. (1993). Unconventional medicine in the United States: Prevalence, costs and patterns of use. *New England Journal of Medicine*, 328(4), 246–252.

Folland, S., Goodman, A. C., & Stano, M. (2001). *The economics of health and health care* (3rd ed.). Upper Saddle River, NJ: Prentice-Hall.

Fox, P. D. (2001). An overview of managed health care. In P. R. Kongsvedt (Ed.), *Essentials of managed health care* (4th ed., pp. 3–16). Gaithersburg, MD: Aspen Publishers, Inc.

Fuchs, V. R. (1993). *The future of health policy*. Cambridge, MA: Harvard Press.

Gabel, J., Levitt, L., Pickreign, J., Whitmore, H., Holve, E., Rowland, D., Dhont, K., & Hawkins, S. (2001). Job-based health insurance in 2001: Inflation hits double digits, managed care retreats. *Health Affairs*, 20(5), 180–186.

Henry J. Kaiser Family Foundation. (2002). *Trends and indicators in the changing health care marketplace 2002*. Menlo Park, CA: Author.

Institute of Medicine. (1999). *To err is human: Building a safer health system*. Washington, DC: National Academy of Science.

Institute of Medicine. (2001). *Crossing the quality chasm: A new health system for the 21st century*. Washington, DC: National Academy of Science.

Levit, K., Cowan, C., Lazenby, H., Sensenig, A., McDonnell, P., Stiller, J., & Martin, A. (2000). Health spending in 1998: signals of change, *Health Affairs*, 19(1),124–132.

Levit, K., Smith, C., Cowan, C., Lazenby, H., Sensenig, A., & Catlin, A. (2003). Trends in U.S. health care spending, 2001. *Health Affairs*, 22(1): 154–164.

Levit, K., Smith, C., Cowan, C., Sensenig, A., Catlin, A., & the Health Accounts Team. (2004). Health spending rebound continues in 2002. *Health Affairs*, 23(1),147–159.

Medicode. (2003). *Almanac of Hospital Financial and Operating Indicators 2003*. Salt Lack City, UT: Ingenix.

National Center for Health Statistics. (1997). *Employer-sponsored health insurance*. Hyattsville, MD: Author.

Park, C. H. (2000). Prevalence of employer self-insured health benefits. *Medical Care Research and Review*, 57(3), 340–360.

Salkever, D. S., & Bice, T. W. (1979). *Hospital certificate-of-need controls: Impact on investment, costs, and use.* Washington, DC: American Enterprise Institute.

Staines, V. S. (1993). Potential impact of managed care on national health spending. *Health Affairs* 12(Suppl), 249–257.

U.S. Bureau of Census (2003). *Health insurance coverage in the United States, 2002.* Washington, DC: Author.

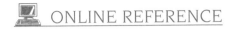 ONLINE REFERENCE

Center for Medicare and Medicaid Services (CMS). Health care system: facts and figures. *http://cms.hhs.gov/charts/healthcaresystem/*

Robin S. Vogt

20
chapter

Protecting the Populace

> Every nation, in every region, now has a decision to make. Either you are with us, or you are with the terrorists.
>
> *George W. Bush, September 20, 2001.*

Chapter Objectives

On completion of this chapter, the reader will be able to:

1. List the five areas of the Centers for Disease Control and Prevention's plan for bioterrorism.
2. List the categories of biologic agents used in bioterrorism and the agents in each category.
3. Define each biologic agent and discuss the symptoms and communicability of the agent.
4. Describe your community's bioterrorism plan.
5. List the categories of chemical agents.
6. Discuss the initial treatment, assessment, and identification of the patient with suspected chemical exposure.

Key Terms

Bioterrorism
Category A Agents
Category B Agents
Category C Agents
Chemical Agents
Smallpox
Anthrax
Plague
Botulism
Tularemia
Filoviruses

Arenaviruses
Q fever
Brucellosis
Glanders
Alphaviruses
Ricinus Communis
Epsilon Toxin of
    Clostridium Perfringens
Enterotoxin B
Nipah Virus
Hantavirus

Tickborne Hemorrhagic
    Fever Viruses
Tickborne Encephalitis
    Viruses
Yellow Fever
Multidrug-Resistant
    Tuberculosis
Chemical Weapons
Personal Protective
    Equipment (PPE)

Historically, there have been numerous attempts at biologic and chemical terrorism. It is documented that as early as 6th century BC, the Assyrians poisoned the wells of their enemies with rye ergot. In the 15th century, during his conquest of South America, Pizarro improved his chances of victory by presenting to the natives, as gifts, clothing laden with the variola virus. In 1767, during the French and Indian War, the English general Sir Jeffrey Amherst gave blankets laced with smallpox to Indians loyal to the French. The epidemic devastated the tribes, resulting in a successful British attack on Fort Carillon. In 1940, the Japanese released plague bacteria at Chuhsien, resulting in the deaths of 21 people. During the Vietnam War in the 1960s, the Vietcong used feces-contaminated spear traps (Eitzen & Takafuji, 1997).

In 1978, Georgi Markov, a Bulgarian exile living in London, was injected in the leg with a steel ball impregnated with ricin. He died 3 days later. In 1995, it was reported that on at least ten occasions, Aum Shinrikyo attempted to disperse anthrax, botulinum toxin, Q fever, and Ebola virus against the mass population and authority figures in Japan; no reported infections occurred. And in 2001, a 38 year-old assistant to NBC anchorman Tom Brokaw, handled a letter containing white powder, which turned out to be the cause of the first case of cutaneous anthrax (Biological Terrorism Response Manual, 2001).

It is a good life for a germ in here ... here in this flask it's very, very sweet .... [B]ugs do what they do best ... Eat and multiply, eat and multiply, over and over. ... Bacillus anthracis ... growing ... trillions of anthrax cells. Taken from the cozy dark they are poured onto a flat tray where warm air blows: a drying cabinet ... it forms spores. When dried and milled into lethal fineness, the resulting powder will be, ounce per ounce, more deadly than any explosive—and "smarter" than the most expertly programmed smart bomb. (Osterholm & Schwartz, 2001)

Biologic terrorism and chemical terrorism are common terms in today's society. Since September 11, 2001, we have realized that these events can and do truly occur. It is critical for the nursing professional to be aware of current threats of terrorism with biologic and chemical agents. As technology and knowledge progress, so do the threats to society. Being educated and knowledgeable on how to handle and identify situations that arise has become necessary as core knowledge for the nursing professional. Nurses can provide leadership to other health-care professionals in the identification and care of patients exposed to biologic and chemical agents.

BIOLOGIC AND CHEMICAL PREPAREDNESS

Nursing leaders recognize the need for preparedness and identification of diseases. English and colleagues (1999) developed a template to help prepare health-care professionals for bioterrorism. After all, health-care clinics and nurses may have the first opportunity to respond to a bioterrorism outbreak. Being informed about the most likely agents used, their symptoms, and immediate treatment will help prepare communities in the fight against terrorism. Being prepared also entails understanding your own community's emergency response system. Such systems vary from locality to locality, depending on investment in public health. Preparedness provides the best civil defense against bioterrorism (Henderson, 1997).

Federal Mandates

Before September 11, 2001, Congress had passed three major laws aimed at preventing the acquisition and use of chemical or biologic weapons:

- The Biological Weapons Act of 1989 made it a federal crime to knowingly develop, manufacture, transfer, or possess any biologic agent, toxin, or delivery system for use as a weapon (Public Law, 101–298).

- The Chemical and Biological Weapons Control Act of 1991 (CBWCA) established a system of economic and export controls preventing the export of goods or technologies used in the development of chemical and biologic weapons to designated nations (Public Law, 102–82).
- The Anti-Terrorism and Effective Death Penalty Act of 1996 expanded the government's powers under CBWCA to cover individuals or groups who attempt or even threaten to develop or use a biologic weapon (Public Law, 104–32).

The Centers for Disease Control and Prevention (CDC) was charged with establishing regulations to supplement and detail these laws. CDC's regulations, which took effect April 15, 1997, identified 24 microorganisms and 12 toxins. Possession of these microorganisms or toxins requires registration with CDC, and their transfer involves filing out of forms by both shipper and receiver (CDC, 1997).

On June 12, 2002, President George W. Bush signed into law the Public Health Security and Bioterrorism Preparedness and Response Act of 2002 (Public Law 107–188).

Military and troop protection has been of greatest concern for risk of bioterrorism. Protecting civilians differs from protecting the military. In the civilian population, there is a wide variation of age groups and health concerns. There may be more vulnerability in foodborne or waterborne terrorism in the civilian population. It is because of these differences that an attack on civilians may have greater consequences than an attack on military personnel. Agencies must work together to plan for public protection in the civilian population.

Building on the USA Patriot Act (Public Law 107–56), the new law was aimed at preventing, preparing for, and responding to a bioterrorist attack against the United States.

Role of the Centers for Disease Control and Prevention

As part of a Congressional initiative started in 1999 to upgrade national public health capabilities for response to acts of biologic terrorism, the CDC was designated the lead agency for overall public health planning. On the basis of the overall criteria and weighting, biologic agents were assigned to one of three priority categories, A through C, for initial public health preparedness efforts.

The CDC has also established a multilevel laboratory response network for bioterrorism that links public health agencies to advanced-capacity facilities for the identification and reporting of critical biologic agents (CDC, 1998). They have established regional chemical terrorism laboratories that will provide diagnostic capacity during terrorist attacks involving chemical agents. And, they have established a rapid-response laboratory within the CDC to provide around-the-clock diagnostic support to bioterrorism response teams and to expedite molecular characterization of critical biologic agents.

The CDC has also created an action plan (1998) focusing on five specific areas:

1. Preparedness and prevention
2. Detection and surveillance
3. Diagnosis and characterization of biologic and chemical agents
4. Response
5. Communication

This chapter concentrates on the third focus by covering the most likely biologic and

---

ONLINE CONSULT

Bioterrorism Readiness and Response: Levels of Personal Protective Equipment.
http://www.unmc.edu/bioterrorism/equipment.htm

chemical threats: their definitions, symptoms, and communicability.

AGENTS

It is important for nurses to be familiar with the agents—both chemical and biologic—that have the greatest potential to be used in an act of terror.

Biologic Agents

> **Bioterrorism** is defined as the use of microorganisms that cause human disease, or the toxins released from them, to harm people or elicit widespread fear or intimidation of society. … Biodefense research is similar to other emerging infectious diseases. It entails research to understand the pathogenesis of these microbes, how the host responds to them, and the translation of this knowledge into useful treatments, diagnostics, and vaccines. (Southwest Regional Center of Excellence for Biodefense, 2003)

Biologic agents used by terrorists are divided into three categories, A, B, and C. They are categorized according to priority (CDC 1998).

Category A agents are "high-priority" agents. They pose a risk because they:

- Can be easily transmitted from person-to-person.
- Cause high mortality and potential for a major public health impact.

- May cause public panic and social disruption.
- Require special action for public health preparedness.

Category B agents, the second-highest-priority agents, pose a risk because they:

- Are moderately easy to disseminate.
- Cause moderate morbidity and low mortality.
- Require specific enhancements of CDC's diagnostic capacity and enhanced disease surveillance.

Category C agents, are the third-highest-priority agents, include emerging pathogens that could be engineered for mass dissemination in the future because of:

- Availability.
- Ease of production and dissemination.
- Potential for high morbidity and mortality and a major health impact.

Examples of agents in all three categories are listed in Table 20–1

Chemical Agents

Chemical agents may range from warfare agents to toxic chemicals commonly used in the industry. "Priority" chemical agents include those that:

 ONLINE CONSULT

Category A, B, and C biologic agents.
http://www.bt.cdc.gov/agent/agentlistcategory.asp

 ONLINE CONSULT

Chemical terrorism agents.
http://www.bt.cdc.gov/agent/agentlistchem.asp
Bioterrorism Readiness and Response: Levels of Personal Protective Equipment.
http://www.unmc.edu/bioterrorism/equipment.htm

TABLE 20–1
Biologic Agents with Potential as Terrorist Weapons

Category A	Variola major (smallpox)
	Bacillus anthracis (anthrax)
	Yersinia pestis (plague)
	Clostridium botulinum toxin (botulism)
	Francisella tularensis (tularemia)
	Filoviruses:
	• Ebola hemorrhagic fever
	• Marburg hemorrhagic fever
	Arenaviruses:
	• Lassa (Lassa fever)
	• Junin (Argentine hemorrhagic fever) and related viruses
Category B	*Coxiella burnetii* (Q fever)
	Brucella species (brucellosis)
	Burkholderia mallei (glanders)
	Alphaviruses:
	• Venezuelan encephalomyelitis
	• Eastern and western equine encephalomyelitis
	Ricin toxin from *Ricinus communis* (castor beans)
	Epsilon toxin of *Clostridium perfringens*
	Staphylococcus enterotoxin B
	Others in this group include pathogens that are food or waterborne.
Category C	Nipah virus
	Hantaviruses
	Tickborne hemorrhagic fever viruses
	Tickborne encephalitis viruses
	Yellow fever
	Multidrug-resistant tuberculosis

- Are chemical agents already known to be used as weapons.
- Are available to potential terrorists.
- Are likely to cause major morbidity or mortality.
- Have potential to cause public panic and social disruption.
- Require special action for public health preparedness.

Chemical agents that have potential to be used by terrorists are listed in Table 20–2.

Hundreds of new chemicals are produced monthly. Varied combinations of chemicals produce new threats each month, making it impossible to keep track of all newly developed chemicals. This situation, as well as the limited capability of antiterrorist groups to detect new chemical weapons, creates an advantage in the use of chemicals for warfare. Treatment of suspected chemical terrorism or exposure should focus on the clinical syndrome rather than the specific agent. Because response plans vary by community, their consideration is beyond the scope of this chapter. One of the most important steps nurses can take to be prepared, however, is to become familiar with biologic and chemical

TABLE 20–2
Chemical Agents with Potential as Terrorist Weapons

Nerve agents	Tabun Sarin Soman GF (cyclohexylmethylphosphonofluoridate) VX (o-ethyl-{S}-{2-diisopropylaminoethyl} methylphosphonothiolate)
Blood agents	Hydrogen cyanide Cyanogen chloride
Blister agents	Lewisite Nitrogen and sulfur mustards Phosgene oxime
Heavy metals	Arsenic Lead Mercury
Volatile toxins	Benzene Chloroform Trihalomethanes
Pulmonary agents	Phosgene Chlorine Vinyl chloride
Incapacitating agents	BZ (3-quinuclidinyl benzilate)
Pesticides, persistent and nonpersistent	Tetraethyl pyrophosphate (TEPP) Parathion
Dioxins, furans, and polychlorinated biphenyls (PCBs)	Organochlorines (industrial byproducts)
Explosive nitro compounds and oxidizers	Ammonium nitrate combined with fuel oil
Flammable industrial gases and liquids	Gasoline Propane
Poison industrial gases, liquids and solids	Cyanides Nitriles
Corrosive industrial acids and bases	Nitric acid Sulfuric acid

agents. These agents are reviewed in detail below.

 BIOLOGIC TERRORISM

Category A, B, and C biologic agents are described here by definition, symptom, and communicability.

Category A Agents

These agents are considered by the CDC to have the highest priority. The following information has been extracted from the CDC Website on bioterrorism.

Smallpox

Definition

Smallpox is a serious, contagious, and often fatal infectious disease caused by the variola virus (CDC, 2003p). There is no specific treatment, and currently, the only prevention is vaccination. The name *smallpox* is derived from the Latin word for "spotted" and refers to the raised bumps that appear on the face and body of an infected person. There are two clinical forms of smallpox, variola major and variola minor. Variola major is the more severe (and more common) form with an extensive rash and higher fever. The fatality rate is 30 percent. Variola minor is a less severe form with only about 1 percent fatality rate.

Symptoms

The normal incubation period for smallpox is 12 to 14 days but may range from 7 to 17 days. First symptoms include, fever (sometimes high [101–104° F]), malaise, head and body aches, and vomiting. The person is usually too sick to engage in normal activities. This "prodrome phase" may last 2 to 4 days.

A rash follows the prodrome phase. It spreads and progresses to raised bumps that crust, scab, and fall off after about 3 weeks, leaving pitted scars. Usually, the greatest concentration of these bumps is on the face and extremities. Most of the lesions are deep-seated, firm, round, and well-defined. The bumps are all in the same stage of development on any part of the body.

Communicability

Generally, direct and fairly prolonged face-to-face contact is required to spread smallpox from one person to another. Smallpox also can be spread through direct contact with infected bodily fluids or contaminated objects, such as bedding and clothing. Rarely, smallpox has been spread through the air in enclosed settings such as buildings, buses, and trains. Humans are the only natural hosts of variola. Smallpox is not known to be transmitted by insects or animals. The person is contagious from the first appearance of the rash until the last scab falls off. If there is an outbreak of smallpox, a person experiencing symptoms of the prodrome should be isolated until the onset of a rash or until smallpox can be ruled out in order to decrease the spread of this disease.

Anthrax

Definition

Bacillus anthracis, the etiologic agent of **anthrax**, is a large, gram-positive, nonmotile, spore-forming bacterial rod. Human anthrax has three major clinical forms: cutaneous, inhalation, and gastrointestinal. If left untreated, anthrax in all forms can lead to septicemia and death (CDC, 2003d).

Symptoms (Divided by Type)

Cutaneous anthrax is the most common naturally occurring type of infection (>95%) and usually occurs after skin contact with contaminated meat, wool, hides, or leather from infected animals. The incubation period ranges from 1 to 12 days. The skin infection begins as a small papule, which progresses to a vesicle in 1 to 2 days and is followed by a necrotic ulcer. The lesion is usually painless, but patients may also have fever, malaise, headache, and regional lymphadenopathy. Most anthrax infections (about 95%) occur when the bacterium enters a cut or abrasion on the skin. Skin infection begins as a raised bump that resembles a spider bite, but (within 1–2 days) it develops into a vesicle and then a painless ulcer, usually 1 to 3 cm in diameter, with a characteristic black necrotic area in the center. Lymph glands in the adjacent area may swell. About 20 percent of untreated cases of cutaneous anthrax result in death. Deaths are rare if patients are given appropriate antimicrobial therapy.

Inhalational anthrax is the most lethal form of anthrax. Anthrax spores must be aerosolized in order to cause inhalational anthrax. The number of spores needed to cause human infection is unknown. The incubation period of inhalational anthrax among humans is unclear, but it is reported to range from 1 to 7 days, possibly up to 60 days. Inhalational anthrax resembles a viral respiratory illness, initial symptoms being sore throat, mild fever, muscle aches, and malaise. These symptoms may progress to respiratory failure and shock, frequently with development of meningitis.

Gastrointestinal anthrax, which usually follows the consumption of raw or undercooked contaminated meat, has an incubation period of 1–7 days. It is associated with severe abdominal distress followed by fever and signs of septicemia. The disease can take an oropharyngeal or abdominal form. Lesions at the base of the tongue, sore throat, dysphagia, fever, and regional lymphadenopathy usually characterize involvement of the pharynx.

Lower bowel inflammation usually causes nausea, loss of appetite, vomiting and fever, followed by abdominal pain, vomiting blood, and bloody diarrhea.

Communicability

Anthrax is not contagious; the illness cannot be transmitted from person to person.

Plague

Definition

Plague is an infectious disease of animals and humans caused by the bacterium *Yersinia pestis.* This bacterium is found in rodents and their fleas and occurs in many areas of the world, including the United States (CDC, 2003k).

Symptoms (Divided by Type)

- *Bubonic plague:* Enlarged, tender lymph nodes, fever, chills, and prostration.
- *Septicemic plague:* Fever, chills, prostration, abdominal pain, shock, and bleeding into skin and other organs.
- *Pneumonic plague:* Fever, chills, cough and difficulty breathing; rapid shock, and death if not treated early.

Communicability

Bubonic plague is usually transmitted to humans by the bites of infected rodent fleas. During rodent plague outbreaks, many animals die and their hungry fleas seek other sources of blood to survive. People and animals that visit places where rodents have

 ONLINE CONSULT

Check the Web site showing state-by-state numbers of individuals vaccinated against smallpox. How does your state compare?
http://www.cdc.gov/od/oc/media/spvaccin.htm

recently died from plague risk getting the disease from fleabites. Persons also can become directly infected through handling of infected rodents, rabbits, or wild carnivores that prey on these animals, when plague bacteria enter through breaks in the skin. House cats are also susceptible to plague. Infected cats become sick and may transmit plague directly to persons who handle or care for them. Also, dogs and cats may bring plague-infected fleas into the home. *Y. pestis* is easily destroyed by sunlight and drying. Even so, when released into air, the bacterium will survive for up to 1 hour, although this period may vary with conditions. Inhaling droplets expelled by the coughing of a plague-infected person or animal (especially a house cat) can result in plague of the lungs (plague pneumonia). Transmission of plague pneumonia from person to person is uncommon but sometimes results in dangerous epidemics that can spread quickly.

Botulism

Definition

Botulism is a muscle-paralyzing disease caused by a toxin made by a bacterium called *Clostridium botulinum*. The three main kinds of botulism are as follows:

- *Foodborne botulism* occurs when a person ingests pre-formed toxin that leads to illness within a few hours to days. Foodborne botulism is a public health emergency because the contaminated food may still be available to other persons besides the patient.
- *Infant botulism* occurs in a small number of susceptible infants each year who harbor *C. botulinum* in their intestinal tracts.
- *Wound botulism* occurs when wounds are infected with *C. botulinum* that secretes the toxin (CDC, 2003f).

Symptoms

The classic symptoms of botulism are double vision, blurred vision, drooping eyelids, slurred speech, difficulty swallowing, dry mouth, and muscle weakness. Infants with botulism appear lethargic, feed poorly, are constipated, and have a weak cry and poor muscle tone. These are all symptoms of the muscle paralysis caused by the bacterial toxin. If untreated, these symptoms may progress to cause paralysis of the arms, legs, trunk, and respiratory muscles. In foodborne botulism, symptoms generally begin 18 to 36 hours after consumption of contaminated food, but they can occur as early as 6 hours or as late as 10 days.

Communicability

Botulism is not spread from one person to another. Foodborne botulism follows ingestion of toxin produced in food by *C. botulinum*. The most common source is home-canned food prepared in an unsafe manner. Wound botulism occurs when *C. botulinum* spores germinate within wounds. Intestinal colonization botulism occurs when *C. botulinum* spores germinate and produce toxin in the gastrointestinal tract.

Tularemia

Definition

Tularemia is an infectious disease caused by a hardy bacterium, *Francisella tularensis*, found in animals (especially rodents, rabbits, and hares) (CDC, 2003n).

Symptoms

Symptoms of tularemia include sudden fever, chills, headaches, muscle aches, joint pain, dry cough, progressive weakness, and pneumonia. People with pneumonia may experience chest pain and bloody spit, and may have trouble breathing or sometimes stop breathing. Other symptoms of tularemia depend on how a person was exposed to the tularemia bacteria. They can include ulcers on the skin or mouth, swollen and painful lymph glands, swollen and painful eyes, and a sore throat. Symptoms usually appear 3 to 5 days after exposure to the bacteria but can take as long as 14 days to manifest.

Communicability

Tularemia is not known to be spread from person to person, so people who have tularemia do not need to be isolated. People who have been exposed to *F. tularensis* should be treated as soon as possible. The disease can be fatal if it is not treated with the appropriate antibiotics. The most common means of contracting the disease is inoculation through the skin or mucous membranes from infected deer flies or ticks or insufficiently cooked rabbit meat.

Viral Hemorrhagic Fevers

Viral hemorrhagic fevers (VHFs) are a group of illnesses caused by several distinct families of viruses. In general, the term *viral hemorrhagic fever* is used to describe a severe multisystem syndrome. Characteristically, the overall vascular system is damaged, and the body's ability to regulate itself is impaired. These symptoms are often accompanied by hemorrhage; however, the bleeding is rarely life-threatening. Although some types of hemorrhagic fever viruses can cause relatively mild illnesses, many cause severe, life-threatening disease. This latter category includes the filoviruses and arenaviruses.

Filoviruses

DEFINITION

Filoviruses belong to a virus family called Filoviridae and can cause severe hemorrhagic fever in humans and nonhuman primates. So far, only two members of this virus family have been identified: *Marburg* virus and *Ebola* virus. Four species of Ebola virus have been identified: Ivory Coast, Sudan, Zaire, and Reston. Ebola-Reston virus is the only known filovirus that does not cause severe disease in humans (CDC, 2003h).

SYMPTOMS

People infected with Ebola virus have sudden fever, weakness, muscle pain, headache, and sore throat, followed by vomiting, diarrhea, rash, limited kidney and liver functions, and both internal and external bleeding. Death rates range from 50 to 90 percent.

Symptoms of Marburg virus occur after an incubation period of 5 to 10 days. The onset of the disease is sudden and is marked by fever, chills, headache, and myalgia. Around the fifth day after the onset of symptoms, a maculopapular rash, most prominent on the trunk, may occur. Nausea, vomiting, chest pain, a sore throat, abdominal pain, and diarrhea then may appear. Symptoms become increasingly severe and may include jaundice, inflammation of the pancreas, severe weight loss, delirium, shock, liver failure, massive hemorrhaging, and multiple-organ dysfunction.

COMMUNICABILITY

Viruses causing hemorrhagic fever are initially transmitted to humans when the activities of infected reservoir hosts or vectors and humans overlap. The viruses carried in rodent reservoirs are transmitted when humans have contact with urine, fecal matter, saliva, or other body excretions from infected rodents. The viruses associated with arthropod vectors are spread most often when the vector mosquito or tick bites a human or a human crushes a tick. However, some of these vectors may spread the virus to animals, such as livestock; humans then become infected when they care for or slaughter the animals.

Once a human is infected, person-to-person transmission is the means by which further infections occur. Specifically, transmission involves close personal contact between an infected individual or their body fluids and another person. During recorded outbreaks of hemorrhagic fever due to filovirus infection, people who cared for or worked very closely with infected individuals were especially at risk of becoming infected themselves. Nosocomial transmission, through contact with infected body fluids via reuse of unsterilized syringes, needles, or other medical equipment contaminated with these fluids, has also been an important factor in the spread of disease. When close contact between uninfected and infected persons is minimized, the number of new filovirus infections in humans usually declines. Although in the laboratory the viruses display some capability of infection through small-particle aerosols, airborne spread among humans has not been clearly demonstrated.

Arenaviruses

DEFINITION

The Arenaviridae family of viruses (**arenaviruses**) is generally associated with rodent-transmitted disease in humans. Each virus usually is associated with a particular rodent host species in which it is maintained. Arenavirus infections are relatively common in humans in some areas of the world and can cause severe illnesses (CDC, 2003e). Lassa fever is the most common type of Arenavirus.

SYMPTOMS

Signs and symptoms of Lassa fever typically occur 1 to 3 weeks after the patient comes into contact with the virus. These include fever, retrosternal pain (pain behind the chest wall), sore throat, back pain, cough, abdominal pain, vomiting, diarrhea, conjunctivitis, facial swelling, proteinuria, and mucosal bleeding. Neurologic problems have also been described, such as hearing loss, tremors, and encephalitis. The symptoms of Lassa fever are so varied and nonspecific, however, that clinical diagnosis is often difficult.

The incubation period of Lassa fever infection is usually between 8 and 13 days. A characteristic biphasic febrile illness then follows. The initial phase, which may last as long as a week, typically begins with any or all of the following symptoms: fever, malaise, anorexia, muscle aches, headache, nausea, and vomiting. Other, less common symptoms are sore throat, cough, and joint, chest, testicular, and

parotid pain. After a few days of remission, the second phase of the disease occurs, consisting of symptoms of meningitis or characteristics of encephalitis.

COMMUNICABILITY

The viruses are shed into the environment in the urine or droppings of their infected hosts. Human infection with arenaviruses is incidental to the natural cycle of the viruses and occurs when an individual comes into contact with the excretions or materials contaminated with the excretions of an infected rodent, such as ingestion of contaminated food, or through direct contact of abraded or broken skin with rodent excrement. Infection can also occur through inhalation of tiny particles soiled with rodent urine or saliva. The types of incidental contact depend on the habits of both humans and rodents.

Some arenaviruses, such as Lassa and Machupo viruses, are associated with secondary person-to-person or nosocomial transmission. This occurs when a person infected by exposure to the virus from the rodent host spreads the virus to other humans, in a variety of ways. Person-to-person transmission is associated with direct contact with the blood or other excretions of infected individuals that contain virus particles. Airborne transmission has also been reported in connection with certain viruses. Contact with objects contaminated with these materials, such as medical equipment, is also associated with transmission.

> *According to the World Health Organization (WHO), 143 cases of Ebola virus had been reported, including 128 deaths, in the districts of Mbomo and Kéllé in the Cuvette Ouest Département by May 2003. Thirteen of the cases were confirmed by laboratory tests, and 130 were epidemiologically linked (WHO, 2003).*

Category B

Category B agents are CDC's next level of priority as illustrated in the following extracts.

Coxiella burnetii (Q Fever)

Definition

Q fever is a zoonotic disease caused by *Coxiella burnetii*, a species of bacteria that is distributed globally. In 1999, Q fever became a notifiable disease in the United States, but reporting cases of Q fever is not required in many other countries. Because the disease is underreported, scientists cannot reliably assess how many cases of Q fever have actually occurred worldwide. Many human infections are not apparent. Cattle, sheep, and goats are the primary reservoirs of *C. burnetii*. Infection has been noted in a wide variety of other animals, including other breeds of livestock and domesticated pets. Humans are often very susceptible to the disease, and very few organisms may be required to cause infection (CDC, 2003f).

Symptoms

Only about half of all people infected with *C. burnetii* show signs of clinical illness. Most acute cases of Q fever begin with sudden onset of one or more of the following: high fevers (up to 104 to 105° F), severe headache, general malaise, myalgia, confusion, sore throat, chills, sweats, nonproductive cough, nausea, vomiting, diarrhea, abdominal pain, and chest pain. Fever usually lasts for 1 to 2 weeks. Weight loss can occur and persist for some time. Thirty to 50 percent of patients with a symptomatic infection experience pneumonia. Additionally, a majority of patients have abnormal results of liver function tests, and some have hepatitis. Most patients recover to good health within several months without any treatment. Only 1 to 2 percent of people with acute Q fever die of the disease.

Communicability

In the United States, Q fever outbreaks have resulted mainly from occupational exposure of veterinarians, workers in meat-processing plants, sheep and dairy workers, livestock farmers, and researchers at facilities housing sheep. Prevention and control efforts should be directed primarily toward these groups and environments.

Coxiella burnetii is a highly infectious agent that is rather resistant to heat and drying. It can become airborne and inhaled by humans. A single *C. burnetii* organism may cause disease in a susceptible person.

Brucella Species (Brucellosis)

Definition

Brucellosis is an infectious disease caused by bacteria of the genus *Brucella*. These bacteria are primarily passed among animals, and they cause disease in many different vertebrates. Various *Brucella* species affect sheep, goats, cattle, deer, elk, pigs, dogs, and several other animals. Humans become infected by coming in contact with animals or animal products that are contaminated with the bacteria. In humans, brucellosis can cause a range of symptoms similar to those of the flu—fever, sweats, headaches, back pains, and physical weakness. Severe infections of the central nervous systems or lining of the heart may occur. Brucellosis can also cause long-lasting or chronic symptoms such as recurrent fevers, joint pain, and fatigue (CDC, 2003g).

Symptoms

Symptoms of brucellosis are extremely variable. Symptoms of the acute form (<8 weeks from illness onset) are nonspecific and "flu-like," including fever, sweats, malaise, anorexia, headache, myalgia, back pain, and, uncommonly, death. In the undulant form (<1 year from illness onset), symptoms include undulant fevers, arthritis, and orchiepididymitis. Neurologic symptoms may occur acutely in up to 5 percent of cases. Symptoms of the chronic form (>1 year from onset) include chronic fatigue syndrome–like, depressive episodes, and arthritis.

Communicability

Transmission of brucellosis is zoonotic, commonly through abrasions of the skin from handling infected mammals. In the United States, transmission occurs more frequently through ingestion of contaminated milk and dairy products. The disease is highly infectious in the laboratory via aerosolization. Direct person-to-person spread of brucellosis is extremely rare. Mothers who are breast-feeding may transmit the infection to their infants. Sexual transmission has also been reported.

Burkholderia mallei (Glanders)

Definition

Glanders is an infectious disease caused by the bacterium *Burkholderia mallei.* Primarily a disease affecting horses, it also affects donkeys and mules and can be contracted naturally by goats, dogs, and cats. Human infection, although not seen in the United States since 1945, has occurred rarely and sporadically among laboratory workers and people in direct and prolonged contact with infected, domestic animals (CDC, 2003i).

Symptoms

The symptoms of glanders depend on the route of infection with the organism. The types of infection are localized, pus-forming cutaneous infections, pulmonary infections, blood-stream infections, and chronic suppurative infections of the skin. Generalized symptoms of glanders include fever, muscle aches, chest pain, muscle tightness, and headache. Additional symptoms are excessive tearing of the eyes, light sensitivity, and diarrhea.

- *Localized infections:* If there is a cut or scratch in the skin, a localized infection with ulceration will develop within 1 to 5 days at the site where the bacteria entered the body. Swollen lymph nodes may also be apparent. Infections involving the mucous membranes in the eyes, nose, and respiratory tract cause increased mucous production from the affected sites.
- *Pulmonary infections:* In pulmonary infections, pneumonia, pulmonary abscesses, and pleural effusion can occur. Chest x-rays show localized infection in the lobes of the lungs.
- *Blood-stream infections:* Glanders blood stream infections are usually fatal within 7 to 10 days. Generally, symptoms are respiratory distress, severe headache, fever, diarrhea, development of pus-filled lesions on the skin, muscle tenderness, and disorientation.
- *Chronic infections:* The chronic form of glanders involves multiple abscesses within the muscles of the arms and legs or in the spleen or liver.

Communicability

Glanders is transmitted to humans through direct contact with infected animals. The bacteria enter the body through the skin or through mucosal surfaces of the eyes and nose. The sporadic cases have been documented in veterinarians, horse caretakers, and laboratory workers. In addition to animal exposure, cases of human-to-human transmission have been reported, including two suggested cases of sexual transmission and several cases in family members who cared for the patients.

Alphaviruses

The **alphaviruses** include Venezuelan encephalomyelitis (VEE) and Eastern and Western equine encephalomyelitis (EEE and WEE, respectively).

Definition

WEE is a member of the antigenically similar group of viruses known as Togaviridae, which encompasses EEE and VEE. These alphaviruses are spherical and have a diameter of 60 to 65 nm (CDC, 2003c).

Symptoms

Diffuse central nervous system involvement characterizes WEE in its more severe stages. The large number of immunologically active cells that enter the brain parenchyma and perivascular areas mediate much of the damage. Focal necrosis is often found in the striatum, globus pallidus, cerebral cortex, thalamus, pons, and meninges. Neutrophils and macrophages may infiltrate the brain parenchyma and cause neuronal destruction, neuronophagia, focal necrosis, and spotty demyelination. Vascular inflammation with endothelial proliferation, small-vessel thrombosis, and perivascular cuffing may also occur. Cell death occurs primarily in the glial and inflammatory cells.

Communicability

WEE, EEE, and VEE are spread primarily via the vector mosquito *Culex tarsalis*. Other mosquitoes (e.g., *Aedes* species) and, occasionally, small wild mammals have also been known to spread the virus. *C. tarsalis*, a mosquito that is often found on the West Coast of the United States, prefers warm, moist environments. In these locations, cycles of wild bird and mosquito interactions and infectivity allow the virus to remain endemic. No known cases of bird transmission of the disease exist, making mosquitoes the primary vector and birds simply the reservoirs. Epidemic outbreaks in the equine or pheasant population often precede human epidemics of WEE.

Ricin Toxin

Definition

The seeds from the castor bean plant, **Ricinus communis**, are poisonous to people, animals, and insects. One of the main toxic proteins is "ricin." Now we know that the agglutination observed with ingestion of the seeds is due to another toxin also present, called RCA (*Ricinus communis* agglutinin). Ricin is a potent cytotoxin but a weak hemagglutinin, whereas RCA is a weak cytotoxin and a powerful hemagglutinin. Poisoning by ingestion of the castor bean is due to ricin, not RCA, because RCA does not penetrate the intestinal wall and does not affect red blood cells unless given intravenously. If RCA is injected into the blood, it will cause the red blood cells to agglutinate and burst by hemolysis (CDC, 2003l).

Symptoms

- *Inhalation*: Within a few hours of inhalation of significant amounts of ricin, the likely symptoms would be coughing, tightness in the chest, difficulty breathing, nausea, and aching muscles. In the next few hours, the body's airways would become severely inflamed, excess fluid would build up in the lungs, breathing would become even more difficult, and the skin might turn cyanotic. Excess fluid in the lungs would be diagnosed on x-ray or by listening to the chest with a stethoscope.
- *Ingestion*: Someone who swallowed a significant amount of ricin would have internal bleeding of the stomach and intestines that would lead to vomiting and bloody diarrhea. Eventually, the liver, spleen, and kidneys might stop working, and death could result.
- *Injection*: Injection of a lethal amount of ricin would at first cause the muscles and lymph nodes near the injection site to die. Eventually, the liver, kidneys, and spleen would stop working, and the person would have massive bleeding from the stomach and intestines. The person would die from multiple organ failure.

Death from ricin poisoning could take place within 36 to 48 hours of exposure, whether by injection, ingestion, or inhalation. If the person lives longer than 5 days without complications, he or she will probably recover. Presentation with the preceding signs and symptoms does not necessarily mean, however, that a person has been exposed to ricin.

Communicability

Contracting ricin could only be the result of a deliberate act to make ricin and use it to poison people. Accidental exposure to ricin is highly unlikely. People can breathe in ricin mist or powder and be poisoned. Ricin can also get into water or food and then be swallowed. Pellets of ricin, or ricin dissolved in a liquid, can be injected into people's bodies. Depending on the route of exposure (such as injection), as little as 500 micrograms of ricin could be enough to kill an adult. A 500-microgram dose of ricin would be about the size of the head of a pin. A much greater amount would need to be inhaled or swallowed to be fatal. Ricin poisoning is not contagious. It cannot be spread from person to person through casual contact. Some reports have indicated that ricin may have been used in the Iran-Iraq war during the 1980s and that quantities of ricin were found in Al Qaeda caves in Afghanistan. Because of the similarity of the symptoms of many biologic and chemical agents, nasal or throat swabs and induced respiratory secretions may be collected for toxin assay. Blood can be collected for serum and toxin assays as well as measurement of antibody response using serum.

Epsilon Toxin of *Clostridium perfringens*

Definition

Epsilon toxin is a potent toxin produced by the bacterium ***Clostridium perfringens***. Each of the types of *C. perfringens* produces a unique spectrum of toxins. Of the five types known (A through E), only B and D produce toxin. These strains have a limited host range, being isolated mainly from sheep and lambs, occasionally from goats and cattle, and rarely from humans. The two strains, along with strain C, are responsible for producing a very severe and often fatal form of enterotoxemia (Northstar Preparedness Network, n.d.).

Symptoms

Diarrhea is accompanied by severe abdominal cramping and bloating. There seems to be little or no information about the effects of epsilon toxin on humans. Extrapolation from studies with experimentally infected animals indicates that neurologic signs or pulmonary edema may be possible in humans. The toxin increases intestinal permeability, ensuring its absorption into the circulation, where it damages vascular endothelium, leading to fluid loss and edema. Stress responses to cerebral edema trigger catecholamine release, resulting in adenylate cyclase activation, hyperglycemia related to cyclic adenosine monophosphate (cAMP), and glycosuria, a common finding in enterotoxemia. Postmortem autolysis is rapid. Subserous and subendocardial hemorrhages and excess fluid in the body cavities are sometimes seen. Cerebral hemorrhaging and degenerative lesions are common in less acute cases.

Communicability

It is possible for the epsilon toxin to be transmitted in contaminated food and water or by aerosol. Specific information is not available for the epsilon toxin. Toxins are not generally transmitted from animal to animal or from animal to people.

> *Because of the similarity of the symptoms of many biologic and chemical agents, nasal or throat swabs and induced respiratory secretions may be collected for toxin assay. Blood can be collected for serum and toxin assays as well as measurement of antibody response using serum.*

Staphylococcal Enterotoxin B

Definition

Staphylococcal **enterotoxin B** (SEB) is one of several exotoxins produced by *Staphylococcus aureus* (CDC, 2003m).

Symptoms

From 3 to 12 hours after aerosol exposure, high fever (103 to 106° F), chills, headache, myalgia and nonproductive cough may appear. Some patients may have shortness of breath and retrosternal chest pain. If pulmonary edema or adult respiratory distress syndrome (ARDS) develops, there may be a cough with frothy sputum. Fever may last 2 to 5 days and cough may persist for up to 4 weeks. Ingestion of the toxin leads to acute salivation, nausea, and vomiting followed by abdominal cramps and diarrhea. Fever and respiratory involvement are not seen in foodborne SEB intoxication. Higher exposure can lead to septic shock and death if left untreated.

Physical findings in SEB intoxication are often unremarkable. Postural hypotension may be present, particularly with ingestion of SEB, because of fluid loss. Conjunctivitis or rale may also be found.

Communicability

SEB toxin is heat stable and water-soluble. The incapacitating dose is 30 ng/person by inhalation. SEB, one of several exotoxins produced by *S. aureus*, may be aerosolized or used to sabotage food supplies. Although it would be effective in causing illness that incapacitates victims for up to 2 weeks, it would not be a weapon likely to produce significant mortality rates.

 ONLINE CONSULT

The New York Health Department has developed a concise table identifying—on the basis of symptoms—different types of biologic terrorism. It includes the testing to be done as well as the treatment.
http://www.health.state.ny.us/nysdoh/bt/pdf/rapid_response_card.pdf

Category C

The agents in Category C are regarded as lower priority by the CDC, as illustrated in the following extracts.

Nipah Virus

Definition

Nipah virus and Hendra virus are newly recognized zoonotic viruses. They are typically grouped together and are members of the *Paramyxoviridae* family. It is currently believed that certain species of fruit bats are the natural hosts of both Nipah and Hendra viruses. Although members of this group of viruses have caused only a few focal outbreaks, the biologic ability of these viruses to infect a wide range of hosts and to produce a disease causing significant mortality in humans has made this emerging viral infection a public heath concern (World Health Organization [WHO], 2001).

Symptoms

The incubation period for Nipah and Hendra viral infections is between 4 and 18 days. In many cases the infection is mild or not apparent, and diagnosis is determined through assays. Treatment is supportive. In symptomatic cases, the onset is usually with "influenza-like" symptoms, with high fever and myalgia. The disease may progress to encephalitis with drowsiness, disorientation, convulsions and coma. Fifty percent of people with clinically apparent infection die.

Communicability

The mode of transmission from animal to animal, and from animal to human is uncertain but appears to require close contact with contaminated tissue or body fluids. Nipah antibodies have been detected in pigs as well as other domestic and wild animals. The role of species other than pigs in transmitting

ONLINE CONSULT

Go to
http://www.cdc.gov/
and review the number of recent outbreaks of SARS and West Nile. When was
the last reported case of smallpox?

infection to other animals has not yet been determined.

It is unlikely that Nipah virus is easily transmitted to humans. Despite frequent contact between fruit bats and humans, there is no serologic evidence of human infection among bat carriers. Pigs were the apparent source of infection in most human cases in the Malaysian outbreak of Nipah virus, but other sources, such as infected dogs and cats, cannot be excluded. Human-to-human transmission of Nipah virus has not been reported.

Hantaviruses

Definition

Hantavirus pulmonary syndrome (HPS) is caused by a hitherto unknown virus, subsequently isolated and named Sin Nombre Virus (SNV). Commonly referred to as hantavirus disease, HPS is a febrile illness characterized by bilateral interstitial pulmonary infiltrates and respiratory compromise usually requiring supplemental oxygen and clinically resembling acute respiratory disease syndrome (ARDS) (CDC, 2003a).

Symptoms

Early symptoms are fatigue, fever, and muscle aches, especially of the large muscle groups—thighs, hips, back, and sometimes shoulders. These symptoms are universal. There may also be headaches, dizziness, chills, and abdominal problems, such as nausea, vomiting, diarrhea, and abdominal pain. Because there have been so few cases of HPS, the "incubation time" is not quite clear. On the basis of limited information, however, it

appears that symptoms may develop between 1 and 5 weeks after exposure to potentially infected rodents and their droppings. Typical clinical laboratory findings are hemoconcentration, left shift in the white blood cell count, neutrophilic leukocytosis, thrombocytopenia, and circulating immunoblasts.

Communicability

Some rodents are infected with a type of hantavirus that causes HPS. In the United States, deer mice (as well as cotton rats and rice rats in the southeastern states and the white-footed mouse in the Northeast) are the rodents carrying the hantaviruses that cause HPS. These rodents shed the virus in their urine, droppings, and saliva. The virus is mainly transmitted to people when they breathe in air contaminated with the virus. This happens when fresh rodent urine, droppings, or nesting materials is stirred up and aerosolized. The types of hantavirus that cause HPS in the United States cannot be transmitted from one person to another; these viruses are not known to be transmitted by any types of animals other than certain species of rodents.

Tickborne Hemorrhagic Fever Viruses

Definition

Crimean-Congo hemorrhagic fever (CCHF), one of the **tickborne hemorrhagic fever viruses**, is a viral hemorrhagic fever of the Nairovirus group. Although it is primarily a zoonosis, sporadic cases and outbreaks of CCHF affecting humans do occur (CDC, 2003j).

Symptoms

The length of the incubation period for the illness appears to depend on the mode of acquisition of the virus. After infection via tick bite, for example, the incubation period is usually 1 to 3 days, with a maximum of 9 days. The incubation period after contact with infected blood or tissues is usually 5 to 6 days, with a documented maximum of 13 days.

Onset of symptoms is sudden, with fever, myalgia, dizziness, neck pain and stiffness, backache, headache, sore eyes and photophobia. There may be nausea, vomiting and sore throat early on, which may be accompanied by diarrhea and generalized abdominal pain. Over the next few days, the patient may experience sharp mood swings and may become confused and aggressive. After 2 to 4 days, the agitation may be replaced by sleepiness, depression, and lassitude, and the abdominal pain may localize to the right upper quadrant, with detectable hepatomegaly.

Communicability

The CCHF virus may infect a wide range of domestic and wild animals. Many birds are resistant to infection, but ostriches are susceptible and may show a high prevalence of infection in endemic areas. Animals become infected with CCHF from the bite of infected ticks. The most important source for acquisition of the virus by ticks is believed to be infected small vertebrates on which immature *Hyalomma* ticks feed. Once infected, the tick remains infected through its developmental stages, and the mature tick may transmit the infection to large vertebrates, such as livestock.

Patients with suspected or confirmed CCHF should be isolated and cared for with the use of barrier nursing techniques. Specimens of blood or tissues obtained for diagnostic purposes should be collected and handled with universal precautions. Sharps and body wastes should be safely disposed through appropriate decontamination procedures. Health-care workers are at risk of acquiring infection from sharps injuries during surgical procedures, and in the past, CCHF infection has been transmitted to surgeons operating on patients to determine the cause of the abdominal symptoms in the early stages of disease.

Tickborne Encephalitis Viruses

Definition

Tickborne encephalitis (TBE), also known as spring-summer encephalitis, is a viral infection of the central nervous system transmitted by bites of certain vector ticks. Human infections follow bites of infected *Ixodes ricinus* ticks, usually in people who visit or work in forests, fields, or pastures. Infection with **tickborne encephalitis viruses** also can be acquired by consuming unpasteurized dairy products from infected cows, goats, or sheep (CDC, 2003j).

Symptoms

Symptoms of TBE include sudden fever, headache, vomiting, photophobia, stiff neck, confusion, drowsiness, and clumsiness. Symptoms requiring emergency treatment are loss of consciousness, stupor, coma, seizures, muscle weakness or paralysis, and sudden severe dementia. TBE is a virus of the central nervous system. Focal epilepsy and flaccid paralysis often characterize this type of encephalitis. Once the virus enters the blood stream it can make its way into the brain, causing inflammation of the brain cells and the surrounding membranes. White blood cells try to fight off the infection, but in the process, they invade the brain tissue. Cerebral edema occurs and can cause destruction of nerve cells, bleeding in the brain, and brain damage.

Communicability

The TBE virus is transmitted by the bite of an infected tick. Ticks and mammals conjoined appear to be the true reservoir. Sheep, deer, rodents, small mammals, and birds serve as sources of tick infection. Humans become infected through the bite of an infective tick or the consumption of milk from certain infected animals. The virus cannot be transmitted from human to human.

Yellow Fever

Definition

Yellow fever is a mosquito-borne viral disease that occurs in tropical and subtropical areas. Yellow fever is seen only in Africa and South America. Sporadic infections occur almost exclusively in forestry and agricultural workers due to occupational exposure in or near forests (CDC, 2003o).

Symptoms

Initial symptoms may be dengue fever–like and include fever, headache, vomiting, and backache. As the disease progresses, the pulse slows and weakens, and gums start to bleed. Bloody urine and jaundice may also occur. The incubation period is usually 3 to 6 days, after which symptoms of fever, malaise, headache, photophobia, nausea, vomiting, and irritability appear. Physical examination at this time shows a patient who is febrile, is toxic in appearance, and has hyperemic skin, injected conjunctiva, coated tongue, and epigastric or hepatic tenderness. Faget's sign, a relative bradycardia with a fever, may be present. After 3 to 5 days, the patient either recovers or goes onto the next stage, fulminant disease.

Fulminant disease consists of significant hepatic injury with jaundice, yielding the name "yellow fever." Renal failure is not uncommon. A hemorrhagic diathesis, consisting of epistaxis, oozing at the gums, petechiae, ecchymosis, hematemesis, melena, hematuria, thrombocytopenia, and disseminated intravascular coagulation, may occur. Myocarditis, encephalopathy, and shock may also ensue. The case fatality rate is 20 to 50 percent. Anyone who survives can expect to recover fully.

Communicability

Yellow fever is a viral disease transmitted to humans by a mosquito. The vector is the *Aedes aegypti* or *Haemagogus* mosquito. *Vertical transmission* occurs when the virus is passed on to the mosquito's ovum. This feature is advantageous for continuation of the life cycle during the dry season, when the eggs may lay dormant. When the rainy season returns, the eggs hatch, allowing the virus to carry on. *Horizontal transmission* occurs when either an animal (typically monkeys) or humans are infected by the mosquito. The mosquito is the true reservoir of the virus; yellow fever is never transmitted from person to person or animal to person.

Multidrug-Resistant Tuberculosis

Definition

Tuberculosis (TB) is an infectious disease caused by a germ called *Mycobacterium tuberculosis*. **Multidrug-resistant tuberculosis** (MDR TB) is a form of tuberculosis that is resistant to two or more of the primary drugs used for the treatment of tuberculosis. Resistance to one or several forms of treatment occurs when the bacteria develop the ability to withstand antibiotic attack and relay that ability to their progeny (CDC, 2003b).

Symptoms

TB primarily attacks the respiratory system, although it can affect other organs as well. The symptoms of TB include fever, night sweats, weight loss, chest pain, and coughing. TB may be fatal, especially for HIV-infected persons.

Communicability

Tuberculosis is spread through the air when a person sneezes, coughs, or breathes. MDR TB is resistant to at least two of the main drugs used to treat TB— isoniazid (INH) and rifampin. Because that entire strain of bacteria inherits the capacity to resist the effects of the various treatments, resistance can spread from one person to another. On an individual basis, however, inadequate treatment or improper use of the antituberculous medications remains an important cause of drug-resistant and multidrug resistant tuberculosis.

There is evidence that a handful of terrorist organizations have been exploring biologic weapons. Producing germs and being able to disseminate them widely among a civilian population requires hundreds of millions of dollars of research. Some groups may have acquired a fundamental biologic weapons capability, and investigation and experimentation with biologic weapons will most likely continue. This does not automatically translate into an ability to conduct a mass casualty attack with a biologic warfare agent. There are many technical hurdles to developing an effective large-scale chemical or biologic weapons program. This task may be so insurmountable that terrorists would choose to remain reliant on more conventional methods of attack.

CHEMICAL TERRORISM

Chemicals weapons are defined as chemical substances intended for use in military operations to kill, seriously injure, or incapacitate people through physiologic effects. Such weapons are generally separated according to

severity of effects: lethal (choking, nerve, and blood agents), blistering, and incapacitating. Chemical agents are also a direct threat as terrorist agents (CDC, 2000). Because hundreds of new chemicals are produced monthly, treatment should focus on clinical syndrome rather than specific agent.

Patient Arrival in the Emergency Department

Typically, the Emergency Department (ED) staff members are the first point of contact for patients who have been partially or not at all decontaminated. When such a patient arrives in the ED, staff should:

- Try to determine the chemical agent's identity on the basis of the symptoms discussed later. Classification into a group of chemicals is helpful. Do not waste time trying to ascertain this information.
- Prepare personal protection equipment (PPE), decontamination supplies, and antidotes.
- Determine whether there is high suspicion of a chemical hazard. If there is, don personal protective equipment and set up a hot line.
- Clear and secure all areas that could become contaminated.
- Secure hospital entrances and grounds.
- Notify local emergency management authorities if needed.
- If a chemical is a military agent, inform the Army.
- If an organophosphate is involved, notify the hospital pharmacy that large amounts of atropine and 2-PAM may be needed.

The term **personal protective equipment** refers to clothing and respiratory apparatus designed to shield an individual from chemical, biologic, and physical hazards. There are different levels of PPE depending on the type of exposure expected.

When the Patient Arrives Without Warning

A contaminated patient may present at an emergency department (ED) or any office or health-care facility without prior warning. In such circumstances, ED staff should:

- Determine whether a chemical hazard exists. If there is no chemical hazard, handle the patient routinely.
- Determine whether there is suspicion or serious risk of a chemical hazard. Look for liquid on the patient's clothes or skin, symptoms in other patients and emergency medical technicians (EMTs), an odor (H, L, phosgene, chlorine), or positive reaction on M-8 paper.
- Keep the patient outside until preparations are complete, and don personal PPE to assist EMTs as necessary.
- If the patient is grossly contaminated (liquid on skin, positive M-8 paper) or if there is any suspicion of contamination, decontaminate the patient before allowing his or her entry into the building.

Treatment and Identification of the Chemical Agent

Here are some general treatment suggestions followed by specific ways to treat exposure to particular chemical agents:

- Establish the airway if necessary
- Give artificial respiration if the patient is not breathing
- Control bleeding if the patient is hemorrhaging

For any patient with symptoms of specific agents, as described later, staff should check for other possible chemical exposures, looking for decreased level of consciousness without head trauma, an odor on the clothes or breath, and specific signs or symptoms of other chemical agents.

Nerve Agent

Symptoms

If the following symptoms are present or there is a suspicion of cholinesterase poisoning, the problem is considered to be a nerve agent.

- Pinpoint pupils
- Difficulty breathing (wheezing, gasping, etc)
- Local or generalized sweating
- Fasciculations
- Copious secretions
- Nausea, vomiting, diarrhea
- Convulsions
- Coma
- Sudden headache

Treatment

Treatment recommendations for contamination with a nerve agent are as follows:

- If there is severe respiratory distress: Intubate and ventilate. Give atropine (Adults: 6 mg IM or IV. Infants/children: 0.05 mg/kg IV) and 2-PAM Cl (Adults: 600–1000 mg IM or slow IV. Infants/children: 15 mg/kg slow IV).
- If there are major secondary symptoms: Give atropine (Adults: 4 mg IM or IV. Infants/children: 0.02–0.05 mg/kg IV) and 2-PAM Cl (Adults: 600–1000 mg IM or slow IV. Infants/children: 15 mg/kg.). Open the IV line.
- Repeat the atropine as needed until the secretions decrease and breathing is easier (Adults: 2 mg IV or IM. Infants/children: 0.02–0.05 mg/kg I.).
- Repeat 2-PAM Cl as needed (Adults: 1.0 gm IV over 20–30 minutes; repeat every 1 hour times 3 as needed. Infants/children: 15 mg/kg slow IV.)
- If there are seizures: Give diazepam (Adults: 10 mg slow IV. Infants/children: 0.2 mg/kg IV).
- Reevaluate every 3–5 minutes. If signs worsen, repeat atropine, 2-PAM Cl, and diazepam. *Note:* Warn the hospital pharmacy that unusual amounts of atropine and 2-PAM may be needed.

Chlorine Agent

Symptoms

If any of the following symptoms is present, the problem is considered to be a chlorine agent.

- Dyspnea or shortness of breath
- Coughing, chest tightness
- Burning sensation in the nose, throat, and eyes
- Watery eyes, blurred vision
- Nausea and vomiting
- Burning pain, redness and blisters if in contact with skin (similar to frostbite)

Treatment

Treatment recommendations for contamination with a chlorine agent are as follows

- If there is dyspnea, try bronchodilators and give oxygen by mask. A chest x-ray will be needed. Pulmonary edema can occur in 2 to 4 hours. The patient will have to be admitted to the hospital.
- Treat other problems and reevaluate (consider phosgene).
- If phosgene poisoning is a possibility, refer to the phosphene agent section.
- Give supportive therapy; treat other problems and/or discharge.

> The most familiar historical use of a chemical agent was by a Japanese cult. In 1995, Aum Shinrikyo released sarin gas, a nerve agent, in the Tokyo subway system, killing 12 people and injuring 5500. The sarin produced by the cult was an impure form and not nearly as lethal as military grade. It is reported that this cult also attempted to develop a biologic agent but was unsuccessful, even with a reported six laboratories and a budget of $300 million.

Lewisite Agent

Symptoms

If there were thermal burns, did they begin within minutes of poisoning? If they did, consider the problem a lewisite agent (can be from vapors or liquids).

- Immediate burning and blistering of any part of the body contacted.

- Burns of eyes—immediate edema of lids, conjunctiva and cornea. Burns can also affect mucous membranes and lungs.
- Skin—immediate burns, erythema within 15 to 30 minutes, and vesication within a few hours. Blisters start small and expand to cover entire site. Maximum blistering may take up to 4 days. Blisters are less fragile than those due to mustard agents.
- Burns usually less severe than with mustard agents.
- Systemically absorbed lewisite, by any route, can cause "lewisite shock," resulting in potential death.

Treatment

Treatment recommendations for contamination with a lewisite agent are as follows:

- Survey the extent of injury.
- Treat the affected skin with British antilewisite (BAL) ointment (if available).
- Treat affected eyes with BAL ophthalmic ointment (if available).
- Treat any pulmonary or severe effects (BAL in oil, 0.5 ml/25 lb body wt. deep IM to max of 4.0 ml. Repeat every 4 hours times 3).
- Give morphine as needed for pain.
- If there is severe poisoning, shorten the interval for BAL injections to every 2 hours.

Mustard Agent

Symptoms

If the patient experienced burns or eye irritation beginning 2 to 12 hours after exposure, consider problem a mustard agent:

- Mild to severe conjunctivitis with 1- to 2-week recovery.
- Mild to severe corneal erosions and necrosis resulting in potential blindness.
- Skin exposure is latent; it may be several hours before lesions are noted (this is the hallmark of mustard agents):
  - Erythema with slight edema and itching is seen 2 to 48 hours after exposure.

- Blisters are uncomfortable and tense and rupture easily.
- Deep burning (up to full-thickness loss) is possible anywhere but most likely in the genital and axillary areas.
- Rhinorrhea, burning throat pain, and hoarseness start 4 to 6 hours later.
- Bone marrow can be depleted, causing leukopenia and aplastic anemia.
- Nausea, vomiting, and diarrhea occur.
- Systemic absorption can cause central nervous system involvement.

Treatment

There is no specific treatment for contamination with a mustard agent; the following measures are recommended:

- The goal of therapy is relieve symptoms, prevent infection, and promote healing.
- If there is airway obstruction, a tracheostomy may be needed.
- If there are large burns, establish an IV line (do not push fluids as for thermal burns).
- Drain vesicles: unroof large blisters and irrigate the area with topical antibiotics.
- Treat other symptoms appropriately.

Phosgene Agent

Symptoms

If the patient has immediate eye pain, respiratory symptoms (immediate if inhaled, later if absorbed through the skin), and skin irritation (white with circular erythema), consider the problem a phosgene agent:

- Immediate skin irritation: Exposed skin turns white and is surrounded by a circular zone of erythema, giving the appearance of a target. Within 24 hours, there is edema, and severe necrosis can develop.
- Inhalation causes immediate respiratory symptoms leading to pulmonary edema. Severe skin exposure can lead to delayed respiratory symptoms and/or pulmonary edema.

Treatment

No specific treatment is available for contamination with a phosgene agent. The following measures are recommended:

- Restrict fluids, perform a chest x-ray, and obtain blood gas measurements.
- If the patient is experiencing dyspnea, oxygen with positive end-expiratory pressure (PEEP) will be needed.
- Observe the patient closely for at least 6 hours. If severe dyspnea develops or x-ray or blood gas findings are consistent with phosgene poisoning, the patient will have to be admitted, with oxygen via PEEP, fluid restriction, and monitoring with chest x-rays and blood gas measurements. The patient will be seriously ill.

CONCLUSION

Keeping abreast of the current biologic and chemical threats is a challenge but is the responsibility of all nursing professionals. Nurses are often on the front lines for identification of the signs, symptoms, and trending of populations with certain types of diseases. Frequently, accessing new and current information in this area is necessary to understand the most up-to-date information and threats that must be considered. Clients look to nurses to know what symptoms to watch for and what to do in the event of a chemical or biologic terrorist act. Having a clear understanding of resources and information to discuss with patients makes the nursing professional invaluable.

Key Points

- Biologic agents used in terrorism are divided into three categories: Category A (high priority), Category B (second-highest-priority), and Category C (third-highest-priority).
- Category A agents pose a risk because they (1) are easily transmitted from person to person, (2) cause high mortality and the potential for a major public health impact, (3) can cause public panic and social disruption, and (4) require special action for public health preparedness.
- Category B agents pose a risk because they (1) are moderately easy to disseminate, (2) cause moderate morbidity and low mortality, and (3) require specific enhancements of CDC's diagnostic capacity and enhanced disease surveillance.
- Category C agents pose a risk because they (1) are readily available, (2) are easily produced and disseminated, and (3) have a potential for high morbidity and mortality as well as a major health impact.
- Chemical agents range from warfare agents to common toxic chemicals used in industries today. Hundreds of new chemicals are produced monthly. Identification and treatment of chemical exposure focuses on the clinical syndrome rather than the specific agent.
- Knowledge of what to do and what not to do is imperative in the treatment of chemical exposure.
- Don personal protection equipment (PPE) prior to decontaminating the patient. Assess and establish the airway after PPE is in place.
- Major groups of chemicals used as weapons are: (1) nerve agents, (2) chlorine agents, (3) lewisite agents, (4) mustard agents, and (5) phosgene agents.

Thought and Discussion Questions

1. The CDC has identified five focus areas for terrorism. The emphasis of this chapter has been on the third focus, diagnosis and characterization of biologic and chemical agents. Discuss what your community has done for focus number one, preparedness and prevention. What has your educational institution done to prepare for a terrorist attack if it should occur while you, as a student, are at a clinical site?
2. Be prepared to discuss the chronology of a chemical terrorist attack in your community. Discuss how to triage patients properly and give your views on allowing patients to expire who are determined to be beyond the ability to save.
3. Review the case study in the Case Study Bank on the Intranet site and be prepared to discuss it in class.
4. Discuss how this story ends: You are working at a hospital. You have been notified that there are two confirmed cases of smallpox at the local school. The city has become aware. The school is in a panic, and the next day, 25 percent of the students are kept at home. You have received eight call-ins for various reasons but realize the underlying fear is exposure. The local supermarket is closed because of staffing issues. What would be your course of action? How would you handle staffing issues? Would you let your children attend school? Would you return to work?

5. Discuss the central nervous system involvement of the Alphaviruses in the severe stages.
6. Discuss how the Nipah virus is transmitted.
7. When a patient arrives with an unknown chemical exposure, how do you know what to treat?
8. Review the Chapter Thought on the first page of the chapter, and discuss your views on how to prevent terrorist attacks and how to deal with countries that do launch such attacks.

Interactive Exercises

1. Go to the Web site for Bioterrorism Nursing Policies: **http://www. hospitalsoup.com/public/bioplan.pdf.** Locate your state's or territory's FBI and Public Health Director phone numbers. (Note: Phone numbers may change; review updates regularly.)
2. Go to the CDC Web site: **http://www.cdc.gov/od/sap/docs/fr96.pdf**. From the Rule, 42 CFR Part 72, list the 13 viruses included as select agents in this list.
3. Draw a table with different modes of transmission as column headings and write the name of each of the Category A biologic agents reviewed in the chapter in the proper column. See the Intranet site for a sample table.
4. Complete the short answer questions listed for this chapter in the Interactive Exercises section of the Intranet site.
5. List three biologic agents, one from each category (A, B, and C), and discuss one reason that each agent might be chosen for use as a biologic weapon for terrorism.
6. Describe the "typical" laboratory findings in the patient with hantavirus pulmonary syndrome by doing some Internet research.
7. Evaluate your own understanding of and preparedness for biologic/chemical terrorism by completing the online Interactive Exercise entitled: Self-Assessment of Biologic/Chemical Terrorism.
8. Begin a reference notebook with contact numbers of whom you should call if you suspect a chemical or biologic event. Update all the numbers twice a year. Include information on the Category A, B, and C biologic agents and their symptoms and communicability. Include information regarding the evaluation and identification of the major chemical agents.

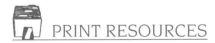

PRINT RESOURCES

References

Centers for Disease Control and Prevention. (1997). *Additional requirements for facilities transferring or receiving select agents.* (42 CFR Part 72/RIN 0905-AE70.) Atlanta: U.S. Department of Health and Human Services.

Centers for Disease Control (1998). *Preventing emerging infectious diseases: A strategy for the 21st century.* Atlanta: Georgia: Author.

Centers for Disease Control and Prevention. (2000) Biological and chemical terrorism: Strategic plan for preparedness and response. Recommendations of the CDC Strategic Planning Workgroup. MMWR, 49.

Eitzen, E. M., & Takafuji, E. T. (1997) *Textbook of military medicine: Medical aspects of chemical and biological warfare* (pp. 415–424). Published by the Office of The Surgeon General, Department of the Army, USA. Washington, DC.

Henderson, D. A. (1997) Bioweapons and bioterrorism. JAMA, 278, 351–370, 389–436.

New Jersey State Health Department (2002). What you should know about Q fever. *http://www.state.nj.us/health/cd/f_qfever.htm*

Osterholm, M., & Schwartz, J. (2001) *Living Terrors: What America needs to know to survive the coming bioterrorist catastrophe.* Belmont, CA: Wadsworth.

Bibliography

Department of Defense. (2001). *21st Century bioterrorism and germ weapons. U.S. Army field manual for the treatment of biological warfare agent casualties (anthrax, smallpox, plague, viral fevers, toxins, delivery methods, detection, symptoms, treatment, equipment).* Washington, DC: Progressive Management.

Federal Emergency Management Agency. (2003) *Guidelines for public sector hazardous materials training.* Washington, DC: Author.

Henderson, D. A., Inglesby, T. V., & O'Toole, T. (Eds.) (2002). *Bioterrorism: Guidelines for medical and public health management.* Chicago, IL: American Medical Association.

U.S. Government. (2002) *2002 Bioterrorism after the anthrax attacks: Complete revised guide to biological weapons and germ warfare, anthrax, smallpox, medicines, treatment, preparedness, White House, Homeland Security, CDC, HHS, FDA, NIH, Military manuals.* Washington, DC: Progressive management.

Venzke, B. (1998) *First responder chem-bio handbook.* Alexandria, VA: Washington, DC: Tempest Publisher.

Vorobyov, A. (1994, April). Criterion rating as a measure of probable use of bio agents as biological weapons. *In: Papers presented to the Working Group on Biological Weapons Control of the Committee on International Security and Arms Control. National Academy of Sciences.* Washington, DC.

ONLINE REFERENCES

Biological Terrorism Response Manual. (2001). *http://www.bioterry.com/History_of_Biological_Terrorism.asp*

Centers for Disease Control (2003a). Public health and emergency preparedness and response: All about hantavirus. *http://www.cdc.gov/ncidod/diseases/hanta/hps/*

Centers for Disease Control (2003b). Public health and emergency preparedness and response: Emerging infectious diseases. *http://www.cdc.gov/ncidod/eid/vol8no11/02–0507.htm*

Centers for Disease Control (2003c). Public health and emergency preparedness and response: Facts about alphaviruses. *http://www.cdc.gov/ncidod/dvbid/arbor/alphavir.htm*

Centers for Disease Control (2003d). Public health and emergency preparedness and response: Facts about Anthrax. *http://www.bt.cdc.gov/DocumentsApp/FactSheet/Anthrax/about.asp*

Centers for Disease Control (2003e). Public health and emergency preparedness and response: Facts about arenaviruses. *http://www.cdc.gov/ncidod/dvrd/spb/mnpages/dispages/arena.htm*

Centers for Disease Control (2003f). Public health and emergency preparedness and response: Facts about botulism. *http://www.bt.cdc.gov/DocumentsApp/FactSheet/Botulism/about.asp*

Centers for Disease Control (2003g). Public health and emergency preparedness and response: Facts about brucellosis. *http://www.cdc.gov/ncidod/dbmd/diseaseinfo/brucellosis_g.htm*

Centers for Disease Control (2003h). Public health and emergency preparedness and response: Facts about filoviruses. *http://www.cdc.gov/ncidod/dvrd/spb/mnpages/dispages/filoviruses.htm*

Centers for Disease Control (2003i). Public health and emergency preparedness and response: Facts about glanders. *http://www.cdc.gov/ncidod/dbmd/diseaseinfo/glanders_g.htm*

Centers for Disease Control (2003j). Public health and emergency preparedness and response: Facts about hemorrhagic fever virus. *http://www.cdc.gov/od/sap/appen1/appdef01.htm*

Centers for Disease Control (2003k). Public health and emergency preparedness and response: Facts about plague. *http://www.bt.cdc.gov/DocumentsApp/FactSheet/Plague/About.asp*

Centers for Disease Control (2003l). Public health and emergency preparedness and response: Facts about ricin. *http://www.bt.cdc.gov/agent/ricin/faq/index.asp*

Centers for Disease Control (2003m). Public health and emergency preparedness and response: Facts about staphylococcal enterotoxin B. *http://www.rivma.org/Staph%20Enterotoxin%20B.doc*

Centers for Disease Control (2003n). Public health and emergency preparedness and response: Facts about tularemia. *http://www.bt.cdc.gov/agent/tularemia/faq.asp*

Centers for Disease Control (2003o). Public health and emergency preparedness and response: Facts about yellow fever. *http://www.cdc.gov/ncidod/dvbid/yellowfever/*

Centers for Disease Control (2003p). Public health and emergency preparedness and response: Smallpox fact sheet. *http://www.bt.cdc.gov/agent/smallpox/overview/disease-facts.asp*

Centers for Disease Control (2003q). Q fever. *http://www.cdc.gov/ncidod/dvrd/qfever/index.htm*

English, J. F., Cundiff, M. Y., Malone, J. D., & Pfeiffer, J. A. (1999) CDC Hospital Infections Program Bioter-rorism Working Group. *http://www.hospitalsoup.com/public/bioplan.pdf*

Northstar Preparedness Network. (n.d.) Clostridium perfringens toxins. *http://www.preparednessnetwork.org/northstar/warfare/cpt.html*

Southwest Regional Center of Excellence for Biodefense and Emerging Infectious Disease Research. (2003). *http://bt.swmed.edu/index.html*

World Health Organization (WHO). (September, 2001). WHO Information Fact Sheets: Nipah virus fact sheet. *http://www.who.int/inf-fs/en/fact262.html*

World Health Organization (WHO). (May, 2003). Communicable Disease Surveillance and Response. *http://www.who.int/csr/don/2003_05_07/en/*

Rose Kearney-Nunnery
Jimmie E. Nunnery

21
chapter

The Political Imperative

> *A political life, I've often said, is a continuing education in human nature, including one's own.*
> Hillary Rodham Clinton

Chapter Objectives

On completion of this chapter, the reader will be able to:

1. Explain why it is important for nurses to possess political efficacy.
2. Discuss the process for the enactment of laws and associated regulations.
3. Identify the major committees at the federal and state levels, especially those that influence health policy.
4. Identify how nurses can influence the passing of legislation.
5. Analyze statutes and regulations governing nursing practice.
6. Examine the roles and activities of nurses and professional associations in influencing health policy decisions.
7. Demonstrate political involvement on a current health policy issue.

Key Terms

Political Efficacy
Government
Law
Bill
Committee Structure
Conference Committee
Regulations

Precedent
Nurse Practice Acts
Title Protection
Lobbying
Grassroots Effort
Political Action
   Committees

Workplace Issues
Community or Civic
   Involvement
Professional
   Organizations
Voice of Agency

Gaston (1998) has observed that "for people engaged in government, politics as a profession is both an art and a science [but] for the rest of us, it is simply the process we use in finding solutions to our everyday personal and community problems" (p. 3). Nurses are engaged in finding solutions to problems on a daily basis. These problems are not restricted to a location or practice area. The nursing professional advocates for the health of people and policies aimed at health protection and promotion. This imperative for change requires a broader view of what is involved in making changes in public policy at the local, state, and national levels. Nurses have become increasingly interested in public policy, realizing that both their personal and their professional lives are significantly influenced by governmental policy and programs.

All of this involves regulation of activities for the public good. How the regulation occurs is the process. Nurses are effective in the political process when they understand the sources of power and are willing to be involved and make a difference. Wilson and DiIulio (1998) have defined **political efficacy** as having two components, internal political efficacy and external political advocacy. Internal political efficacy is personal competence or the "ability to understand and take part in political affairs" (Wilson and DiIulio, 1998, p. 102). External political advocacy is the "ability to make the system respond to the citizenry" (Wilson and DiIulio, 1998, p. 102). Nurses must develop their internal political efficacy by being increasingly able to take part in the political process. This will further the external political efficacy of the nursing profession. These two components are the political imperative of the profession. External political efficacy is possible by virtue of the number of nurses in the profession who are skillful in promoting change. In addition, we see the active involvement of nursing organizations in political initatives to effect change in health policy. As described by Leininger (2002), "political aspects of nursing are now a dominant and frequent topic in hospitals and schools of nursing in the current era" (p. 189).

Both internal efficacy and external political efficacy are growing as the involvement of nurses develops. As noted by Mason and colleagues (2002), "patient care is indeed a political endeavor—one that is influenced by politics developed at all levels of government and by the private sector, including health care institutions" (pp. 1–2). The first step in the development of political efficacy is understanding the political process in goverment.

STRUCTURE AND FUNCTION OF GOVERNMENT

When we think of the term *government,* different images may come to mind. We may be thinking of the federal structure with its three components, executive, legislative, and judicial. Or, at the local level, we may be envisioning the organizational, local, and state influences on the operation of the health-care unit. **Government** is merely the controlling entity that has the authority to make decisions and regulations for the public good. Milstead (2003) describes government as an "iron triangle" of congresspeople, bureaucratic staff, and interest groups. Nursing has the responsibility to contribute to the decisions by providing the information needed and offering support for wise policy decisions that protect the public and the profession. To participate most effectively in the political process, one must understand the structure of government at each level. Because government structures do vary, it is essential to be familiar with your local, state, and national or federal governing bodies.

Branches of Government

Each branch of government plays a significant role in the development and implementation of health policy. The federal government and most state governments have three branches: legislative, executive, and judicial. The powers of the three federal branches are vested in accordance with the U.S. Constitution.

Executive Branch

At the federal level, the executive branch consists of the President, the cabinet-level departments, and regulatory agencies. The executive branch is responsible for the administration of government and the laws enacted. The President sets the legislative agenda for Congress and the annual budget for the nation. The President's budget influences the funding available for health-care programs, reimbursement, and education. In addition, the agenda set by the President determines what programs have a high priority for the administration. The President can recommend legislation and can approve or veto legislation passed by Congress. It is also the executive branch that makes appointments to government departments, boards, and committees, as with the appointment of the Surgeon General or the Secretary of Health and Human Services. The Consitution mandates that certain executive appointments be confirmed by the legislative branch.

Legislative Branch

The legislative branch comprises the two houses or chambers of Congress, the Senate and the House of Representatives. Congress is responsible for lawmaking, representation, and administrative oversight, including oversight of the agencies of the executive branch. Congress also provides the operational funding for the administrative agencies. The composition of and qualifications for the U.S. Congress are listed in Table 21–1. Compare these qualifications with those for the President. Also consider the reelection cycle and how the priorities, policies, and laws can be influenced by executive and legislative agendas and majority control.

Judicial Branch

The judicial branch includes the Supreme Court, which interprets laws and, through their judicial review process, can declare an act of Congress or the President unconstitutional. The nine federal Supreme Court Justices are appointed for life by the President after their selection has been confirmed by the Senate. The federal system also comprises lower courts and appellate or circuit courts. Federal judges are also nominated by the executive branch and confirmed by the Senate. This system of checks and balances manages to create an equilibrium, vesting limited power in each branch with oversight by another branch.

State and Local Systems

State government structures are similar to those described at the federal level. They also receive their mandates from the U.S. Constitution and their respective state constitutions. Like the President, the governor can sign legislation into law and use the power of the veto. State legislatures can also override a governor's veto. In some states, members of the state board of nursing, or other important health commissioners, are appointed by the governor. As with the federal government, some legislative branches must confirm selected executive appointments. State Supreme Courts and lower courts interpret the law and render decisions under judicial review.

County government generally entails a board of supervisors, elected board of commissioners, county executive or county manager, or mixed county board. Cities, towns, and villages also have a variety of elected officials similar to those of county government. Local health policies and politics must be consistent with state and federal law but can also have a profound influence on the health and welfare of a community, as with public utitlties and local programs.

Although nurses are most often involved with the legislative branch of government, the executive branch and the judicial branch can also be of great importance to nursing and

TABLE 21–1
Qualifications for Service in the U.S. Congress or Executive Office

	Senate	House of Representatives	Presidency
Number	100 senators (two from each state) Equal representation Senior Senator (elected first) and Junior Senator	435 Members Representation based on state population; minimum of 1 from each state with reapportionment every 10 years based on the U.S. Census The House also includes delegates from the District of Columbia, Guam, the Virgin Islands, American Samoa, and Puerto Rico, who have voting rights in committees but not in matters before the full House of Representatives	1 In the case of the inability of the President to fulfill his or her role, succession of power occurs as follows: Vice President as second in line, then Speaker of the House, and then President Pro Tempore of the Senate
Terms	Elected for a term of 6 years, on alternate schedule	Elected for a term of 2 years	Elected for a term of 4 years
Reelection	Every 2 years, one third of senators face reelection	Entire membership is up for reelection every 2 years	Eligible for re-election once (two-term limit)
Qualifications	At least 30 years of age Citizen of United States for 9 years Resident of the state represented when elected	At least 25 years of age Citizen of United States for 7 years Resident of the state represented when elected	At least 35 years of age A natural-born citizen of the United States and a resident for at least 14 years

health care. It is essential that nurses understand the functions of the different branches of govenment and how laws and regulations are enacted and implemented.

HOW LAWS ARE MADE

A **law** is a mandate of prescribed conduct, grants certain rights, requires certain responsibilities, or a combination of these attributes. A law can come from a constitution, from the legislature, or from the courts. Administrative agencies promulgate regulations, which supplement and further develop the laws. Consider the types of laws and regulations identified in Table 21–2.

The idea for a law may originate with an individual, a professional group, a legislator, or the executive branch. *Statutory law* is legislation that has been approved by both legislative houses of Congress and signed by the executive branch. The legislation starts as a **bill** or a proposal for a law authored or sponsored by either a representative or a sen-

TABLE 21–2
Types of Law

Type	Description	Example
Constitutional	Specific guarantees granted by the U.S. Constitution	Freedom of speech
Statutory	Formal laws enacted by federal, state, and local legislative branches of government	Nurse practice acts
Administrative	Regulations created by administrative agencies under the direction of the executive branch of government	Regulations associated with nurse practice acts to assist with implementation
Court, case or common law	Laws created from judicial decisions Judgments create a precedent on which future decisions are based	"Miranda Rights" must be read to an arrestee before he or she is taken into custody

ator, who introduces it after it has been written in appropriate language by the legislative counsel of either the House or the Senate. A bill may also be introduced from a legislative committee. A bill proposed in the Senate is designated "S." followed by a number, and a bill introduced in the House of Representatives is designated "H.R." followed by a number.

Congressional Committees

At the federal level, bills are referred to full committee and sometimes to a subcommittee, because of the thousands of bills introduced each year. The U.S. Senate has 16 standing committees, with a variable number of associated subcommittees, depending on the scope and work of the committee, and four select or special committees. The House of Representatives has 19 standing committees and additional special or select committees. There are also four joint committees, staffed by both houses, that focus on common oversight functions for printing, taxation, the Library of Congress, and economics.

It is within the **committee structure** that most of the work of Congress takes place, at both the federal and state level. Committee action is perhaps the most important phase of the congressional process because it is at this phase that proposed measures are given the most intensive consideration and people have an opportunity to provide testimony for consideration and incorporation into the record. The committee or subcomittee level is where nursing can have a powerful impact. The subcommittee studies the issues contained in each bill carefully, holds hearings, and reports back to the full committee with recommendations. Each committee has jurisdiction over certain subjects. Some of the committees identified in Table 21–3 focus specifically on health-related issues.

States operate much like the federal government. In a particular state, there are also specific committees and subcommittees that handle selected topics. For example, in South Carolina, the Medical, Military, Public, and Municipal Affairs Committee for the House and the Medical Committee of the Senate generally handle the topics of concern to nursing and health care. But state structures differ, and it is important to be aware of the differences and to know the committees in which the issues of major concern to nursing arise. Appointment to the committees is often based on seniority or priority. Members often have special interests in an area. Because these members represent their constituents, it is important to know on which committees your congressperson serves and that they have valid information, resources, and background to address your concerns. Testimony, either written or in person, provides valu-

TABLE 21–3
Major Committees of the U.S. Congress

Senate

Standing committees (16)	Agriculture, Nutrition & Forestry
	Appropriations*
	Armed Services
	Banking, Housing & Urban Affairs
	Budget*
	Commerce, Finance & Transportation
	Energy & Natural Resources
	Environment & Public Works
	Finance*
	Foreign Relations
	Governmental Affairs
	Health, Education, Labor & Pensions*
	Judiciary
	Rules & Administration
	Small Business & Entrepreneurship
	Veteran's Affairs*
Select, special, & other committees (4)	Indian Affairs*
	Aging*
	Ethics
	Intelligence

House

Standing committees (19)	Agriculture
	Appropriations*
	Armed Services
	Budget*
	Education & the Workforce*
	Energy & Commerce*
	Financial Services
	Government Reform
	House Administration
	International Relations
	Judiciary
	Resources
	Rules
	Science
	Small Business
	Standards of Official Conduct
	Transportation and Infrastructure
	Veteran's Affairs*
	Ways and Means*
Select or special committees	Aging*
	Children, Youth & Families*
	Homeland Security
	Intelligence

*Frequently addresses health-related matters.

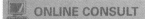

ONLINE CONSULT

American Nurses Association.
http://www.nursingworld.org/gova
U.S. Government Web Portal.
http://firstgov.gov
THOMAS, U.S. Congress on the Internet.
http://thomas.loc.gov
And visit your own state legislature online.

> *Committee action is perhaps the most important phase of the congressional process, because it is at this phase that proposed measures are given the most intensive consideration.*

able information to the committee member, whether information from constituents, special interest groups, experts, or other public officials.

How a Bill Becomes a Law

Consider a bill, for instance, that has been sponsored by your legislator, a member of the House of Representatives. It has been sent to the applicable subcommittee or committee for review. After consideration by the full committee, several things may happen to this bill:

- It may be reported out of committee favorably and be scheduled for debate by the full House.
- It may be reported out favorably, but with amendments or "markups" to the bill.
- It may be reported out unfavorably or not acted upon at all; thus, it is "killed" or "dies in committee."

Generally, once the bill has been reported favorably out of a House committee, it goes to the Rules Committee, which schedules bills and determines (1) how much time will be spent on debate and (2) whether or not amendments will be allowed. A written report is drafted, including a summary of the bill along with impact statements. Bills are then placed on the calendar and scheduled for action. After a bill is debated under the procedural rules of the House, possibly amended, voted upon, and passed, it is sent to the Senate, where it goes through the same procedure. If the bill also passes the Senate without any changes, it is sent to the President or governor for signature. If minor changes were made in the Senate, it is referred back to the originating chamber (in this case the House of Representatives) for concurrence before submission to the executive branch. If significant changes were made to the bill in the Senate, the bill is sent to a **conference committee,** composed of representatives of both chambers, who reconcile differences and prepare a conference report for approval by both chambers. If it does not get approved, the bill dies. After the conference report, the bill must be accepted or rejected, because no further amendments can be made.

If the bill is approved in both houses, it goes to the executive branch. If the President or governor signs the bill, it becomes law, and the Congress is notified. If the bill is vetoed, it is referred back to the House and Senate. A two-thirds vote by both chambers is required to override the veto. The bill may also become law if the President or governor fails to veto or return the bill to Congress with objections within a specified time.

Once the bill is signed or passes, it becomes an act, and is *enacted* into law. Laws are enforceable only if they do not violate the Constitution. They are mandates based on the Constitution, enacted by federal or state legislatures and interpreted by the courts. Once a law is passed, it is assigned to the appropriate department of the executive branch of gov-

1. Concerned party contacts legislator, bill drafted

2. Sponsors obtained, introduced to House and/or Senate

3. To committees for recommendation/ammendments

4. Debate on floor

5. Vote and recommendation to other chamber

6. Consideration in a similar manner by the other chamber

7. Passage or to Conference Committee

8. Back to both houses for concurrence

9. If agreement by both chambers, to president or governor for signature

10. If executive veto, back to chambers for potential override with a 2/3 vote of Congress or the legislature.

FIG. 21–1. The legislative process.

ernment, where the process of developing regulations to interpret the law takes place. The department studies the law and drafts the regulations for implementation. Administrative agencies, governed by the executive branch, promulgate **regulations** or rules, which serve the pupose of detailing and applying the laws. For example, the Health Insurance Portability and Accountability Act (HIPAA) was enacted as Public Law 104–191 in 1996. The Department of Health and Human Services (HHS) published a final Privacy Rule in December 2000 with a general compliance date of April 14, 2003, and a compliance date of April 14, 2004 for small health plans. All of this activity involved detailing regulations for application of the law.

The legislative process is sometimes long and seemingly endless, especially when the bill stays in committee, perhaps during a recess or between legislative sessions. In addition, proposed regulations from the judicial branch may require public hearings for input prior to finalization and enforcement of statute. A legislative session spans a 2-year period, with the 109th Congressional session, for example, running from January 1, 2005, through December 31, 2006.

Laws and regulations govern behavior and relationships with others in society. Consider the impact of laws that have been passed

and their effect on nursing. When the federal government implemented diagnosis-related groups (DRGs) for Medicare reimbursement, patients began to be discharged from hospitals "sicker and quicker." Although this law applied only to Medicare clients, it set a precedent that other insurance carriers followed. In law, a **precedent** is merely a decision or verdict from a prior case that becomes the example in future cases.

Awareness of laws and regulations governing health care is essential in professional nursing practice so that nurses can help to influence the making of policy and laws. Nurses can and do play a significant role at several points in the legislative process, whether through lobbying or providing testimony or information to legislators or regulatory bodies (Box 21–1).

REGULATING NURSING PRACTICE

Nursing practice and education are also regulated by law. Nurse practice acts are contained in state statute (laws) and associated regulations that dictate practice parameters. As part of the statute, nursing education programs in different forms are regulated. For example, most states require a new, beginning nursing program to receive approval from the board of nursing according to specified standards before it can open. These standards ensure that the organization, curriculum, faculty, and services are appropriate for preparation of students and protection of the public. Nursing education is further regulated indirectly through the accrediting bodies that are authorized by the Department of Education.

> *The State Boards of Nursing and their asssociated practice acts define the scope of practice; establish the requirements for licensure, entry into practice, continuing competency, and advanced practice; create and empower a board of nursing; and identify grounds for disciplinary action.*

Nurse Practice Acts

Nurse practice acts are developed by each state to protect the public health, safety, and welfare. The various state boards of nursing and their associated practice acts define the scope of practice; establish the requirements for licensure, entry into practice, continuing competency and advanced practice; create and empower a board of nursing; and identify grounds for disciplinary action. An important component in many practice acts is **title protection**. This is a part of the law that maintains the use of the title *nurse* only for the licensee authorized by the board. The term *nurse* is used in some contexts outside professional practice, and more states are moving to protect the integrity and identity of this title.

Nurse practice acts can be revised or completely eliminated through a single legislative action, so the prospect of "opening the practice act" in the legislature can cause great anxiety. Although state practice acts (statute and regulations) are specific to the state, there is general content common to many acts. For example, the National Council of State Boards of Nursing (NCSBN) has a model act and model rules that illustrate standard contents of the legislation and associated reg-

**BOX 21–1
NURSES' INVOLVEMENT
IN THE LEGISLATIVE PROCESS**

- Meeting with legislators, their aides or staff to influence the introduction of a bill as private citizens or as members of a professional organization
- Providing information to assist in drafting the bill and gathering support for legislators or bill sponsors on the proposed legislation
- Providing testimony in committee or subcommittee hearings about their position on the bill
- Contacting legislators to support or not support proposed legislation, both in the home district and the capitol
- Contacting either the President or the governor to sign or veto the proposed legislation
- Responding to requests for comments, either written or verbal testimony, by regulatory agencies or committees
- Submission of an *Amicus Curiae* (friend of the court) brief for consideration by the court

ulations for implementation (Box 21–2). In addition, in 1998 a mutual recognition model for interstate practice among the "compact states" was introduced. This mutual recognition model requires further specific language to be incorporated into state law to allow a nurse to have one license (in the state of residency) and to practice in other states that are members of the compact. However, the nurse is required to practice in accordance with each state's specific practice law and regulations. Because state laws differ in accordance with their state constitution and associated powers, it is important for nurses to understand the laws regulating their practice.

Appointments to a state board of nursing are often made by the governor. The state board should be composed of a variety of members who represent practice throughout all areas of nursing. In four states, there are separate boards for licensed practical nurses–licensed visiting nurses (LPNs/LVNs) and registered nurses (RNs), but the boards are combined in the remaining jurisdictions. RN boards address both professional nursing and advanced practice nurses (APRNs). APRN regulations may also be addressed in the respective practice acts of other health professions such as the Board of Medicine. In addition, the Board of Nursing may have advisory committees or practice committees that research issues for recommendations to the board on practice or policy issues. Review your state's practice act for the composition of members on the board or perhaps seek a seat on the board. In many cases, serving on the Board of Nursing is both a humbling and an enlightening experience, and allows you to serve your state and your profession.

Because regulatory changes proposed by a state board can lead to statutory law and rules that have the same force as law, it is imperative for nurses to remain aware of the activi-

ties of the board that regulates practice within their state. The American Nurses Association (ANA) provides recent updates to practice acts and the status of proposed legislation on its Web site. In addition, some states issue advisory opinions; although such opinions do not have the same impact as law, they do guide acceptable standards of practice. Nurses are often unaware that changes are even being proposed. Some states distribute the state nurses association newsletter to all registered nurses, whether or not they hold membership in the ANA or the state association. Many of the newsletters issues contain periodic informational alerts concerning changes in or interpretations to the statute or advisory opinions by the board.

State boards and their respective members are concerned about nurses' current understanding of their respective state law. To encourage and increase nurses' knowledge about their respective practice acts, several states award continuing education credits for specific courses. These courses and the multiple-choice post-tests of 20 to 22 questions specific to the state are available through the NCSBN at *http://www.ncsbn.org*. It is vital that nurses understand the content of their respective practice acts. This understanding must be ongoing, beyond the point of original licensure or title recognition. Put a bookmark in your computer's Internet browser with the Web site of your nursing board(s) to give yourself quick information and links to related resources.

Additional State and Federal Laws Affect Nursing Practice

Many states have passed laws, for example, allowing some nurses to be directly reimbursed by clients or insurers. Legislation varies from state to state, but APRNs, particularly nurse anesthetists, nurse practitioners, and nurse midwives, are most commonly covered. Almost 200,000 APRNs are providing essential health-care services as certified nurse midwives, certified registered nurse anesthetists, nurse practitioners, and clinical nurse specialists (ANA , 2003a).

BOX 21–2
NURSE PRACTICE ACTS

General content for both statute and regulations:

- Title and purpose
- Definitions, scope, and standards of practice
- Board of nursing—authority and how it functions
- Application of other state statutes and the state's administrative law act
- Licensure
- Titles and abbreviations
- Approval of nursing education programs
- Violations and penalties
- Discipline and proceedings
- Emergency relief for public protection
- Reporting requirements
- Exemptions
- Revenue and fees
- Implementation of the statute and regulations

State laws that affect practice can be passed with the support of nursing. Some states have passed laws to allow registered nurses to pronounce death. Others are addressing safe practice through staffing requirements, tort reform, and prohibitions on mandatory overtime. Still others are addressing delegation to assistive personnel. Public protection is a concern at all levels of government. In the area of advanced practice, for example, states differ in level of supervision or collaboration and prescriptive authority for advanced practice nurses. Nurses must be politically astute and must continue to develop their internal political efficacy and the external efficacy of the profession.

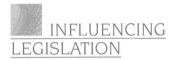

INFLUENCING LEGISLATION

As mentioned previously, the idea for a law may originate from a concerned citizen or special interest group, a legislator, a professional group, or the executive branch to address a community problem or a public policy issue. However, many laws originate from the legislature, which is composed of individuals who are elected by constituents with specific interests, needs, and concerns. Legislators' knowledge and recognition of particular needs and concerns come about through influence. For instance, special interest groups representing large numbers of the voting public can have a lot of influence on legislators. Special interest groups have become more politically savvy at influencing the creation of public policy, and more controls have emerged, as with campaign financing reforms. Special interest groups influence legislators through lobbying activities, professional lobbyists, professional organizations, political action committees, and grassroots efforts. Each of these groups represents the dollars and votes of a particular special interest group, and each group uses expert communication and interpersonal skills to influence change.

Lobbying

Activities to influence legislators vary from formal to informal and often take the form of lobbying. **Lobbying** may be defined as attempting to persuade a legislator or legislative aide of the merits of your viewpoint in order to influence legislation. Individuals may "lobby" through face-to-face interviews, letter writing, telephone calls, faxes, e-mails, letters to the editor, and testimony (verbal or written). Valuable clues on and guidelines for letter writing are provided by professional associations that recognize the value of individual constituents' contacting their elected legislators. These professional organizations often provide special alerts or suggestions to the members to assist with lobbying activities. For example, some professional organizations provide an alert when congresspersons are on recess and should be contacted in their home states. Other organizations may include lobbying tips on their Web sites, along with background issues and talking points to assist in lobbying activities.

But there is definitely an art at getting your point across. The bottom line is that numbers mean something to the legislative aide or legislator, especially from constituents. There are other considerations, however, such as

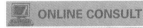

ONLINE CONSULT

ANA: Government Affairs.
http://www.nursingworkd.org
National League for Nursing: Policy.
http://www.nln.org

time. The impact of a well-composed, factual, meaningful, and succinct letter far outweighs the form letter that has less impact or a letter that rambles on. Another consideration is the form of the correspondence. Postal delays cannot compete with the immediacy of e-mail, for instance. For a personal appointment, be aware of the congressional calendar, and do not be disappointed if you meet with a legislative aide. The aide may be more knowledgeable about your issue and can be persuaded to communicate the information to the legislator.

The professional lobbyist is a person on the staff of a professional association or organization who has outstanding skills in persuasion, in-depth knowledge of the organization, and an acute sense of the intricacies of the political system. These professionals understand the legislators and their political agendas. The professional lobbyist is present at the appropriate time with the correct message, especially in the case of the undecided legislator. The role of the professional lobbyist is to provide the facts and the support base to persuade the legislator. The ANA has several professional lobbyists working at the federal level. A significant number of constituent state associations (CNAs) and specialty professional organizations also hire professional lobbyists.

Lobbying is especially effective when there is an associated strong **grassroots effort** that responds with mobilization of a group to provide additional correspondence and support on the position presented to the legislator or legislative aide. This approach has been used effectively by many professional organizations to influence public policy. Various nursing and other grassroots networks have been established to lobby in support of the legislative goals and objectives of the state nurses associations. There are specific channels of communication for response to a key issue. Key contacts for each legislator or legislative district must be active and ongoing. ANA's N-STAT is an example of this grassroots lobbying system. Established in 1993, N-STAT continues to grow, with more nurses providing a rapid response on legislative and policy issues. Nurses can register online, receive periodic alerts, and take an active step toward political efficacy. Sign up today, or periodically refer to the ANA Web site for particular national and state initiatives and legislative alerts at *http://www. nursingworld.org.*

Professional Organizations

Nurses have always had a great deal of potential power by virtue of numbers, but have now begun to use their power collectively. This is one important reason to join **professional organizations**. Only through united efforts will nurses be seen as a powerful group and will their voices be recognized in the policy arena. This has been demonstrated continually by many vocal and powerful organizations readily visible on Capitol Hill, on surrounding streets in Washington, DC or in your state capitol, such as the American Medical Association (AMA) and the American Hospital Association (AHA). In a study conducted in 2003, the ANA was listed along with the AMA and the AHA in the top 20 of groups with most influence on Capitol Hill (Heaney, 2003). And consider the number of professional nursing organizations with headquarters located in the Washington, DC area (refer to the professional organizations listed on the Intranet site).

The ANA and its 53 constituent state members are also associated with the Washington, DC area organizational affiliate members. The legislative or political arm of the ANA is known as the Department of Governmental Affairs. It actively advocates for legislation and works with administrative agencies on regulations for implementation of laws and health policy. ANA regularly monitors the work of more than a dozen federal agencies that affects health-care policy, like the Centers for Medicare and Medicaid Services (CMS) and the Agency for Health Research and Quality (AHRQ). The ANA (2002), in association with other affiliated nursing organizations, also promoted an *Agenda for the Future: A Call to the Nation*, that identified the following ten areas as of concern and demanding action:

- Leadership and planning
- Delivery systems
- Legislation/regulation/policy
- Professional/nursing culture
- Recruitment/retention
- Economic value
- Work environment
- Public relations/communication
- Education
- Diversity (p. 7)

To address this agenda in addition to its lobbying activities, ANA establishes legislative and regulatory initiatives for each session of Congress. For example, for the 108th Congress, the ANA (2003b) specified an advocacy agenda for nurses that focused on the following issues: the nursing shortage, appropriate staffing, workplace rights, health and safety, and patient safety and advocacy. These are broad-based initiatives with well-developed statements of the issue, background, and the ANA position.

The ANA's Department of Government Affairs also contains the political action unit N-STAT, made up of the grassroots lobbying network that functions through the activities of Congressional district coordinators, Senate coordinators, and the ANA's political action committee (ANA-PAC).

Political Action Committees

As a result of campaign reform in the 1970s, restrictions were placed on contributions made by individuals or organizations to a candidate for a federal office. This campaign financing reform also allowed for the creation of **political action committees** (PACs), through which organizations could make openly reported contributions. Wilson and DiIulo (1998) have observed that although any organization can form a PAC, more than half of PACs are sponsored by corporations, about a tenth by labor unions, and a growing number by ideological groups (p. 259). It is a political reality that legislators are more likely to see and listen to a group of people who have contributed money to their campaign.

Political campaigns can be quite costly because of the money spent on media coverage. Campaign reforms have continued with the Bipartisan Campaign Reform Act (BCRA) of 2002, including an increase on permissible contributions from individuals, a ban on contributions by minors, limitations on and disclosure of contributions made for issue advertisements presented through the media, and a contribution increase for non–multi-candidate PACs. The act also called for new disclaimer requirements in electioneering communications. These regulations include a "Millionaire Amendment," to allow an increase in contribution limits for candidates facing an opponent with a great deal more campaign resources as expenditures of personal funds.

The ANA (2004) formed a PAC more than three decades ago to create power and influence for the nursing profession. Contributions to the ANA-PAC support pro-nursing candidates, current legislators, and legislation. It is bipartisan, supporting candidates of both national parties. The PAC is focused on the public office and the candidate for that office, whether incumbent or opponent. Endorsements and financial contributions are based on the candidates' support for the ANA legislative agenda and stance on health policy. In addition, some state constituents of ANA have separate state-associated PACs working on behalf of nursing issues in their particular states and at the federal level. Other specialty professional nursing organizations have PACs as well, representing issues critical to their respective missions.

GAINING SKILL IN POLITICAL EFFICACY

The initial step in developing political efficacy is understanding the process and having the willingness to be involved. But even more basic is possessing an understanding of people and policy needed for public health and welfare. This understanding of people and their health-care needs is basic to nursing practice. The next prerequisite to political efficacy is an understanding of the issues involved. It is vital that nurses use their voices and individual power to empower nurses and nursing. As Milstead (2003) has observed, "involvement in policy making is not an option for a professional nurse—it is a necessity" (p. 15). This is your imperative for action. Nurses can influence change in the workplace, in their communities, in professional organizations, and in government.

Workplace Issues

As illustrated with management in the organizational setting, the workplace is a significant area for nurses to promote policy changes, particularly regarding workplace advocacy and client safety and advocacy. Nurses are highly regarded by clients and the public. In addition, they have the five general bases of power identified by Mintzberg (1983): control of resources, control of a technical skill, control of a body of knowledge, exclusive rights or privileges to impose choices (legal prerogatives), and access to people who have and can be relied on for the other four. To be influential, nurses must take an active role in institutional decision-making, either at the unit level or by volunteering to serve on various committees. To contribute to policy decisions, they must remain current on health policy issues and must provide factual information. This involvement with **workplace** issues provides the basis for the improvements needed in the delivery of care and positive outcomes for both clients and the profession.

Community or Civic Involvement

A prime responsibility for all citizens is to be part of the electorate—to be registered and to vote in local, state, and national elections. Nurses have traditionally been involved in the community, whether serving on committees like the local school or hospital board or helping out with a local health fair. These activities constitute **community or civic involve-**

ment. In the community, nurses can identify potential health hazards that require the attention of local officials or businesspersons, and can intervene in the case of health risks or hazards. Nurses are adept at understanding community issues, and active involvement of professional nurses in community or civic activities is truly an imperative.

Professional Organizations

Active involvement in professional organizations provide both constant development and valuable information. As illustrated with the governmental functions of the ANA, professional organizations offer policy analysis and updates, and they can lead effective campaigns to influence policy change. As already described, Nursing's Agenda for the Future (ANA, 2002) addresses many policy areas that the ANA and the 18 other professional organizations on the steering committee are committed to addressing. From the steering group of 19 organizations, more than 60 nursing organizations became united in collaboration on these issues (ANA, 2002, p. 19). Nurses should remain knowledgeable about the positions of the professional organizations on issues that are likely to come before Congress. This awareness can assist with needed action on health policies and legislation through participation in grassroots efforts of the organization. It can also lead to service in elected and appointed positions or opportunities to provide testimony on behalf of the organization.

Government

Be aware of who your legislators and other elected or appointed officials are at local, state, and national levels. Keep yourself informed on how they support the issues, especially those related to health policy. Communicate with these officials. Nurses have the expertise in the care for clients and they witness the impact of health policy on a daily basis. Legislators want to hear the concerns of their nurse constituents and will appreciate the information you provide to help address the concerns of all their consitutents. Often, legislators' only view of the health-care arena is through the care they or a family member receives and the views imparted to them by their legislative aides and constituents. At times, this perspective can be narrow and very personal. The issues being confronted by federal, state, and local legislators on health policy can have long-term and wide-ranging effects on both the profession and care of clients. Nurses are serving in growing numbers in important roles to assist with the passage of health policy for the good of both the public and the profession.

At the state level, nurses have successfully lobbied to enact legislation that allows them to bill insurance companies directly for the care they provide. Prescriptive authority, interstate practice, amendments or revisions to practice acts, and safe staffing requirements are current issues in many state legislatures. To have legislation enacted, individual nurses or a nursing organization can seek a sponsor and co-sponsors to introduce it. Once the legislation is introduced, nurses must lobby legislators to provide information on how passage of the bill will benefit the legislator's constituents. Nurses elected to leadership positions and appointed to serve on boards at the state government level are becoming more common, but there is a great need to increase the numbers who are willing and prepared to serve in these roles. Often it is through involvement at the local level that nurses gain experience and the confidence to move on to state positions.

COMMUNICATING WITH LEGISLATORS

To effectively influence policy, nurses must establish a relationship with legislators and their legislative aides whenever possible. These officials are elected to serve—and are concerned about the needs of—their constituents. They expect constituents to inform

them of their concerns. Watch the interactions that occur at your next community or state function attended by a legislator. It may not be an election year, but the legislator is present because the particular function is of importance to a group the legislator represents. A nurse's offer to serve as a personal resource is frequently welcomed by the legislator and his or her staff. This is particularly true at the local and state levels, at which legislators may not have extensive staff to assist with legislation involving health policy. Nurses can also be valuable in providing testimony for regulatory change. However, practice and preparation are needed for developing proficiency, effectiveness, and ease in these activities, particularly in dealing with the media. Being knowledgeable and articulate in both subject matter and presentation is essential.

CONCLUSION

Nurses must be part of the process, whether providing needed facts and background on the issues or serving in an office. Buresch and Gordon (2000) describe this as the **voice of agency,** "a strong and authentic voice that accurately represents and honors the experience of illness as well as the experience of those who care for the sick and vulnerable" (p. 34). Nurses must increasingly be involved in advocating beyond the hospital or health-care unit environment. We have unique insights and the knowledge base to effect change and improve health care and health policy. This is the political imperative: be involved, be active, continue to develop interpersonal and political skills, and continue to understand the evolving needs of people and the profession. The issues for action with public policy are further discussed in Chapter 22. However, act now on current legislation and consider the information provided in Box 21–3 on tips for communicating with your legislator and Box 21–4 on tips for presenting testimony before a committee or regulatory body.

BOX 21–3
TIPS FOR TALKING TO LEGISLATORS

- Before meeting with your legislator, get to know as much as possible about his or her background, special interests or initatives, voting record, committee assignments, and involvement with health policy issues.
- Prepare your position, including a list of talking points to assist you during the discussion.
- Investigate both sides of the issue but stay focused on the facts.
- Request a meeting of at least 15 to 30 minutes.
- Practice your presentation with a friend or colleague to gain comfort with the content and to anticipate questions that may arise.
- If the legislator is not available, meet with the legislative aide or staff member who has a good knowledge of the issues.
- Be on time, and be professional.
- Introduce yourself and thank the legislator or legislative aide for his or her time and interest.
- Be prepared to explain what you do as a nurse, your philosophy of care, and the impact of pending legislation on health care and care delivery for the legislator's constituents.
- Use concise and explicit examples from your practice to illustrate your position.
- Be prepared to offer additional information or solutions, but stick to the facts.
- If the legislator or legislative aide indicates support for your position, ask what you can do to reach other legislators or sponsors.
- Provide an opportunity to answer any questions and offer any additional assistance on the circumstances of the proposed legislation or regulation.
- Send a follow-up thank you note for the time spent, in which you restate your position.
- And you may even want to follow your interview with a well-worded letter on your position to the editor of the local newspaper—and perhaps gain further support among other constituents.

BOX 21–4
TIPS FOR PRESENTING TESTIMONY

- Be prepared, with:
  - A full, well-developed written statement and talking points.
  - An understanding of the committee process and regulatory structure.
  - An anticipation of any follow-up questions that may be asked of you.
- Be on time.
- Be confident in your abilities and knowledge base, and remain calm.
- Be flexible; you may not have the time for your presentation that you were told you would.
- Recognize the members of the body ("Mr./Madam Chairperson and members of the _____ Committee") and thank them for allowing you the opportunity to address them.
- Introduce yourself and be respectful.
- Do not read your written testimony; ask to have it placed in the record.
- Use the talking points to present your case and focus on the facts.
- Again, try to use concise and explicit examples from your practice to illustrate your position.
- Do not go over your allocated time.
- Leave time at the end of your presentation for any questions from the members.
- Thank the committee for the opportunity to present your testimony at the end.

Key Points

- Internal political efficacy is personal competence or the "ability to understand and take part in political affairs," and external political advocacy is the "ability to make the system respond to the citizenry" (Wilson and DiIulo, 1998, p. 102).

- Laws are mandates based on the Constitution, enacted by federal or state legislatures, and interpreted by the courts. Administrative agencies, governed by the executive branch, promulgate regulations or rules, which serve the pupose of detailing and applying the laws.

- The enactment of a law begins with introduction of the bill by the sponsoring legislator to either the House or the Senate. Then, it is referred to committee for recommendations and amendments.

- Common law is created by judicial decisions that form a precedent upon which future decisions are based.

- Nurse practice acts are statutory law with associated administrative regulations developed by each state to protect the public health, safety, and welfare. They define the scope of practice; establish requirements for licensure, entry into practice, continuing competency and advanced practice; create and empower a board of nursing to oversee licensees; and identify grounds for disciplinary action.

- Title protection is the part of the nursing practice act that protects and restricts the use of the term *nurse* to the licensee authorized to practice by the board.

- Activities to influence legislators vary from formal to informal. Lobbying may be defined as attempting to persuade a legislator or legislative aide of merits of your viewpoint and to influence legislation.

- Lobbying is especially effective when there is an associated strong grassroots effort that responds with mobilization of a group that provides additional correspondence and support on the issues.

- Special interest groups have become more politically savvy at influencing the creation of public policy, and more controls have emerged, as with campaign financing reforms. One form of a special interest group is the political action committee (PAC).

- Buresch and Gordon (2000) define a voice of agency as "a strong and authentic voice that accurately represents and honors the experience of illness as well as the experience of those who care for the sick and vulnerable" (p. 34). Nurses can influence change in the workplace, the community, professional organizations, and government.

Thought and Discussion Questions

1. Consider the laws allowing direct reimbursement of nursing services by insurance companies. Discuss the processes that led to passage of these laws.
2. Identify how you will demonstrate both internal and external political efficacy. Be prepared to participate in a discussion in class or online to be scheduled by your instructor.
3. Select a current issue of concern and develop an action plan to present your views to a legislator.
4. Review the Chapter Thought located on the first page of the chapter, and discuss it in the context of the contents of the chapter.

Interactive Exercises

1. Locate one example of each type of law (constitutional, statutory, administrative, and common) relevant to health-care or health policy.

2. Complete the interactive exercise on the Intranet site on the practice act in your state of licensure and a state that has mutual recognition. Compare and contrast the information obtained for each state. Be prepared to participate in an online discussion, to be scheduled by your instructor, on the information you identify.

3. Locate a professional organization of interest on the Intranet site. Describe the information on political involvement provided by the organization. Investigate the current political initiatives and the activities of the organization.

4. Complete the interactive exercise on the Intranet site on communicating with your elected member of Congress, outlining your concerns over one of the major health-care issues presented in the ANA legislative and regulatory agenda, using the identified resources to support your position. Be prepared to participate in an online discussion, to be scheduled by your instructor, before sending your e-mail.

5. Prepare to provide testimony before a legislative committee. Identify proposed legislation or regulation at the state level of interest to you. Using the guidelines provided on the Intranet site, complete your research, present your testimony, and evaluate the results.

6. Using the form on the Intranet site, identify the steps you will now take to demonstrate your internal and external political efficacy.

PRINT RESOURCES

References

American Nurses Association Government Affairs Department. (2003b). *Legislative and regulatory initiatives for the 108th Congress* (pub. Number LR123CM6). Washington, DC: American Nurses Publishing.

Buresh, B., & Gordon, S. (2000). *From silence to voice: What nurses know and must communicate to the public.* Ottawa, Ontario: Canadian Nurses Association.

Clinton, H. R. (2003). *Living history.* New York: Simon & Schuster.

Gaston, M. A. (1998). The value of politics [editorial]. *Journal of Dental Hygiene, 72*(3), 3–4.

Heaney, M. T. (2003, October 1). PhRMA tops health groups with most pull on Hill. *The Hill,* Special Section: Health Care.

Leininger, M. (2002). Cultures and tribes of nursing, hospitals, and the medical culture. In M. Leininger & M. R. McFarland, *Transcultural nursing: Concepts, theories, research, and practice* (3rd ed.) (pp. 181–204). New York: McGraw-Hill.

Mason, D. J., Chaffee, M. W., & Leavitt, J. K. (2002). *Policy and politics in nursing and health care* (4th ed.). Philadelphia: WB Saunders.

Mintzberg, H. (1983). *Power in and around organizations.* Englewood Cliffs, NJ: Prentice-Hall.

Wilson, J. Q., & DiIulio, J. J. (1998). *American government: Institutions and policies.* Boston: Houghton Mifflin.

Bibliography

Johnson, C. W. (1998). *How our laws are made.* Washington, DC: U.S. Government Printing Office.

Oleszek, W. J. (2001). *Congressional procedures and the policy process.* Washington, DC: CQ Press.

ONLINE RESOURCES

References

American Nurses Association. (2004). American Nurses Association Political Action Committee (ANA-PAC).

Legislative Branch. *http://vocusgr.vocus.com/grconvert1/webpub/ana/Profile.asp?Entity=PRAsset&EntityID=…*

American Nurses Association. (2003a). *Nursing facts.* Washington, DC: American Nurses Publishing. *http://nursingworld.org/readroom/fsdemogrpt.htm#summ*

American Nurses Association. (2002). Nursing's agenda for the future. *http://www.nursingworld.org/readroom/rnagenda.htm*

Milstead, J. A. (2003). Interweaving policy and diversity. *Online Journal of Issues in Nursing,* 8(1). *http://www.nursingworld.org/ojin/topic20//tpc20_4.htm.*

Resources

Federal Election Commission (2003). FAQ and the BRCA and other new rules. *http://www.fec.gov.*

Official Government Web Portal. *http://www.firstgov.gov.*

U.S. Constitution. *http://www.usconstitution.net/const.html*

U.S. Department of Health and Human Services. (2003). Summary of the HIPAA Privacy Rule. *http://www.hhs.gov/ocr/privacysummary.pdf.*

THOMAS, U.S. Congress on the Internet. *http://thomas.loc.gov*

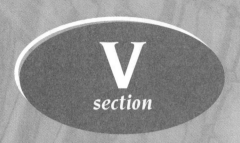

Health-Care Issues in the New Millennium

Sister Rosemary Donley

22
chapter

Nursing's Health-Care Agenda

> *Nursing in its broadest sense may be defined as an art and a science which involves the whole patient—body, mind, and spirit; promotes his spiritual, mental, and physical health by teaching and by example; stresses health education and health preservation, as well as ministration to the sick; involves the care of the patients' environment—social and spiritual as well as physical; and gives health service to the family and community as well as to the individual.*
>
> Sr. M. Olivia Gowan, founding Dean, The Catholic
> University of America, School of Nursing, June, 1944

Chapter Objectives

On completion of this chapter, the reader will be able to:

1. Discuss the issues that are on nursing's health-care agenda.
2. Describe the interaction between the issues.
3. Discuss how the nursing shortage influences nursing's ability to influence change.

Key Terms

Surgicenters and
  Urgicenters
Niche Services
Staffing Ratios
Best Practices
Cost-Benefit-Burden Ratio

Tiered Payments
Breakthrough Drugs
Technological
  Imperative
Health Disparities
Medicare Parts A, B, C, D

S-CHIP
Prescription Drug Act
  of 2003
The Nurse Reinvestment
  Act

In the past 20 years, nurses have become interested and engaged in health-care policy. Most schools of nursing teach classes or entire courses in health policy. Professional and specialty nursing organizations monitor federal and state legislation, provide information about health or nursing issues, lobby members of Congress or state legislators, and make financial contributions to or enter into funding programs to support candidates who embrace nursing and its legislative and policy agenda. Many factors contribute to nurses' interest in policy and politics. Recent events in the world, the tragic events of September 11, 2001, and threats of bioterrorism have made nurses aware of their positions as first- and second-line responders. The nursing shortage, the uninsured, and changes in the health-care delivery system and modes of reimbursement have altered the practice of nursing and the nursing care of patients in all health-care settings. Nurses realize that many of the problems that affect the health of all Americans can be addressed only by informed and collective action. In the 21st century, policy awareness and advocacy are professional responsibilities. This chapter addresses current issues on the nursing policy agenda, specifically:

- Health care as a business
- Health-care costs
- Uninsured persons
- Health disparities
- Medicare, Medicaid, and S-CHIP
- Nursing shortage

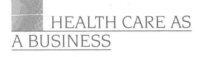

HEALTH CARE AS A BUSINESS

The United States is the only first-world country without a universal program of health insurance sponsored by its government. Heath care is intertwined with the U.S. government in several ways. Although the federal government is involved in health care at many levels, it is important to remember that health care in the United States is a business partnership between the public (government) and the private sector. One way the government is involved in health care is research. The federal government contributes to research and development in health. Scientists at the National Institutes of Health (NIH), located in Bethesda, Maryland, conduct clinical studies within their own clinical center. The major research thrust financed and supported by NIH, however, is carried out around the United States, most notably in the nation's medical schools and academic health centers. Other federal agencies also sponsor extramural research, scientific studies conducted outside the walls of the funding agency. The Centers for Disease Control (CDC), the Centers for Medicare and Medicaid Services (CMS), the Agency for Healthcare Research and Quality (AHRQ), the Substance Abuse and Mental Health Services Administration (SAMHSA), and the Center for Nursing Research (CNR) are just a few of the federal agencies that support studies to improve the health of the nation.

The federal government and some state governments also provide scholarships and loans to students who study nursing and medicine. In some cases, these loans are forgiven if physicians or nurses work in the state or, in the case of federal grants, in underserved areas after graduation.

The federal government's most extensive involvement in health care is through its insurance programs: Medicare, Medicaid, and the State Children's Health Insurance Program (S-CHIP). In fact, when most people talk about the federal government and health care, they think of Medicare. Anyone interested in pubic policy is interested in Medicare, Medicaid, and S-CHIP because these programs pay for the care of persons older than 65 years, for the poor and disabled, and for poor children.

Public/Private Model of Healthcare

In America, health care contributes significantly to the economic well being of the

494

country. America is a model of private and public (government) collaboration around health. For some eligible persons— military personnel on active duty, their dependents, and retirees, veterans with service connected illnesses or disabilities, Native Americans, and prisoners—the federal government operates its own health system and provides direct care. This service program is significant; the Veterans' Administration Nursing Service is the largest nursing service in the United States. Some public hospitals and long-term care facilities are also run by state or local governments. The Cook County Hospital is one example of a public hospital that provides care to underserved people in Chicago.

Most people in this country, however, receive health care in the private sector: physicians' offices, clinics, ambulatory care centers, and hospitals run as either for-profit or not-for-profit operations. Although both state and federal governments play a role in the private sector by licensing health-care providers, such as doctors and nurses, and establishing and maintaining safety and health standards in institutions, the responsibility of providing preventative, therapeutic, or rehabilitative care is in the hands of doctors and nurses who are not employees of the government. These health professionals participate as an integral part of the private sector economy.

Because this public-private model of health care is unique among first-world nations, it is often cited in discussions of health-care costs and health-care outcomes. The United States spends close to 15% of its gross domestic product (GDP) on health care. It ranks above Japan, Great Britain, and the countries of Western Europe in health-care expenditures. Yet when health outcomes, as measured by public health indicators such as mortality, morbidity, infant mortality, low-birth-weight babies, and immunizations, are examined, the United States ranks behind other countries that spend less money on health care (U.S. Dept. of Health and Human Services [DHHS], 2000).

Supporters of the private sector involvement in health care note that America's health-care system is the envy of the world. Its technology and expertise are exported to many countries; its medical and nursing schools and hospitals are the training sites for many multinationals; the United States is a major developer of new drugs; and its biomedical researchers contribute to international journals. Closer to home, hospitals are often the largest employers in communities, employing a wide range of workers. Physicians and nurses with graduate degrees are at one end of the spectrum. At the other end, hospitals offer jobs and career advancement opportunities to persons who have not completed high school. Hospitals often have desirable benefit packages for all employees that include health insurance, retirement benefits, on-the-job training and staff development, and tuition support programs. Hospitals fuel local economies. Health careers are sought after; places in medical school are coveted; and jobs in the health-care sector seem to be stable even in periods of recession.

Some critics of this public/private American

FOR-PROFIT VERSUS NOT-FOR-PROFIT

The majority of hospitals in America are not-for-profit. Profit, the positive difference between income and expenditures, that is generated by not-for-profit hospitals is re-invested in the hospitals or in their local communities. In for-profit institutions, most nursing homes, some hospitals, and most clinics and ambulatory care centers, profit is shared among the investors. In the for-profit health sector, the focus is upon making the business (health care) profitable, competitive, and therefore attractive to investors. Individuals in private or group practices—physicians and some advanced practice nurses—must run profitable health-care operations to stay in business.

plan blame rising health-care costs and the failure to achieve good outcomes on business involvement in health care. These critics address the link between employment and health insurance, the for-profit nature of health care, and the placing of efficiency and economic gain above the care of patients. In the United States, health-care providers are entrepreneurs. This fact is most evident in the practice of medicine, in which most physicians are self-employed or share a medical partnership with a group of doctors. Because most physicians are not employed by institutions, they earn income according to the number of patients they see and the nature of their practices. Specialist physicians earn more than primary care physicians, and surgeons earn more than internists. American physicians have adjusted their practices to the financial incentives present in their communities. In fee-for-service medicine, physicians perform more tests and examinations than are absolutely necessary to diagnose and treat the patients' illnesses, because physicians are paid according to the number and type of services provided.

When managed care became the dominant form of health insurance, physicians learned that the financial incentives for the practice of medicine had changed (Relman, 1992). They realized that they could make more money by providing fewer tests and referrals. Managed care companies offered special financial incentives to physicians who used less expensive tests and treatments and were able to keep their patients out of hospitals. Managed care's control of tests, procedures, and treatments has had some effect on health-care costs and the practice protocols of physicians. It has also intensified the underlying business reality that physicians in managed care systems are working for themselves as well as their patients. The traditional idea that physicians are agents of their patients has been distorted in contemporary health care. Patients and families are no longer certain whether medical advice represents the patients' best interest or the financial well-being of the doctors. This conflict of interest has caused a loss of trust in doctors and the health-care system itself.

Competition in Health Care

American health care operates in a competitive market. Competition exists between physicians and nurses, especially physicians and advanced practice nurses, between hospitals and physicians, between hospitals, and among hospitals and insurance companies. In a true marketplace, competition drives down prices and allows the most competent and efficient to survive. Health care is not the best example of a marketplace. Patients are often ill and unable to do the research or make the judgments that are in their best interests. The health-care industry is regulated. In many states, medical societies have influence over state legislators. Revision of practice acts to permit more independence for advance practice nurses, nurse practitioners, nurse anesthetists, clinical specialists, and midwives is often blocked. Although studies have demonstrated the competence and cost-effectiveness of nurse practitioners, the role that advance practice nurses could play in lowering the cost of health care without affecting its quality has never been tested because of the control that physicians and their lobbyists have on state legislatures.

Physician competition with hospitals is more complex. The simplicity and availability of technology, changes in reimbursement for hospitals and physicians, and the pressure to limit hospital admissions and provide care in less expensive settings have encouraged many physicians to join together and set up freestanding ambulatory care businesses that compete with hospitals. Physicians and nurses in these **surgicenters and urgicenters** can safely perform procedures, biopsies, cataract surgery, many orthopedic procedures, and some gynecologic and urologic procedures in attractive and convenient settings. Insurance companies recognize that these centers operate without the high overhead costs of hospitals because they do not provide costly services, such as emergency and intensive care. Ambulatory centers are one type of **niche services** that meet particular needs.

Hospitals have engaged in significant competition with one another. Before the changes in reimbursement for Medicare initiated during the early 1980s, hospitals competed by offering amenities such as family-centered maternity care. However, after diagnostic related groups (DRGs) became the standard of payment for inpatient care, hospitals began to compete on price. Price competition enabled hospitals that could provide quality care within the DRG payment structure to reduce their costs. These efficient hospitals competed with other hospitals for managed care contracts. Hospitals that could not compete on price experienced lower occupancy rates. Because DRGs caused patients to be admitted late and discharged early, all hospitals, even efficient ones, experienced reduced occupancy. Hospitals responded by decreasing their numbers of beds.

This downsizing also triggered a reduction in nursing and support staff. Some commentators trace the current nursing shortage to staffing decisions made by hospitals in the mid-1980s. When downsizing did not help the bottom line, hospitals re-organized. The decade of the eighties saw many hospitals merge or become organized into health systems. *Vertical organization* became the term in the hospital literature to describe hospital systems that organized along similar service lines. As an alternative to vertical organization, some hospitals built integrated service networks that combined into one organization all the health services that patients might need. These sophisticated *horizontal organizations* included services as acute care, home care, extended care, durable medical equipment providers, and pharmacies. Hospitals that joined horizontal organizations hoped that they could compete more successfully for managed care contracts because they could offer patients a form of one-stop shopping. Other values that encouraged hospitals to merge or form systems as a way of competing were economies of scale and access to capital for expansion, acquisition of new services including physician practices, and the enlarging of the system itself.

The last form of competition occurred between insurance companies and hospitals. In some cases, hospitals became insurance companies, and in others, insurance companies bought hospitals and physician practices.

The idea behind these business arrangements was to lower the costs and control the delivery of health care within communities.

Business Influence on Health Care

The relationship of private and public sectors in the area of health care has been expanded in the past 20 years. The influence of business is evident in the adoption of the language and ethics of business. It is not uncommon for patients to be described as "consumers" or "market share" and for health or nursing care to be described as "product lines." Nurses have not been immune to the influence of business on their practices. Some have tried to learn or at least adapt to the business model in providing health care. Others have tried to practice what they believe is important to the care of patients. Some have joined unions or advocated for legislation to mandate **staffing ratios** to ensure a sufficient number of nurses to care for patients, especially those who are hospitalized.

One positive influence of the business community on health care is its insistence that outcomes are more important than processes. For years, the health-care community relied on structure and process to ensure quality of care. The business community wants health-care outcomes that show some demonstrable change or benefit to the patient and some positive cost-benefit ratio to society. The professional community, especially physicians and nurses, has responded to these mandates. This response has caused nurses and other health-care professionals to examine the outcomes or results of their interventions and to base their practice on evidence. There is also a growing interest in the health community in finding and then using the **best practices**. Simply put, a *best practice* is something that works, that accomplishes the goal. Discovering and sharing best practices is one mode, research is another, of basing nursing practice on evidence. Evidence-based practice is increasingly important to the professional practice of nursing. Health professionals have added another factor to businesses' concern with cost-benefit ratios: the **cost-benefit-**

burden ratio. Considerations of *burden* look at the patient's perception and experience of planned diagnostic or therapeutic interventions. This approach puts the patient at the center of clinical decision-making.

> *The business community wants health-care outcomes that show some demonstrable change or benefit to the patient and some positive cost-benefit ratio to society.*

HEALTH-CARE COSTS

Health-care costs are always on nursing's policy agenda, probably because these costs have risen for more than 40 years. As medical technology and drug therapy have become more sophisticated, people live longer, and the "baby boomer" generation nears retirement, there is renewed concern because no system or method consistently reduces health expenditures in the United States. In the 1990s, policy makers and the Congress of the United States had great hope that managed care would control rising health-care costs. The United States spends, on average, $5440 per person for health care per year, approximately twice what is spent in European countries (Levit et al., 2004). Initially, policy makers were encouraged because health costs increased by only 5 to 5.3 percent from 1996 to 1998. Since then, however, costs have begun to rise. A report released early in 2004 revealed that health-care spending grew by 9.3 percent in 2002, the sixth straight year of reported increases (Brown, 2004). The authors of this report, researchers at the CMS, identified the following explanatory factors for the growth of expenses in 2002:

- Technology, especially those technologies delivered in acute care hospitals
- Physician services
- Home health care
- Prescription drugs (Levit et al., 2004).

The last category, cost of prescription drugs, rose 15 percent in 2002. This increase, notable in itself, is of particular interest because of the new prescription drug benefit enacted under Medicare. In 2002, retail prescription spending alone accounted for 10.5 percent of the health expenditures (Levit et al., 2004).

Rising health-care expenditures confirm that managed care has lost its ability to control health-care costs. Why did this happen? The American public, physicians, and hospitals became tired of the second-guessing of clinical decisions and the control exerted by managed care officials. There was a public outcry against practices such as the same-day discharge of new mothers, which some called "drive-by deliveries." People believed that their health providers, not their insurance companies, should make health-care decisions. Managed care companies responded to public and legal pressure and gave patients more choice of primary care providers and greater access to certain specialists.

Most companies have responded to increases in both the cost of health care and the cost of providing health insurance to employees by changing payment and benefit structures. Employees now pay higher deductibles (the amount the person must pay before the insurance pays) and more in co-payments for any health service: medical visits, tests, visits to the emergency room, therapy, and drugs. Many plans have **tiered payments** so that patients pay one fee to visit their primary care providers and a higher fee to visit specialists. This same pattern applies to prescription drugs:

- Generic drugs have a small co-payment.
- Mid-range drugs have a higher co-payment.
- New, **breakthrough drugs** have the highest co-payment.

The employer is sharing or passing on increases in health insurance to employees through deductibles and co-payments (Feldstein, 2003).

"High-Tech" Acute Care

American style health care is expensive because it emphasizes acute care rather than prevention or primary care. In the other countries, where health-care costs are less, there is more emphasis on primary care.

Because Americans have invested in high-technology medicine, they are caught up in many technologic revolutions, medical and informational. Hospitals are familiar with the need to upgrade and advance their medical technology. However because of managed care, Medicare regulations, and the multiple settings of health care, the health-care system has become increasingly dependent on informational technology, its infrastructure, and security systems. Medical and computer-assisted technologies, too numerous to enumerate, explain why America is the leader in health care. The costs of high-technology medicine must be weighed in light of benefit and burden. Used wisely, these technologies benefit providers and patients. They give providers rapid access to medical records and reports of diagnostic tests. Many of these technologies:

- Reduce length of stay (e.g., laparoscopic surgery).
- Shorten time in surgery (e.g., lens implants).
- Avoid painful, intrusive, and sometimes dangerous tests (e.g., magnetic resonance imaging).

High-technology medicine does not occur in a vacuum. Americans are pragmatic and want results and innovation. These cultural factors support America's investment in technologic medicine. At another level, many health providers perceive losing a patient to disease as failure. In the American medical psyche, there is an impetus to treat, to try another intervention, not to give up. Because technology is so readily available, there is **a technologic imperative**: If the technology is there, it should be used. Some patients undergo more technologic interventions than they want or perhaps need. It is not by chance that the majority of health expenditures for Medicare recipients are incurred in the last 6 months of a patient's life.

Medical Error

Another factor associated with increased costs is error. Nurse practitioners and physicians, especially physicians in certain specialties,

recognize the cost of malpractice insurance and the effect of malpractice claims on their reputation and practice patterns (Wilensky, 2004). There is now greater sensitivity to the cost of unnecessary interventions and the cost of error (Leape, 1992). Several studies by the Institute of Medicine (IOM) have alerted the public and providers about the frequency, seriousness, and cost of medical error. One IOM study, *To Err is Human: Building a Safer Health System* (Kohn et al., 2000), recognizes the role of the health team in contemporary practice. It also addresses the importance of developing a culture of safety in preventing error. A second IOM study, *Crossing the Quality Chasm: A New Health System for the 21st Century* (Committee on Quality Health Care, 2001) presents recommendations to reduce error and enhance the quality of health care.

 ## THE UNINSURED

Many of the issues on nursing's policy agenda are interrelated. There is a connection between the role that health care plays in the economy, the cost of health care, and the number of people in the United States who do not have health insurance. As has been stated earlier in this text, health insurance in America is not a right associated with citizenship. Lacking a system of national health insurance, Americans either must qualify for a government program because they fit entitlement categories—military (Veterans, Tri-Care), age (Medicare) or poverty (Medicaid or S-CHIP)—or must be employed by a company that offers health insurance benefits. The insurance structure in the United States, which effectively connects health-care coverage to employment, does not protect 43 million **uninsured** people from illness or trauma. When the uninsured become injured or ill, they seek care in hospital emergency departments. Uninsured people contribute to the rising cost of health care because their care is not compensated in other words, or paid to the provider by health insurance. Another IOM panel has estimated that the cost to society of having over 43 million people uninsured is between $43 billion and $130 billion a year (Committee on the Consequence of Uninsurance [CCU], 2004).

The quality of care that uninsured people receive is also significant. The IOM panel discussed the health consequences of being an uninsured working adult with common illnesses, such as cancer, diabetes, human immunodeficiency virus (HIV) infection and acquired immunodeficiency syndrome (AIDS), heart and kidney disease, mental illness, trauma, and heart attacks. The main findings of the report are that uninsured working age people (roughly 30 million, or 1 in 7 workers):

- Receive too little medical care.
- Receive it too late.
- Are sicker.
- Die sooner.
- Receive poorer care, even when hospitalized for trauma (CCU, 2004).

It is relevant to note that the number of uninsured people is rising. This figure increased by 5.7 percent (from 14.6 percent) in 2002, when an estimated 15.2 percent of the population, or 43.6 million people, were without health insurance for the entire year (U.S. Dept. of Census, 2004). The 2002 Census data reveal some interesting information about uninsured Americans:

- Young adults (18 to 24 years old) were less likely to be insured than other age groups.
- Poor workers were less likely to have insurance than non-workers.
- Hispanics (67.6 percent) were less likely to have health insurance.
- Although Medicaid insured 14 million people, another 10.5 million people (some 30.4 percent of the poverty population) had no insurance.
- The percentage of people covered by employment-based insurance dropped from 62.2 percent to 61.3 percent.
- The number covered by governmental programs, notably Medicaid, rose slightly, from 25.3 to 25.7 percent.
- The number of uninsured children remained at 11.6 percent of all children, or 8.5 million.

The AHRQ (2003) indicates that from 1998 to 2001, three measures of the uninsured seemed to remain stable: between 21 and 31 million people were uninsured all year; at any point in time, about 40 million people were uninsured; and during some part of the year, 60 million people were uninsured. In America, the problem of the uninsured does not go away.

 HEALTH DISPARITIES

The Surgeon General's report, *Healthy People 2010*, establishes two ambitious goals (DHHS, 2000):

- Increase quality and years of healthy life
- Eliminate **health disparities**

In discussing the second goal, the elimination of health disparities, the report states that socioeconomic status, race, ethnicity, and access to care must be considered along with disease in understanding and addressing differences in health status in Americans. It also identifies a list of leading health indicators that are helpful in assessing the health status of individuals and populations. These factors should be integrated into nursing assessments:

- Physical activity
- Overweight and obesity
- Tobacco use
- Substance abuse
- Responsible sexual behavior
- Mental health
- Injury and violence
- Environmental quality
- Immunization
- Access to health care

The idea that factors other than biology or genetics contribute to health status, severity of disease, response to treatment, and even death is not new. Representations of the significance and the interplay of factors that explain health, like the one presented in FIG. 22–1, are well documented in the community health and public health literature. What is new and exciting is that the Surgeon General's report highlights the importance of assessing the person's lifestyle and environment.

> *The idea that factors other than biology or genetics contribute to health status, severity of disease, response to treatment, and even death is not new.*

It is also significant that the message of *Healthy People 2010* reminds nurses of the 1948 World Health Organization's definition of *health* as more than the absence of disease. An interesting source of information on health disparities can be found in the IOM's study,

Unequal Treatment: Confronting Racial and Ethnic Disparities in Health Care (Smedley et al., 2003).

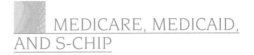

MEDICARE, MEDICAID, AND S-CHIP

Because uninsured people have limited access to care and suffer greater health disparities than people who do have health insurance, the contemporary practice of professional nursing requires that nurses understand how care is financed. This section addresses three

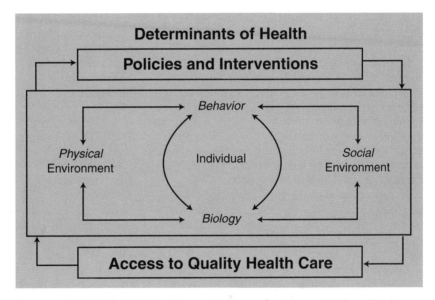

Source: U.S. Dept. Of Health and Human Services, 2000, p. 7.

FIG. 22–1. Determinants of health. (From U.S. Dept. of Health and Human Services. [2000]. *Healthy People 2010* [p. 7]. Washington, DC: U.S. Government Printing Office.)

 ONLINE CONSULT

The Healthy People Web site, www.healthypeople.gov, provides information about the 28 focus areas where health disparities exist and presents tool kits to help nurses and other health professionals address the gaps in health care and health status in this country.

governmental programs: Medicare, Medicaid, and S-CHIP.

Medicare

Medicare, a federal health insurance program that primarily serves (1) the elderly and (2) disabled people younger than 65 years who receive Social Security cash payments and have fulfilled the two-year waiting period, has changed little since 1965 (Feldstein, 2003). Most of the amendments made to Medicare were efforts to reduce health-care costs, limit utilization, and refine the method of payment. There are some exceptions. In 1972, persons with end-stage renal disease were made eligible for Medicare regardless of age. In 1983, Congress added a hospice benefit.

In late 2003, President George W. Bush signed the Medicare Prescription Drug Improvement and Modernization Act of 2003 (**Prescription Drug Act of 2003**) which will significantly change Medicare after 2010. In that year, a demonstration project in six metropolitan areas will put Medicare in competition with private health insurance plans. The theory is that because Medicare serves an older, sicker, and more expensive population, the costs of traditional Medicare will force more people into private plans and Medicare will be privatized (Understanding the New Medicare, 2003).

Because the cost of prescription drugs became an issue early in the 2004 presidential campaign, the press has publicized the prescription drug benefit component of the law. This benefit, effective in 2006 with an interim prescription drug discount card available in 2004, adds a costly and complex Medicare benefit. The implementation of this benefit will be difficult and confusing to the beneficiaries. As it stands, after the beneficiary has paid a premium and an annual deductible of $250, the plan will pay 75 percent of his or her drug bill. The beneficiary will cover the remaining 25 percent until expenses reach $2250. At this point, the coverage stops and the beneficiary is responsible for drug costs until they reach $5100. Then catastrophic coverage begins (the beneficiary has spent $3600 out-of-pocket). For the rest of the year, beneficiaries pay a flat co-payment of $2 for each generic and $5 for each brand-name drug. There is no rationale for what is described as the "doughnut hole," the start-stop-start again insurance benefit. The payment scheme was an attempt to reduce the cost of the benefit and keep it within the $400 billion ceiling set by President Bush. Most beneficiaries do not understand the complexities of the Prescription Drug Act. Some commentators believe that the real winners are the drug companies and the managed care industry (Understanding the New Medicare, 2003).

As of the beginning of 2004, the Medicare program had four parts, each offering different benefits and using different financing mechanisms. **Part A** provided hospital insurance (HI), **Part B** provided supplemental medical insurance (SMI), and **Part C** offered Medicare beneficiaries a choice of a variety of managed health plans rather than traditional Medicare. People enrolled in **Medicare Part C** had prescription drug benefits. The new Prescription Drug Act is **Part D**.

Medicaid

Medicaid, a means-tested health program for the poor, pays for medical and long-term care to more than 15 percent of the population. The Medicaid population consists of five groups: pregnant women, adults in families with dependent children, children, persons with disabilities, and the poor elderly (CMS, 2004). It is administered by each state, but the policy is shared by the federal government, which pays between 50 and 76 percent in matching funds on the basis of each state's financial capacity (per capita income) (Feldstein, 2003). These federal dollars make Medicaid a less expensive approach for the states to use in expanding access to medical care to persons of low income. The states may expand eligibility beyond the five federally mandated population groups, but to qualify for federal matching funds, they must offer the following benefits: inpatient care, outpatient care, laboratory services, early and periodic screening, diagnoses, and treatment

(EPSDT) for children, and other services such as prescriptions and home health.

S-CHIP

The State Children's Health Insurance Program (S-CHIP) is a newcomer to federal investment in health care. This program, Title XXI of the Social Security Act, was originally passed as part of the Balanced Budget Act of 1997. In many ways, S-CHIP has a policy structure similar to that of Medicaid, but it is targeted to children. It is designed to help states expand health coverage to uninsured children, especially those whose family income is above the federal poverty line or too high to qualify them for Medicaid in the various states. The federal poverty level is the standard used to determine whether people qualify for programs like Medicaid and S-CHIP. Most Medicaid programs cover people whose income is at 100 to 150 percent of the federal poverty level. The latest federal poverty level (FPL) for a family of four is $18,400 (DHHS, 2003). S-CHIP covers children who live in families with higher incomes, usually at 200 percent of the FPL ($36,800).

NURSING SHORTAGE

The current nursing shortage represents a failure in both recruitment and retention (Donley et al., 2002). Nursing has failed to project a contemporary image of professional practice and career opportunities to school counselors, other health professionals, and the public (Nurses for Healthier Tomorrow, n.d.). Consequently, stereotypes and myths about practice are passed on. Many young people do not see nursing as an attractive career option (Steinbrook, 2002). It is perceived as too demanding, too dangerous, and too undervalued. For others, nursing is an exciting, meaningful, and socially relevant profession. Although failure to project an attractive image of contemporary professional nursing to the public is not the only cause of the shortage, there is a documented 6-year decline in enrollment in all levels of nursing

education—diploma, associate, and baccalaureate degrees (Nursing Faculty Shortage Fact Sheet, 2002). Concern about low enrollment is intensified by a shortage of teachers and by the age of the current nurse faculty (Spratley et al., 2001). Faculty shortage has limited enrollment in schools around the country (Nursing Faculty Shortage Fact Sheet, 2002).

Even the most optimistic do not expect that the number of nursing students will increase to fill the positions of nurses required by the baby boomer generation. The population cohort is smaller, and the current career opportunities for women (who account for 90 percent of registered nurses) are much more numerous than they were for women born in the mid-1940s. The positive side of the nursing shortage is that new graduates will have a wide choice of jobs, the opportunity to enter specialty practice immediately, higher salaries, and an enhanced ability to move up the career ladder. It is a good time to be a nursing student (Johnson & Johnson Health Care Systems, 2002).

Although nursing shortages are not new to the profession, this particular shortage has been troublesome. It has called attention to the practice of nursing and the nursing workforce. Nurses, especially hospital nurses, have expressed dissatisfaction with many issues (Steinbrook, 2002; Norrish & Randall, 2001):

- Poor staffing ratios that affect patient safety and quality of care
- Mandatory overtime
- A workplace culture that is not respectful of the nurses' knowledge or experience
- Poor communication with administrators and physicians
- Over-reliance on agency staff or travel nurses, especially in specialty areas
- Lack of opportunities for job advancement
- Lack of involvement in decisions that affect nurses and their patients

The public, the federal government, physicians, the hospital industry, health workers unions, and nurses themselves have responded to the crisis in nursing (AHA Commission, 2002; JCAHO, 2002; Tri-Council for Nursing, 2001; SEIU, 1993) by developing white papers, commissioning studies, and presenting testimony to Congress advocating for:

- More scholarships for students of nursing
- Demonstration projects to address retention and nurse satisfaction
- Involvement of professional nurses in governance structures in their places of work
- Loan forgiveness programs for nurses who study to be teachers

There is also a movement within nursing to promote magnet hospitals (McClure & Hinshaw, 2002). In fact, the American Nurse Credentialing Center (ANCC) (2004) has a program to accredit magnet hospitals, institutions that demonstrate the following attributes:

- Professional nursing practice
- Programs of nursing excellence in the delivery of patient care
- Vehicles to disseminate successful nursing practices and strategies
- Positive patient outcomes

In 2002, the President signed **the Nurse Reinvestment Act,** Public Law 107–205. This visionary piece of legislation addresses the nursing shortage from the viewpoint of recruitment: public image programs; scholarships and loan forgiveness programs; and support for the advanced nursing education of clinical specialists, teachers, administrators, and practitioners. It also addresses the nursing shortage from the retention side: demonstration funds to support innovation in practice and career ladder programs. As the title of the public law indicates, the country has reinvested in nursing and nurses as a national resource.

 CONCLUSION

Nurses are needed at policy tables. The issues on the nursing agenda, outlined in this chapter, address many of the domestic issues in the country. They affect the health of the public and the future of professional nursing. You can play a role in advocating for the nursing agenda as students and as practitioners. Get informed and get involved.

Key Points

- Health care in the United States is a business partnership between the public sector and the private sector and is a model of collaboration around health.
- Some critics of the public/private American plan blame rising health-care costs and the failures to achieve good outcomes on business involvement in health care and the link between employment and health insurance, the for-profit nature of health care, and the placing of efficiency and economic gain above the care of patients.
- The simplicity and availability of technology, changes in reimbursement for hospitals and physicians, and the pressure to limit hospital admissions and provide care in less expensive settings have encouraged the development of surgicenters and urgicenters as freestanding ambulatory care businesses and niche services that compete with hospitals.
- Values that encouraged hospitals to merge or form systems as a way of competing were: economies of scale and access to capital for expansion, acquisition of new services including physician practices, the enlarging of the system itself, and the concept of one-stop shopping for patients.
- The influence of business is evident in the adoption of the language and ethics of business. Two recent influences from the business community are its insistence that outcomes are more important than processes and the use of best practices.
- Legislation to mandate staffing ratios has been introduced in an effort to ensure a sufficient number of nurses to care for patients. *(continued)*

(*continued*)

- Most companies have responded to rises in both the cost of health care and the cost of providing health insurance to employees by changing payment and benefit structures.
- American-style health care is expensive because it emphasizes acute care rather than prevention or primary care and contains a technologic imperative.
- Uninsured Americans have limited access to care and suffer greater health disparities than people who do have health insurance.
- Medicare, a federal health insurance program that primarily serves the elderly and disabled people younger than 65 years who receive Social Security, has four Parts, each offering different benefits and using different financing mechanisms.
- Medicaid is a means-tested health program that pays for medical and long-term care for five indigent groups: pregnant women, adults in families with dependent children, children, persons with disabilities, and the poor elderly.
- S-CHIP is a federal health insurance program designed to help states expand health coverage to uninsured children.
- The current nursing shortage represents a failure in both recruitment and retention. The Nurse Reinvestment Act, Public Law 107–205, is designed to address nurses as a national resource by promoting both recruitment and retention.

THOUGHT AND DISCUSSION QUESTIONS

1. A classmate, not a nursing student, asks you whether she should buy health insurance. She is a 29-year-old single mother with two preschool-age children. Everyone in the family is healthy.
   - How would you advise your classmate?
   - Give reasons for your advice using the cost-benefit-burden equation.
   - What governmental programs may be helpful to this woman and her children?
2. What populations are most at risk for health disparities?
3. Explain how you can integrate the leading health indicators into your assessments of patients.
4. Identify 3 factors associated with recruitment and retention in nursing.
5. Review the Chapter Thought located on the first page of the chapter, and discuss it in the context of the contents of the chapter.

Interactive Exercises

1. Conduct an online search and identify the populations most at risk for health disparities. Start with the information available on the Healthy People Web site (**www.healthypeople.gov**). Examine available health insurance coverage for these individuals.
2. The Nurse Reinvestment Act was signed into law in 2002. Conduct an online search for the provisions of this law and results demonstrated since its enactment. Start with Health Resources Services Administration Bureau of Health Professions Web site (**http://bhpr.hrsa.gov/nursing/reinvestmentact.htm**). Select additional resources from the chapter's Online References.

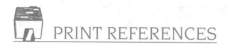

PRINT REFERENCES

AHA Commission on Workforce for Hospitals and Health Systems (April 2002). *In our hands now: How hospital leaders can build a thriving workforce.* Chicago: American Hospital Association.

Brown, D. (January 9, 2004). Health care spending increases for 6th year. *Washington Post*, Health section, A3.

Committee on the Consequences of Uninsurance. (2004). *Insuring America's health: Principles and recommendations.* Washington, DC: The National Academy Press.

Feldstein, P. (2003). *Health policy issues.* Chicago: Health Administration Press.

Institute of Medicine (2001). *Crossing the quality chasm: A new health system for the 21st century.* Washington, DC: The National Academy Press.

Joint Commission on Accreditation of Healthcare Organizations (JCAHO). (2002). *Health care at the crossroads: Strategies for addressing the evolving nursing crisis.* Chicago: Author.

Kohn, L. T., Corrigan, J. M., & Donaldson, M. S. (Eds.) (2000). *To err is human: Building a safer health system.* Washington, DC: National Academy Press.

Leape, L. L. (1992). Unnecessary surgery. *Annual Review of Public Health*, 13, 363–383.

Levit, J., Smithe, C., Cowan, C., Sensenig, A., Cathlin, A., & the Health Accounts Team. (2004). Health spending rebound continues in 2002. *Health Affairs*, 23(1),147–159.

McClure, M. L., & Hinshaw, A. S. (Eds.) (2002). *Magnet hospitals revisited: Attraction and retention of professional nurses.* Washington, DC: American Nurses Association.

Norrish, B. R., & Randall, T. G. (March 2001). Hospital restructuring and the work of registered nurses. *The Milbank Quarterly*, 79(1), 55–79.

Relman, A. S. (1992). What market values are doing to medicine. *The Atlantic Monthly*, 269, 99–106.

Service Employees International Union (SEIU) (1993). *The national nurse survey: 10,000 dedicated healthcare professionals report on staffing, stress and patient care in U.S. hospitals and nursing homes.* Washington, DC: SEIU, AFL-CIO.

Smedley, B. D., Stith, A. Y., & Nelson, A. R. (Eds.). (2003). *Unequal treatment: Confronting racial and ethnic disparities in health care.* Washington, DC: The National Academies Press.

Spratley, E., Johnson, A., Sochalski, J. Fritz, M., & Spencer, W. (September 2001). *The Registered Nurse Population*, March
2000, Chart 17. Rockville, MD: Health Resources and Service Administration, Bureau of Health Professions, Division of Nursing.

Steinbrook, R. (May 30, 2002). Nursing in the crossfire. *New England Journal of Medicine*, 346(22), 1757–1766.

U.S. Dept. Health and Human Services (2000). *Healthy People* 2010. Washington, DC: U.S. Government Printing Office.

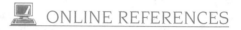

ONLINE REFERENCES

Agency for Health Care Research and Quality (n.d.). The uninsured in America—1996–2002, Statistical Brief No. 24. *www.ahrq.gov*

American Association of Colleges of Nursing. (2002). Nursing Faculty Shortage Fact Sheet (2002). *www.aacn.nche.edu/media/backgrounders/facultyshortage.htm*

American Nurses Credentialing Center (2004). ANCC magnet program. *http://nursingworld.org/ancc/magnet*

American Association of Colleges of Nursing. (2001). Tri-Council for Nursing. Strategies to reverse the new nursing shortage. *http://www.aacn.nche.edu/Publications/positions/tricshortage.htm*

Center for Medicare and Medicaid Services (2004). State Children's health insurance program (S-CHIP). *http://www.cms.gov/schip/*

Donley, Sr. R., Flaherty, Sr. M. J., Sarsfield, E., Taylor, L., Maloni, H., & Flanagan, E. (December 12, 2002). What Does the Nurse Reinvestment Act Mean to You? *Online Journal of Issues in Nursing*, 8(1), Manuscript 5. *http://nursingworld.org/ojin/topic14/tpc14_5.htm*

Johnson & Johnson Health Care Systems, Inc. (2002). Discover nursing. *www.discovernursing.com*

Nurses for a Healthier Tomorrow (n.d.) Campaign news. *http://www.nursesource.org/campaign_news.html*

Understanding the new Medicare prescription drug benefit (November 25, 2003). *www.info@familiesusa.org*

U.S. Dept. of Census (2004). *http://www.census.gov*

U.S. Dept. Health and Human Services (2003). The 2003 HHS Poverty Guidelines. *http://aspe.hhs.gov/poverty/03poverty.htm*

U.S. Dept. Health and Human Services (2000). Healthy People 2010. *http://www.healthypeople.gov*

Wilensky, G. (January 28, 2004). Health cost drivers and the uninsured. Testimony presented to Committee on Health, Education, Labor and Pensions. *www.health.senate.gov/bills/035*

Rose Kearney-Nunnery

Expanding the Vision

There is no security on this earth; there is only opportunity.

General Douglas MacArthur, 1880–1964

Chapter Objectives

On completion of this chapter, the reader will be able to:

1. Evaluate trends in professional practice.
2. Continue to evaluate her or his personal philosophy.
3. Envision personal competencies in professional nursing practice.
4. Develop personal strategic initiatives for future contributions to professional nursing practice.

Key Terms

Competencies
Collaboration
Collegiality

Continued Competence
Continued Professional
    Nursing Competence

Involvement

We have seen nursing and health care change radically in the past few years. With restructuring of health care, nursing professionals have responded with refinements, advancements, and innovations. Nursing has moved from the functional service mode of the mid-1900s to a cost-, community-, quality-, and consumer-focused orientation. It is no longer the nursing care plan for the patient, but is now the collaborative care plan of the client. And this care must be framed in the context of safety and client involvement in an environment with shortages of health-care providers, especially nursing professionals.

To address the health of people, all health professions are now faced with the challenges of transformation, innovation, and collaboration. We have options and challenges ahead. Collegiality and collaboration extend beyond the structural walls of a single institution or the boundaries of a community. In a global society, we can reach out to colleagues and clients physically or electronically. Critical components of professional practice continue to expand and be enhanced through technology. And we continually strive to envision the challenges ahead. It is now time to expand the vision and address the challenges ahead.

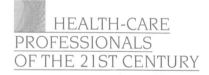

HEALTH-CARE PROFESSIONALS OF THE 21ST CENTURY

Several initiatives have lead to the changes in practice and the profession during the last decade.

The Pew Health Professions Commission

The Pew Charitable Trust Foundation established the Pew Health Professions Commission, which worked from 1989 to 1999 to address issues of health-care reform and health policy across the professions. At that time, the health-care industry was in the midst of redesigning services and roles and containing costs with declining resources. The Commission identified 17 specific competencies for health professionals for the year 2005 (Box 23–1). **Competencies** are those qualities that illustrate effectiveness and appropriateness in our respective professional roles. In 1995, reports from the commission produced strong reactions and responses throughout the professional communities, with predictions for redesign needed in education and health care and for a rapid transformation in the health professions workforce. The four "r"s were redesign, re-regulate, right-size, and restructure. The view of the health-care system presented by the commission was market-driven and integrated with more managed and primary care. In addition, this health-care system and its professionals would be more accountable to the public and responsive to consumers; would be more efficient, effective, and innovative; and would focus primarily on education, prevention, and care management rather than treatment (Finocchio et al., 1995).

The work of the Pew Commission continued, concentrating on the assets and needs of each of the health professions to address the nation's health. The commission proposed five strategies to prepare nurses with the professional competencies that would be essential in the year 2005. Further, the Commission made ten recommendations aimed at state regulation for protecting and promoting the public's health concerning the following areas:

- Standardization of terms and regulations
- Entry-to-practice requirements
- Scopes of practice
- Assessment of continuing competence and disciplinary processes
- Professional boards
- Providing information and public accountability
- Data collection
- Evaluation processes
- Development of partnerships to streamline regulation

> ## BOX 23–1
> ## TWENTY-ONE COMPETENCIES FOR THE 21ST CENTURY
>
> 1. Embrace a personal ethic of social responsibility and service.
> 2. Exhibit ethical behavior in all professional activities.
> 3. Provide evidence-based, clinically competent care.
> 4. Incorporate the multiple determinants of health in clinical care.
> 5. Apply knowledge of the new sciences.
> 6. Demonstrate critical thinking, reflection, and problem-solving skills.
> 7. Understand the role of primary care.
> 8. Rigorously practice preventive health care.
> 9. Integrate population-based care and services into practice.
> 10. Improve access to health care for those with unmet health needs.
> 11. Practice relationship-centered care with individuals and families.
> 12. Provide culturally sensitive care to a diverse society.
> 13. Partner with communities in health-care decisions.
> 14. Use communication and information technology effectively and appropriately.
> 15. Work in interdisciplinary teams.
> 16. Ensure care that balances individual, professional, system, and societal needs.
> 17. Practice leadership.
> 18. Take responsibility for quality of care and health outcomes at all levels.
> 19. Contribute to continuous improvement of the health-care system.
> 20. Advocate for public policy that promotes and protects the health of the public.
> 21. Continue to learn and help others learn.
>
> From O'Neil, E. H., & the Pew Health Professions Commission. (1998). *Recreating health professional practice for a new century: The fourth report of the Pew Health Professions Commission*. San Francisco: Pew Health Professions Commission.

The recommendations directed at the profession of nursing involved public accountability, recognition of our assets, the need for clarity in our roles and functions, and the need to meet the demands of the marketplace.

The final major report of the commission detailed professional characteristics of nursing, stating that "over the past 50 years, nursing has changed substantially from a largely supportive role in health care to one with many independent and complex responsibilities in care delivery" (O'Neil & Pew Health Professions Commission, 1998, p. 61). Recommendations presented for nursing professionals included: the need to develop a more diverse and younger workforce; specific competencies through educational mobility and advancement; educational curricula addressing differentiated practice, learning experiences, advanced education and skills; and faculty experience in clinical practice and research (O'Neil, 1998a).

As a result of the findings of the commission and the associated reactions from different professional groups, O'Neil (1998b) identified strategic directions for nursing that included addressing differentiated practice, curricula changes, core competencies, a commitment to research, the creation of strategic partnerships, and enhanced leadership. Later that year, however, the focus changed from the future competencies of health professionals to a call for immediate attention to client safety

The Institute of Medicine Quality Chasm

The health professions came under fire with the release of two reports from the Institute of Medicine (IOM) of the National Academies on the high incidence of medical errors, changing the focus from the future of health care to the current need to improve safety to clients. The IOM is a nonprofit organization designed to provide science-based advice as a public service. Its quality initiative is described as "the degree to which health services for individuals and populations increase the likelihood of desired health outcomes and are consistent with current professional knowledge" (IOM, 2003a, p. 1). The 2001 report from the IOM, *Crossing the Quality Chasm*, proposed ten rules for the health system in the 21st century for quality health care (see Chapter 1 Box 1–4). The six overall aims—that care should be safe, effective, patient-centered, timely, efficient, and equitable—underlay the ten rules (IOM, 2003a, p. 1). A further report after a Health Professions Education Summit led to the identification of the five core competencies for all health professionals:

- Provide patient-centered care
- Work in interdisciplinary teams
- Employ evidence-based practice
- Apply quality improvement
- Utilize informatics (Greiner & Knebel, 2003)

Client safety and effectiveness of outcomes became major national objectives and directed additional attention to nursing. Research by the Agency for Healthcare Research and Quality (AHRQ) (2002) focused on expanding the knowledge base on how the quality of the health-care workplace affects the quality of health-care provided, especially in the areas of workload and working conditions, effects of stress and fatigue, reducing adverse events, and the organizational climate and culture. Client outcomes were now being investigated, along with nursing-sensitive indicators and factors that promote safe and effective practice.

In late 2003, nursing itself was the focus of the IOM in their report, *Keeping Patients Safe: Transforming the Work Environment of Nurses*. The IOM's Committee on the Work Environment and Patient Safety provided specific recommendations to both acute care and long-term care organizations on issues of management practices, workforce capability, work design, and the organizational safety culture (IOM, 2003b, p.1). The following risk factors were identified for patient safety in nursing work environments:

- More acutely ill patients
- Shorter hospital stays
- Redesigned work
- Frequent patient turnover
- High staff turnover
- Long work hours
- Rapid increases in new knowledge and technology
- Increased interruptions and demands on nurses' time (Page, 2004, pp. 37–45)

Although these facts were no surprise, their identication as risk factors to clients was significant. Nurses have been reporting these factors but now they were included in a major national report. This committee also documented the national shortages of both nurses and nursing assistants. Recommendations to nursing leadership and management on how to address the deficiencies in the documented work environments called attention to the following areas:

- Leadership, communication skills, collaborative decision-making, and resources

- Emphasis on safety goals *along with* productivity and financial goals
- Management practices promoting safety, trust, change, engagement, and learning collaboratives
- External support for evidence-based management practices

In addition, at the staff level the committee found "strong evidence that nurse staffing levels, the knowledge and skills level of nursing staff, and the extent to which workers collaborate in sharing their knowledge and skills affect patient outcomes and safety" (Page, 2004, p. 161). This finding provides further support for the need to incorporate the five core competencies into professional nursing practice on a consistent basis. Nurses consistently strive to provide client-centered care but, for positive client outcomes, this must also be done in light of the other core competencies, given the nature of the health-care environment. Evolving technologies, evidence-based collaborative practice, and continued competence are essential components for quality improvement in the delivery of health care to consumers.

The Professional Nursing Practice Environment

Changes in the practice environment have received serious attention with the focus on safety and client outcomes. The IOM Committee on the Work Environment and Patient Safety (Page, 2004) identified necessary client safeguards in the environment (Box 23–2). These recommendations call for leadership, collaboration, and action.

Leadership in the practice enviroment is essential for client safety but also for the satisfaction, involvement, and commitment of dedicated health-care professionals. One area that is receiving serious consideration is adequacy of staffing. The focus on productivity and appropriate staffing has led to a renewed emphasis on quality outcomes. Indicators that are nursing sensitive, like infection rates, client satisfaction, and nursing hours per

---

ONLINE CONSULT

Agency for Healthcare Research & Quality. (AHRQ).
www.ahrq.gov
Institute of Medicine (IOM).
http://www.iom.edu

BOX 23–2
NECESSARY CLIENT SAFEGUARDS IN THE WORK ENVIRONMENT

- Governing boards that focus on safety
- Leadership and evidence-based management structures and processes
- Effective nursing leadership
- Adquate staffing
- Organizational support for ongoing learning and decision support
- Mechanisms that promote interdisciplinary collaboration
- Work design that promotes safety
- Organizational culture that continually strengthens patient safety

From Page, A. (Ed.). (2004). *Keeping patients safe: Transforming the work environment of nurses.* Washington, DC: National Academies Press.

patient day, are being studied in relation to staffing. A study on turnover rates and productivity in the hospital setting considered the relationship between profitability and patient outcomes. The researchers reported that the average costs to replace a medical surgical nurse and an intensive care nurse were $46,000 and $64,000 respectively (VHS Center for Research, and Innovaion 2002, p. 6). They also proposed that the "true currency of a strong work force is leadership, vision, commitment, and energy" (VHS Center for Research and Innovation, 2002, p. 15). These components are vital in the practice environment.

The American Association of Colleges of Nursing has identified selected characteristics of work environments that support professional nursing practice (AACN, 2002):

- Magnet status
- Preceptorships and residencies
- Differentiated practice
- Interdisciplinary collaboration

Recognition as a magnet hospital requires that applicant health-care organizations meet specific eligibility criteria, including strong nursing leadership in line with national standards of practice. The self-assessment requirement for the institution applying for magnet recognition is described as revealing and "creating opportunities for organizational advancement, team building, and enhancement of individuals' professional self esteem" (American Nurses Credentialing Center [ANCC], 2003, p. 1). Retention and appropriate staffing are characteristics of magnet organizations. Further, the Joint Commission on Accreditation of Healthcare Organizations (JCAHO) has released a position paper on the nursing shortage recommending the creation of "organizational cultures of retention" modeled on the successes in magnet hospitals (JCAHO, 2003, p. 9).

The importance of retention is further enhanced when professionals have had an opportunity to expand their knowledge base and skills with a rapidly changing practice environment through preceptorships for students and residencies for graduates. Joel (2002) correlates this to the student teacher, resident, or law clerk engaging in hands-on

experiences that are intended "to socialize the neophyte into the field and provide a transition to professional accountability" (p. 6). Mentorship is an important component to advance the skills of the neophyte and of the seasoned clinician. Matching the knowledge and skills of the professional with the requirements of the position is an ongoing consideration. This can be promoted through activities for continuing education and competency and differentiated practice.

Differentiated nursing practice (see Chapter 15), the third characteristic identified by AACN in the supportive practice environment, is illustrated through advancement structures in the organization based on experience, additional education, certification, or other identified indicators of excellence (AACN, 2002, pp. 6–7). Implementation of differentiated practice has historically been difficult; the combination of skills matched to the position requirements must be delineated. As Nelson (2002) has proposed, it is not feasible to try to differentiate practice along current educational points of entry when the roles have not been translated into the practice setting (p. 7).

Interdisciplinary collaboration, illustrated through teamwork, trust, shared responsibility, and respect, also enhances client outcomes. The AACN (2002) proposed eight hallmarks of excellence in the professional nursing practice environment. Consider how these hallmarks for the practice environment (Table 23–1) also address the core competencies for all health professionals identified by the IOM. Note the focus on quality care for clients, collaboration, competency, and leadership throughout.

COLLABORATION AND COLLEGIALITY

Essential activities of contemporary practice include strategic partnerships, leadership, and collaboration. This collaboration and collegiality must both occur within the profession and be interdisciplinary. The initial step in collaboration and collegiality is valuing our colleagues who provide clinical nursing care,

TABLE 23–1
Hallmarks of Professional Practice and Core Competencies

Hallmarks of the Professional Nursing Practice Environment*	Core Competencies for Health Professionals†			
	Provide Patient-Centered Care	Work in Interdisciplinary Teams	Employ Evidence-Based Practice	Apply Quality Improvement
Manifest a philosophy of clinical care emphasizing quality, safety, interdisciplinary collaboration, continuity of care, and professional accountability.	☑	☑	☑	☑
Recognize contributions of nurses' knowledge and expertise to clinical care quality and patient outcomes.	☑	☑	☑	☑
Empower nurses' participation in clinical decision-making and organization of clinical care systems.	☑	☑	☑	☑
Promote executive-level nursing leadership	☑	☑	☑	☑
Maintain clinical advancement programs based on education, certification, and advanced preparation.	☑	☑	☑	☑
Demonstrate professional development support for nurses.	☑	☑	☑	☑
Create collaborative relationships among members of the health-care provider team.	☑	☑	☑	☑

*From American Association of Colleges of Nursing (AACN). (2002). *Hallmarks of the professional nursing practice environment.* Washington, DC: Author.
†From Greiner, A.C., & Knebel, E. (Eds.). (2003). *Health professions education: A bridge to quality.* Washington, DC: Institute of Medicine.

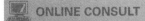 **ONLINE CONSULT**

American Association of Colleges of Nursing (AACN).
http://www.aacn.nche.edu
American Nurses Credentialing Center (ANCC).
http://nursingworld.org/ancc/magnet/facilities.html
Joint Commission on Accreditation of Healthcare Organizations (JCAHO).
http://www.jcaho.org

specialty care, advanced clinical practice, education, or administration. Collaboration and collegiality are both intradisciplinary, within the discipline of nursing, and interdisciplinary, among other health-care professionals.

Collaboration

The health-care team is an ideal example of collaboration. **Collaboration** involves actively working together to meet some identified goal, such as the client's treatment goals. Within the discipline, nurses from each area of nursing contribute to that goal—the admission nurse or discharge planner, the student in a clinical rotation, the operative nurse, the acute care nurse practitioner, and other professional nurses providing care to raise the client's level of well-being. In times of limited staffing and growing responsibilities, seeing the broader picture with collaboration is necesssary to ensure effective client outcomes.

A cooperative spirit with collaboration will bring more efficient achievement of goals and greater personal reward for both colleagues and clients. Questions of authority and responsibility arise with this cooperative or collaborative spirit, such as who is the leader of the team and who is responsible for insuring quality client outcomes. This ownership of responsibility must be shared in a true collaborative relationship rather than create "turf" issues in a more competetive environment. The goal is the effectiveness of the client outcomes with collaboration as the means to get to the goal. Effective communication and clinical skills, along with trust, leadership, and collegiality, are important attributes of the health-care professional collaborating with other health-care professionals. These skills are critical for the efficient use of scarce human and physical resources in a consumer environment that is focused on effectiveness of client outcomes and overall safety.

Collegiality

Collegiality is sharing responsibility and authority to achieve a goal or prescribed out-

come. Power and responsibility for outcomes related to clients' health and well-being are invested in more than one person. Mutual respect and collaboration are important components of a collegial relationship. All colleagues contribute to the intended goals and are accountable for the outcomes.

Collaboration and Collegiality in Practice

Both collaboration and collegiality are specified by the American Nurses Association as standards of professional performance in its document *Nursing: Scope and Standards of Practice*. As identified in Chapter 1, the document contains six standards of practice and nine standards of professional performance, with objectives and measurement criteria (ANA, 2004 pp. 21–45). The standards of practice reflect the steps of the nursing process, whereas the standards of performance are those behaviors expected of the professional. Collaboration is measured by virtue of communication, consultation, documentation, and referrals within and outside the nursing discipline. Measures of collegiality include sharing knowledge and skills, providing constructive feedback, enhancement of practice, and creating and supporting a learning and work environment. In the revised standards, additional measurement criteria have been added for the advanced practice nurse and speciality nurse to accommodate the additional expectations in interdisciplinary practice.

Nursing professionals also are responsible for promoting collaboration and collegiality among the professions. As described throughout this text, health-care delivery systems are becoming more and more integrated and interdisciplinary. In our present multidisciplinary health-care system, collaboration must be effective among all members of the various health professions and care disciplines. Collegiality between professionals is also critical for the team to function effectively.

In 1998, the President's Advisory Commission on Consumer Protection and Quality in the Health Care Industry reported that "the challenge for industry leaders is to harness the tremendous talent, energy, and commitment of the 10 million people who have been drawn to work in the health-care industry because of its strong sense of mission" (President's Advisory Committee, 1998, p. 197). Since then, the IOM report *Keeping Patients Safe* has recommended that health-care organizations "should take action to support interdisciplinary collaboration by adopting such interdisciplinary practice mechanisms as interdisciplinary rounds, and by providing ongoing formal education and training in interdisciplinary collaboration for all health-care professionals on a regularly scheduled, continuous basis" (IOM, 2003b, p. 216). The IOM also identified necessary precursors to collaboration (IOM, 2003b):

- Individual clinical competence
- Mutual trust and respect
- Shared understanding of goals and roles
- Effective communication
- Shared decision-making
- Conflict management (IOM, 2003b, p. 213)

In addition to these characteristics is the necessary ingredient of continued competence to maintain safety and quality care for the client and effective interdisciplinary practice.

COMPETENCE

The issue of competence is a vital issue to all professionals. Although not restricted to nursing, professional competence has received greater attention after the reports from both the Pew Health Professions Commission and the IOM. Professional competence is of great concern to health professionals, their regulatory bodies, and consumers. It is an issue of definition, ownership, policy development, and demonstration. Regulatory bodies are required to assure the public of safe and competent professional practice by the professionals they regulate. But definitions vary by statute, and measurement issues are complex. Consider two different ways in which competence can be measured: by continuing practice and through continuing education.

But then the following question arises: Is the continuing practice safe and effective in meeting appropriate client outcomes using evidence-based practice? Or, in the case of continuing education, are the programs or sessions selected directed at the area of practice to improve and enhance practice or merely counting hours toward license renewal without a focus on clients and responsible professional practice? In fact, measurement issues are further complicated by the different levels of practice that must be regulated—student, continued practice, and advanced practice.

Entry into practice occurs through licensure on the basis of performance on a psychometrically sound instrument, the National Council Licensure Exam (NCLEX). Advanced practice is regulated differently in the various jurisdictions but often through the certification process. But, how should the regulators monitor continued professional competence for the clinician not governed by specialty practice certification?

The issue of **continued competence** is not restricted to state and federal regulatory bodies. As described in *Nursing's Social Policy Statement* (ANA, 2003), regulation of practice also includes the following:

- Self-regulation, as personal accountability and through peer review
- Professional regulation, with education requirements and a defined scope of practice
- Legal regulation, through statutory and regulatory requirements

Glaser (1999) has stated that "the primary goal of continued competence is to assure safe, *quality*, nursing care/practice to clients/the public" (p.1). The National Council of State Boards of Nursing (NCSBN) has illustrated a collaborative model for continued competence that includes the individual nurse, the employer, the regulatory body, the educator, and the consumer of nursing care (NCSBN, 1996). Although continued competence is ultimately the professional responsibility of the individual clinician, the professional education level must be appropriate to the defined scope of practice and professional standards, the health-care employer must ensure the competence in the practice setting, and the client must be assured (and should assure himself or herself) of safe and effective practice.

The professional performance standard of education of the *Scope and Standards of Practice* states that for continued competence, "the nurse attains knowledge and competency that reflects current nursing practice" (ANA, 2004, p. 35). In addition, nurses are required to be "lifelong learners," taking advantage of appropriate, adequate, and innovative learning opportunities and solutions (ANA, 2004, p. 20). Ongoing educational activities occur through continuing education—formal, non-credit (CE), and on-the-job. However, in research conducted by the NCSBN, respondents "rated contributions of work experience, initial professional education, and mentors above the contributions of CE in assisting them to their current levels of ability" (Smith, 2003, p. 25). Concerning continued learning in the work environment, the IOM report *Keeping Patients Safe* recommended that health-care organizations should "dedicate budgetary resources equal to a defined percentage of the nursing payroll to support nursing staff in their ongoing acquisition and maintenance of knowledge and skills" (IOM,

2003b, p. 210). Further, the concept of a learning environment is extended beyond its start in an educational setting to one encouraged in the practice setting. A learning environment in the practice setting supports the core competencies and ongoing professional competence. The individual professional must determine, seek, and utilize resources to maintain his or her continued competence in the safe and effective performance of nursing practice activities.

After the report of a special panel, the ANA has defined **continuing professional nursing competence** as the "ongoing professional nursing competence according to level of expertise, responsibility, and domains of practice as evidenced by behavior based on beliefs, attitudes, and knowledge matched to and in the context of a set of expected outcomes as defined by nursing scope of practice, policy, *Code of Ethics*, standards, guidelines, and benchmarks that assure safe performance of professional activities" (Whittaker et al., 2000, p. 1). This definition of competence requires demonstration of skillful, effective, and evidence-based practice both in nursing and interdisciplinary endeavors, with a view of the core competencies and the challenges ahead.

 CHALLENGING PRACTICE

The recommendations and changes in the health-care environment present all nurses with additional career opportunities and responsibilities, whether they are in acute, ambulatory, home, or long-term care settings or in a nontraditional setting as a clinician,

> *Although continued competence is ultimately the professional responsibility of the individual clinician, the professional education level must be appropriate to the defined scope of practice and professional standards, the health-care employer must ensure the competence in the practice setting, and the client must be assured of safe and effective practice.*

 ONLINE CONSULT

National Council of State Boards of Nursing (NCSBN).
http://www.ncsbn.org/public/resources/ncsbn_competence.htm
American Nurses Association (ANA).
http://www.nursingworld.org
American Nurses Credentialing Center (ANCC).
http://nursingworld.org/ancc/

case manager, researcher, administrator, consultant, educator, advanced practice nurse, or nurse entrepreneur. These challenges in your future are dynamic and evolve daily as we address the themes of safety, quality client outcomes, evolving technology, and interdisciplinary practice. Consider the implications of the following challenges in the workforce or in a specific delivery setting:

• A culture supportive of safe and quality client outcomes
• Appropriate staffing patterns and skill mixes
• Training and supervision of unlicensed assistive personnel
• Competencies and continued knowledge development of professionals
• Differentiated practice
• Coordination of care across practice settings
• Changes in populations and health-care needs
• Strategies to improve health and eliminate health disparities
• Cost containment
• Evidence-based interdisciplinary practice
• Consumer satisfaction
• Using information technologies and quality-based indicators

The challenges in your future truly depend on you, your practice environment, colleagues, and future initiatives.

And then comes the consideration of specialty practice as an advanced practice nurse (APRN). Consider the APRN practice roles of nurse practitioner, clinical nurse specialist, nurse anesthetist, or nurse midwife. As the knowledge base grows, evidence-based practice is guided by the specialty area. Nevertheless, we are experiencing a shortage of nurses active in generalist staff practice settings as well as a critical shortage of nursing faculty. Although we have seen an increase in the numbers of nurses prepared at the master's and doctoral levels (ANA, 2003), graduate education has been directed at clinical practice in four areas: nurse practitioner, clinical nurse specialist, nurse anesthetist, and nurse midwife. Since the 1980s, education tracks in graduate programs have declined, and the average age of nursing faculty continues to rise. As the National League for Nursing

(NLN) observes, "while being a good clinician is essential, it is not sufficient for the educator role" (NLN, 2002, p. 2). "Nursing faculty at all levels must be current, clinically competent, and sound in the art and science of teaching" (AACN, 2002a, p 2). Additional skills in curriculum development and evaluation, teaching and learning, and interdisciplinary education are required in the nurse educator role. A nurse educator has a futher practice opportunity in involvement in the preparation of skilled professionals.

The main challenges ahead in professional practice are ongoing professional development and involvement for engagement in the delivery of client-centered care with a focus on safety, efficacy, and quality through the use of informatics and evidence-based practice and leadership in the interdisciplinary practice setting, whether nurses are in practice, education, research, or administration. This involvement reflects the core competencies of health professionals and advances practice, client outcomes, and the profession.

INVOLVEMENT

When we think of **involvement**, we think of our function as advocates and health-care providers for our clients. These functions are one form of involvement. Our professional involvement focuses on the individual attributes, needs of, and outcomes for our clients, the consumers of nursing and health care. This involvement, as individual professionals with the clients and families who are the consumers of evidence-based, quality nursing care, must address all core competencies.

Our involvement as one of the core competencies is also as members of the health-care team. Collaboration and collegiality have been described in relation to nursing and interdisciplinary practice. This book also discussed the importance of group dynamics and group skills, and the art of negotiation in leading and managing. All of these functions relate to active involvement with a defined group to attain specified goals for the consumers of health care.

A third form of professional involvement is

as a member of the professional group. This form of involvement requires time and commitment for advancement of the profession. Professional contributions result from participation in professional organizations, research, publications, theory evaluation, and promotion of the further development of the profession. Personal contributions in professional practice occur through your education, competency, ethical behaviors, use of theory and evidence-based interventions, and communication, political efficacy, client advocacy, and leadership.

Both professional and personal contributions are the ingredients of your professional career. However, skills, which are the ingredients of professional nursing practice require ongoing refinement. The International Leadership Institute of Sigma Theta Tau, International Honor Society of Nursing (2000), has proposed eight skills (Box 23–3) to be used as guideposts by the nurse navigating a "healthy career," from before entry into nursing education and nursing to obtaining further credentials, demonstrating career growth, and moving into an active retirement. Notice that these skills include those in the practice setting as well as personal life. These skills are also not restricticed to nursing or health care. Your own demonstration of these skills is defined by your views on practice, the client, the environment, health, and nursing.

BOX 23–3
SKILLS FOR A HEALTHY CAREER

- Develop your personal self.
- Locate special resources.
- Become financially astute.
- Become a futures thinker.
- Navigate any organization.
- Become technologically savvy.
- Position yourself for recognition.
- Retire actively.

From International Leadership Institute, Sigma Theta Tau International. (2000). Eight skills for a healthy career. *Reflections on Nursing Leadership*, *26*(1), 20–21.

REVISITING YOUR PHILOSOPHY OF NURSING

Now is the time to reflect on your personal contributions to and philosophy of nursing. Nurses are talented, creative, and visionary—when they allow themselves to be. They are frequently viewed as leaders and risk takers as they advocate for the perceived good of their clients. But what skills required of professionals do we need to refine? Step back and think of the vital and basic skills needed to demonstrate our professional competencies. These skills are what we continually strive to refine:

- Our knowledge base
- Critical thinking skills
- Technical skills
- Interpersonal skills
- Articulation skills

Clinical practice requires these skills for provision of client-centered care, involvement in interdisciplinary and evidence-based practice, and the use of informatics and emerging technologies for quality improvement and effective client outcomes. These skills are enhanced through the professional attributes of collaboration, collegiality, continued competence, and involvement in the health promotion of society. Concern for the health of people, whether individual clients, families, communities, or groups in their environment, is the core of professional nursing. Individuals like you are dedicated and exemplify those characteristics of a professional described here. Your philosophy of nursing will evolve and develop, just as you do as a professional.

 ## EMBRACING CHANGE

The recent focus on the health professions and the evident shortages of professionals has had the beneficial effect of opening up the discussion for needed changes in the health-care system and the professions. Discussions have been held at national, state, and local meetings, and debate and discussion on the issues continue in professional newsletters and journals as well as online. Communication and critical thinking are taking place. The restraining and driving forces of change are present. We see that practice and education can no longer serve the needs of the consumers without change. All professionals are shareholders in the process of improving the health of society at large.

Technology continues to expand our horizons and challenge our practice. Improved equipment and technologies are developing at a rapid pace. Information is available immediately. Colleagues readily communicate at a distance using e-mail, instant messaging, ListServs, and news groups. Computer-adaptive testing for licensure and certification is a given. Re-engineering has become a common occurrence in practice settings, as have cost containment, measurement of client outcomes, evidence-based practice, and a focus on consumer satisfaction.

The topics that you have embraced through this book have presented you with some of the issues involved in this time of rapid change in the profession and in practice. Facing the responsibilities inherent in professional practice is a way of revisiting our present roles and considering how they meet the needs of our clients and the intent of our profession. The student role provides the setting for analyzing information related to current practices. Theories that guide practice continue to be tested and refined as appropriate to their utility in practice, education, and research. Communication and critical thinking are vital components of this activity as we function as leaders, managers, and care providers in organizations and communities. We function as change agents, teachers, and group leaders in practice settings. Knowledge of research and the political process give us direction, as change agents, for addressing the changes needed for a healthier society. The focus remains on clients, their safety, needs, and healthy outcomes.

Current health-care initiatives must be evaluated for applicability, acceptability, and appropriateness for meeting the needs of the population, with due consideration given to economic and quality indicators. All these issues are addressed within the ethical parameters of professional nursing practice.

The information presented here has been designed to address the challenge of the book's title, *Advancing Your Career: Concepts of Professional Nursing*. We are all challenged to advance our professional practice.

Key Points

- The Pew Health Professions Commission (1995) described the emerging health-care system and focused on four themes: redesign, re-regulate, right-size, and restructure. The commission further specified 21 competencies for health professionals in the 21st century.
- Competencies are those qualities that illustrate effectiveness and appropriateness in our respective professional roles. The Health Professions Education Summit led to the identification of the five core competencies for all health professionals:
  • Provide patient-centered care.
  • Work in interdisciplinary teams.
  • Employ evidence-based practice.
  • Apply quality improvement.
  • Utilize informatics (Greiner & Knebel, 2003).
- The IOM's Committee on the Work Environment and Patient Safety identified the following necessary client safeguards in the practice environment (Page, 2004):
  • Governing boards that focus on safety
  • Leadership and evidence-based management structures and processes

(continued)

(*continued*)
  • Effective nursing leadership
  • Adquate staffing
  • Organizational support for ongoing learning and decision support
  • Mechanisms that promote interdisciplinary collaboration
  • Work design that promotes safety
  • Organizational culture that continually strengthens patient safety

- The AACN (2002) has proposed eight hallmarks of excellence in the professional nursing practice environment based on selected characteristics of work environments that support professional nursing practice.

- Collaboration involves actively working together to meet some identified goal, such as the client's treatment goals.

- Collegiality is the sharing of responsibility and authority to achieve a goal or prescribed outcome. Respect and collaboration are important components of a collegial relationship.

- Continued competence is of great concern to health professionals, their regulatory bodies, and consumers.

- The ANA has defined ongoing *continuing professional nursing competence* "according to level of expertise, responsibility, and domains of practice as evidenced by behavior based on beliefs, attitudes, and knowledge matched to and in the context of a set of expected outcomes as defined by nursing scope of practice, policy, *Code of Ethics*, standards, guidelines, and benchmarks that assure safe performance of professional activities" (Whittaker et al., 2000, p. 1).

- A nurse's involvement as a professional takes three forms:
  • As an individual professional with clients, families, and communities who are the consumers of nursing care
  • As a group member or leader of an interdisciplinary health-care team
  • As an active member of the professional group

- Professional contributions result from participation in professional organizations, research, publications, theory evaluation, and promotion of the further development of the profession.

- Vital and basic skills needed and continually refined by professionals include expanding one's knowledge base, critical thinking, and technical, interpersonal, and articulation skills.

 Thought and Discussion Questions

1. Identify additional challenges for improvements in the delivery of quality health care.
2. Describe your plans for two specific personal contributions to professional nursing practice that you will attempt during the next 10 years.
3. Develop three personal goals to be met in your professional nursing practice during the next 5 years.
4. Review the Chapter Thought located on the first page of the chapter, and discuss it in the context of the contents of the chapter.

Interactive Exercises

1. Complete the exercise on the Intranet site entitled Meeting Professional Competencies to develop your plan to address the core competencies for health professionals.

2. Given that professionalism is an attribute in constant refinement, reassess your professional status by completing the exercise on Professionalism in Nursing on the Intranet site. Do not refer back to your original assessment until you have completed the inventory.

3. To evaluate what is expected from you in professional practice in your state, complete the exercise on the Intranet site entitled Continued Competency Expectations.

4. After the report of a special panel, the ANA defined *continuing professional nursing competence*. Use the ANA's definition and the format provided on the Intranet site to identify how you can document and enhance your continued competence.

5. Refine your personal philosophy of nursing using the format provided on the Intranet site. Be prepared to participate in an online discussion, to be scheduled by your instructor, in which you will discuss and explain any changes in your views since the start of this course.

6. Develop your professional resumé using the format provided on the Intranet site.

7. Using the format provided on the Intranet site, develop your plan to address the eight skills for a healthy career identified by the International Leadership Institute of Sigma Theta Tau International (2000).

8. Locate a ListServ using one of the resources provided by ANA (at *http://www.nursingworld.org/ listserv/index.htm*), and communicate with a colleague on the core competencies needed by registered nurses in your practice area.

PRINT RESOURCES

References

American Association of Colleges of Nursing (AACN). (2002). *Hallmarks of the professional nursing practice environment*. Washington, DC: Author.

American Nurses Association. (2004). *Nursing: Scope and standards of practice* (Publication No. 03SSNP). Washington, DC: American Nurses Publishing.

American Nurses Association. (2003). *Nursing's social policy statement* (2nd ed.). (Publication No. 03NSPS 15M 09/03). Washington, DC: Author.

Finocchio, L. J., Dower, C. M., McMahon, T., Gragnola, C. M., & Taskforce on Health Care Workforce Regulation. (1995). *Reforming health care workforce regulation: Policy considerations for the 21st century*. San Francisco: Pew Health Professions Commission.

Greiner, A. C., & Knebel, E. (Eds.). (2003). *Health professions education: A bridge to quality*. Washington, DC: Institute of Medicine.

International Leadership Institute, Sigma Theta Tau International. (2000). Eight skills for a healthy career. *Reflections on Nursing Leadership*, 26(1), 20–21.

Joint Commission on Accreditation of Healthcare Organizations (JCAHO). (2003). New Release: Nursing shortage poses serious health care risk: Joint Commission expert panel offers solutions to national health care crisis. *http://www.jcaho.org/news+room/news+release+archives/ nursing+shortage.htm*

National League for Nursing. (2002). *Position statement: The preparation of nurse educators*. New York: Author,

O'Neil, E. (1998a). The changing health care environment. In E. O'Neil & J. Coffman (Eds.), *Strategies for the future of nursing* (pp. 3–7). San Francisco: Jossey-Bass.

O'Neil, E. (1998b). Nursing in the next century. In E. O'Neil & J. Coffman (Eds.), *Strategies for the future of nursing* (pp. 211–224). San Francisco: Jossey-Bass.

O'Neil, E. H., & Pew Health Professions Commission. (1998).

Recreating health professions practice for a new century: Fourth report of the Pew Health Professions Commission. San Francisco: Pew Health Professions Commission.

Page, A. (Ed.). (2004). *Keeping patients safe: Transforming the work environment of nurses*. Washington, DC: National Academies Press.

Pew Health Professions Commission. (1995). *Critical challenges: Revitalizing the health professions for the twenty-first century*. San Francisco: UCSF Center for the Health Professions.

The President's Advisory Commission on Consumer Protection and Quality in the Health Care Industry. (1998). *Quality first: Better health care for all Americans* [Final report to the President of the United States]. Columbia, MD: Consumer Bill of Rights.

Smith, J. (2003). *Report of findings: Exploring the value of continuing education mandates*. Chicago: National Council of State Boards of Nursing.

Bibliography

American Nurses Association. (2002). *Nursing Facts: Nursing-sensitive indicators for community-based non-acute care settings and ANA's safety and quality initiative*. Washington: Author.

American Nurses Association. (2002). *Nursing Facts: Nursing-sensitive quality indicators for acute care settings and ANA's safety and quality initiative*. Washington: Author.

Berwick, D.M. (2002). *Escape fire: Lessons for the future of health care*. New York: Commonwealth Fund.

Corrigan, M. S., Donaldson, M. S., Kohn, L. T., Maguire, S. K., & Pike, K. C. (2001). *Crossing the quality chasm: A new health system for the 21st century*. Washington, DC: National Academy Press.

Miller, B. K., Adams, D., & Beck, L. (1993). A behavioral inventory for professionalism in nursing. *Journal of Professional Nursing*, 9, 290–295.

Miller, T. (2003). *Building and managing a career in nursing: Strategies for advancing your career*. Indianapolis: Sigma Theta Tau and NurseWeek Publishing.

Owens, J. K., & Patton, J. G. (2003). Take a chance on nursing mentorships: Enhance leadership with this win-win strategy. *Nursing Education Perspectives*, 24, 198–204.

Pesut, D. J. (2002). Differentiation: Practice versus services. *Journal of profesional nursing*, 18 (3), 118–119.

Safriet, B .J. (2002). Closing the gap between can and may in health care providers' scopes of practice: A primer for policy makers. *Yale Journal on Regulation*, 19(2), 301–334.

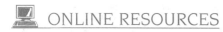 ## ONLINE RESOURCES

Online References

Agency for Healthcare Research and Quality (AHRQ). (2002). *Impact of working conditions on patient safety*. Fact sheet (AHRQ Publication No. 03-P003). Rockville, MD: Author. *http://www.ahrq.gov/news/workfact.htm*

American Association of Colleges of Nursing. (2002a). Certification and regulation of advanced practice nurses. *http://www.aacn.nche.edu/Publications/positions/cerreg.htm*

American Association of Colleges of Nursing (AACN). (2002b). *Hallmarks of the professional nursing practice environment*. Washington, DC: Author. *http://www.aacn.nche.edu/Publications/positions/hallmarks.htm*

American Association of Colleges of Nursing. (2002c). Position statement on defining scholarship for the discipline of nursing. *http://www.aacn.nche.edu/Publications/positions/scholar.htm*

American Association of Colleges of Nursing. (2002d). A vision of baccalaureate and graduate nursing education: The next decade. *http://www.aacn.nche.edu/Publications/positions/vision.htm*

American Nurses Association (ANA). (2003). Nursing Facts: Today's registered nurses—numbers and demographics. *http://www.nursingworld.org/readroom/fsdemogrpt.htm*

American Nurses Credentialing Center (ANCC). (2003). The Magnet application and appraisal process. *http://nursingworld.org/ancc/magnet/process.html*

Glaser, G. (1999). The policy and politics of continued competence. *Online Journal of Issues in Nursing*. *http://www.nursingworld.org/ojin/tpclg/leg_8.htm*

Institute of Medicine (IOM). (2003a). Crossing the quality chasm: The IOM Health Care Quality Initiative. *http://www.iom.edu/focuson.asp?id=8089*

Institute of Medicine (IOM). (2003b). Keeping patients safe: Transforming the work environment of nurses. *http://www.iom.edu/report.asp?id=16173*

Joel, L. A. (2002). Education for entry into nursing practice: Revisited for the 21st century. *Online Journal of Issues in Nursing* (Manuscript 4), 7 (2), 1–9. *http://www.nursingworld.org/ojin/topic18/tpc18_4.htm*.

Joint Commission on Accreditation of Healthcare Organizations (JCAHO). (2003). Health care at the crossroads: Strategies for addressing the evolving nursing shortage. *http://www.jcaho.org/about+us/public+policy+initiatives/health+care+at+the+crossroads.pdf*

National Council of State Boards of Nursing (NCSBN). (2003). About NCSBN. *http://www.ncsbn.org/public/about/about_index.htm*

National Council of State Boards of Nursing (NCSBN). (1996). Assuring competence: A regulatory responsibility. National Council position paper, 1996. *http://www.ncsbn.org/public/resources/ncsbn_competence.htm*

Nelson, M. A. (2002). Education for professional nursing practice: Looking backward into the future. *Online Journal of Issues in Nursing* (Manuscript 3), 7 (3), 1–13. *http://www.nursingworld.org/ojin/topic18/tpc18_3.htm*.

VHA Center for Research and Innovation. (2002). The business case for work force stability. *http://www.vha.com/research/public/stability.pdf*

Whittaaker, S., Carson, W., & Smolenski, M. C. (2000). Assuring continued competence—policy questions and approaches: How should the profession respond? *Online Journal of Issues in Nursing. http://nursingworld. org/ojin/topic10/tpc10_4.htm.*

 ONLINE RESOURCES

American Association of Colleges of Nursing. (2003). AACN white paper: Faculty shortages in baccalaureate and graduate nursing programs: Scope of the problem and strategies for expanding the supply. *http://www.aacn.nche.edu/Publications/WhitePapers/FacultyShortages. htm.*

American Association of Colleges of Nursing. (2000). The baccalaureate degree in nursing as minimal preparation for professional practice. *http://www.aacn.nche.edu/Publications/positions/baccmin.htm.*

Donley, R., & Flaherty, M. J. (2002). Revisiting the American Nurses Association's first position on education for nurses. *Online Journal of Issues in Nursing* (Manuscript 1), 7 (2), 1–17. *http://www.nursingworld.org/ojin/topic18/tpc18_1.htm.*

Kany, K. (2004) "Nursing in the Next Decade: Implications for Health Care and for Patient Safety" *Online Journal of Issues in Nursing.* Vol. #9 No. #2, Manuscript 3. Available: *www.nursingworld.org/ojin/topic24/tpc24 3.htm.*

National Council of State Boards of Nursing. (2003). Nursing regulation. *http://www.ncsbn.org/public/regulation/regulation_index.htm.*

National Council of State Boards of Nursing. (2002). Alternative regulatory nurse licensure models: NCSBN reaffirms support for single state and mutual recognition models of state nurse licensure. *http://www.ncsbn.org/public/news/res/Position_Altern_Reg_Models_102202.pdf.*

National Council of State Boards of Nursing. (2001). NCBSN position statement: Nurse shortage. *http://www.ncsbn.org/public/news/ncsbn_position_nurse_shortage.htm.*

National Council of State Boards of Nursing. (1997). Position paper on telenursing: A challenge to regulation. *http://www.ncsbn.org/public/resources/ncsbn_telenursing.htm.*

National Council of State Boards of Nursing (NCSBN). (1998). Using nurse practitioner certification for state nursing regulation: A historical perspective. *http://www.ncsbn.org/public/regulation/licensure_aprn_practitioner.htm*

National League for Nursing. (2003). Position statement: Innovation in nursing education: A call to reform. *http://www.nln.org/aboutnln/PositionStatements/innovation.htm.*

National League for Nursing. (2003). NLN's role in continuing education in nursing. *http://www.nln.org/aboutnln/PositionStatements/conted01.htm.*

VHA Center for Research and Innovation. (2004). 50 way to change the role of the registered nurse. *http://www.vha.com/research/workforce/public/cno_changingroles.asp.*

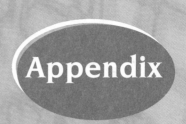

PROFESSIONAL NURSING ORGANIZATIONS

Academy of Medical Surgical Nurses (AMSN)
East Holly Avenue, Box 56
Pitman, NJ 08071-0056
(856) 256-2323
(856) 589-7463 (FAX)
http://www.medsurgnurse.org

Air & Surface Transport Nurses (ASTNA)
[National Flight Nurses Association]
9101 E. Kenyon Avenue, Suite 3000
Denver, CO 80237
(800) 897-NFNA (6362)
(303) 770-1812 (FAX)
http://www.astna.org

American Academy of Ambulatory Care Nursing (AAACN)
East Holly Avenue, Box 56
Pitman, NJ 08071-0056
(800) AMB-NURS
(856) 589-7463 (FAX)
http://www.aaacn.org/cgi-bin/WebObjects/AAACNMain
http://www.aacn@ajj.com

American Academy of Nurse Practitioners
P.O. Box 12846
Austin, TX 78711
(512) 442-4262
(512) 442-6469 (FAX)
http://www.aanp.org

American Assembly for Men in Nursing (AAMN)
%NYSNA
11 Cornell Rd
Latham, NY 12110
(518) 782-9400 ext. 346
aamn@aamn.org

American Association of Colleges of Nursing (AACN)
1 Dupont Circle, NW, Suite 530
Washington, DC 20036
(202) 463-6930
(202) 785-8320 (FAX)
http://www.aacn.nche.edu

American Association for Continuity of Care (AACC)
P.O. Box 532
Dunedin, Florida 34697
(800) 816-1575
(727) 738-8099 (FAX)
http://www.continuityofcare.com

American Association for the History of Nursing (AAHN)
Lanoka Harbor, NJ 08734
(609) 693-7250
(609) 693-1037 (FAX)
http://www.aahn.org/

American Association of Critical-Care Nurses (AACN)
101 Columbia
Aliso Viejo, CA 92656-1491

(800) 899-2226
(949) 362-2000
(949) 362-2020
http://www.aacn.org

American Association of Diabetes Educators (AADE)
100 W. Monroe, Suite 400
Chicago, IL 60603
(800) 338-3633
(312) 424-2427
http://www.aadenet.org

American Association of Legal Nurse Consultants (AALNC)
401 N. Michigan Avenue
Chicago, IL 60611
(877)402-2562
Fax: (312)673-6655
http://www.aalnc.org

American Association of Managed Care Nurses (AAMCN)
4435 Waterfront Drive, Suite 101
Glen Allen, VA 23060
(804) 747-9698
(804) 747-5316 (FAX)
http://www.aamcn.org

American Association of Neuroscience Nurses (AANN)
4700 W. Lake Avenue
Glenview, IL 60025-1485
(888) 557-2266
(877) 734-8677 (FAX)
http://www.aann.org

American Association of Nurse Anesthetists (AANA)
222 South Prospect Avenue
Park Ridge, IL 60068-4001
(847) 692-7050
(847) 693-6968 (FAX)
http://www.aana.com

American Association of Nurse Attorneys
7794 Grow Drive
Pensacola, FL 32514
(877) 538-2262
(850) 484-8760 (FAX)
http://www.taana.org

American Association of Occupational Health Nurses (AAOHN)
2920 Brandywine Road, Suite 100
Atlanta, GA 30341
(770) 455-7757
(770) 455-7271 (FAX)
http://www.aaohn.org

American Association of Office Nurses (AAON)
109 Kinderkamack Road
Montvale, NJ 07645
(800) 457-7504
(201) 573-8543 (FAX)
www.aaon.org

American Association of Spinal Cord Injury Nurses (AASCIN)
75-20 Astoria Boulevard
Jackson Heights, NY 11370-1177
(718) 803-3782
(718) 803-0414 (FAX)
http://www.aascin.org

American College of Healthcare Executives
One North Franklin Street, Suite 1700
Chicago, IL 60606-4425
(312) 424-2800
(312) 424-0023
www.ache.org

American College of Nurse-Midwives (ACNM)
818 Connecticut Avenue, NW, Suite 900
Washington, DC 20006
(202) 728-9860
(202) 728-9897 (FAX)
http://www.acnm.org

American College of Nurse Practitioners (ACNP)
1111 19th Street, NW, Suite 404
Washington, DC 20036
(202) 659-2190
(202) 659-2191 (FAX)
http://www.nurse.org/acnp

American Holistic Nurses Association (AHNA)
P.O. Box 2130

Flagstaff, AZ 86003-2130
(800) 278-2462
http://www.ahna.org

**American Medical Informatics
Association (AMIA)**
4915 St. Elmo Avenue, Suite 401
Bethesda, MD 20814
(301) 657-1291
(301) 657-1296 (FAX)
http://www.amia.org/

**American Nephrology Nurses'
Association (ANNA)**
ANNA National Office
East Holly Avenue, Box 56
Pitman, NJ 08071-0056
(888) 600-2662
(856) 256-2320 (FAX)
http://anna.inurse.com

American Nurses Association (ANA)
600 Maryland Avenue, SW, Suite 100 West
Washington, DC 20024-2571
(800) 274-4262
(202) 651-7001 (FAX)
American Academy of Nursing (800) 274-
4262
American Nurses Foundation (ANF) (800) 274-
4262
American Nurses Credentialing Center (AACC)
(800) 284-2378
Ethnic/Racial Minority Fellowship Program (800)
274-4262
http://www.nursingworld.org

**American Nursing Informatics
Association (ANIA)**
PMB 105
10808 Foothill Blvd. Suite 160
Rancho Cucamonga, CA 91730
http://www.ania.org

**American Organization of Nurse
Executives**
Liberty Place, 325 Seventh Street, NW
Washington, DC 20004
(202) 626-2240
(202) 638-5499 (FAX)
One North Franklin, 32nd Floor
Chicago, IL 60606
(312) 422-2800

(312) 422-4503 (FAX)
http://www.hospitalconnect.com/aone/
about

**American Psychiatric Nurses
Association (APNA)**
1555 Wilson Blvd., Suite 515
Arlington, VA 22209
(703) 243-2443
(703) 243-3390 (FAX)
http://www.apna.org

**American Public Health Association
(APHA)**
Public Health Nursing Section
800 I Street, NW
Washington, DC 20001-3710
(202) 777-2742
(202) 777-2532 (FAX)
http://www.apha.org/sections

**American Radiologic Nurses Association
(ARNA)**
7794 Grow Drive
Pensacola, FL 32514
866-486-2762
850-484-8762 (FAX)
http://www.arna.net

**American Society for Parenteral and
Enteral Nutrition (A.S.P.E.N.)**
8630 Fenton Street, Suite 412
Silver Spring, MD 20910
(301) 587-6315
(301) 587-2365 (FAX)
http://www.clinnutr.org

**American Society of Ophthalmic
Registered Nurses, Inc. (ASORN)**
P.O. Box 193030
San Francisco, CA 94119
(415) 561-8513
(415) 561-8531 (FAX)
http://webeye.ophth.uiowa.edu/asorn

**American Society of PeriAnesthesia
Nurses (ASPAN)**
10 Melrose Ave, Suite 110
Cherry Hill, NJ 08003-3696
(877) 737-9696
(856) 616-9601 (FAX)
http://www.aspan.org

American Society of Plastic Surgical Nurses (ASPSN)
P. O. Box 56
Pitman, NJ 08071-0056
(856) 256-2340
(856) 589-7463 (FAX)
http://www.aspsn.com

American Thoracic Society, Assembly on Nursing
61 Broadway
New York, NY 10006-2755
(212)315-6440
http://www.thoracic.org/assemblies/nur/
nur@thoracic.org

Association for Professionals in Infection Control and Epidemiology (APIC)
1275 K Street, NW, Suite 1000
Washington, DC 20005-4006
(202) 789-1890
(202) 789-1899 (FAX)
http://www.apic.org

Association of Camp Nurses (ACN)
8630 Thorsonveien NE
Bemidji, MN 56601
218-586-2633
http://www.campnurse.org

Association of Nurses in AIDS Care (ANAC)
3538 Ridgewood Road
Akron, Ohio 44333
(800) 260-6780
(330) 670-0109 (FAX)
http://www.anacnet.org

Association of Operating Room Nurses (AORN)
2170 S. Parker Road, Suite 300
Denver, CO 80231-5711
(800) 755-2676
(303) 755-6300
http://www.aorn.org

Association of Pediatric Oncology Nurses (APON)
4700 W. Lake Avenue
Glenview, IL 60025-1485

(847) 375-4724
(847) 375-8755 (FAX)
http://www.apon.org

Association of Rehabilitation Nurses (ARN)
4700 W. Lake Avenue
Glenview, IL 60025-1485
(800) 229-7530
(877) 734-9384 (FAX)
http://www.rehabnurse.org

Association of Women's Health, Obstetric & Neonatal Nurses (AWHONN)
2000 L Street, NW, Suite 740
Washington, DC 20036
(800) 673-8499 (US)
(800) 245-0231 (Canada)
(202) 728-0575 (FAX)
http://www.awhonn.org

Canadian Intravenous Nurses Association
4433 Sheppard Avenue E., Suite 200
Agincourt, Ontario, Canada M1S IV3
(416) 292-0687
(416) 292-1038 (FAX)
http://web.idirect.com/csotcina

Canadian Nurses Association
50 Driveway
Ottawa, Ontario, Canada K2P 1E2
(800) 361-8404
(613) 237-3520 (FAX)
http://www.cna-nurses.ca

Commission on Graduates of Foreign Nursing Schools (CGFNS)
3600 Market Street, Suite 400
Philadelphia PA 19104
(215) 349-8767
(215) 662-0425 (FAX)
http://www.cgfns.org

Dermatology Nurses' Association (DNA)
East Holly Avenue, Box 56
Pitman, NJ 08071-0056
(800) 454-4362
(856) 589-7463 (FAX)
http://dna.inurse.com

Developmental Disabilities Nurses Association (DDNA)
1733 H St, Suite 330, PMB 1214
Blaine, WA 98230
(800) 888-6733
(360) 332-2280
http://www.ddna.org

Emergency Nurses' Association (ENA)
915 Lee Street
Des Plaines, IL 60016-6569
(800) 900-9659
(847) 460-4001 (FAX)
http://www.ena.org

Health Ministries Association
980 Canton Street Building 1, Suite B
Roswell, Georgia 30075
(800) 280-9919
(770) 640-1095 (FAX)
http://www.hmassoc.org

Home Healthcare Nurses Association (HHNA)
228 7th Street, SE
Washington, DC 20003
(202) 546-4754
(202) 547-3540 (FAX)
http://www.hhna.org

Hospice and Palliative Nurses Association (HPNA)
Penn Center West One, Suite 229
Pittsburgh, PA 15276
(412) 787-9301
(412) 787-9305 (FAX)
http://www.hpna.org

Infusion Nurses Society (INS)
220 Norwood Park South
Norwood, MA 02062
(781) 440-9408
(781) 440-9409 (FAX)
http://www.insl.org

International Association of Forensic Nurses
East Holly Avenue, Box 56
Pitman, NJ 08071-0056
(856) 256-2425

856-589-7463 (FAX)
http://www.iafn.org

International Council of Nurses (ICN)
3 Place Jean Marteau
1201 – Geneva, Switzerland
http://www.icn.ch

International Nurses Society on Addictions
P.O. Box 10752
Raleigh, NC 27605
Tel (919) 821-1292
FAX (919) 833-5743
http://intnsa.org

International Nurses Transplant Society
1739 East Carson Street, Box 351
Pittsburgh, PA 15203
(412) 343-ITNS
(412) 343-3959
http://www.itns.org

International Society of Nurses in Genetics (ISONG)
2593 West 15th St. South
Newton, IA 50208-8500
janderson@isong.us
http://www.globalreferrals.com/isong.html

International Society of Psychiatric-Mental Health Nurses (ISPN)
Association of Child and Adolescent Psychiatric Nurses (ACAPN)
International Society of Psychiatric Consultation Liaison Nurses (ISPCLN)
Society of Education and Research in Psychiatric-Mental Health Nursing (SERPN)
Adult and Geropsychiatric-Mental Health Nurses (AGPN)
1211 Locust Street
Philadelphia, PA 19107
(800) 826-2950
(215) 545-8107 (FAX)
http://www.ispn-psych.org/html/contact.html

National Association of Clinical Nurse Specialists (NACNS)
3969 Green Street
Harrisburg, PA 17110

Phone (717) 234-6799
Fax (717) 234-6798
http://www.nacns.org

**National Association of Directors of
Nursing Administration in Long Term
Care (NADONA/LTC)**
10101 Alliance Rd., #140
Cincinnati, OH 45242
(800) 222-0539
(513) 791-3699 (FAX)
http://www.nadona.org

National Association of Hispanic Nurses
1501 16th Street, NW
Washington, DC 20036
(202) 387-2477
(202) 483-7183 (FAX)
http://www.thehispanicnurses.org

National Association of Neonatal Nurses
4700 W. Lake Avenue
Glenview, IL 60025-1485
(800) 451-3795
(888) 477-6266 (FAX)
http://www.nann.org

**National Association of Nurse Massage
Therapists (NANMT)**
P.O. Box 24004
Huber Hts, OH 45424
(800) 262-4017
http://www.nanmt.org

**National Association of Nurse Practi-
tioners in Women's Health (NPWH)**
503 Capitol Court, N.E., Suite 300
Washington, DC 20002
(202) 543-9693
(202) 543-9858 (FAX)
http://www.npwh.org

**National Association of Orthopaedic
Nurses (NAON)**
NAON National Office
401 N. Michigan Avenue, Suite 2200
Chicago, IL 60611
(800) 289-6266
(312) 527-6658 (FAX)
http://www.orthonurse.org

**National Association of Pediatric Nurse
Practitioners (NAPNAP)**
20 Brace Road, Suite 200
Cherry Hill, NJ 08034-2633
(856) 857-9700
(856) 857-1600 (FAX)
http://www.napnap.org

**National Association of School Nurses
(NASN)**
Eastern Office
P.O. Box 1300
Scarborough, ME 04070-1300
(877) 627-6476
(207) 883-2683 (FAX)
Western Office
1416 Park Street, Suite A
Castle Rock, CO 80109
(866) 627-6767
(303) 663-0403 (FAX)
http://www.nasn.org

**National Black Nurses Association
(NBNA)**
8630 Fenton St, Suite 330
Silver Spring, MD 20910-3803
(301) 589-3200
(301) 589-3223 (FAX)
http://www.nbna.org

**National Conference of Gerontological
Nurse Practitioners**
P.O. Box 232230
Centreville, VA 20120-2230
(703) 802-0088
(703)802-1436 (FAX)
http://www.ncgnp.org

**National Council of State Boards of
Nursing (NCSBN)**
111 East Wacker Drive, Suite 2900
Chicago, Illinois 60601
(312) 525-3600
(312) 279-1032 (FAX)
http://ncsbn.org

**National Gerontological Nursing
Association (NGNA)**
7794 Grow Drive
Pensacola, FL 32514-7072

(800) 723-0560
(850) 484-8762 (FAX)
http://www.ngna.com

National League for Nursing (NLN)
61 Broadway
New York,NY 10006
(800) 669-1656
(212) 812-0393 (FAX)
http://www.nln.org

National Nursing Staff Development Organization (NNSDO)
7794 Grow Drive
Pensacola, FL 32514
(800) 489-1995
http://www.nnsdo.org

National Organization of Nurse Practitioner Faculties (NONPF)
1522 K Street, NW, Suite 702
Washington, DC 20005
(202) 289-8044
(202) 289-8046 (FAX)
http://www.nonpf.com

National Rural Health Association (NRHA)
One West Armour Blvd., Suite 203
Kansas City, MO 64111
(816) 756-3140
(816) 756-3144 (FAX)
http://www.nrharural.org

North American Nursing Diagnosis Association (NANDA)
1211 Locust Street
Philadelphia, PA 19107
(215) 545-8105
(215) 545-8107 (FAX)
http://www.nanda.org

Nurse Practitioner Associates for Continuing Education of Advanced Practice Clinicians (NPACE)
209 West Central Street, Ste. 302
Natick, MA 01760
(508) 907-6424
(508) 907-6425 (FAX)
http://www.npace.org

Nurses Organization of Veterans Affairs (NOVA)
1726 M Street, NW, Suite 1101
Washington, DC 20036
(202) 296-0888
(202) 833-1577 (FAX)
http://www.vanurse.org

Oncology Nursing Society (ONS)
125 Enterprise Drive
Pittsburgh, PA 15275-1214
(866) 257-4ONS
(877) 369-5497 (FAX)
http://www.ons.org

Pediatric Endocrinology Nursing Association
P.O. Box 2933
Gaithersburg, MD 20886-2933
http://www.pens.org

Philippine Nurses Association
1663 F.T. Benitez Street,
Malate, Manila, Philippines
http://www.filnurse.com/pna

Preventative Cardiovascular Nurses Association
613 Williamson St. Suite 205
Madison, WI 53703
(608) 250-2440
http://www.pcna.net

Respiratory Nursing Society
c/o NYSNA
11 Cornell Rd.
Latham, NY 12110
(518) 782-9400 Ext. 286
rns@nysna.org
http://www.respiratorynursingsociety.org

Sigma Theta Tau International
550 West North Street
Indianapolis, IN 46202-3191
(888) 634-7575 (US & Canada)
(800) 634-7575-1 (International)
(317) 634-8188 (FAX)
http://www.nursingsociety.org

Society for Vascular Nursing
7794 Grow Drive

Pensacola, FL 32514
(888) 536-4786
(850) 484-8762 (FAX)
http://www.svnnet.org

**Society of Gastroenterology Nurses &
Associates (SGNA)**
401 North Michigan Avenue
Chicago, IL 60611-4267
(800) 245-7462
(312) 527-6658 (FAX)
http://www.sgna.org

**Society of Otorhinolaryngology & Head-
Neck Nurses, Inc. (SOHN)**
116 Canal St, Suite A
New Smyrna Beach, FL 32168
(386) 428-1695
(386) 423-7566 (FAX)
http://www.sohnnurse.com

Society of Pediatric Nurses
7794 Grow Drive
Pensacola, FL 32514
(800) 723-2902
(850) 484-8762 (FAX)
http://www.pedsnurse.org

Society of Trauma Nurses
PMB 300 223 N. Guadalupe
Santa Fe, NM 87501
(505) 983-4923 FAX (505) 983-5109
http://www.traumanursesoc.org

**Society of Urologic Nurses & Asso-
ciates (SUNA)**
East Holly Avenue, Box 56
Pitman, NJ 08071-0056
888-827-7862
(856) 589-7463 (FAX)
http://www.suna.org

Transcultural Nursing Society
36600 School Croft Road
Livonia, MI 48150
(888) 432-5470
(734) 432-5463 (FAX)
http://www.tcns.org

**Wound, Ostomy and Continence Nurses
Society (WOCN)**
4700 W. Lake Ave
Glenview, IL 60025
(888) 224-WOCN
866-615-8560 (FAX)
http://www.wocn.org

Index

Note: Page numbers in *italics* indicate a figure, "b" indicates a box, "t" indicates a table.

Educational settings, informatics positions in, 414, 414b
Educational streamlining, 39–40
Effectiveness, 434
Elder abuse, 369, 370
Embryo splitting, 322
Emergency Department, patient arrival in, in chemical terrorism, 464–465
Empirical research, 136–138
Encephalitis, tickborne, 462–463
Encephalomyelitis, Eastern equine, 457, 458
Venezuelan, 457, 458
Western equine, 457, 458
Encoder, 154
End-of-life decisions, 319–320
Endurance, of negotiator, 274
Enrollees, in managed care, 428
Enterotoxin B, staphylococcal, 459–460
Environment, external, organizations and, 256–257
Environmental quality, 363
Environmental risks, in aging, 368
Epsilon toxin, 459
Erikson, E.H., eight ages of man, 58, *58*
Ethical codes, 132
Ethical principles, 306b, 306–308
Ethical rights, 308
Ethical systems, 308–311
Ethical theories, 311–315
Ethics. *See also* Professional ethics
code of, 7, 7b, 12, 315
decision-making model in, 311–315, 312b, *313*
Euthanasia, 317–318
Evidence-based practice, 15, 139–141, 145–146, 410
Executive, as term, 267
Exercise, interactive. *See* Interactive exercise
Experimental designs, 143
Explanations, as leadership task, 243–244
Eye contact, in communication, 163

F

Facial expressions, in communication, 164
Families, resources for, 37–38
Fayol, Henri, 266, 267
Fee-for-service (FFS) payment system, 426, 429
Feelings, interpretation of, 199
Fidelity, 307
Field theory, 284–285, *285*
Filoviruses, 454
Financial aid, 35
Financing of health care, 425–427

Flat organized structures, 263
Fletcher, Joseph, 309
Flow charts, 393, *394*
Formal goals, 264
Formalistic system, 310
Framework, definition of, 50
Functional health patterns, 117b
Functional nursing, 339–340
Functional structure, 260, *260*

G

Gandhi, 236
Gaston, M.A., 472
Gebelein, S.H., 273
General system theory, 63, *63*
General Systems Framework, 75–76
Genetic manipulation, cloning and, 322–324
Gestalt theory, 210
Glanders, 457
Goals, attainment of, 177
envisoning of, 240, 240b
organizational, 255–256, 264
personal, setting of, 22–23
Government, branch(es) of, 472–474
executive, 473
judicial, 473
legislative, 473
Executive Office, qualifications for service in, 474t
involvement of nurses in, 484–485
legislative process, *478*
nurses' involvement in, 479b
state and local systems of, 473–474
structure and function of, 472–474
U.S. Congress, major committees of, 476–477t
qualifications for service in, 474t
Grades, 24–25
Graduate nursing education, 517
Grand theories, 53, 87–91
Great man leadership theory, 238–239
Grohar-Murray, M.E., 280
Group(s), adjourning of, 180
characteristics of, 174–178
composition of, 175
difficult people in, 186, 186b
effective, 176–177
effectiveness of, evaluation of, 177
focus, 175–176
forming of, 179
functional group-building roles of, 183–185, 184t
functional task roles of, 183t, 183–185